CYTOKINES
STRESS AND IMMUNITY
Second Edition

CYTOKINES
STRESS AND IMMUNITY
Second Edition

EDITED BY
Nicholas P. Plotnikoff, Robert E. Faith,
Anthony J. Murgo, and Robert A. Good

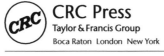

CRC Press
Taylor & Francis Group
Boca Raton London New York

CRC Press is an imprint of the
Taylor & Francis Group, an **informa** business

CRC Press
Taylor & Francis Group
6000 Broken Sound Parkway NW. Suite 300
Boca Raton. FL 33487-2742

First issued in paperback 2019

ISBN-13: 978-0-8493-2074-3 (hbk)
ISBN-13: 978-0-367-39015-0 (pbk)

Library of Congress Cataloging-in-Publication Data

Cytokines : stress and immunity / edited by Nicholas P. Plotnikoff ... [et al.].
  -- 2nd ed.
    p. cm.
  Includes bibliographical references and index.
  ISBN 0-8493-2074-7 (alk. paper)
  1. Cytokines. 2. Stress (Physiology) 3. Stress (Psychology) 4. Immunity. 5.
Psychoneuroimmunology. I. Plotnikoff, Nicholas P. II. Title.

QR185.8.C95C996 2006
616.07'9--dc22   2006040583

Visit the Taylor & Francis Web site at
http://www.taylorandfrancis.com

and the CRC Press Web site at
http://www.crcpress.com

Table of Contents

In Memoriam: Robert A. Good

by Diana Pickett, M.D., Ph.D., and Noorbibi Day-Good, Ph.D.

> Quid edit beificium taceat; narret qui accepit. *(*Let him who has done a good deed be silent; let who has received it tell it.*)*

INTRODUCTION

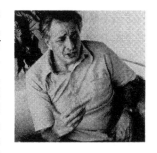

Robert A. Good, B.A., M.D., Ph.D., D.Sc., FACP, the father of modern immunology and cellular engineering, will always be remembered for his extensive studies of X-linked agammaglobulinemia bisecting the immunological universe, the universe of the lymphoid system, and the universe of viruses. He identified and defined numerous primary immunodeficiencies of humans, and especially identified and defined chronic granulomatous disease (CGD) of childhood. His research achievements include the discovery of the function of the thymus and the definition of the two distinct major cellular components of the immunity system, and performance of the first successful bone marrow transplantation in a human.

Good was like Paul Bunyan, the legendary figure who hailed from his home state of Minnesota: super sized in all that he did. If ever the field of medicine and medical research needed a recruitment model to induce bright young minds to follow a career in the sciences, the life and legend of Bob Good would be a great choice.

> Ab ovo usque ad mala. (To the stars through difficulties.)

He overcame the death of his father at an early age and a crippling bout of Guillain–Barré that left him partially paralyzed. He turned the challenge of hours when he was unable to play sports into an advantage and used them to study science and medicine. He demanded the best from himself and others and yet was always supportive, seemingly when needed most. He out-published, out-worked, and out-shined most of his colleagues but it did not turn his head; instead, his feet were planted, in those famous tennis shoes, firmly on the ground. He said he felt more at home and in his element patting the fontanels and rubbing the abdomens of his little patients than on stage giving a speech. Good loved every minute of life and life returned the compliment. Bob Good has not left us; he has merely gone on ahead, as he always has.

THE TRANSLATIONAL PHYSICIAN SCIENTIST

Good is considered one of the greatest figures in 20th century medicine and medical research. He was one of the very first "translational physician scientists" to set the standard beginning at bedside, by observation and conversation, with his patients, his greatest teachers. Information gleaned and questions posed were taken to both the clinical and experimental laboratories for dissection and analyses. Results were gathered and returned via translation to the patient's bedside, with answers, treatments, and many times cures for their illnesses.

All life is an experiment.

Ralph Waldo Emerson

SCIENTIFIC COMPASS, TENACITY, AND "EXPERIMENTS OF NATURE"

Good was a visionary who could seemingly see around scientific corners and intuitively know in which direction research in immunology was headed and what were the important and necessary issues to explore at that particular moment in time. He maintained his theories and interests even if it sometimes meant temporarily setting them aside on a "mental bench." He never gave up until all avenues had been explored and exhausted. The story of his theory, formed in 1953, on the role of the thymus in mammalian immunity and the two different sets of rabbit thymectomy experiments, separated by a pregnant pause, was a perfect example of step-wise experiments and Good's tenacity in staying the scientific course until the answer was forthcoming.

You'll have to repeat that experiment. That's why we call it RE-search!

Robert A. Good

He was able to visualize and analyze unwell areas in body systems responsible for "dis-ease" in his patients, and then connect the dots leading from the clinical presentation to the diagnosis, etiology, treatment, and, in many cases, cure. He wanted to be able to understand it all: how, why, when, and where immunity was responsible in defining health and disease. Questions developed from observing and conversing with patients regarding these fabled "experiments of nature," a term used by one of Good's first mentors, Irving McQuarrie at the University of Minnesota, when he gave the young Bob Good advice on how he should approach his career in medicine and medical research by becoming a pediatrician and observing "experiments of nature." Bob was so impressed by that intriguing and eloquent description of illness that from that moment forward "experiments of nature" became his hallmark signature phrase.

THE GOOD METHODOLOGY: IN PURSUIT OF EXCELLENCE

Salus populi suprema lex esto. (Let the welfare of the people be the supreme *law.*)

Good's methodology of placing the patient first and his or her welfare as the focus and driving force of his research steered his research and clinical efforts. Tenacity;

incisive questioning over and again; challenging current dogma and those who proposed it; voluminous reading, writing, and publishing; critiquing theories and results; innate intelligence and 20-hour workdays led Bob Good to become one of the finest pediatricians and clinical and basic immunologists of all times.

CONTINUING TRADITION

We are what we repeatedly do. Excellence, then, is not an act, but a habit.

Aristotle

Bob Good was the consummate people person, professor, mentor, team player, and even better team leader. He trained over 300 young scientists worldwide, many of whom distinguished themselves as professors, chairmen, heads of departments and institutions, and leaders in their fields. Good was extremely pleased to see his former students and fellows, whom he affectionately called his intellectual children and grandchildren, develop their own careers and become distinguished professionals. Bob, to his credit, gave female scientists the respect of not being treated differently from their male counterparts; for him, the only criterion was the degree of excellence.

Good practiced the adage that sharing is strength, learning from and sharing with others throughout his entire life. He generously gave to others as he received, in kind, from his own mentors, E. Lyon, I. McQuarrie, L. Thomas, H. Kunkel, Mac McCarthy, professors, colleagues, and students. As a young professor at the University of Minnesota, Good said of his own dean:

> Harold S. Diehl conveyed this heritage [the "Golden Age" of scholarship at the University of Minnesota] to me as my dean, and I shall always think of him in this role. A fine scholar in his own right, he cherished good research. He opened many doors for me, created innumerable opportunities, and fostered my development as a student, young faculty member, and ultimately professor.

EDUCATION AND ACADEMIC OPPORTUNITIES

Education and academic opportunity were the cornerstones of Good's upbringing and would become his constant, welcome, and challenging companions throughout his lifetime. Good was a straight A student and completed all his pre- and post-graduate studies at the University of Minnesota in Minneapolis. After receiving a bachelor's degree in 1944, he continued his academic studies by matriculating concurrently in both the medical and graduate schools in the first honors M.D./Ph.D. program at the university. Good studied and worked in the laboratory day and night throughout the year. In 1947, a short three years after beginning the programs, he graduated with honors and became the first student at the University of Minnesota to receive both degrees in the same ceremony.

The pursuit of excellence in all that he did was his true North Star. Encouraging others to do better than they think they can do was the scientific mantra he repeated over and over again to remind others as well as himself to continue their efforts. He never talked down to people nor did he confront them, even when their performances were lacking. He gave everyone the opportunity to rise to a challenge and self-correct.

He believed in working hard — if at first you don't succeed, then keep at it until you do. Making the best use of time, as exemplified by his own daily schedule and monumental scientific work product, was important to him.

His intellectual capacity, creativity, and sheer volume of professional accomplishment were more than vast. His work at the bench and with patients spanned almost 60 years; it was prodigious in both depth and scope. He cast his intellectual, clinical, and scientific nets far and wide. He captured many "experiments of nature" first observed at his patients' bedsides and brought them to the laboratory bench to analyze and solve their mysteries for the benefit of his patients. His encyclopedic knowledge and recall of pediatric and adult medicine were well known among his colleagues and yet he always made the time to listen to patients, colleagues, and students. Good never thought he knew all there was to know on a subject and was always willing and eager to learn something new and fill any existing lacunae in his knowledge base. In fact, two of his famous sayings were:

> All I can say is that the last word has not been written on the subject.

> A medical problem can always be analyzed in terms of how it fits into phylogeny, ontogeny, or pathology.

INFLUENCE ON OTHERS

Nowhere are the character of Bob Good and his influence on others better portrayed than in the quotes of students, colleagues, and others whose lives he touched.

> In our lives, we meet many people and they all influence us in one way or another. However, the person who influenced me most is my dear teacher, Dr. Robert A. Good, one of the greatest medical scholars in the world. Dr. Good taught me how to do research and how to approach it. He encouraged me to study hard and not to be afraid of making mistakes. When I would make a mistake, he warmly told me not to become discouraged but instead to learn from my experience. He said we will all succeed in the end, if we do not give up.

Chih-Hsin Chen, M.D.

Good was known to often give sage and direct advice, based on his own productive life and decades-long career:

> Experiential docet. (Experience teaches.)

> Be selfish. Think of your own career first. No one else will!

> Some of my fondest memories are when we get together and discuss science and ideas and we keep on working right through lunchtime.

> We are so very lucky.

> This is no kitten ball game.

Good always made sure he gave everyone credit, both orally and in publications. He never made an unkind comment about anyone and always found something positive to say about everyone:

That fellow's feelings of inferiority are totally justifiable. I cannot praise him highly enough!

Good told his students, as he was told by his mentors, that to stand out from the crowd one must ask critical questions, accept only definitive answers, put both mind and body to the task, and proceed.

Trahimur omnes laudis studio. (We are all led on by our eagerness for praise.)

Good also said that he was told by one of his mentors that a little bit of acclaim is good as long as you don't swallow it!

Carpe diem. (Seize the day.)

It was hard to catch Good for one-on-one time. He started his days at 4 A.M., worked at home, and saw his fellows for early morning meetings until 8 A.M. He then went on rounds at the hospital to see his patients and worked in his lab. Evening schedules were just as tight. More than one colleague has told of how he exchanged cutting Good's hair for a morning appointment because of Good's active schedule! Another told of a breakfast meeting in New York and his astonishment when the breakfast menu consisted of steak and French fries. When he commented on the menu, Good retorted that it was already lunchtime! These are only a few of the many stories about the long and fulfilled days in the life of Robert A. Good.

UNIVERSITY OF MINNESOTA, 1944

Outstanding people have one thing in common: an absolute sense of mission.

Zig Ziglar

Good's dual careers as a clinician and clinical and basic researcher spanned almost 60 years, from 1944 to 2003. He remained at his alma mater, which always held a special place in his heart and mind, in his beloved home state of Minnesota, for 28 years. He served on the medical school faculty from 1950 to 1972 as an instructor, assistant professor, associate professor, American Legion Memorial research professor, professor of pediatrics, professor of microbiology, and professor and head of the Department of Pathology. His greatest scientific accomplishments were fostered during his time in that exceptional clinical and teaching environment.

Good wanted to be remembered foremost as a pediatrician, immunologist, and teacher. In following his own scientific trail, as he did so eloquently when writing about E. Lyon, one can see exactly how he fosters independence and originality as well as sharing and inviting others to join him in generating excitement, and pursuing ideas, concepts, and theories among his colleagues and medical and graduate students.

Keywords in Good's Scientific Lexicon

It is always the challenge of a new day, this feeling of excitement.

Robert A. Good

Were Good able, in 1944, to see his future scientific trajectory spread out before him, the core of his research legacy and scientific contributions would certainly be the dense, compact, and mysterious immune system. Much like fission, the nuclear core would explode into myriad discrete areas of the human immune response to be explored; described by a string of keywords that would have been, with each learning experience and observed "experiment of nature," added to the increasing fund of knowledge to help solve the puzzle and balance the equation between ease and dis-ease.

To the student interested in analyzing Good's scientific opus, the titles of his early papers incorporate the seminal and recurring themes found throughout the corpus of his vast bibliography. Plasma cells, bone marrow, inflammation, allergic reactions, reticuloendothelial system, kidney and liver disease, autoimmune disorders, pathology viewed by the electron microscope, and hypersensitivity were Good's constant themes. He worked at relating them to each other, bit by bit to connect the dots and form matrices bridging the gaps and providing answers and treatment cures caused by malfunctioning immunological systems. His scientific course was set after only a dozen papers published before he was 27 years old!

SCIENTIFIC CONTRIBUTIONS

Throughout the centuries there were men who took first steps down new roads, armed with nothing but their own vision.

Ayn Rand

Plasma Cells and Antibody Production, 1944

Beginning with the armature of the immune system and in particular, the plasma cell, Good contributed to the further understanding of its function beginning in 1944 on work published as the subject of his doctoral dissertation in 1947. He demonstrated that plasma cells were indeed the major antibody-producing cells in the immune system. His investigations were independent of but contemporaneous with contributions of Astrid Fagraeus of Sweden. This knowledge was soon applied to patients with X-linked agammaglobulinemia. Good discovered that these patients lacked both plasma cells and germinal centers but had normal lymphocyte numbers and cell-mediated immunities. The study of the plasma cell would become the core of research throughout Good's life. His studies of patients with severe agammaglobulinemia showed that not only do two distinct immunological systems exist (later called T and B cell systems), but his patient's "experiments of nature" were examples of bisections of the bacterial, viral, lymphoid, and immunologic universes (1954–1956) — a most amazing and insightful observation made by Good.

ROCKEFELLER INSTITUTE, 1949

As a recipient of a Helen Hay Whitney Fellowship, Good was obliged to take a year of training away from the University of Minnesota. This would be the first time Good spent living outside his beloved home state. The world was waiting for him and him for it. He chose, upon the recommendation of McQuarrie, the Rockfeller Institute — a veritable Mt. Olympus or prestigious ivory tower. He joined the rheumatic fever laboratory of Maclyn McCarty, of DNA fame. New York City energized Good and vice versa. In fact, New York was probably the only city that could keep pace with Good as he began to cut a wide scientific and clinical path for himself and others. He loved the culture, music, art, food, and most of all the incredibly interesting people he met there.

LESSONS LEARNED FROM HODGKIN'S AND MULTIPLE MYELOMA PATIENTS

Good did not initially find his own unique scientific niche in those first few months at the Rockefeller, but thanks to a circuitous route that included Henry Kunkel, an early mentor, who happened to need large amounts of myeloma serum to continue immunochemical studies on proteins, Good was brought into contact with a myeloma patient and the characteristics of that particular disease. Good was known in some circles as a very successful plasma cell hunter and obtained all the sera Kunkel needed. In exchange for sera contributions, Kunkel taught the young Bob Good about the emerging fields of immunochemistry and serum globulin proteins. Good still had not found the perfect fit or research area to which he could devote his time and make a contribution.

Al Stetson suggested that Good crystallize CRP which presumably would have made Maclyn McCarty, Good's boss in the rheumatic fever laboratory, happy. David Karnofsky of the newly established Sloan-Kettering Institute recommended using pleural and peritoneal effusions from Hodgkin's patients as copious sources of CRP as starting materials. This led Good to see another spectrum of diseases involving the immune system in Hodgkin's patients whose susceptibilities were completely opposite to those found in myeloma patients.

Quod erat demonstrandum. (Which was to be proved.)

These were the scientific happenstances and underpinnings that combined to create the critical mass that would precipitate the major focus of Good's long-standing research interests: T and B cells, their progenitors, and their progeny. Good would find his own niche and embark on what would become his own particular course in an area he would later term "clinical immunology" steadied by the keel and rudder in the form of the plasma cell and cell-mediated immunity and the two "experiments of nature": multiple myeloma and Hodgkin's disease, whose secrets he would later decipher in collaboration with his colleagues and students when he returned to his clinical work and laboratory in Minnesota.

Organized activity and maintained enthusiasm are the wellsprings of power.

Paul J. Meyer

Trying to get one's arms around and grasp Good's research and the clinical issues in which Good was involved is like reading several books at the same time. One must be able to follow parallel paths and remember the plots and characters of each scientific study when reading his bibliography. His research as seen from a distance was much like a symphony: "Variations on a Theme of Immunology in G Major," played by an orchestra of different instruments with Good as the conductor most of the time, co-conductor some of the time, or sitting in the back giving support and advice to others. There were many "first violins" brought up through the ranks along the way — promising young and brilliant scientists who today are prominent in their fields. Good published over 2,100 publications, many times shared with over 1,200 co-authors, along with 50 books, countless articles and abstracts, and other contributions to the communities where he lived and worked.

BEGINNING OF GOOD'S GOLDEN YEARS

Every great institution is the lengthened shadow of a single man. His character determines the character of the organization.

Ralph Waldo Emerson

THE GENESIS (1944) AND DEMONSTRATION (1965) OF THE TWO-COMPONENT SYSTEM OF CELL-MEDIATED AND HUMORAL IMMUNITY

Good's studies of patients with severe agammaglobulinemia showed that two distinct immunological systems, later designated T and B cells, existed. Also, the expression of his patient's diseases bisected the bacterial/viral microbial universe divided into the high grade encapsulated bacterial pathogen and the acid-fast bacilli, fungi, and some viruses.

In 1952, before discovering the role of the thymus in immunology, Good showed through his investigations of agammaglobulinemia, Hodgkin's disease, and multiple myeloma, that two major arms of immunity exist. Antibody production based on plasma cells was shown to represent the major defense against encapsulated bacterial pathogens; the other thymus-dependent arm of immunity based on lymphocytes represented the major defense against many viruses, fungi, and facultative intracellular bacterial pathogens. A work Good published in 1964 with senior fellow Ray Peterson and Max Cooper, a young fellow in Good's laboratory, clearly delineated and demonstrated Good's 1952 theory of a two-component immune system consisting of humoral and cell-mediated immunity. Peterson and Cooper brought the proof of that theory to fruition in experiments with chickens. Unlike other animal models, chickens provided an excellent opportunity to tease out the two-component theory of immunity in that they have two morphologically and distally separate lymphoid organs: a cell-mediated thymus-dependent system and a bursa that was found to be responsible for humoral immunity.

Good, his colleagues, fellows, and student associates were about to make scientific history again. Their findings were published in *Immunologic Deficiency Diseases in Man* under the title of "The two-component concept of the lymphoid system," authored by Cooper, Perey, Peterson, Gabrielsen, and Good.

In addition to receiving the first E. Meade Johnson Award and performing otherwise recognized work on the Shwartzman phenomenon, Good was about to begin one of the most exciting and challenging periods of his career. He opened his green pediatric journal one day in 1952 and read about Col. Ogden Bruton's 8-year-old male pediatric patient whose serum electrophoretic pattern was void in the pattern area of gamma globulin.

Extending Col. Bruton's initial findings, Good was eager to test his plasma cell theory that certain immunologically challenged patients would not develop plasma cells. The anticipated opportunity to test his theory was soon presented to him by three of his own pediatric patients. Two were brothers, which suggested a genetic component to their agammaglobulinemic illness. He found, as he predicted, neither plasma cells nor gamma globulin Schlieren patterns in the sera of the children. Germinal centers were absent as was the development of lymphocytes. Good extended his studies to include patients from neighboring hospitals and soon had a dozen patient profiles. He was to call this syndrome Bruton's agammaglobulinemia to "recognize the unique contributions made by Col. Ogden Bruton."

Good found several different types of agammaglobulinemia within the patient population, including XLA, hypogammaglobulinemia, and delayed allergic reactions.

GOOD'S SYNDROME: THYMOMA WITH IMMUNODEFICIENCY, 1953

A most telling experiment of nature.

Robert A. Good

In 1953, Good was asked to consult on an adult patient who had previously presented to Richard Varco's chest clinic in 1951 with far too many recurrent bouts of pneumonia. Soon thereafter, Varco extirpated a 565-g benign stromal epithelial anterior mediastinal tumor. Removal of the tumor did not restore the patient's immunological response. Good tested the patient's serum and found the presence of "some" plasma cells, indicating hypogammaglobulinemia, rather than an XLA patient devoid of all plasma cells and agammaglobulinemic. This led Good to question the role played by the thymus, if any, in the immune response. He postulated, based on both patient and experimental observations, that it did play an essential part in immunity, but confirmation of that theory would be left to the rabbits; however, the glory did not go to the class of 1954, the 4- to 5-week old group, but to the class of 1959; the "hot little newborns," as Good called them.

This was the beginning of a lifetime of study of immunodeficiency diseases in humans with the ogammaglo bulinemic patient providing a challenging and perplexing "experiment of nature."

In order to experimentally test Good's theory regarding the thymus, 4- to 5-week old rabbits were thymectomized to test for their subsequent ability to produce antibodies, thus demonstrating the role of the thymus. Laboratory findings for that particular experimental construct were published from 1954 through 1957. While the instant experiments confirmed the 1945 published work of Harris, they did not demonstrate Good's theory that the thymus was intimately involved in the immune response and that thymectomy would disrupt that process. Successful and promising results of subsequent rabbit experiments were submitted to the American Association of Immunologists (AAI) in December of 1960, demonstrating that, indeed, the thymus was found to be critical to the immune process when thymectomy in rabbits was performed during the neonatal period.

How the Rabbit Experiments Began, 1954

Good, one of Varco's fellows named L.D. MacLean, and Sol Zak, a medical student of Good, set about doing that first set of unremarkable rabbit thymectomy experiments in 1954 and 1955. The experimental design was based upon earlier publications beginning with Bruton's 1952 paper on his agammaglobulinemic patient and Good's plethora of papers on agammaglobulinemia, plasma cells, and thymoma. Based on the evidence, it was reasonable to assume that a difference should be demonstrated by thymectomized rabbits.

Good was familiar with the immunological states of newborn humans, rabbits, and other experimental animals. What was not calculated then was the timing of maturity of the rabbit's immune system. Thymectomy at 4 to 5 weeks of age seemed a sound supposition physiologically and ontogenetically, but it was too late in immunological development to show the desired effect of thymectomy. Had the experiments been done in mice whose immunological apparatus matured later than those of rabbits at the 4- to 5-week-old mark, the defining history of the crucial role played by the thymus in mammalian immunity might have been told at an earlier date.

In their 1956 paper titled "Thymic tumor and acquired agammaglobulinemia: a clinical and experimental study of the immune response," MacLean, Zak, Varco, and Good boldly began by stating with great conviction and logic that

the simultaneous occurrence of acquired agammaglobulinemia and benign thymoma in humans suggested that the thymus might participate in the control of antibody formation.

Despite what were disappointing results, they continued to insist that

the thymus does not participate in the control of the immune response under the conditions described herein is indicated by the experimental findings. In spite of the data obtained in this investigation, which indicate that the normal thymus does not exercise a controlling influence on the immune response in the rabbit, it still seems likely that some essential relationship exists between the thymic tumor and the acquisition of acquired agammaglobulinemia.

Those final words do not seem to be ones reflective of a mindset of surrender in deciphering the mysteries of the thymus. Indeed, the authors, in closing, entreat further research in the area: "Determination of the nature of the relationship awaits further investigation." And just like MacArthur and others with determination, the authors did return in 1959 to complete the mission.

Definitive Second Rabbit Experiments, 1959

In 1959, at a spring meeting of the Federation of American Societies for Experimental Biology (FASEB), Harold Wolfe, a friend and colleague, sought Good out after a presentation to tell him about a 1956 paper by Glick et al., unknown to most immunologists. The paper discussed the effects of neonatally bursectomizing chickens and their subsequent failure to produce antibodies. This was, indeed, important news. Wolfe also told Good about his own recent laboratory findings in Wisconsin with Mueller and Meyer that confirmed Glick's work and extended their own studies in bursectomized chickens.

Good said he then knew what the problem had been with the earlier rabbit experiments. The rabbits were thymectomized too late in their immunological development! Ben Papermaster, a fellow in Good's lab with whom Good had published work on antibody production in neonatal chickens, went to visit Wolfe in his Wisconsin lab to learn more about the lab's bursectomy experiments. When Papermaster returned, Good, his colleagues, and his students began a series of neonatal thymectomy experiments in rabbits, mice, and other animal models.

Exciting New Results, 1960

As an AAI member, Good communicated the results of the first animal experiments in abstract format. He directed the work of master's student Olga K. Archer and James C. Pierce, Varco's surgical fellow. The abstract was submitted in December of 1960, published in *Federation Proceedings* in March of 1961, and orally presented by Archer in April of 1961 at the FASEB meeting in Atlantic City, New Jersey. The title of the abstract was "Role of [the] thymus in [the] development of the immune response." The bottom line of the abstract was that "the thymus is necessary for the normal development of the immune response in the rabbit." After the presentation, Good, who chaired the session, presented an in-depth report on their latest experimental results with co-authors John Kersey, Carlos Martinez, Gus Dalmasso, and Ben Papermaster. The report covered findings with rabbits, chickens, and mice and clearly indicated that thymectomy or prevention of thymus development very early in life prevented the normal development of both humoral and cell-mediated immunities.

Additional Evidence

Their evidence also showed that thymectomy prevented homograft or allograft rejection of normal tissues and prevented rejection of both allogeneic and syngeneic tumors. Graft versus host reaction (GVHR) was inhibited due to surgical or hormonal thymectomy. Good also discussed their extensive and convincing research on skin graft rejection across multiple minor and major histocompatibility barriers. These celebrated findings led Good to state in his usually audacious way that at long last they had established the essential function of the thymus! A series of more than twenty papers flowed on the subjects of the thymus and the demonstration of the two-component system of immunity from Good and his colleagues and fellows.

IMMUNODEFICIENCY DISEASES

Chronic Granulomatous Disease, 1957

Good said that one of the most rewarding and challenging areas of his work came from opportunities offered by observing and conversing with patients and learning about "experiments of nature," evidenced by the different forms of genetically determined and acquired immunodeficiency diseases. He was dedicated to every one of his patients and called them his best teachers. Studying the various forms of immunodeficiency diseases afforded a means to dissect immunological development and function. Good identified and provided the initial descriptions of at least eight distinct varieties of primary immune deficiency disease (PIDD) in humans in clinical and pathological detail. One was chronic granulomatous disease (CGD) of childhood. He linked hypergammaglobulinemic disease to phagocytes and established that this disease was based on a failure of phagocytic cells to kill ingested catalase-positive bacteria and generate hydrogen peroxide, one of the activated states of oxygen. Because CGD patients exhibited increased susceptibility to infection by catalase-positive bacteria, but not to catalase-negative bacteria, Good looked once again to the bisected microbial universe for answers, according to the specific mechanism of bodily defense toward potential pathogens.

PHYLOGENY, ONTOGENY, PATHOLOGY, AND COMPLEMENT, 1964

Good's seminal and elegant work, beginning in 1964, on the phylogeny and ontogeny of the origins and development of the immune system using the lamprey, hagfish, and other species showed that immunity including the complement system appeared much earlier in evolution than had been imagined — dating back 400 million years. Good, despite the belief among certain members of the Boston group that isolated complement deficiencies were not associated with disease, was the first to refute that and demonstrate that patients with infections and collagen-like diseases most certainly had isolated complement deficiencies. These early observations by Gewurz, Pickering, and Day were followed by many more studies of additional patients with complement deficiencies.

> A medical problem can always be analyzed in terms of how it fits into phylogeny, ontogeny, or pathology.
>
> **Robert A. Good**

TRANSPLANTATION: GENESIS, 1955

Good's first published manuscript on transplantation in humans was a February of 1955 *JAMA* article titled "Successful homograft of skin in a child with agammaglobulinemia." One of Good's patients, it was reported, kept a skin graft for more than a year while others vigorously rejected them. This led Good to begin experiments on the transferability of delayed allergic responses from agammaglobulinemic patients to normal recipients. Good was beginning to fine tune the different types of immunodeficient patients, based upon their clinical presentations and the courses of their diseases. The title of one of Good's papers published in 1963 with co-authors Martinez and Gabrielsen gave another hint of how close the possibility of success was: "Progress toward manipulation of the transplantation barrier."

Good was keenly interested and active in the area of transplantation many years before success could be claimed. Carefully planned research, insights derived from solid education and training in several disciplines, constant contacts with patients that focused on "experiments of nature," a network of colleagues and students to inspire and from whom to receive inspiration and lessons all led to the promise of success once the theoretical feasibility of organ transplantation had been established.

CELLULAR ENGINEERING AND TRANSPLANTATION, 1967

Good coined the phrase *cellular engineering* to describe a methodology for treating disorders of the immune system and was the first to successfully use fetal liver cells and bone marrow transplantation as examples.

FIRST BONE MARROW TRANSPLANTATION PATIENT, 1968

In August of 1968, Good and a group of his fellows put into practice his earlier published theory of the possibility of curing an X-linked congenital form of severe combined immunodeficiency disease (SCID) by bone marrow transplantation (BMT). The first successful transplantation and the first cure of an X-linked SCID by cellular engineering were achieved. The 4-month-old male SCID patient developed aplastic anemia, a complicating acquired immunodeficiency disorder that compromised the initial successful transplant necessitating in November of the same year a second allogeneic bone marrow transplantation with the same matched (B, C, D loci) sibling donor. This second BMT corrected and subsequently cured the acquired aplastic anemia developed, most likely Good said, from an A antigen mismatch between donor and recipient in the first BMT.

DETAILS OF FIRST BMT

Jerome L'Heureux, a pediatrician in Meriden, Connecticut, knew of Good's work and interest in immunodeficiency diseases and the promising area of BMT. L'Heureux was convinced that Bob Good held the only chance for the survival of his 4-month-old male patient. Eleven male babies on the child's mother's side of the family succumbed to this SCID before their first birthdays. No male child had survived in eight years. L'Heureux's patient had already faced several bouts of life-threatening pneumonia, each one staved off by antibiotics. He gave the child little hope of survival unless Bob Good had an idea that would save the child from a certain and early death.

The child was found to be suffering from the X-linked form of SCID. He had four healthy sisters but he was getting weaker every day. Good examined the child and determined that he was a likely candidate for BMT as an effort to try to cure the X-linked SCID (XSCID) from which he suffered. If a reasonable major histocompatibility complex (MHC) matched donor could be found, they would proceed with the transplant.

Only one of the patient's sisters appeared compatible enough to allow doctors to attempt the procedure, but one chance was all that was needed. Good assembled the transplant team. Richard Hong was an independent colleague and associate professor who helped Good train fellows clinically and in the laboratories and treated children with both primary and secondary immunodeficiency diseases. Edmond Yunis had become director of the University of Minnesota blood bank and brought the group to the cutting edge of research on lymphoid and hematopoietic transplants in experimental animals. Carlos Martinez and Yunis had earlier shown that it was possible to achieve lymphoid cell transplants without producing GVHD — a critical factor in successfully transplanting bone marrow and having it engraft in the recipient without killing him. Hilaire Meuwissen, a senior fellow interested in carrying out transplants of stem cells from marrow to treat SCID, would supervise the surgery. Richard Gatti had just joined Good's group as a research fellow. Gatti, with assistance from Hugh Allen, a clinical resident, would make history by actually performing the transplant.

The patient and his sister were later shown to be less compatible than previously thought, by a single antigen attributed to an A locus mismatch due to a previous genetic cross-over event in the recipient. No prophylactic myeloablative treatment was used. The transplant was deemed a success. Both T and B cells were reconstituted within the recipient within a month. The second part of the story is well known in that the first BMT, while successful in curing the XSCID, created a complicating and life-threatening aplastic anemia due to an antigenic mismatch unknown at the time of the first transplant. The majority opinion was to destroy the first transplant that caused the anemia, but Good felt that would bring the patient back to ground zero — still suffering from the fatal XSCID that would soon claim another victim. Good's reasoning prevailed and with the family's consent a second bone marrow transplant was performed in November of 1968 in an attempt to cure the fatal anemia that developed as a result of the first transplant. The same brave little sibling donor was asked to donate more of her bone marrow to her ailing brother. This time, the little patient was completely cured; neither XSCID nor aplastic anemia was present after the second transplant. Good described his young patient's new immune system thus:

Mature red blood cells, white blood cells, and platelets promptly appeared in the circulating blood. The patient's red blood cell type switched over entirely from cells of the patient's genetic A type to production of red cells from the marrow that were now entirely of donor origin-blood group O cells.

Now, almost 40 years later, the patient is completely cured of his congenital and acquired diseases, is married, and has two healthy twin sons.

BMT, a form of cellular engineering, has been applied to more than 75 otherwise fatal diseases. It has been demonstrated to be a viable method of reconstituting a hereditarily defective immunological system and to correct both structure and function of a hematopoietic system affected by an acquired disease.

RECOGNITION BY ESTEEMED COLLEAGUES

Good was nominated many times for the Nobel Prize, which he no doubt should have won for myriad clinical and scientific contributions and discoveries in various areas over the span of his six-decade-long career. The committee, in 1990, however, favored Dr. E. Donnell Thomas and Dr. Joseph Murray to share the prize in medicine and physiology for Thomas's perfection of bone marrow transplantation and Murray's first successful kidney transplant from one identical twin to the other. Good was, nonetheless, brought before that august podium in Stockholm, if not in person, then by everlasting words spoken by his colleague and friend E. Donnell Thomas, upon delivery of his Nobel Lecture on December 8, 1990:

> In November of 1968* Dr. Robert Good and his colleagues carried out the first marrow transplant from a matched sibling for an infant with an immunological deficiency disease.** Our team carried out our first transplant using a matched sibling donor for a patient with advanced leukemia in March 1969.

Good was held in such high esteem by his colleagues that when it came time to select the keynote speaker for the special lecture honoring Thomas at his own institution in Seattle, Good it was often said, received the popular vote. People needn't have been worried whether Good, who did not receive the Prize for the BMT he was the first to perform, would be upset to be asked to congratulate his competitor and recipient of the prize. Good said that he felt honored to be able to laud the successes of his colleague and friend, Don Thomas, for his accomplishments in the field of marrow transplantation in leukemia. Seattle gave Good his own award by naming the conference room where the event was held in his honor.

NEW YORK AND SLOAN-KETTERING INSTITUTE 1973

CANCER

Good's extensive work in the fields of congenital, acquired, and/or induced oncological diseases meant it was time to create a separate section in his research portfolio. He delineates the relationship of cancer and immunity in an editorial article titled "The cancer–immunity interface in a hospital practice."

CANCER AND IMMUNODEFICIENCY DISEASES

In 1973, Good became president of the Sloan-Kettering Research Institute. He appeared on the cover of *Time* and was featured in the March 19 issue of the magazine. Good noted in the article that he and his co-workers observed a high

---

* The first BMT was actually performed in August of 1968; the second was in November of 1968.
** Gatti, R.A., Meuwissen, H.J., Allen, H.D., Hong, R., and Good, R.A., *Lancet* ii, 1366–1369 (1968).

correlation between cancer and the immunodeficiency diseases and that "in order for cancer to occur and persist, there must be a failure of the immunological process." These "failures" provided the stimulation for Good to devote his life to the study and understanding of immunological "experiments of nature," finding ways to correct the imbalances and relieve the suffering of all creatures, large and small. He said:

> Understanding the immune system will enable us to do far more than treat allergies or immunodeficiency diseases or to control cancer; it will enable us to understand the basic processes of life.

NUTRITION, CALORIE RESTRICTION, LONGEVITY, AUTOIMMUNITY, AND CANCER

Good, with colleagues Day and Engelman, analyzed in detail the molecular biology, cellular biology, and virology of the bases by which calorie restriction inhibits development of breast cancer in mice. Most striking were the observations that calories, on energy intake restriction, control and reduce proliferation of vegetative cell systems and reproductive organs while enhancing cell proliferation essential during immune responses and tissue regeneration. In studies extending over a 24-year period, Good and his students and younger colleagues were at the forefront in making many important contributions to analyses of the influence of nutrition, impacts of individual nutriments on immune function, and the development of immunologically based diseases. In addition, Good and Gabriel Fernandes showed reduced calorie consumption made it consistently possible to double, often triple, and occasionally quadruple the life spans of genetically short-lived autoimmune-prone mice and prevent the immunologic involution that occurs with aging in these animals. Using diets high in both calories and saturated fats, Good and his colleagues produced striking models of arthrosclerosis and arteriosclerosis in autoimmune-prone mice, but not in autoimmune-resistant strains.

ADDITIONAL SIGNIFICANT CONTRIBUTIONS

Good, his colleagues, and his fellows made other important contributions in the areas of nutrition and immunity, longevity and cancer, autoimmune diseases, systemic lupus erythematosus (SLE), kidney and liver diseases, virology, and other areas of interest.

- Good was the first to publish in-depth research demonstrating the immunosuppressive qualities of viruses.
- A 1973 paper on pneumocystis carinii pneumonia that Good co-authored with Burke is still considered a classic in the field of medicine.
- Among the most important contributions was the definitive analysis of the crucial role played by zinc in thymic function and in the development and maintenance of immunologic functions of both T and B cells.

PUBLICATIONS AND AWARDS

Good published more than 2,100 scientific papers. He authored, co-authored, or edited more than 50 books and wrote countless articles in his almost 60-year career at the laboratory bench and the patient's bedside. Good literally supported the pencil industry by writing all of his works in long hand in pencil. His archives house thousands of pages of handwritten papers, notes, articles, and other memorabilia. He was lauded as the most cited scientist in any discipline during a 15-year period from 1961 to 1976 by the Citation Index.

He was the recipient of more than 250 awards, honors, and recognitions including the Albert Lasker Clinical Medical Research Award; the Emperor's Sacred Treasure; the Gold and Silver Star, the highest honor Japan can bestow on a non-Japanese scientist; the prestigious Canadian Gairdner Foundation Award; the Claude Bernard Prize; the E. Meade Johnson Award; the Lila E. Gruber Award for his work on the Shwartzman phenomenon; the Parke-Davis Award; the Borden Award; the International Bone Marrow Transplant Registry 25th Anniversary Award; the John Howland Award, the highest honor granted by the American Pediatric Association; the David Karnofsky award for cancer research; and the Ronald McDonald Award of Excellence, to name but a few. Good was a generous patron of local and national charities and often donated his prize monies to charities.

Good received 13 honorary doctorates from Hahnemann Medical College; Catholic Medical College of Seoul, South Korea; University of Uppsala, Sweden; New York Medical College; Medical College of Ohio, Toledo; College of Medicine and Dentistry of New Jersey; University of Chicago; University of Rome; St. John's University; Chicago Medical School; Miami Children's Hospital; University of Minnesota; and Shinshu University School of Medicine. His research throughout his long career was funded by the National Institutes of Health, the American Cancer Society, and other agencies. His last honor was a merit award from the National Institutes of Health. He also served for several years on study sections of the NIH, NCS, and other agencies.

MEMBERSHIPS AND CONTRIBUTIONS TO THE COMMUNITY

Good was a founder and/or member of myriad professional organizations. He served as president of the American Association of Immunologists, the American Association of Pathologists, the American Society for Clinical Investigation, the American Society for Experimental Biology and Medicine, and the International Society for Preventive Oncology, among others. Good was a charter member of the Institute of Science and when he arrived in Florida in 1985, he was the only member of the National Academy of Sciences in the Department of Medicine at the University of South Florida. He sat on over 40 editorial boards and served as an untiring consultant to many others. He was in demand as a lecturer and was able to present science in its simplest terms to lay audiences.

National Marrow Donor Program and Registry

Good was honored before the Congress of the United States by the Hon. Bill Young of Florida in 1994 for his pivotal, seminal, and sustaining role in establishing the first National Bone Marrow Registry Program in the U.S. in 1987. To date, over 93 million potential donors have been registered under this program and over 4 million transplants have been performed under the National Marrow Donor Program.

Bone Marrow Transplantation Programs

Good started the first BMT programs at the University of Minnesota, New York's Sloan-Kettering Institute, the University of Oklahoma, and All Children's Hospital in St. Petersburg, Florida. Mrs. Eleanor Naylor Dana donated $1 million toward the transplant unit in New York. She also named Good a trustee of the Eleanor Naylor Dana Trust and he served on the board for 28 years.

CELEBRATIONS AND ENDOWED CHAIRS

Hines Chair

Good was a recipient of the Hines Chair at All Children's Hospital in St. Petersburg Florida and the University of South Florida (USF) at Tampa. He generously gave up the chair to recruit a molecular geneticist for the Department of Pediatrics at the university.

Fifty Years of Medicine and Medical Research

In May of 1994, in St. Petersburg, Florida, on the occasion of his 78th birthday and 50 years in medicine and medical research, Dr. Good was honored by USF in a three-day celebration, organized by Professor Richard Lockey, director of the Allergy and Immunology Program, and attended by distinguished leaders in the fields of medicine and medical research. Over 500 colleagues, and members of academic and professional societies to which he belonged joined in the celebration. The highlight of the event was an important scientific symposium entitled: Perspectives in Immunology and Medicine I: A Symposium in Honor of Dr. Robert A. Good, 1944–1994.

Robert A. Good "Super" Chair

The University of South Florida again honored Good by establishing the Robert A. Good Chair in immunology. The Dana Foundation contributed a second million dollars in support of continuing the legacy of Bob Good and his research efforts. Both contributions were matched by the state and the university to become a phenomenal $5.2 million "super" chair in immunology.

HONORED BY THE U.S. CONGRESS

The Hon. Bill Young, a member of the House of Representatives, honored Dr. Good on the floor of the U.S. Congress for his outstanding contributions and pioneering role in establishing the National Marrow Donor Program in 1987. The President of the University of South Florida; Ambassador and Mrs. Marker; the President of All Children's Hospital, Dennis Sexton; and many others also paid tribute to the man who inspired and infused the university and hospital through his talent and generosity.

TRIBUTE OF DR. EDMOND YUNIS

Dr. Edmond Yunis, a celebrated colleague and good friend, honored Good with a special tribute — a poem excerpted below:

When I was young we walked
through the wooded fields
near the tall trees close to the night,
when the loon sang distant songs.
Other times when was cold
the winter evenings with the bright snow
and the moon giving certain blue taint
showed lights covering the ground.
But, it was at dawn when often
we shared precious moments
of excitement and inquiry; new questions
and the challenge for answers.

We have all been there
and again we are here,
a gathering of the young and not so young
with binding forces like chains.
Today, we celebrate his life
one half a century, a triumph.
A natural contingency,
a miraculous chance.
Fifty years and more will come
and, when we meet again
we shall look at the sea,
and the warm breeze near our faces
with invisible birds above,
will fly together unfinished trips
beyond shadows and winds.

Then a toast to Robert, the scientist
our friend, the teacher and the physician.

THE ROBERT A. GOOD LECTURE SERIES

In February of 2001, the University of South Florida College of Medicine at Tampa honored Good in a special three-day tribute. The endowed annual Robert A. Good Lecture was established to carry on the legacy he established at the university and within the state of Florida.

PERSONAL GLIMPSES

Robert Good was a physically commanding, attractive, larger-than-life, warm, brilliant, eccentric, generous, optimistic, constantly energized, impressive, and charismatic man. He slept fewer than four hours a night throughout his life. What daylight did not give freely he stole from the night. It was quite normal for him to start his day at 4 A.M. by meeting with colleagues, fellows, and students at home over a pot of coffee. He often said:

Your day can always be expanded at the front end, i.e., get up a little earlier!

If you can't sleep, then get up and work!

I can think of no greater punishment than to be made to stay in bed till 7 A.M.!

EARLY YEARS, MINNESOTA, 1922

Good was born on May 21, 1922, in Crosby, Minnesota, a small town north of Minneapolis, with a population of 2,065. He was the second of four sons born to educators Roy Homer Good and Ethel Whitcomb, both born in Hennepin County, Minnesota. Good's paternal grandparents, Charles and Emma Good, moved from Canada to Wisconsin and then to Minnesota before his father was born in 1861. Charles Good's family emigrated to Canada from England in 1874. Emma Good was born in England in 1866. Her family emigrated to Canada from England in 1864.

Roy Homer Good was completing his Ph.D. program in education in 1927 when he died of testicular cancer at the age of 37. Bob Good was only 5 then; his three brothers were all under 7 years of age. His mother decided not to remarry and continued to teach school while raising and supporting her four boys, all of whom grew up to become outstanding doctors. Bob collaborated with his brother Tom, a dermatologist, in writing several papers.

GUILLAIN–BARRÉ, 1941

In June of 1941, at age 19, during his pre-med university years, Good suffered a mild case of what Good later said was Guillain–Barré (GB) — not polio nor amyotrophic lateral sclerosis. At the time of diagnosis, doctors did not know whether Good would ever be able to walk again or, what surely must have been a worse prognosis, be able to continue his university studies and realize his dream of becoming a doctor and helping to cure cancer — a promise he made to his father when he was only 5 years old.

The illness started suddenly and quickly left him paralyzed from the neck down, but did not necessitate the use of artificial ventilation or an "iron lung" as the device was known in the days of polio epidemics that crippled lives as well as bodies. Fortunately, Good suffered only a mild case of GB and gradually regained control of his muscles. The illness resolved within the year but left him with paralysis below the knees and lacking knee jerk reflexes. This led to his early and understandable interest in the two-nerve two-axon studies he conducted in Berry Campbell's neurophysiology lab while he was still a graduate student, before Fred Kolouch wooed him away with alluring studies of plasma cells.

Good, always an A student, was among the first 14 students to be selected for admission to medical school in March of 1943. Upon hearing of Good's illness, the dean arbitrarily deleted Good's name from the list. When Good found out, he naturally went to see the dean and ask why his name had been eliminated. The dean said he "assumed" Good would not be entering medical school because he had Lou Gehrig's disease. Good's minor paralytic disease left him lame below the knees, not above the neck, and certainly did not preclude him from thinking and writing! The dean put Good's name back on the roster and the rest is history. Good's lameness necessitated his somewhat eccentric but vastly more comfortable wearing of tennis shoes instead of more elegant oxfords.

FAMILY LIFE

Good married and had five children, beginning in 1948 with Robert Michael, followed by Mark Thomas, Alan Maclynn, Margaret Eugenia, and Mary Elizabeth. As of 2003, his children had presented him with 14 grandchildren. He acquired three more grandchildren from the family of his wife, Noorbibi Day-Good, for a total of 17 little children to spoil and read to. Good said with so many children and grandchildren he memorized the stories so that he could be ready at a moment's notice when a little face was upturned toward his and asked for a story. One of his granddaughters is carrying on the family pediatrician tradition.

Good, divorced from his first wife, remarried and divorced a second time. He found happiness both professionally and privately when he married his long-time friend and colleague, Noorbibi Day, Ph.D., a Kenyan of Indian descent and a well-known scientist in her own right. They had known each other since 1957 when she interviewed with Good for a position in his laboratory. He said that she was welcome to work but asked if she had to work wrapped up in those swaddling clothes. Noorbibi said the garment was a sari and that she was used to working in one. Noorbibi went to work with Good and wore her sari. Bob and Bibi both had families of their own then and were professional colleagues and friends. When they married years later, their families including Bibi's two sons Kahlil Day and Selim Day melded together very nicely. The two families still remain in close contact. Life is unpredictable. While it may not offer an entire lifetime of happiness, it provided several decades' worth in Bob and Bibi's case.

Noorbibi Day-Good published her first paper from Good's laboratory in 1958. Their professional relationship continued more than 45 years and produced more than 175 papers along with a dozen books and articles. They shared 20 years as husband and wife. They were usually the first on the dance floor and the last to sit down. Theirs was a good marriage based on a lifetime of friendship and respect.

Memories of Bob Good

Bob loved animals, especially dogs. His personal library contains many books about dogs. A photo of his last cocker spaniel, KD (the dog was a gift from Kahlil Day, and Bob named the dog in Kahlil's honor) remains on display in the library along with photos of family members, friends, and colleagues. He loved American football, especially when his hometown team, the Tampa Bay Buccaneers, won the Super Bowl in Tampa! He loved classical music, opera, and poetry, especially that of Robert Frost, good conversation, and gourmet food he prepared. Good was convinced that all great scientists must by nature be great chefs! He loved to travel the world and see all that could be seen by one man who lived life to the hilt.

The End of a Chapter

Robert A. Good retired from his lab and from this life on Friday, June 13, 2003, after 81 revolutions around the sun. He died at home, surrounded by his family, friends, and one of his student fellows. This was the end of a chapter but not the end of the book that has yet to be written about Bob Good. He suffered but never complained during a long and valiant battle with esophageal cancer, a fatal "experiment of nature" diagnosed in 1997. Despite three surgeries, radiation treatments and all that goes with battling such illness, he nevertheless continued to work, teach courses, attend lectures and events, and mentor his beloved students and fellows. His body was wearing down, but his mind was razor sharp until the end. He was reading a book on DNA on his terrace in St. Petersburg, Florida, looking east at the vast expanse of the blue-green waters of the Gulf of Mexico he loved so well. Boats were in the harbor and small private planes were taking off and landing at Albert Whitted airport in front of his 23rd floor condominium. The sky was brilliantly blue and cloudless on the day Bob died. He never tired of being alive until the very end when he was told that the cancer returned with a vengeance and nothing more could be done. When his wife asked whether there was anyone he wanted to see, he replied, "my students." Bob closed his book and as the sun set, called it a Good day and a Good life. He never forgot us and we will never forget him.

Memorials

Two memorial services honored Good. The first one was in June of 2003 at All Children's Hospital in St. Petersburg. The second one was held in November of 2003 at All Souls Unitarian Church in New York City and was followed by a major memorial symposium at Rockefeller University — the site of Bob's early work in Maclyn's lab that allowed him to find his own scientific niche studying myeloma and Hodgkin's patients. The symposium was sponsored by Bob's long-time friends

Fred and Vicki Modell, who founded the Jeffrey Modell Foundation in honor of their son who died of PIDD. Scientists and dignitaries from around the world, friends, and family members gathered to remember and pay their respects to a man who had given his life to the well-being of others.

The Modells, generous patrons who have devoted their lives to finding cures for diseases like the one that stole their son, are building an impressive state-of-the-art immunology center at Harvard Medical School to commemorate the 20th anniversary of their foundation. The library at the center will be named in Bob Good's honor as testimony to his contributions to the field of immunology. It is hoped that bright young minds will find inspiration by learning about the life of Robert A. Good and that the torch he has passed to others will not be extinguished and will burn even more brightly in years to come.

Fred Rosen

One keynote speaker at Good's memorial service was Fred Rosen, who passed away in May of 2005. Rosen was a favorite of Good's, a good friend, erudite scholar, exceptional physician scientist, and healthy competitor, hailing from Harvard and the Boston group. Rosen spoke thus of Bob Good:

Fred Rosen's Tribute to Good

In 1865, in his *An Introduction to the Study of Experimental Medicine*, Claude Bernard wrote:

> Great men may be compared to torches shining at long intervals, to guide the advance of science. They light up their time, either by discovering unexpected and fertile phenomena, which open up new paths and reveal unknown horizons, or by generalizing acquired scientific facts and disclosing truths, which their predecessors had not perceived.

How can I sum up the career of one such great man, Bob Good, in one thousand words, without shortchanging his memory and his larger-than-life presence in the medical science arena for half a century? Many things have been said of Bob Good since he left us, but there is one word that I have not heard. He was, after all is said and done, extremely intelligent. His scintillating, smart mind dominated any assembly where he was present. An example of this occurred in the early 1950s.

Gitlin and Janeway, my mentors, had presented at a meeting of the Society for Pediatric Research in Atlantic City an abstract on children with susceptibility to infection and hypergammaglobulinemia. On the spot he pointed out that this was absurd, that the latter was a consequence of the former and not the cause. He went home and quickly demonstrated in a similar cohort of patients that this phenomenon was due to a phagocyte defect, namely chronic granulomatous disease. Along with his colleague Beulah Holmes, he showed that this disease results from a fault in bacterial killing and that the hypergammaglobulinemia was the consequence of persistent antigenic stimulation. In one stroke, he opened a new field of scientific endeavor in the economics of phagocytic function that provided scientific employment for many who proceeded to exploit this extraordinary observation. The time allotted to me does not allow further digressions to illustrate this point. It happened over and over again.

Bob was deeply humanistic and perhaps because of his own infirmities he always expressed his personal and caring concerns to others. He harassed me for years about all my bad habits, about smoking and being overweight, and I never took offense at his telling me these things because they were expressed with compassionate concern. Of course, his feelings for his own patients bore the same imprimatur of commitment and caring, He was after all a consummate physician.

He had a puckish sense of humor, sometimes eliciting the prankster in him. Once many years ago, while seated next to him at a meeting in St. Pete Beach, Florida, we listened to one of his research fellows present a talk, which I thought was awful. When he was done, I leaned over to Bob and said, "This guy is a preacher, not a scientist." Later that day, at a cocktail reception, this young man approached me and said, "Bob Good says you think I'm a preacher!" Slowly I felt myself sinking into the woodwork, thinking, "How could Bob have been so callous as to transmit my harsh opinion of this guy?" when suddenly the young man in question perked up and added, "How perceptive of you, Dr. Rosen. I am a graduate of the Louisiana Baptist Seminary!"

Those of us who knew him will always remember him as a tireless scribe, always sitting in the front row on the center aisle, taking copious notes of everything that was said. His storehouse of immunologic knowledge was immense. He was the outstanding immunopathophysiologist of his time and he had no equal in that regard. I see him now, shuffling hundreds of slides, overflowing into yet another carousel, as he entranced many listeners with his experiments of nature, and those of us who were fortunate enough to have shared his cup of knowledge and were inspired by his tireless, inquiring mind will never forget him.

In the first act of Chekhov's *Uncle Vanya*, Dr. Astrov, who has just returned from a village where epidemic typhus was raging, asks the nursemaid, "Will those who live a hundred or two hundred years after us and for whom we have prepared the way, will they remember us with a kind word?" And the nursemaid answers, "No, people don't remember. That is why God remembers." In Bob Good's case, they will remember for generations and generations to come.

And you too, Fred Rosen, as well as all the other illuminating pathfinders, those medical scientists who have gone on before us, will be remembered by your colleagues, students, and friends for your contributions.

Editors

Nicholas P. Plotnikoff, Ph.D., is a professor of pharmacology at the College of Pharmacy, College of Medicine, and Graduate College at the University of Illinois in Chicago. His principal research interest is in the area of psychoneuroimmunology with special emphasis on stress hormones and cytokines (enkephalins and endorphins). His current research focuses on the clinical effects of methionine enkephalin in the treatment of cancer and AIDS patients. In 1999, together with Robert E. Faith, Anthony J. Murgo, and Robert A. Good, he helped organize an update of the state-of-the-art *Cytokines: Stress and Immunity* (CRC Press LLC).

Robert E. Faith, D.V.M., Ph.D., is the associate dean for veterinary medicine and director of the Biomedical Resource Center of the Medical College of Wisconsin. He earned a D.V.M. from Texas A&M University in 1968 and a Ph.D. in immunology from the University of Florida in 1979 and pursued residency training in laboratory animal medicine at the University of Florida from 1968 to 1971. From 1974 to 1978, Dr. Faith served as staff fellow and senior staff fellow at the National Institute of Environmental Health Sciences. He was director of the Biomedical Research Center at Oral Roberts University from 1978 to 1984, director of Animal Care Facilities at the University of Houston from 1984 to 1990, associate director of the Center for Comparative Medicine at Baylor College of Medicine from 1990 to 1997, and director of the Center for Comparative Medicine at Baylor from 1997 to 2002. He joined the Medical College of Wisconsin in 2002.

Anthony J. Murgo, M.D., M.S., FACP, is a medical oncologist and an adjunct professor of medicine at the Uniformed Services University of the Health Sciences F. Edward Hébert School of Medicine in Bethesda, Maryland. Dr. Murgo received his M.D. and M.S. in pathology and immunology in 1975 from the State University of New York Downstate Medical Center. He completed medical residency training at Maimonides Medical Center in Brooklyn and a fellowship in hematologic oncology at Memorial Sloan-Kettering Cancer Center in New York City. Dr. Murgo is board certified in internal medicine and medical oncology and is a fellow of the American College of Physicians. He was on the medical faculty at the Oral Roberts University School of Medicine from 1980 to 1983. He later joined the faculty of the West Virginia University School of Medicine where he was a professor of medicine in the Section of Hematology and Oncology until 1989. He subsequently was a medical officer at the U.S. Food and Drug Administration's Division of Oncologic Drug Products from 1989 to 1996 and then joined the National Cancer Institute specializing in investigational drug development and clinical trials.

Robert A. Good, Ph.D., M.D. D.Sc., FACP, earned graduate degrees from the University of Minnesota in the early 1950s. He was the physician-in-chief at All

Children's Hospital in St. Petersburg, Florida, and a distinguished research professor at the University of Florida College of Medicine. His remarkable career includes service as the president and director of the Sloan-Kettering Institute for Cancer Research in New York; professorships in pediatrics, pathology, and medicine at Cornell University; head of cancer research at the Oklahoma Medical Research Foundation; and head of research at Memorial Hospital in New York.

He distinguished himself with major contributions to both basic and clinical immunology. His research achievements include discovery of the function of the thymus and definition of the two distinct major components of the immune systems. Dr. Good was the recipient of 13 honorary doctorates and more than 100 major citations and awards. He wrote and edited more than 50 books and book chapters.

Dr. Good had been president of the American Association of Immunologists, Association of American Pathologists, Central Society for Clinical Research, American Society for Clinical Investigation, Reticuloendothelial Society, and Society for Experimental Biology and Medicine. In 1978, he was recognized by Citation Index as the most cited scientist in the world over a 10-year period.

Contributors

Massimo Alfano
Department of Immunology
  and Infectious Diseases
and
Center of Excellence on
  Physiopathology of Cell
  Differentiation
San Raffaele Scientific Institute
Milan, Italy

Tihomir Balog
Department of Molecular Medicine
Rudjer Bošković Institute
Zagreb, Croatia

Istvan Berczi
Department of Immunology
Faculty of Medicine
The University of Manitoba,
Winnipeg, Manitoba, Canada

Jos A. Bosch
Department of Periodontics
University of Illinois
Chicago, Illinois, U.S.A.
and
School of Sports and Exercise Sciences
University of Birmingham
Birmingham, U.K.

Stanley A. Brod
Department of Neurology
The University of Texas Medical School
and
The University of Texas Graduate
  School of Biomedical Sciences
Houston, Texas, U.S.A.

Peter John Cabot
School of Pharmacy
The University of Queensland
St. Lucia, Queensland, Australia

John T. Cacioppo
Chicago Center for Cognitive and
  Social Neuroscience
and
Department of Psychology
University of Chicago
Chicago, Illinois, U.S.A.

Edith Chen
Department of Psychology
University of British Columbia
Vancouver, British Columbia, Canada

Maurice Corcos
Départment de Psychiatrie de l'Enfant
  de l'Adolescent
Institut Mutualiste Montsouris
Paris, France

Nachum Dafny
Department of Neurobiology
  and Anatomy
The University of Texas Medical School
Houston, Texas, U.S.A.

Robert Day
Départements de Pharmacologie
  et de Biochimie
Université de Sherbrooke
Sherbrooke, Quebec, Canada

Adrian J. Dunn
Department of Pharmacology,
  Toxicology, and Neuroscience
Louisiana State University Health
  Sciences Center
Shreveport, Louisiana, U.S.A.

Yogesh Dwivedi
Department of Psychiatry
University of Illinois
Chicago, Illinois, U.S.A.

Christopher G. Engeland
Department of Periodontics
University of Illinois
Chicago, Illinois, U.S.A.

Robert E. Faith
Biomedical Resource Center
Medical College of Wisconsin
Milwaukee, Wisconsin, U.S.A.

Paolo Falaschi
Faculty of Medicine
University of Rome La Sapienza
Rome, Italy

Sivia Franchi
Department of Pharmacology
University of Milan
Milan, Italy

Olivier Guilbaud
Départment de Psychiatrie de l'Enfant
  de l'Adolescent
Institut Mutualiste Montsouris
Paris, France

Helena Haberstock-Debić
Department of Molecular Medicine
Rudjer Bošković Institute
Zagreb, Croatia

Margaret D. Hanson
Department of Psychology
University of British Columbia
Vancouver, British Columbia, Canada

Louise C. Hawkley
Chicago Center for Cognitive
  and Social Neuroscience
and
Department of Psychology
University of Chicago
Chicago, Illinois, U.S.A.

Thomas K. Hughes, Jr.
Microbiology, Immunology,
  and Pathology
University of Texas Medical Branch
Galveston, Texas, U.S.A.

Philippe Jeammet
Départment de Psychiatrie de l'Enfant
  de l'Adolescent
Institut Mutualiste Montsouris
Paris, France

Jennifer Kelschenbach
Department of Pharmacology
University of Minnesota
Minneapolis, Minnesota, U.S.A.

Margaret E. Kemeny
Department of Psychiatry
University of California
San Francisco, California, U.S.A.

Kalman Kovacs
Department of Pathology
St. Michael's Hospital
University of Toronto
Toronto, Ontario, Canada

Ziad Kronfol
Department of Psychiatry
University of Michigan
Ann Arbor, Michigan, U.S.A.

Catherine Liu
Department of Molecular Genetics,
  Microbiology, and Immunology
Robert Wood Johnson Medical
  School
University of Medicine and Dentistry
  of New Jersey
Piscataway, New Jersey, U.S.A.

Horace H. Loh
Department of Pharmacology
University of Minnesota
Minneapolis, Minnesota, U.S.A.

Tatjana Marotti
Department of Molecular
  Medicine
Rudjer Bošković Institute
Zagreb, Croatia

Antonio Martocchia
Faculty of Medicine
University of Rome La Sapienza
Rome, Italy

Cataldo Martucci
Department of Pharmacology
University of Milan
Milan, Italy

Phillip T. Marucha
Department of Periodontics
University of Illinois
Chicago, Illinois, U.S.A.

Aron D. Mosnaim
Department of Cellular and Molecular
  Pharmacology
Rosalind Franklin University
The Chicago Medical School
Chicago, Illinois, U.S.A.

Rama Murali
Department of Psychology
University of British Columbia
Vancouver, British Columbia, Canada

Anthony J. Murgo
Uniformed Services University
  of the Health Sciences
Edward Hébert School of Medicine
Bethesda, Maryland, U.S.A.

Ghanshyam N. Pandey
Department of Psychiatry
University of Illinois
Chicago, Illinois, U.S.A.

Carmine Pariante
Stress, Psychiatry, and Immunology
  Laboratory
Institute of Psychiatry
London, U.K.

Nicholas P. Plotnikoff
Department of Biopharmaceutical
  Sciences, College of Pharmacy
and
Department of Psychiatry, College of
  Medicine
University of Illinois
Chicago, Illinois, U.S.A.

Guido Poli
Department of Immunology
  and Infectious Diseases
and
Center of Excellence on
  Physiopathology of Cell
  Differentiation
and
School of Medicine
San Raffaele Scientific Institute
Milan, Italy

Javier Puente
Department of Biochemistry
  and Molecular Biology
University of Chile
Santiago, Chile

Andres Quintanar-Stephano
Department of Physiology
  and Pharmacology
Autonomous University of
  Aguascalientes
Aguascalientes, Mexico

Gopinath Ranjith
Maudsley and Bethlem Royal Hospitals
London, U.K.

Arthur I. Roberts
Department of Molecular Genetics,
  Microbiology, and Immunology
Robert Wood Johnson Medical School
University of Medicine and Dentistry of
  New Jersey
Piscataway, New Jersey, U.S.A.

Sabita Roy
Department of Pharmacology
University of Minnesota
Minneapolis, Minnesota, U.S.A.

Paola Sacerdote
Department of Pharmacology
University of Milan
Milan, Italy

Michel Salzet
Laboratoire de Neuroimmunologie
 des Annélides
Université des Sciences et Technologies
 de Lille
Villeneuve d'Ascq, France

Suzanne C. Segerstrom
Department of Psychology
University of Kentucky
Lexington, Kentucky, U.S.A.

Yufang Shi
Department of Molecular Genetics,
 Microbiology, and Immunology
Robert Wood Johnson Medical School
University of Medicine and Dentistry of
 New Jersey
Piscataway, New Jersey, U.S.A.

Eric M. Smith
Psychiatry and Behavioral Sciences
and
Microbiology, Immunology,
 and Pathology
University of Texas Medical Branch
Galveston, Texas, U.S.A.

Sandra Sobočanec
Department of Molecular Medicine
Rudjer Bošković Institute
Zagreb, Croatia

Erwei Sun
Department of Molecular Genetics,
 Microbiology, and Immunology
Robert Wood Johnson Medical School
University of Medicine and Dentistry of
 New Jersey
Piscataway, New Jersey, U.S.A.

Višnja Šverko
Department of Molecular Medicine
Rudjer Bošković Institute
Zagreb, Croatia

Huolin Tu
Microbiology, Immunology, and
 Pathology
University of Texas Medical Branch
Galveston, Texas, U.S.A.

M. Antonieta Valenzuela
Department of Biochemistry and
 Molecular Biology
University of Chile
Santiago, Chile

Lixin Wei
Department of Molecular Genetics,
 Microbiology, and Immunology
Robert Wood Johnson Medical School
University of Medicine and Dentistry of
 New Jersey
Piscataway, New Jersey, U.S.A.

Marion E. Wolf
International Neuropsychiatry
 Consultants
Highland Park, Illinois, U.S.A.

Pamela B. Yang
Department of Neurobiology
 and Anatomy
The University of Texas Medical School
Houston, Texas, U.S.A.

1 Behavioral Effects of Cytokines: A Psychiatrist's Perspective

Ziad Kronfol

CONTENTS

INTRODUCTION

The notion that cytokines play an important role as mediators between the immune and nervous systems is now well established. It is also well established that this interaction is bidirectional, with products of activated immune cells (cytokines) interacting with cells of the nervous system and products of nerve cells (neurotransmitters) interacting with various immune cells.[1] The resulting complex dialogue is meant to help protect the organism and prolong survival of the species. However, as with every biological system, malfunctions can occur and resulting pathology follows.

In this chapter, we will first review some of the behavioral effects of cytokines commonly found in psychiatric patients. These effects include disturbances in sleep, appetite, mood, cognition, energy and fatigue levels, and sex drive. This will be followed by a critical review of the cytokine hypothesis of major depression. The roles of cytokines as mediators in depression and other major illnesses such as infection, cancer, cardiovascular disease, and AIDS will then be discussed. We will also address the issue of behavioral toxicity associated with cytokine treatment for conditions such as hepatitis C and malignant melanoma. Thus, we hope to briefly cover most of the issues associated with cytokines and cytokine treatment from the perspective of the clinical psychiatrist.

BEHAVIORAL EFFECTS OF CYTOKINES

The observation that cytokines are associated with specific behavioral symptoms dates back at least a decade or two. Animal studies revealed that rats and mice injected with phytohemagglutinin (PHA) or lipopolysaccharide (LPS), substances that stimulate the production of different cytokines, exhibited symptoms of lethargy, fatigue, anorexia with decreased preference for sweetened water, decreased grooming, and decreased sexual activity — a clinical picture that prompted certain investigators to label sickness behavior because of its resemblance to the behavior of animals that were sick with infections.[2] We will therefore start by providing an overview of the relationship between specific cytokines and specific behavioral symptoms, both in animals and in humans.

Sleep

Sleep is a complex physiological process that is important for the survival of a species. Mammals exhibit at least two stages of sleep: non-rapid eye movement (NREM) and rapid eye movement (REM) sleep. The administration of exogenous interleukin-1ß (IL-1ß) or tumor necrosis factor (TNF) to mice or rats enhanced NREM sleep.[3] Substances that enhance the production of IL-1ß or TNF (such as bacterial or viral products) enhance sleep, while substances that inhibit the production of IL-1ß or TNF inhibit sleep.[4] Furthermore, the inhibition of IL-1ß or TNF inhibits the sleep induced by muramyltripeptide, a bacterial cell wall product, implicating these cytokines in the sleep responses associated with bacterial infection.[5]

In addition, clinical conditions associated with excessive sleepiness or fatigue seem to involve TNF. This, for example, is true for HIV patients who have disrupted TNF rhythms,[6] sleep apnea patients,[7,8] and chronic fatigue patients[9] with excessive plasma TNF levels as well as cancer patients receiving TNF.[10] Patients with postdialysis fatigue also have elevated levels of TNF.[11,12] Treatment of rheumatoid arthritis patients with etanercept, a soluble TNF receptor, alleviated the fatigue.[13] In major depression, most reports point toward an association between severity of depression and levels of TNF.[14,15] These cytokines, particularly TNF, seem to play a role in the fatigue and sleep disturbances seen in psychiatric patients and in medical patients with psychiatric symptoms.

APPETITE

Appetite changes and accompanying weight gain or loss are major symptoms of both medical (e.g., infection, cancer) and psychiatric (e.g., depression, anorexia, bulimia) illnesses. The physiology of appetite and feeding behavior is very complex and involves neuroanatomical, neurophysiological, and neurochemical pathways that have not been completely elucidated. Recent evidence suggests that pro-inflammatory cytokines such as IL-1, IL-2, IL-6, IL-8, TNF, and interferon (IFN) suppress appetite.[16] Furthermore, conditions such as infection,[17] inflammation,[18] cancer,[19–24] and possibly advanced age[25–28] that are usually associated with increased cytokine production have also been associated with anorexia and weight loss.

This, however, has not always been the case. For instance, increases in circulating cytokine levels have not been found in all cancer patients[29,30] and may be associated with certain forms of cancers, (e.g., pancreatic cancer)[23] but not others.[30] Similarly, the cachexia or weight loss may correlate with one cytokine (e.g., IL-6)[23] but not another.[31] Similar reservations have been mentioned for the association of cytokines with appetite and weight changes in other medical and/or psychiatric conditions. In eating disorders such as anorexia and bulimia nervosa, cytokine measures have been made but the results appeared inconsistent[32–34] and, therefore, the clinical significance remains doubtful.

MOOD

As mentioned earlier, cytokines are associated with sickness behavior, a series of well coordinated but non-specific symptoms generally associated with infection or inflammation.[35] These symptoms include sleep and appetite disturbance, lethargy, anhedonia, depression, and a state of amotivation, usually accompanied by fever and an increase in hypothalamic pituitary adrenal activity. The purpose of the increased adrenal activity is to mobilize the organism's energy to combat infection by enhancing heat production (which in turn stimulates the proliferation of immune cells and interferes with the growth of many pathogens) and changing behavior to maximize the ability to fight the invading organism.

The behavioral changes in experimental animals included decreased food and water intake,[36,37] conditioned taste aversion,[38,39] decreased social exploration,[40–42] decreased grooming behavior, decreased motivational activities, and decreased spatial learning.[35] While the mood and affect of an animal cannot be directly and accurately measured, the symptoms described above have been compared to the symptoms of depression in humans.[43] In fact, human volunteers who received endotoxin injections in a double-blind, placebo-controlled manner to stimulate cytokine production reported increases in depression and anxiety only in the endotoxin-stimulated group.[44]

The authors reported significant positive correlations between cytokine secretion and endotoxin-induced anxiety and depression. In addition, treatment with cytokines

(IL-2 for cancer, IFNα for hepatitis C or malignant melanoma, IFNβ for multiple sclerosis) was associated with a high incidence of depressive adverse effects varying from 5% to as high as 40% of patients treated.[45]

MEMORY AND COGNITION

Memory and cognitive disturbances are central to various neurological and psychiatric conditions. While the etiology of such cognitive impairment can differ and includes various structural and metabolic elements, the realization that cytokines can produce such an effect is new. The first hint that cytokines can influence memory in humans probably dates back to the cognitive effects of IL-2 in the treatment of certain forms of cancer.[46,47] Further observations revealed that cognitive disturbance was also a major adverse effect in the treatment of hepatitis C patients with IFN immunotherapy.[48]

There were also reports of cognitive disturbances associated with IFN in the treatment of multiple sclerosis. Experimental studies in human volunteers revealed that endotoxin injections that stimulated the release of various cytokines were associated with both verbal and non-verbal memory disturbances in treated patients compared to controls.[44] Animal studies support these findings and, in particular, point toward a significant role of the hippocampus in these interactions.[49,50] Furthermore, chronic dosing of IL-2 in aging mice produced memory deficits along with neuronal damage that seemed to affect the hippocampus selectively.[51]

SEX DRIVE

The relationship of neurocircuitry, neurohormones, gonadal hormones, and sex drive is very complex and not completely understood. Until recently, sexual behavior was thought to be driven almost exclusively by central neural pathways (e.g., serotonergic or dopaminergic systems)[52] and gonadal hormones such as androgens that modulate sexual behavior both in males and females. However, with the development of the sickness behavior model in association with different cytokines, the suspicion is growing that various cytokines may directly affect sex drive the same way they affect sleep, appetite, and other neurovegetative functions.

Avitsur and colleagues[53] investigated this possibility in female rats. They showed that IL-1 inhibits sexual activity, motivation, and attractivity in female but not in male rats following central or peripheral administration. They also showed that TNF may also have a synergetic effect on this activity.[54] They concluded that from an evolutionary and adaptive standpoint, females are less likely to conceive during an infection, thus reducing the chances for development of an abnormal fetus, while males are less affected by IL-1 because reproduction during an infection is less risky for them than for their female counterparts.[55]

FATIGUE AND LETHARGY

Fatigue and lethargy are common symptoms of both psychiatric diseases and medical illnesses as well. Major depression and anxiety are frequently associated with fatigue. Schizophrenic patients are often lethargic. Fatigue and lethargy are also common symptoms of cancer and cardiovascular disease.[56] The underlying pathophysiology in all of these conditions has not been adequately investigated. Different explanations range from purely psychological (e.g., being overwhelmed with a condition) to purely biological (e.g., changes in the levels of hormones or neurotransmitters).[57]

Several investigators have recently advanced the hypothesis that fatigue, at least in cancer patients, may be attributed to excessive secretion of pro-inflammatory cytokines brought about by immune activation.[58,59] The immune activation may be in response to a tumor or to the treatments for the disease. To test this hypothesis, Bower and colleagues compared specific cytokine markers in 20 fatigued and 20 non-fatigued breast cancer survivor controls. Their results showed significantly higher levels of markers of pro-inflammatory cytokines in the fatigued group, including IL-1 receptor antagonist (IL-1ra), soluble tumor necrosis factor receptor type II (sTNF.r2), and neopterin.[60] They also noted lower levels of plasma cortisol in the fatigued group. They concluded that pro-inflammatory cytokines may play a role in the fatigue reported by some breast cancer survivors. Similar data have been reported for other types of cancers.

CYTOKINES AND MAJOR DEPRESSION

PSYCHOBIOLOGICAL FEATURES OF MAJOR DEPRESSION

Major depressive episode (MDE) is characterized by distinct clinical and biological features. Clinically, MDE is associated with persistent sadness or anhedonia (decrease in pleasurable activities). Other important clinical features are disturbed sleep (insomnia or hypersomnia), often with early morning awakening; disturbed appetite with increased or decreased weight; fatigue; psychomotor retardation or agitation; feelings of worthlessness, hopelessness, and guilt; difficulty concentrating; and suicidal ideation.

The biological features are more controversial. They include increased hypothalamic pituitary adrenal activity (manifested by increased ACTH and cortisol secretion, probably secondary to increased levels of CRH)[61] and defects in feedback mechanisms associated with cortisol.[62] Other biological markers include altered noradrenergic[63] and serotonergic[64] functions, the latter often associated with impulsivity and suicidal behavior. Sleep EEG findings are characterized by shortened REM latency and decreases in delta sleep.[65] Immunological characteristics of depression include neutrophilia and lymphocytopenia, decreased lymphocyte response to mitogen stimulation, decreased natural killer cell activity, and increased secretion of pro-inflammatory cytokines such as IL-1 and IL-6.[66] Other inflammatory markers that are increased in depression include C-reactive protein (CRP), neopterin, and haptoglobin.[67]

CYTOKINE HYPOTHESIS OF MAJOR DEPRESSION

Because of the similarities between sickness behavior in animals and major depression in humans[43] and because both seem to be associated with stress, some investigators have proposed that depression may be the result of an exaggerated immune response to stress.[68,69] The hypothesis states that in genetically predisposed individuals, stress (either past or present) will stimulate certain components of the immune system, resulting in excessive secretion of pro-inflammatory cytokines such as IL-1 and IL-6. These cytokines, directly or indirectly, will activate specific areas of the brain, leading to the appearance of sickness behavior along with other features of depression, such as neurochemical and neuroendocrine changes.[70]

What is the evidence in favor of this hypothesis? As mentioned earlier, one line of evidence is the similarity between cytokine-induced sickness behavior and the symptoms of major depression. The symptoms include disturbances in sleep, appetite, mood, cognition, level of energy, and sex drive and all of them have been reported in conjunction with the administration of cytokines in both humans and in animal models.[71]

The other line of evidence is concerned with the neurochemical and neuroendocrine changes associated with cytokines. Animal studies revealed that intraperitoneal injections of PHA or PLS are often accompanied by changes in neurotransmitter turnover in specific areas of the brain — areas associated with mood disorders. IL-1, for example, has been shown to increase the brain concentrations of norepinephrine and serotonin, but not dopamine. IL-2 increased the levels of serotonin only.[72] Similarly, animal studies revealed that intraperitoneal injections of cytokine (IL-1) activated the HPA axis, resulting in increased secretions of CRH, ACTH, and cortisol.[73] Increases in both neurotransmitter turnover and activation of the HPA axis have been described in depression.[61-64]

Perhaps the most direct line of evidence comes from immunological studies in depressed patients presented in a previous publication.[66] In summary, studies of cytokine in depression can be divided into two categories: (1) studies measuring plasma and CSF concentrations of cytokines and/or soluble cytokine receptors in patients with major depression compared to healthy controls and (2) studies measuring cytokine production in stimulated leukocyte cultures in these groups. The results of studies of serum and CSF concentrations revealed increases in IL-1β,[74] IL-2R,[75] IL-6,[75-78] and SIL-6R[75] in serum and an increase in IL-1β but not IL-6 in CSF.[79] Unfortunately, the results are inconsistent and some results are contradictory.[80] Furthermore, many studies are plagued with methodological flaws, such as sensitivity, diurnal variations, heterogeneity of study populations, and medication status of subjects.

Cytokine production studies tend to be more informative, but they are fewer in number and vary in methodology (tissue used, nature of stimulus, duration of culture, type of control). Again, results vary. Maes and colleagues reported an increase in IL-1β production in response to PHA[81] while Weizman's group reported a decrease in IL-1β production in response to LPS.[82] Seidel and Kronfol did not find significant changes in IL-1β in response to PHA[83] or LPS.[84] The increase in IL-6 secretion, however, seemed to be a robust finding.[84] Similarly, the increase in IFN production seemed well replicated.[85,86]

CRITIQUE OF CYTOKINE HYPOTHESIS

The cytokine hypothesis of major depression, at first glance, can explain many of the behavioral, neurochemical, and neuroendocrine features of depression as described above. Furthermore, stressful life events that often trigger depressive episodes can also activate the immune/inflammatory system, leading to excess secretion of cytokines.[69] There are also occasional reports of decreases in cytokine secretion in conjunction with the use of antidepressant medications.[87,88] While all these factors support the hypothesis, they provide only circumstantial evidence of a role for cytokines in the pathology of major depression. Direct evidence would ideally come from the assessment of cytokine activities in various areas of the brain in depressed patients and normal controls. However, since the technology to perform such testing is not yet available, testing of the hypothesis will have to rely on measurement of circulating cytokines or *ex vivo* cytokine production in serum or blood samples, knowing well that the results may not reflect actual values in key areas of the brain associated with clinical depression.

Another problem is the varying and often contradictory results reported in the literature for different cytokines in depressed and control subjects. This is particularly worrisome because the results come from a very small number of laboratories and are often not confirmed by other laboratories. However, even with more independent confirmations of the results, other challenges must be confronted before the cytokine hypothesis becomes universally accepted as a plausible and serious explanation for major depression. The challenges include discrepancies between common clinical features of depression such as insomnia and the clinical effects of cytokines, mostly fatigue and hypersomnia. Another controversy relates to the subtype of depression affected. The cytokine hypothesis predicts that many vegetative signs such as sleep and appetite disturbances and HPA hyperactivity are associated with severe or melancholic depression, while according to recent reports, cytokine abnormalities have been mostly associated with dysthymia,[89] a milder form of depression.

CYTOKINES AS MEDIATORS BETWEEN DEPRESSION AND MEDICAL ILLNESS

While immunological abnormalities in patients with major depression are now well documented,[66,71] the clinical role these reported immunological aberrations play in the physical and mental health of an individual is not clear. We have already addressed the relationship of cytokines and mental health, particularly depression. This section will address the relationship of immune dysregulation, cytokines, and specific medical illnesses such as infection, cancer, coronary artery disease, and AIDS.

INFECTION

Infection is usually the result of a complex interaction between invasive organisms (most commonly bacteria or viruses) and a host. Animal models have shown that stress increases susceptibility to viral infection by altering the immune response.[90] Human studies looking at the relationship of stress, infection, and immune function are rare. Cohen and colleagues, in a landmark study, experimentally inoculated healthy volunteers with five different strains of common cold viruses and conducted extensive psychosocial assessments of these individuals. Their results indicated a positive association between the intensity of the psychosocial stressor and frequency and severity of the infection.[91]

In another study, the same group of investigators inoculated healthy volunteers with the influenza A virus and monitored upper respiratory symptoms and nasal levels of IL-6.[92] They found a significant association of stress, severity of upper respiratory symptoms, and nasal levels of IL-6. Kiecolt-Glaser and colleagues found that spousal caregivers of dementia patients — a group considered chronically stressed — showed poorer antibody responses to influenza vaccination than non-stressed age- and sex-matched controls.[93]

CANCER

Several recent epidemiologic reports suggest an association between depression and the development of cancer.[94,95] Although not all studies agree,[96] at least one meta-analysis seemed to confirm a small but statistically significant association between depression and the risk of developing cancer.[97] Another research question that has led to some controversy is whether mood states in general and depression in particular are associated with poorer prognoses in patients already diagnosed with cancer. Ben-Eliyahu and colleagues[98] used animal models to show that stress leads to faster and wider metastasis of implanted tumors in stressed animals compared to controls. They also found that stress-induced declines in immune parameters could explain, at least in part, the more rapid progression of the illness. Human studies, however, have not been that convincing. Spiegel and colleagues investigated the role of group psychotherapy in the quality of life in women with breast cancer. An incidental finding that generated a lot of interest was the increased survival in women who participated in support groups.[99] Although these studies could not be confirmed by other investigators,[100] the relation of depression, social support, immune function, and cancer survival remains a subject of great theoretical and practical interest for people working in this field.

CORONARY ARTERY DISEASE

The notion that inflammation plays a role in the etiology of coronary artery disease has recently gained ground.[101] Increased levels of the inflammatory marker C-reactive protein have been associated with increased cardiac morbidity and mortality in both cardiac patients and healthy individuals.[102,103] Increased levels of the IL-1β and IL-6 pro-inflammatory cytokines have also been reported to be increased in unstable angina,[104] along with reports of an association between increased IL-6 levels and mortality in this disease.[105] Epidemiological studies have shown an association between depression and the risk of developing coronary artery disease on the one hand and between depression and increased mortality following myocardial infarction on the other.[106,107]

Unfortunately, a link among depression, immune dysregulation, and survival following myocardial infarction has not been firmly established. Large-scale multi-center studies (ENRCHD) failed to underline the value of behavioral therapy following myocardial infarction.[108] Similarly, large-scale multicenter studies also failed to show any protective effect of an SSRI antidepressant (sertraline) on future cardiac events in depressed patients following myocardial infarction.[109]

AIDS

Psychosocial research involving AIDS patients has focused primarily on the impact of the illness and coping skills. Several investigators have also examined the effects of depression and stress on progression of the disease. The hypothesis is that depression and stress can alter immune function, thus leading to higher morbidity and mortality for individuals infected with HIV. Lesserman and colleagues found that depressive symptoms affected the overall distribution of lymphocyte subsets in HIV-infected men.[110] They postulated that more depression and stress and less social support are important factors in the progression from HIV infection to full-blown AIDS.[111]

There have also been reports of an association between depressive symptoms and an increase in mortality among AIDS patients,[112] but these reports have not always been confirmed.[113,114] In most of these studies, the emphasis has been on stress-related changes in the CD4+ cells.[113] The role of cytokines as mediators of psychosocial effects in HIV and AIDS has not been adequately investigated.

ADVERSE PSYCHIATRIC EFFECTS OF TREATMENT WITH CYTOKINES

One of the major tenets of the cytokine hypothesis of depression described above is the psychiatric clinical picture presented by many patients receiving cytokines to treat their medical conditions. Cytokines — and interferons in particular — have served as the treatments of choice for several medical illnesses such as infection with hepatitis C virus, malignant melanoma, and multiple sclerosis.[45] While cytokines have proven very effective in the treatment of these conditions, side effects have been common and often severe enough to necessitate reduction of dose or cessation of use.[115]

Perhaps the most widely prescribed cytokine treatment is the use of interferon alpha (IFNα) for infection with the hepatitis C virus.[116] IFNα has been associated with various adverse effects including flu-like symptoms such as fever, tachycardia, headache, and arthralgia. The effects tend to appear early in treatment.[116] The adverse neuropsychiatric effects usually occur later.[117] Their frequency in those receiving treatment ranges from 5% to 35%. Fatigue is one of the most common side effects. It is dose-related and tends to remit when treatment is discontinued.

Other neuropsychiatric side effects include mood changes (depression, anxiety, irritability, even suicidal behavior) and cognitive changes (decreased concentration, poor memory, confusion, delirium). Psychosis is rare, but can occur.[118] Recent evidence indicates that the depression is responsive to antidepressant treatment (e.g., an SSRI), can be prevented by pre-treatment with an SSRI, and is more likely to be seen in patients with histories of psychiatric illness, namely depression.[119, 120]

IFNα has been used in the treatment of chronic myelogenous leukemia, renal cell carcinoma, and metastatic melanoma. IFNβ is used in multiple sclerosis. IFNα,

IL-1, and TNF are used in advanced cancer. Fatigue, depression, somnolence, anorexia, and cognitive impairment are common side effects with all these modalities. Interestingly, when anticytokines, for example, anti-TNF antibodies for rheumatoid arthritis, are used, no such side effects have been reported.

CONCLUSION

In addition to their inflammatory and immunological effects, cytokines have behavioral effects that contribute to the sickness behaviors of infected or injured animals. These behavioral effects include neurovegetative symptoms such as changes in sleep, appetite, level of energy, and sex drive. In humans, these symptoms are reminiscent of the clinical picture of major depression. These observations led to the formulation of the cytokine hypothesis of major depression. Data have been presented in support of this hypothesis. A critical assessment has also been provided. With the therapeutic use of cytokines for different medical conditions on the rise, future research should provide more insight into the various epidemiological, pathophysiological, and clinical issues discussed in this chapter.

REFERENCES

1. Ader R., Felten D., and Cohen N., Eds. *Psychoneuroimmunology*, 3rd ed., Academic Press, San Diego, 2001.
2. Dantzer R. Cytokine-induced sickness behavior: where do we stand? *Brain, Behav. Immunit* 2001; 15: 7.
3. Krueger J.M., Obal F. Jr., Fang J., et al. The role of cytokines in sleep regulation. *Ann. NY Acad. Sci.* 2001; 933: 211.
4. Krueger J.M. and Majde J.A. Microbial products and cytokines in sleep and fever regulation. *Crit. Rev. Immunol.* 1994; 14: 355.
5. Krueger J.M., Fang J., Majde J.A. Sleep in health and disease, in *Psychoneuroimmunology*, 3rd ed., Ader B., Felten D., and Cohen N., Eds., Academic Press, San Diego, 2001, p. 667.
6. Darko D.F., Miller J.C., Gallen C., et al. Sleep electroencephalogram delta-frequency amplitude, night plasma levels of tumor necrosis factor alpha, and human immunodeficiency virus infection. *Proc. Natl. Acad. Sci. USA* 1995; 92: 12080.
7. Entzian P., Linnemann K., Schlaak M., et al. Obstructive sleep apnea syndrome and circadian rhythms of hormones and cytokines. *Am. J. Respir. Crit. Care Med.* 1996; 153: 1080.
8. Vgontzas A.N., Papanicolaou D.A., Bixler E.O., et al. Elevation of plasma cytokines in disorders of excessive daytime sleepiness: role of sleep disturbance and obesity. *J. Clin. Endocrinol. Metab.* 1997; 82: 1313.
9. Moss R.B., Mercandetti A., and Vojdani A. TNF-alpha and chronic fatigue syndrome. *J. Clin. Immunol.* 1999; 19: 314.
10. Eskander E.D., Harvey H.A., Givant E., et al. Phase I study combining tumor necrosis factor with interferon-alpha and interleukin-2. *Am. J. Clin. Oncol.* 1997; 20: 511.
11. Dreisback A.W., Hendrickson T., Beezhold D., et al. Elevated levels of tumor necrosis factor alpha in postdialysis fatigue. *Int. J. Artif. Organs* 1998; 21: 83.

12. Sklar A.H., Beezhold D.H., Newman N., et al. Postdialysis fatigue: lack of effect of a biocompatible membrane. *Am J. Kidney Dis.* 1998; 31: 1007.

13. Franklin C.M. Clinical experience with soluble TNF p75 receptor in rheumatoid arthritis. *Semin. Arthritis Rheum.* 1999; 29: 172.

14. Suarez E.C., Lewis J.G., Krishnan R.R., and Young K.H. Enhanced expression of cytokines and chemokines by blood monocytes to *in vitro* lipopolysaccharide stimulation is associated with hostility and severity of depressive symptoms in healthy women. *Psychoneuroendocrinology* 2004; 29: 1119.

15. Suarez E.C., Krishnan R.R., and Lewis J.G. The relation of severity of depressive symptoms to monocyte-associated proinflammatory cytokines and chemokines in apparently healthy men. *Psychosom. Med.* 2003; 65: 362.

16. Lanhaus W. and Hrupka B. Cytokines and appetite, in *Cytokines and Mental Health*, Kronfol Z., Ed., Kluwer Academic Publishers, San Diego, 2003, Ch. 9.

17. Arsenijevic D., Girardier L., Seydoux J., et al. Altered energy balance and cytokine gene expression in a murine model of chronic infection with *Toxoplasma gondii*. *Am. J. Physiol.* 1997; 272: E908.

18. Cooper A.L., Brouwer S., Turnbull A.V., et al. Tumor necrosis factor-alpha and fever after peripheral inflammation in the rat. *Am. J. Physiol.* 1994; 36: R1431.

19. Barton B.E. IL-6-like cytokines and cancer cachexia: consequences of chronic inflammation. *Immunol. Res.* 2001; 23: 41.

20. Bossola M., Muscaritoli M., Bellantone R., et al. Serum tumour necrosis factor-alpha levels in cancer patients are discontinuous and correlate with weight loss. *Eur. J. Clin. Invest.* 2000; 30: 1107.

21. Ikemoto S., Sugimura K., Yoshida N., et al. TNF alpha, IL-1 beta and IL-6 production by peripheral blood monocytes in patients with renal cell carcinoma. *Anticancer Res.* 2000; 20: 317.

22. Mantovani G., Maccio A., Mura L., et al. Serum levels of leptin and pro-inflammatory cytokines in patients with advanced-stage cancer at different sites. *J. Mol. Med.* 2000; 78: 554.

23. Okada S., Okusaka T., Ishii H., et al. Elevated serum interleukin-6 levels in patients with pancreatic cancer. *Jap. J. Clin. Oncol.* 1998; 28: 12.

24. Zhang G.J. and Adachi I. Serum interleukin-6 levels correlate to tumor progression and prognosis in metastatic breast carcinoma. *Anticancer Res.* 1999; 19: 1427.

25. Bruunsgaard H., Pedersen A.N., Schroll M., et al. TNF-alpha, leptin, and lymphocyte function in human aging. *Life Sci.* 2000; 67: 2721.

26. Pedersen B.K., Bruunsgaard H., Ostrowski K., et al. Cytokines in aging and exercise. *Int. J. Sports Med.* 2000; 21: S4.

27. Malaguarnea L., Ferlito L., Imbesi R.M., et al. Immunosenescence: a review. *Arch. Gerontol. Geriatr.* 2001; 32: 1.

28. Yeh S.S. and Schuster M.W. Geriatric cachexia: the role of cytokines. *Am. J. Clin. Nutr.* 1999; 70: 183.

29. Moldawer L.L., Rogy M.A., and Lowry S.F. The role of cytokines in cancer cachexia. *J. Parent. Ent. Nutr.* 1992; 16 (Suppl.): 43S.

30. Noguchi Y., Yoshikawa T., Matsumoto A., et al. Are cytokines possible mediators of cancer cachexia? *Surg. Today* 1996; 26: 467.

31. Saurwein T.M., Blasko I., Zisterer K., et al. An imbalance between pro- and anti-inflammatory cytokines, a characteristic feature of old age. *Cytokine* 2000; 12: 1160.

32. Raymond N.C., Dysken M., Bettin K., et al. Cytokine production in patients with anorexia nervosa, bulimia nervosa, and obesity. *Int. J. Eating Disord.* 2000; 28: 293.

33. Brambilla F., Bellodi L., Brunetta M., et al. Plasma concentrations of interleukin-1 beta, interleukin-6 and tumor necrosis factor-alpha in anorexia and bulimia nervosa. *Psychoneuroendocrinology* 1998; 23: 439.

34. Nakai Y., Hamagaki S., Takagi R., et al. Plasma concentrations of tumor necrosis factor-alpha (TNF-alpha) and soluble TNF receptors in patients with bulimia nervosa. *Clin. Endocrinol.* 2000; 53: 383.

35. Dantzer R., Cytokines and sickness behavior, in *Cytokines and Mental Health*, Kronfol Z., Ed., Kluwer Academic Publishers, San Diego, 2003, Ch. 7.

36. Kent S., Bret-Dibat J.L., Kelley K.W., et al. Mechanisms of sickness-induced decreases in food-motivated behavior. *Neurosci. Biobehav. Rev.* 1995; 20: 171.

37. Plata-Salaman C.R. Cytokines and ingestive behavior: methods and overview, in *Methods in Neuroscience*. De Souza E., Ed. Academic Press. Orlando, 1993, p. 152.

38. Tazi A., Dantzer R., Crestani F., et al. Interleukin-1 induces conditioned taste aversion in rats: a possible explanation for its pituitary-adrenal stimulating activity. *Brain Res.* 1988; 473: 369.

39. Tazi A., Crestani F., and Dantzer R. Aversive effects of centrally injected interleukin-1 are independent of its pyrogenic activity. *Neurosci. Res. Commun.* 1990; 7: 159.

40. Bluthé R.M., Dantzer R., and Kelley K.W. Effects of interleukin-1 receptor antagonist on the behavioral effects of lipopolysaccharide in rats. *Brain Res.*1992; 573: 318.

41. Bluthé R.M., Crestani F., Kelley K.W., et al. Mechanisms of the behavioral effects of interleukin-1: role of prostaglandins and CRF. *Ann. NY Acad. Sci.*1992; 650: 268.

42. Bluthé R.M., Pawlowski M., Suarez S., et al. Synergy between tumor necrosis factor alpha and interleukin-1 in the induction of sickness behavior in mice. *Psychoneuroendocrinology* 1994; 19: 197.

43. Yirmiya R. Endotoxin produces a depressive-like episode in rats. *Brain Res.* 1996; 711: 163.

44. Reichenberg A., Yirmiya R., Schuld A., et al. Cytokine-associated emotional and cognitive disturbances in humans. *Arch. Gen. Psychiatr.* 2001; 58: 445.

45. Kronfol Z. and Remick D. Cytokines and the brain: implications for clinical psychiatry. *Am. J. Psychiatr.* 2000; 157: 683.

46. Denicoff K.D., Rubinow D.R., Papa M.Z., et al. The neuropsychiatric effects of treatment with interleukin-2 and lymphokine-activated killer cells. *Ann. Int. Med.* 1987; 107: 293.

47. West W.H., Tauer K.W., Yannelli J.R., et al. Constant-infusion recombinant interleukin-2 in adoptive immunotherapy of advanced cancer. *New Engl. J. Med.* 1987; 316: 898.

48. Duscheiko G. Side effects of alpha interferon in chronic hepatitis C. *Hepatology* 1997; 26: 1125.

49. Schneider H., Pitossi F., Balschun D., et al. A neuromodulatory role of interleukin-1b in the hippocampus. *Proc. Natl. Acad. Sci. USA* 1998; 95: 7778.

50. Li A., Katafuchi T., Oda S., et al. Interleukin-6 inhibits long term potentiation in rat hippocampal slices. *Brain Res.* 1997; 748: 30.

51. Nemni R., Iannaccone S., Quattrini A., et al. Effect of chronic treatment with recombinant interleukin-2 on the central nervous system of adult and old mice. *Brain Res.* 1992; 591: 248.

52. Kelly A.E. and Berridge K.C. The neuroscience of natural rewards: relevance to addictive drugs. *J. Neurosci.* 2002; 22: 3306.

53. Avitsur R., Weidenfield J., and Yirmiya R. Cytokines inhibit sexual behavior in female rats: II. Prostaglandins mediate the suppressive effects of interleukin-1 beta. *Brain Behav. Immun.* 1999; 13: 33.

54. Avitsur R. and Yirmiya R. Cytokines inhibit sexual behavior in female rats: I. Synergistic effects of tumor necrosis factor alpha and interleukin-1. *Brain Behav. Immun.* 1999; 13: 14.

55. Avistur R, Cohen E., and Yirmiya R. Effects of interleukin-1 on sexual attractivity in a model of sickness behavior. *Physiol. Behav.* 1999; 63: 25.

56. Andrykowski M.A., Curran S.L., and Lighner R. Off-treatment fatigue in breast cancer survivors: a controlled comparison. *J. Behav. Med.* 1998; 21: 1.

57. McEwen B.S., Biron C.A., Brunson K.W., et al. The role of adrenocorticoids as modulators of immune function in health and disease: neural, endocrine, and immune interactions. *Brain Res. Rev.* 1997; 23: 79.

58. Greenberg D.G., Gray J.L., Mannix C.M., et al. Treatment-related fatigue and serum interleukin-1 levels in patients during external beam irradiation for prostate cancer. *J. Pain Symptom Mgt.* 1993; 8: 196.

59. Rigas J.R., Hoopes P.J., Meyer L.A., et al. Fatigue linked to plasma cytokines in patients with lung cancer undergoing combined modality therapy. *Proc. Am. Cancer Soc.* 1998; 17: 68.

60. Bower J.E., Ganz P.A., Aziz, N., et al. Fatigue and proinflammatory cytokine activity in breast cancer survivors. *Psychosom. Med.* 2002; 64: 604.

61. Owens M.J. and Nemeroff C.G. The role CRF in the pathophysiology of affective disorders: laboratory and clinical studies. *Ciba Found. Symp.* 1993; 172: 293.

62. Young F.A, Vazquez D. Hypercortisolemia, hippocampal glucocorticoid receptors, and fast feedback. *Mol. Psychiatr.* 1996; 1: 149.

63. Wong M.L., Kling M.A., Munson P.J., et al. Pronounced and sustained central hyper-noradrenergic function in major depression with melancholic features: relation to hypercortisolism and corticotropin-releasing hormone. *Proc. Natl. Acad. Sci. USA* 2000; 97: 325.

64. Maes M. and Meltzer H.Y. The serotonin hypothesis of major depression, in Bloom F.E. and Kupfer D., Eds., *Psychopharmacology: The Fourth Generation of Progress.* Raven Press, New York, 1995, p. 933.

65. Reynold C., Collin J., and Kupfer D. Sleep and affective states, in *Psychopharmacology: The Third Generation of Progress,* Meltzer, H., Ed., Raven Press, New York, 1987, p. 647.

66. Kronfol Z. Depression and immune dysregulation: a critical review of existing evidence. *Int. J. Neuropsychopharmacol.* 2002; 5: 333.

67. Zorrilla E.P., Luborsky L., McKay J.R., et al. The relationship of depression and stressors to immunologic assays: a meta-analytic review. *Brain Behav. Immun,* 2001; 15: 199.

68. Maes M., Smith R., and Scharpe S. The monocyte–T lymphocyte hypothesis of major depression. *Psychoneuroendocrinology* 1995; 20: 111.

69. Dantzer R., Wollman E.E., and Yirmiya R., Eds. *Cytokines, Stress, and Depression,* Kluwer Academic Publishers, New York, 1999.

70. Dantzer R., Vitkovic L., Wollman E.E., et al. Cytokines and depression: fortuitous or causative association? *Mol. Psychiatr.* 1999; 4: 328.

71. Kronfol Z. *Cytokines and Mental Health,* Kluwer Academic Publishers, San Diego, 2003.

72. Dunn A.H. Effects of cytokines in cerebral neurotransmission and potential relationship to function, in *Cytokines and Mental Health*, Kronfol Z., Ed., Kluwer Academic Publishers, San Diego, 2003, p. 55.

73. Besedovsky H.O. and del Rey A. Immune neuroendocrine interactions: facts and hypotheses. *Endocr. Rev.* 1996; 17: 64.

74. Maes M., Bosmans E., DeJongh R., et al. Increased serum IL-6 and IL-1 receptor antagonist concentrations in major depression and treatment-resistant depression. *Cytokine* 1997; 9: 853.

75. Maes M., Meltzer H., and Bosmans E. Increased plasma levels of interleukin-6, soluble interleukin-6, soluble interleukin-2 and transferin receptors in major depression. *J. Affect. Dis.* 1995; 34: 301.

76. Sluzewska A., Rybakowski J., Bosmans E., et al. Indicators of immune activation in major depression. *Psychiatr. Res.* 1996; 64: 161.

77. Frommberger U.H., Bauer J., Haselbauer P., et. al. Interleukin-6 (IL-6) plasma levels in depression and schizophrenia: comparison between the acute state and after remission. *Eur. Arch. Psychiatr.* 1997; 247: 233.

78. Lu S.J., Shiah I.S., Yatham L.N., et al. Immune inflammatory markers in patients with seasonal affective disorder: effects of light therapy. *J. Affect. Dis.* 2001; 63: 27.

79. Levine J., Barak Y., Chengappa K.N., et al. Cerebrospinal cytokine levels in patients with acute depression. *Neuropsychobiology* 1999; 40: 171.

80. Brambilla F. and Maggione M. Blood levels of cytokines in elderly patients with major depressive disorder. *Acta Psychiatr. Scand.* 1998; 97: 309.

81. Maes M., Bosmans E., Meltzer H.Y., et al. Interleukin-1: a putative mediator of HPA-axis hyperactivity in major depression. *Am. J. Psychiatr.* 1993; 150: 1189.

82. Weizman R., Laor N., Podliszewski E., et al. Cytokine production in major depressed patients before and after chlorimipramine treatment. *Biol. Psychiatr.* 1994; 25: 42.

83. Seidel A., Arolt V., Hunstiger M., et al. Cytokine production and serum proteins in depression. *Scand. J. Immunol.* 1995; 41: 434.

84. Kronfol Z., Aziz M., and Remick. D. Increased LPS-stimulated levels of IL-6 in patients with major depression. *Am. Psychiatr. Assn. New Res.* Abstract 273, 2002.

85. Maes M., Scharpe S., Meltzer H.Y., et al. Increased neopterin and interferon gamma secretion and lower L-troptophan levels in major depression: further evidence for immune activation in severe depression. *Psychiatr. Res.* 1994; 54: 143.

86. Kronfol Z. Cytokine regulation in major depression, in *Cytokines and Mental Health*, Kronfol Z., Ed., Kluwer Academic Publishers, San Diego, 2003, p. 257.

87. Sluzewska A., Rybakowski J.K., Laciak M., et al. Interleukin-6 serum levels in depressed patients before and after treatment with fluoxetine. *Ann. NY Acad. Sci.* 1995; 762: 474.

88. Kubera M., Symbirse A., Basta-Kaim A., et al. Effect of chronic treatment with imipramine on interleukin 1 and interleukin 2 production by splenocytes obtained from rats subjected to a chronic mild stress model of depression. *Pol. J. Pharmacol.* 1998; 48: 503.

89. Anisman H., Ravindran A., Griffith J., et al. Endocrine and cytokine correlates of major depression and dysthymia with typical or atypical features. *Mol. Psychiatr.* 1999; 4: 182.

90. Sheridan J., Dobbs C., Brown D., et al. Psychoneuroimmunology: stress effects on pathogenesis and immunity during infection. *Clin. Microbiol. Rev.* 1994; 7: 200.

91. Cohen S., Tyrell D.A.J., and Smith A.P. Psychological stress and susceptibility to the common cold. *New Engl. J. Med.*1991; 325: 606.
92. Cohen S., Doyle W.J., and Skoner D.P. Psychological stress, cytokine production, and severity of upper respiratory illness. *Psychosom. Med.* 1999; 61: 175.
93. Kiecolt-Glaser J., Glaser R., Gravenstein S., et al. Chronic stress alters the immune response to influenza virus vaccine in older adults. *Proc. Natl. Acad. Sci. USA* 1996; 93: 3043.
94. Friedman G.A. Psychiatrically diagnosed depression and subsequent cancer. *Cancer Epidemiol. Biomarkers Prev.* 1994; 3: 11.
95. Penninx B., Guraluik M., Pahor M., et al. Chronically depressed mood and cancer risk in older persons. *J. Natl. Cancer Inst.* 1998; 90: 1888.
96. Zonderman A., Costa P., and McCrae R. Depression as a risk for cancer morbidity and mortality in a nationally representative sample. *JAMA*, 1989; 262: 1191.
97. McGee R., Williams S., and Elwood M. Depression and the development of cancer: a meta-analysis. *Soc. Sci. Med.* 1994; 38: 187.
98. Ben-Eliyahu S., Yirmyia R., Liebeskind J.C., et al. Stress increases metastatic spread of a mammory tumor in rats: evidence for mediation by the immune system. *Brain Behav. Immun.* 1991; 5: 193.
99. Spiegel D., Bloom J.R., Kraemer H.C., et al. Effect of psychosocial treatment on survival of patients with metastatic breast cancer. *Lancet* 1989; 2: 888.
100. Goodwin P., Leszcz M., Ennis M., et al. The effect of group psychological support on survival in metastatic brain cancer. *New Engl. J. Med.*, 2001; 345: 1719.
101. Ross R. Atherosclerosis: an inflammatory disease. *New Engl. J. Med.* 1999; 340: 115.
102. Mendall M.A., Strahan D.P., Butland B.K., et al. C-reactive protein: relation to total mortality, cardiovascular mortality and cardiovascular risk factors in men. *Eur. Heart J.* 2000; 21: 1584.
103. Ridker P.M., Kennekens C.H., Buring J.E., et al. C-reactive protein and other markers of inflammation in the prediction of cardiovascular disease in women. *New Engl. J. Med.* 2000; 342: 836.
104. Biasucci L.M., Vitelli A., Liuzzo G., et al. Elevated levels of interleukin-6 in unstable angina. *Circulation* 1996; 94: 874.
105. Lindmark E., Diderholm E., Wallentin L., et al. Relationship between interleukin-6 and mortality in patients with unstable coronary artery disease. *JAMA* 2001; 286: 2107.
106. Hemingway H. and Marmot M. Evidence-based cardiology: psychosocial factors in the aetiology and prognosis of coronary heart disease: systematic review of prospective cohort studies. *Br. Med. J.* 1999; 318: 1460.
107. Smith T. and Ruiz J. Psychosocial influences on the development and course of coronary heart disease: current status and implications for research and practice. *J. Consult. Clin. Psychol.* 2002; 70: 548.
108. Writing Committee for ENRICHD Investigators. Effects of treating depression and low perceived social support on clinical events after myocardial infarction: the enhancing recovery in coronary heart disease (ENRICHD) patients randomized trials. *JAMA*, 2003; 289: 3106.
109. Glassman A., O'Connor C., and Califf R. Sertraline treatment of major depression in patients with acute MI or unstable angina. *JAMA* 2002; 288: 701.
110. Leserman J., Petitto J.M., Perkins D.O., et al. Severe stress, depressive symptoms, and changes in lymphocyte subsets in human immunodeficiency virus-infected men. *Arch. Gen. Psychiatr.* 1997; 54: 279.

111. Lesserman J., Jackson E., Petitto J., et al. Progression to AIDS: the effects of stress, depressive symptoms and social support. *Psychosom. Med.* 1999, 61: 397.
112. Mayne T.J., Vittinghoff E., Chesney M.A., et al. Depressive affect and survival among gay and bisexual men infected with HIV. *Arch. Intern. Med.* 1996; 156: 2233.
113. Burack J.H., Barrett D.C., Stall R.D., et al. Depressive symptoms and CD4 lymphocyte decline among HIV-infected men. *JAMA* 1993; 270: 2568.
114. Lyketsos C.G., Hoover D.R., Guccione M., et al. Depressive symptoms as predictors of medical outcomes in HIV infection. *JAMA* 1993; 270: 2563.
115. Loftis J.M. and Housier P. The pharmacology and treatment of interferon-induced depression. *J. Aff. Disord.* 2004; 8: 175.
116. Renault P.F., Hoofnagle J.H., Park H., et al. Psychiatric complications of long term interferon alpha therapy. *Arch. Intern. Med.* 1987; 147: 1577.
117. Meyers C., Scheibel R., and Forman A. Persistent neurotoxicity of systemically administered interferon-alpha. *Neurology* 1991; 41: 672.
118. Janssen H.L., Brouwer J.T., van der Mast R.C., et al. Suicide associated with alfa-interferon therapy for chronic viral hepatitis. *J. Hepatol.* 1994; 21: 241.
119. Capuron L. and Ravaud A. Prediction of the depressive effects of interferon alfa therapy by the patient's initial affective state. *New Engl. J. Med.* 1999; 340: 1370.
120. Musselman D.L., Lawson D.H., Gummick J.F., et al. Paroxetine for the prevention of depression induced by high dose interferon-alfa. *New Engl. J. Med.* 2001; 344: 961.

2 Worried to Death? Stress, Worry, and Immune Dysregulation in Health and HIV

Suzanne C. Segerstrom and Margaret E. Kemeny

CONTENTS

INTRODUCTION

Ample evidence points to a relationship between psychological stressors and the human immune system such that chronic stressors associate with decrements in immune function, and the more chronic the stressor, the more aspects of the immune system are affected (Segerstrom & Miller, 2004). However, this literature has focused mainly on environmental events, and relatively little attention has been paid to internally generated stressors — that is, cognitive representations of environmental threats — and their physiological consequences. Worry is a style of repetitive thought that generates perceptions of threat where no threat exists, exacerbates perceptions of existing threat, and contributes to physiological dysregulation. In essence, people who worry create and exacerbate their own internal stressors, and these stressors may consequently affect the immune system.

Tongue-in-cheek definitions of worry include "wasting energy over something you have no control over" and "the act of planning something more than once."

These sardonic definitions capture much of what is unhealthy about worry, which could be more scientifically described as repetitive, uncontrollable rehearsal of potential negative events. Although worry can serve an effective problem solving or planning purpose when it is brief and controlled, it has a pathological quality when it becomes intrusive, uncontrollable, and prolonged and does not lead to solutions. Pathologically excessive and prolonged worry is the defining characteristic of generalized anxiety disorder (GAD), in which severe worry is accompanied by cognitive and somatic symptoms such as sleep disturbance and difficulty concentrating (American Psychiatric Association, 1994). Although anxious mood typically accompanies worry, worry defines a cognitive phenomenon characterized by negative thoughts about a number of different potential threats, difficulty controlling those thoughts, and pervasiveness of the thoughts.

Whether worry is brief and controlled or chronic and pathological depends more on the person doing the worrying than environmental events. For example, both GAD patients and non-anxious controls worried about relationships, achievements, and daily problems (e.g., mishaps, punctuality), but GAD patients were more likely to worry without recognizable precipitants, had less control over their worries, and were less successful in their attempts to reduce their worries (Craske, Rapee, Jackel, & Barlow, 1989). Worry, therefore, is not a proxy for stressful environmental events but is a quality of the way that people think about both major and minor stressors. Furthermore, worry is common. Although the 1-year prevalence of GAD is relatively low [1%; American Psychiatric Association (APA), 1994], pathological worry is best conceptualized as a continuous individual difference dimension (Ruscio, Borkovec, & Ruscio, 2001). Measures of pathological worry, such as the Penn State Worry Questionnaire, are normally distributed in the population around means that reflect moderate levels of worry (Molina & Borkovec, 1994). In addition to being common, worry is also chronic. Test–retest reliability for measures of pathological worry is .75 to .92 over 2 to 10 weeks, and the course of GAD is typically chronic (APA, 1994; Molina & Borkovec, 1994).

WORRY AND HEALTH

Because worry is both chronic and common, it has the potential for widespread impact on well-being. In particular, persistent, uncontrollable worry has been associated with risk for health problems and for physiological dysregulation in addition to its negative consequences for psychological health. For example, among men in the Normative Aging Study, higher worry was associated with an increased incidence of non-fatal myocardial infarct (heart attack) and total coronary heart disease. Those in the highest worry group faced a risk of myocardial infarct 2.5 times higher than those in the lowest (Kubzansky et al., 1997). Worry also may affect women's health. Worry during pregnancy about potential negative outcomes (e.g., baby's health, delivery, taking care of a new baby) predicted shorter length of gestation after controlling for other risk factors and life circumstances (Rini et al., 1999).

Poor health outcomes in worriers may be attributable to physiological dysregulation, particularly in the autonomic nervous system. A number of studies have found autonomic irregularities in both experimentally induced and naturally occurring worry. Studies comparing heart rate reactivity to threat when preceded by worry or relaxation found less increase in heart rate when threat imagery was preceded by worry, which was attributed to a "blunting" effect of worry (e.g., Borkovec & Hu, 1990). However, more recent evidence indicates that worrying causes physiological reactivity (i.e., increased heart rate and muscle tension) that *anticipates* actual onset of a threat, creating an illusion of blunting. Changes from a pre-worry baseline show equal reactivity (Peasley-Milkus & Vrana, 2000). Furthermore, the only studies to find blunting of reactivity from baseline used GAD patients (Hoehn-Saric, McLeod, & Zimmerli, 1989; Lyonfields, Borkovec, & Thayer, 1995), suggesting that worry is so pervasive in GAD that an unworried baseline is difficult if not impossible to achieve.

In addition to anticipatory physiological reactions, worry may also increase the frequency of reactions because more stimuli are interpreted as threatening. Worry increases reactivity (i.e., increased skin conductance and decreased cardiac vagal control) to ambiguous stimuli, suggesting that worriers are more likely to attach threat to these stimuli (Castaneda & Segerstrom, 2004). In a community sample, trait worry predicted higher waking cortisol responses on workdays but not weekends, suggesting that worrying exaggerated daily stress (Scholtz, Hellhammer, Schulz, & Stone, 2004; cf., Smyth et al., 1998).

Finally, worry may create threat where none exists. In an ambulatory study, worry episodes elevated blood pressure to the same degree as environmental hassles, the only difference being that worry occurred more often than hassles (Brosschot & Thayer, 2004). Chronically elevated sympathetic activity in worriers may occur because of deficient parasympathetic control over sympathetic arousal. Both worry and GAD are associated with low heart rate variability, an index of cardiac parasympathetic control via the vagus nerve (Lyonfields et al., 1995; Thayer et al., 1996). Worry, therefore, is capable of creating physiological reactivity that anticipates actual threat; exacerbating physiological reactivity to ambiguous stimuli that are not necessarily threatening; when severely pathological as in GAD, initiating a physiological reaction where no threat exists; or some combination thereof.

WORRY AND IMMUNE SYSTEM

Because of the close connections between the autonomic and immune systems, it is not surprising in light of the autonomic dysregulation in worry that the immune system is also dysregulated. As was true in the studies focusing on autonomic parameters, worry appears to be capable both of exacerbating responses to existing threat and of generating threat on an ongoing basis, with negative consequences for the immune system.

The 1994 Northridge earthquake in Los Angeles posed a significant ongoing threat to residents of the area. We assessed the relationship between worry and immunity in 47 employees of a Veteran's Administration hospital located approximately 0.5 mile from the epicenter of the earthquake (Segerstrom et al., 1998). In addition to ongoing aftershocks, residents also had to cope with changes to the structures of their lives, including disruptions in their living situations caused by damage to dwellings and belongings, obstacles to mobility caused by damage to infrastructure, and occupational uncertainty caused by damage to their workplaces. Throughout the study period (10 to 100 days after the earthquake), individuals high in trait worry had significantly fewer NK cells (CD3– CD16/56+) in peripheral blood than individuals low in trait worry. Furthermore, when these values were compared with laboratory control values from a demographically matched group, high worriers had significantly fewer NK cells than controls during the entire study period, whereas low worriers had fewer NK cells only at the last time point. These results were consistent with worry causing the threat of the aftermath of the earthquake to have more profound immune effects on individuals with high propensities to worry: They had significantly fewer NK cells earlier in the study and ended the study with the lowest values, at about 60% of laboratory control values.

Dysregulated NK cell response to a stressor was also observed in a laboratory study of the immune effects of exposing phobic individuals to a snake or spider (Segerstrom et al., 1998). Participants had blood drawn before a 5-minute exposure to the feared animal, immediately after the exposure, and at 20- and 40-minute follow-ups. In a group of subjects selected for normal levels of worry, the exposure caused a significant increase in the percent of NK cells in peripheral blood, from about 6% to about 10%. This increase is consistent with a number of other studies that observed an increase in NK cells during brief stressors that evoke a fight-or-flight response. This redistribution of NK cells into the bloodstream is thought to be an adaptive mechanism that prepares the organism for wounding during fight-or-flight stressors such as predation (Dhabhar & McEwen, 2001; Futterman et al., 1994; Segerstrom & Miller, 2004). A group of subjects selected for high worry showed a much abbreviated version of this potentially adaptive change, with an increase in percent NK cells from about 7.5% to about 9%. This abbreviated change was similar to that occurring in a resting control group that was not exposed to a feared animal. Therefore, high worry appears to blunt potentially adaptive immune changes in response to threat.

An apparent lack of immune response to threat exposure might be attributed to reactivity that anticipates actual exposure to threat (Peasley-Miklus & Vrana, 2000). In the phobic fear study, high worriers had non-significantly higher NK percentages than low worriers at a resting baseline (7.5% versus 6%), potentially lending some support to this notion. However, worriers and non-worriers showed significant and equal heart rate and skin conductance reactivity during the exposure, so anticipatory autonomic arousal was apparently not the mechanism for the lack of NK response.

An alternative interpretation invokes the effect of increased arousal due to worry on adrenergic receptors on NK cells. A history of higher or more frequent sympathetic reactivity to daily stressors could desensitize adrenergic receptors that mediate stress-induced increases in NK cells (Benschop et al., 1994). NK cells would therefore respond more weakly to acute sympathetic inputs in people with histories of high worry than in those without such histories.

In the previous studies, worry in normal research volunteers affected immune parameters only during stressors, but the most severe worry may cause tonic as well as phasic irregularities in the immune system. Extremely high levels of pathological worry such as those associated with GAD essentially create a chronic stressor via near-constant anticipation of imagined or exaggerated threat. Consistent with the immunosuppressive effects of chronic stressors, GAD patients showed evidence of impaired cellular immune function and poorer immunity against viruses in a cross-sectional comparison of GAD patients and non-anxious controls (La Via et al., 1996). Specifically, GAD patients had significantly smaller increases in CD25 expression (i.e., interleukin-2 receptor expression) after lymphocyte stimulation with anti-CD3 than controls. This difference was attributable to their more frequent experience of intrusive, uncontrollable thoughts. It is notable that the relationship between intrusive and uncontrollable thoughts and CD25 expression was linear across patients and controls ($r = .33$), so that even among controls, higher levels of worrisome thought were associated with reduced CD25 expression. Furthermore, CD25 expression was related to the number of upper respiratory infections reported over the previous year. Lower levels of IL-2 receptors on T cells could reduce their capability to proliferate in response to viral infection, resulting in a less than adequate population of antigen-specific cells. This immunological consequence of worry may have affected viral immunity and left GAD patients — and worried controls as well — more vulnerable to viral illness.

WORRY, HIV, AND HELPER T CELLS

Upper respiratory infections, although annoying, are rarely life-threatening to young, otherwise healthy individuals. To answer whether a person might be literally "worried to death," we examined the relationship between pathological worry and number of CD4 helper T cells in the context of HIV infection. Because the HIV virus selectively targets helper T cells, their decline is both indicative of the stage of HIV disease and prognostic for complications due to immunosuppression, such as opportunistic infections, and mortality. A relationship between worry and immunity in this population therefore suggests that worry could affect health via its effects on the immune system.

Prolonged and frequent sympathetic arousal is a likely mechanism by which worry would contribute to faster progression in HIV. *In vitro*, norepinephrine accelerated HIV replication in infected cells by suppressing antiviral cytokine production (Cole et al., 1998). *In vivo*, individuals with high sympathetic reactivity had higher HIV viral load and less virologic and immunologic response to highly active anti-retroviral therapy (HAART) (Cole et al., 2003). Because worry predisposes toward more frequent and prolonged sympathetic reactivity and suppresses parasympathetic inhibition of sympathetic arousal, it could accelerate the course of HIV via sympathetic pathways.

Examining the effects of worry on the immune system in HIV infection is also important if worry is conceptualized as a form of internally generated stressor. The effects of stressors on the immune system appear to be greatest in those who are already immunologically vulnerable due to age or disease (Segerstrom & Miller, 2004). Although previous studies have demonstrated effects of worry on the immune system in healthy samples (LaVia et al., 1996; Segerstrom et al., 1998, 1999), these effects may be both more clinically meaningful and more pronounced in a vulnerable sample such as people infected with HIV.

THE NATURAL HISTORY OF AIDS PSYCHOSOCIAL STUDY

The Natural History of AIDS Psychosocial Study (NHAPS; Kemeny et al., 1994) contains a subset of participants from the Multicenter AIDS Cohort Study (MACS; Kaslow et al., 1987), a longitudinal cohort study of the epidemiology and natural history of AIDS in gay and bisexual men that began in 1984. When serostatus testing became available, 49.5% of the MACS sample was found to be seropositive for HIV, so the study included both HIV seropositive and HIV seronegative men. NHAPS participants complete questionnaires at 6-month intervals, timed with medical evaluations that they undergo as part of the MACS. In 1994 and 1995, the NHAPS questionnaire contained a measure of pathological worry, consisting of the nine highest-loading items from the Penn State Worry Questionnaire (Meyer et al., 1990) and the meta-worry subscale from the Anxious Thoughts Inventory (Wells, 1994); these were highly correlated ($r = .85$) and so combined into a single score. The present sample included 27 HIV+ and 40 HIV− men who completed the worry questionnaire and had MACS data including medications and CD4+ helper T cell counts for some portion of the 2 years following questionnaire completion. The sample was predominantly white (92%), with the remainder primarily Hispanic, and ages ranged from 30 to 60 (mean = 43 for HIV+ men and 42 for HIV− men). At the time the worry questionnaire was administered, only 4 HIV+ men reported symptoms of HIV, including diarrhea, weight loss, thrush, night sweats, or fever.

RELATIONSHIP OF WORRY TO HELPER T CELLS IN NHAPS

Because participants contributed different lengths and numbers of follow-up data waves, we used multilevel modeling to assess the relationship of worry to number of CD4 cells at up to five waves: baseline (i.e., the time at which worry was assessed) and up to four 6-month follow-ups (i.e., up to 2 years after completing the worry questionnaire). Multilevel modeling (Singer & Willett, 2003) begins with a within-person model of the observations from each person (e.g., CD4 count as a function of an individual's initial CD4, changes over time, and time-varying covariates such as medication use). Varying numbers of observations can contribute to the within-person parameters, but estimates from individuals with more observations will contribute more heavily. The within-person models are then nested in a between-person model that predicts variance in the estimates of within-person models from between-person predictors (e.g., the effects of worry on CD4 means and changes over time).

HIV+ men contributed a mean of 3.8 observations (range = 1 to 5), and HIV− men contributed a mean of 4.2 observations. For HIV+ men, antiretroviral and HAART use was entered as a covariate at each wave. However, medication use was the exception rather than the rule, with at most nine participants using antiretroviral medication at any time point, and at most three using HAART. The number of follow-up data waves were not truncated by deaths, since no one in the sample died during the study period.

For HIV− men, there was no significant relationship between worry and CD4+ helper T cell numbers. However, for HIV+ men, there was a trend for worry to be associated with fewer helper T cells, as well as a significant worry-by-time interaction

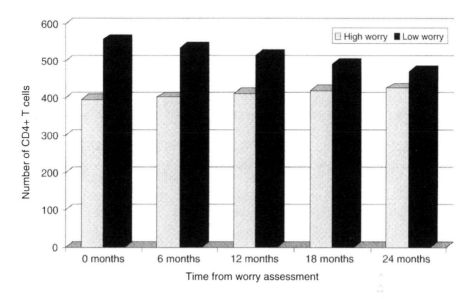

FIGURE 2.1 Number of CD4+ T cells in HIV+ high (+1 SD) and low (−1 SD) worriers.

(F (1,77) = 3.94, p = .05). That is, higher worry predicted lower average CD4+ cell counts, and worry also contributed to differences in how CD4+ cell counts changed over time. Figure 2.1 shows predicted values from the model for high (+1 SD) and low (−1 SD) worriers, including the effects of covariates. At all time points, worry was associated with a lower CD4 count, although this difference diminished over time.

The negative relationship between worry and CD4 count, as well as the change in this relationship over time, could be attributable to a number of different mediators, such as health behavior or anxious affect. In this sample, worry was associated with higher tension–anxiety as reported on the Profile of Mood States (McNair et al., 1971) and less exercise, but also less unprotected anal receptive sex (a behavior that could increase viral load). To examine the roles these factors may have played, the statistical model was repeated after including each factor as a time-varying covariate to see what proportion of the variance in the initial effect (η^2 = .05) could be accounted for. Controlling for anxious mood actually increased the effect size (η^2 = .08). This is consistent with the results of the earthquake study, in which controlling for anxious affect also increased the worry effect size. Similarly, controlling for exercise and unprotected anal receptive sex did not diminish the variance accounted for by worry and, in the case of exercise, also increased it.

Several factors that we could not test could have contributed to the diminution of the worry effect over time. First, worry is a relatively stable construct in this sample as in others. A single true–false worry item from the Taylor Manifest Anxiety Scale administered in 1987 ("I frequently find myself worrying about something") correlated .47 (p <.0001) with the worry scale administered in 1994 and 1995. Controlling for this item reduced the worry effect size (η^2 = .03), so the trait-like propensity to worry statistically accounted for about half of the effect. However, state worry may have also contributed, so that the relationship between worry and helper T cells was stronger at the contemporaneous assessment than at later time points. Another factor may have been the advent of HAART in the latter half of the study. The availability of an effective medication regimen for HIV was associated with a decline of distress and hopelessness among HIV+ men regardless of whether they were actually using the therapy (Rabkin, Ferrando, Lin, Sewell, & McElhiney, 2000). If the advent of HAART changed the degree to which HIV+ participants worried, the predictive power of the earlier worry assessment would decrease.

Second, worry may have been affected by helper T cell counts rather than the other way around. All participants in the MACS can get the results of their immunological assessments, which might have led participants with lower helper T cell counts to worry more than those with higher counts. However, the effect of trait worry measured years earlier suggests that worry prospectively influenced immunity, and the research with non-HIV samples suggests a relationship between worry and the autonomic and immune systems that is not predicated on knowing one's immune parameters, so either or both directions of effect may be correct.

Third, worry may have contributed to more protective health behaviors, with cautious worriers behaving in ways that maintained their CD4 counts relative to incautious non-worriers. In one study, worry about breast cancer was beneficial in that it motivated women to get mammograms (Diefenbach, Miller, & Daly, 1999). Among young heterosexuals, worry about contracting a sexually transmitted disease was associated with less risky sexual behavior (Cochran & Peplau, 1991). Similarly, in the present study, worry was associated with less risky sexual behavior. Although controlling for the health behaviors associated with worry did not diminish the effect, we cannot entirely rule out the possibility that health behaviors that we did not assess contributed to changes in CD4 counts.

REPETITIVE THOUGHT AND IMMUNITY

Taken together, studies of worry and the immune system demonstrate immunological dysregulation associated with worry under varying circumstances: acute and chronic stressors as well as daily life, which severe worry can transform into a chronically threatening circumstance. Furthermore, these results illustrate the role that cognition can take in physiological regulation and dysregulation above and beyond environmental events and emotional reactivity. Although stressful events may lead one to worry more, worry cannot be reduced to environmental events. Even under circumstances where all participants experienced roughly the same event (i.e., the earthquake) or exactly the same event (i.e., experimental exposure to a feared object), worry associated with immunological dysregulation.

Furthermore, although positive and negative affect modulated immune responses, affect actually acted as a suppressor variable with regard to worry. The anxious affect associated with worry is not responsible for its effects on the immune system, and that component of worry that is not affective (i.e., the cognitive component) has the strongest relationship to immune parameters. This is demonstrated by the increases in the worry effect size after controlling for anxious affect:

With regard to the relationship between worry and immune parameters, the affective variance in worry is "noise," and removing it makes the relationship stronger.

Worry is also not the only kind of cognition that may affect the immune system. On the contrary, it is only one example of what is called repetitive thought, that is, a prolonged or frequent thought or, colloquially, having something on your mind. Other examples of repetitive thought that could also be associated with immunological dysregulation include rumination, intrusive thoughts, and depressive rumination. All of these forms of repetitive thought have in common repetitive focus on negative topics: Worry usually constitutes attention to multiple domains of threatening uncertainty; rumination has a focal concern, often a failure or loss; and depressive rumination consists of attending to one's own depressive symptoms and their meanings and consequences (Segerstrom et al., 2003). Thought intrusions are common to several of these forms of repetitive thought and reflect the uncontrollability and undesirability of the thoughts (York et al., 1987).

There is evidence for physiological dysregulation accompanying several forms of negative repetitive thought. For example, trait rumination predicted higher cortisol secretion during an examination (Roger & Najarian, 1998) and increased sympathetic activity, including elevated blood pressure and skin conductance, in several studies (see Siegle & Thayer, 2004 for a review). People who experienced intrusive thoughts (whether as part of worry or some other form of negative repetitive thought) had more pronounced immune changes accompanying a number of different stressors, including natural disaster, cancer, and bereavement. The most reliable change was a decrease in natural killer cell cytotoxicity associated with more intrusive thoughts (see Segerstrom & Miller, 2004 for meta-analytic findings).

Although worry and related forms of repetitive thought have negative effects on the immune system, it is incorrect to conclude that all forms of repetitive thought are dysfunctional. In fact, positive repetitive thought commonly occurs and may have different consequences than negative repetitive thought. Examples of positive repetitive thought include planning, reflection, savoring, and cognitive and emotional processing (Segerstrom et al., 2003). While negative repetitive thought creates chronic stress by creating, exacerbating, anticipating, or prolonging the experience of threat, positive repetitive thought can ameliorate or contain experiences of threat and promote positive experiences such as growth. For example, Bower and colleagues (1998) examined the effects of cognitive processing on the psychological and physiological consequences of bereavement among HIV+ NHAPS participants. About two thirds of the sample engaged in some kind of cognitive processing, defined as deliberate, effortful, or long-lasting thinking about the death. Although some of this thinking may have been negative (e.g., rumination), about half of the men who engaged in cognitive processing found meaning in their bereavement, suggesting positive consequences of their repetitive thought.

These positive consequences included new appreciation for others, commitment to enjoying life, self-understanding, and enhanced spirituality or faith. Positive consequences were virtually absent in the men who did not engage in cognitive processing. Finally, men who both engaged in cognitive processing and found meaning had higher numbers of CD4 cells and lower mortality during a 2- to 3-year follow-up period. Although this study did not examine the exact nature of the cognitive processing, other evidence shows that repetitive thought that seeks positive reinterpretations of negative events can lead to finding meaning (Sears et al., 2003). Note that positive repetitive thought does not have to be about positive events; although positive thoughts such as reminiscing, savoring, or planning can be adaptive, repetitive thought about negative events such as bereavement can also be adaptive when it takes the form of cognitive processing rather than worry or rumination.

CONCLUSIONS

A large body of research associates stressful environmental events with changes in the immune system. However, a focus on the environment misses the rich and varied ways in which people anticipate, perceive, and process events in their environments and even imagine events that are not present. People who are prone to worry create for themselves a state of threat that is physiologically dysregulating and includes changes in the immune system: a lack of acute immune response to threat, an exaggerated immune response to chronic threat, and the potential for ongoing dysregulation that increases vulnerability to both major and minor illness. Furthermore, there is reason to believe that various repetitive thought styles (e.g., rumination, cognitive processing) can have their own diverse consequences. To date, the research remains only suggestive as to how this variety of repetitive thought impacts on the immune system, but this is a rich area of inquiry that has the potential to explain how people's inner and outer lives intersect to affect their immune systems and their health.

ACKNOWLEDGMENT

The National History of AIDS Psychosocial Project was supported by the National Institutes of Health (MH42918 and N01-A1-72631).

REFERENCES

American Psychiatric Association, *Diagnostic and Statistical Manual of Mental Disorders*, 4th ed., American Psychiatric Association, Washington, D.C., 1994, 432.

Benschop, R.J., Nieuwenhuis, E.E., Tromp, E.A., Godaert, G.L., Ballieux, R.E., and van Doornen, L.J., Effects of beta-adrenergic blockade on immunological and cardiovascular changes induced by mental stress, *Circulation*, 89, 762, 1994.

Borkovec, T.D. and Hu, S., The effect of worry on cardiovascular response to phobic imagery, *Beh. Res. Ther.*, 28, 69, 1990.

Bower, J.E., Kemeny, M.E., Taylor, S.E., and Fahey, J.L., Cognitive processing, discovery of meaning, CD4 decline, and AIDS-related mortality among bereaved HIV-seropositive men, *J. Consult. Clin. Psychol.*, 66, 979, 1998.

Brosschot, J.F. and Thayer, J.F., Worry, perseverative thinking, and health, in *Emotional Expression and Health: Advances in Theory, Assessment, and Clinical Applications*, Nyklicek, I., Temoshok, L., and Vingerhoets, A.J.J.M., Eds., Taylor & Francis, London, 2004, chap. 6.

Castaneda, J.O. and Segerstrom, S.C., Effect of stimulus type and worry on physiological response to fear, *J. Anx. Dis.*, 18, 809, 2004.

Cochran, S.D. and Peplau, L.A., Sexual risk reduction behaviors among young heterosexual adults, *Soc. Sci. Med.*, 33, 25, 1991.

Craske, M.G., Rapee, R.M., Jackel, L., and Barlow, D.H., Qualitative dimensions of worry in DSM-III-R generalized anxiety disorder subjects and nonanxious controls, *Behav. Res. Ther.*, 27, 397, 1989.

Dhabhar, F.S. and McEwen, B.S., Bidirectional effects of stress and glucocorticoid hormones on immune function: possible explanations for paradoxical observations, in *Psychoneuroimmunology*, 3rd ed., Ader, R., Felten, D.L., and Cohen, N., Eds., Academic Press, San Diego, 2001, chap. 10.

Diefenbach, M.A., Miller, S.M., and Daly, M.B., Specific worry about breast cancer predicts mammography use in women at risk for breast and ovarian cancer, *Health Psychol.*, 18, 532, 1999.

Futterman, A.D., Kemeny, M.E., Shapiro, D., and Fahey, J.L., Immunological and physiological changes associated with induced positive and negative mood, *Psychosom. Med.*, 56, 499, 1994.

Hoehn-Saric, R., McLeod, D.R., and Zimmerli, W.D., Somatic manifestations in women with generalized anxiety disorder, *Arch. Gen. Psychiatry*, 46, 1113, 1989

Kaslow, R.A., Ostrow, D.G., Detels, R., Phair, J.P., Polk, B.F., and Rinaldo, C.R., The Multicenter AIDS Cohort Study: rationale, organization, and selected characteristics of the participants, *Am. J. Epidemiol.*, 126, 310, 1987.

Kemeny, M.E., Weiner, H., Taylor, S.E., Schneider, S.G., Visscher, B.R., and Fahey, J.L., Repeated bereavement, depressed mood, and immune parameters in HIV seropositive and seronegative homosexual men, *Health Psychol.*, 13, 14, 1994.

Kubzansky, L.D., Kawachi, I., Spiro, A., Weiss, S.T., Vokonas, P.S., and Sparrow, D., Is worrying bad for your heart: a prospective study of worry and coronary heart disease in the Normative Aging Study, *Circulation*, 95, 818, 1997.

La Via, M.F., Munno, I., Lydiard, R.B., Workman, E.W., Hubbard, J.R., Michel, Y., and Paulling, E., The influence of stress intrusion on immunodepression in generalized anxiety disorder patients and controls, *Psychosom. Med.*, 58, 138, 1996.

Lyonfields, J.D., Borkovec, T.D., and Thayer, J.F., Vagal tone in generalized anxiety disorder and the effects of aversive imagery and worrisome thinking, *Beh. Ther.*, 26, 457, 1995.

McNair, D.M., Lorr, M., and Droppleman, L.F., *Profile of Mood States*, Educational & Industrial Testing Service, San Diego, 1971.

Meyer, T.J., Miller, M.L., Metzger, R.L., and Borkovec, T.D., Development and validation of the Penn State Worry Questionnaire, *Beh. Res. Ther.*, 28, 487, 1990.

Molina, S. and Borkovec, T.D., The Penn State Worry Questionnaire: psychometric properties and associated characteristics, in *Worrying: Perspectives on Theory, Assessment, and Treatment*, Davey, D.C.L., and Tallis, F., Eds., Wiley, New York, 1994, chap. 11.

Peasley-Miklus, C. and Vrana, S.R., Effect of worrisome and relaxing thinking on fearful emotional processing, *Beh. Res. Ther.*, 38, 129, 2000.

Rabkin, J.G., Ferrando, S.J., Lin, S.H., Sewell, M., and McElhiney, M., Psychological effects of HAART: a 2-year study. *Psychosom. Med.*, 62, 413, 2000.

Rini, C.K., Dunkel-Schetter, C., Wadhwa, P.D., and Sandman, C.A., Psychological adaptation and birth outcomes: role of personal resources, stress, and social–cultural context in pregnancy, *Health Psychol.*, 18, 333, 1999.

Roger, D. and Najarian, B., The relationship between emotional rumination and cortisol secretion under stress, *Person. Individ. Diff.*, 24, 531, 1998.

Ruscio, A.M., Borkovec, T.D., and Ruscio, J., A taxometric investigation of the latent structure of worry, *J. Abnormal Psychol.*, 110, 413, 2001.

Scholz, W., Hellhammer, J., Schulz, P., and Stone, A.A., Perceived work overload and chronic worrying predict weekend-weekday differences in the cortisol awakening response, *Psychosom. Med.*, 66, 207, 2004.

Sears, S.R, Stanton, A.L., and Danoff-Burg, S., The yellow brick road and the Emerald City: benefit finding, positive reappraisal coping, and post-traumatic growth in women with early-stage breast cancer, *Health Psychol.*, 487, 2003.

Segerstrom, S.C., Glover, D.A., Craske, M.G., and Fahey, J.L., Worry affects the immune response to phobic fear, *Brain Behav. Imm.*, 13, 80, 1999.

Segerstrom, S.C. and Miller, G.E., Psychological stress and the human immune system: a meta-analytic study of 30 years of inquiry, *Psychol. Bull.*, 130, 601, 2004.

Segerstrom, S.C., Solomon, G.F., Kemeny, M.E., and Fahey, J.L., Relationship of worry to immune sequelae of the Northridge earthquake, *J. Behav. Med.*, 21, 433, 1998.

Segerstrom, S.C., Stanton, A.L., Alden, L.A., and Shortridge, B.A., A multidimensional structure for repetitive thought: what's on your mind, and how, and how much? *J. Person. Social Psychol.*, 85, 909, 2003.

Siegle, G.J. and Thayer, J.F., Physiological aspects of depressive rumination, in *Depressive Rumination: Nature, Theory, and Treatment*, Papageorgiou, C. and Wells, A., Eds., Wiley, New York, 2004, chap. 5.

Singer, J.D. and Willett, J.B., *Applied Longitudinal Data Analysis: Modeling Change and Event Occurrence*, Oxford University Press, New York, 2003.

Thayer, J.F., Friedman, B.H., and Borkovec, T.D., Autonomic characteristics of generalized anxiety disorder and worry, *Biol. Psychiatry*, 39, 255, 1996.

Wells, A., A multi-dimensional measure of worry: development and preliminary validation of the Anxious Thoughts Inventory, *Anx. Stress Coping*, 6, 289, 1994.

York, D., Borkovec, T.D., Vasey, M., and Stern, R., Effects of worry and somatic anxiety on thoughts, emotion, and physiological activity, *Behav. Res. Ther.*, 25, 523, 1987.

3 Psychological Stress and Its Relationship to Cytokines and Inflammatory Diseases

Rama Murali, Margaret D. Hanson, and Edith Chen

CONTENTS

STRESS, TH1/TH2 CYTOKINES, AND INFLAMMATORY DISEASE

The role of psychological stressors in health and disease has been a dominant topic of research in health psychology and psychoneuroimmunology. Much of the early research in this field focused on the immunosuppressive consequences of stress on the immune system.[1,2] However, the past decade has seen the evolution of theories regarding stress and the immune system. The theories account for the different conceptualizations of stress (acute versus chronic) and diverse immune parameters (complements and cytokines). Consequently, they present a more complex view of the relationship between stress and immunity that moves away from seeing stress as solely immunosuppressive and sees it as immunomodulatory as well.[3-6]

The goal of this chapter is to discuss the relationship between psychological stress and the group of cytokines known as Th1 and Th2. We will present some basic biological information that will discuss the structures and functions of Th1 and Th2 cytokines and their interactions with hormones such as glucocorticoids. We will review studies that assessed specific types of stressors and the differential effects of these stressors on Th1 and Th2 cytokines and discuss the implications of these relationships for inflammatory diseases. In particular, we will describe the role of these cytokines in asthma and rheumatoid arthritis and demonstrate how shifts or dysregulations of these cytokines during stress affect these diseases. Finally, we will discuss some future research directions with regard to stress, Th1/Th2 cytokines, and inflammatory diseases.

TH1/TH2 CYTOKINES: BRIEF IMMUNOLOGICAL BACKGROUND

Cytokines are protein molecules secreted by white blood cells to regulate the immune response. They have a wide range of biological functions that include attracting cells to sites of injury and infection, activating and suppressing various cellular functions, and inducing proliferation and differentiation. Th1 and Th2 cytokines gain their names from the fact that they are secreted by T helper (Th) cells to serve different functions during an immune response. Th1 cytokines generally regulate cell-mediated immunity (responses to intracellular pathogens that involve activation of cells such as cyotoxic T cells and natural killer cells), and include molecules such as interleukin-2 (IL-2), tumor necrosis factor alpha (TNF-α), and interferon-gamma (IFN-γ). In contrast, Th2 cytokines play an important role in regulating humoral immunity (responses to extracellular pathogens that involve activation of B cells and antibody production), and include molecules such as IL-4, IL-5, IL-9, IL-10, and IL-13.[7-10]

Although researchers sometimes refer to white blood cells as Th1 or Th2, it is important to remember that this distinction is functional and not morphological, that is, cells are grouped in this way because of the cytokines they generally (but not always) secrete, not because they have observable structural differences. In fact, researchers have had little success in documenting morphological differences between cells that have Th1 versus Th2 cytokine secretion profiles.

The role of the above cytokines also extends beyond the scope of Th1- and Th2-related immune functions. However, based on our interest in implications for inflammatory diseases noted in this chapter, we will restrict our discussion to the roles of Th1 and Th2 cytokines.

Recent research has shown that both psychological and biological (glucocorticoid) components of stressful experiences can influence the expression of Th1 and Th2 cytokines.[3,9,11] In turn, Th1 and Th2 cytokines play a role in the pathophysiology of inflammatory diseases such as asthma and rheumatoid arthritis. Individuals with asthma have marked predominances of Th2 cytokine profiles. Patients with rheumatoid arthritis are shifted toward a Th1 cytokine profile.[3,4,12–15] Focusing on Th1 and Th2 cytokines will allow us to discuss the implications of psychological stress on the exacerbation and progression of these diseases.

DIFFERENTIATION AND CROSS-REGULATION

Th1 and Th2 cells are derived from the same precursors: Th0 cells. These naïve Th0 cells are undifferentiated CD4+ helper T cells that become polarized and develop into Th1 or Th2 cells via cytokines and stress hormones that are present at the time of differentiation (in addition to other immune components such as antigen-presenting cells, that will not be discussed in this chapter).[9] Th0 cells require the presence of IL-12, a cytokine produced by activated monocytes or other antigen-presenting cells, to polarize to Th1 cells.[3,9,11] In contrast, IL-4 must be present for Th2 polarization.[9]

Interestingly, Th1 and Th2 cells do not exist independently; they cross-regulate or counterbalance each other via their respective cytokine production mechanisms.[9] For example, IFN-γ suppresses the secretion of IL-4, the cytokine responsible for the differentiation of Th0 cells to Th2.[9] In addition, IL-4 and IL-10 inhibit the secretion of IFN-γ and IL-12, the cytokine responsible for differentiation to Th1.[9] It is important to note that not all Th1 and Th2 cytokines regulate Th0 cell development. For example, IL-13 (a Th2 cytokine) does not drive the differentiation of Th0 cytokines to Th2, as its IL-4 Th2 companion is known to do.[10]

MEASUREMENT OF TH1 AND TH2 CYTOKINES IN STRESS STUDIES

Before reviewing stress and Th1/Th2 cytokine studies, it is important to comment on the measurement of these cytokines in human psychological stress studies. The Th1 and Th2 cytokines discussed in the following sections are generally difficult to detect in basal concentrations because they degrade quickly in tissue and do not spill over into peripheral blood (where immune processes are typically assessed in human subjects) in large quantities.[16] Thus, an alternative methodological approach to investigating the role of stress in cytokines is the stimulation of human lymphocytes *in vitro* with a mitogen (i.e., lipopolysaccharide [LPS] or phytohemagglutinin [PHA]).

Over the course of a 24- to 48-hour incubation period, lymphocytes will then secrete cytokines in response to the mitogen, and researchers can measure levels of mitogen-stimulated cytokines in culture supernatant. When interpreting research in this area, it is critical to remember that important conceptual and methodological differences exist in these approaches to cytokine measurement. With measures of basal cytokine in circulation, researchers ask whether stress influences the expression of cytokines in peripheral blood at a particular moment in time. With stimulated-cytokine measures, the question is whether stress influences the ability of white blood cells to produce cytokines when they are challenged *in vitro*.

Apart from asking different types of questions about stress and immunity, these procedures also reveal differing strengths and weaknesses related to internal and external validity. A person's basal concentration of cytokine can be influenced by many factors — an ongoing infection, exposure to allergens, a recent injury or surgery — but in most cases it is impossible to definitively identify the stimulus. Hence, basal measures are subject to multiple influences that a researcher cannot control, and this introduces the possibility of alternative explanations for any links between stressors and cytokines. Much less ambiguity surrounds cytokines produced following mitogenic stimulation. The culturing conditions are standardized across subjects and tightly controlled, and any differences in cytokine production can be attributed to individual differences such as stressor exposure. That said, the true meaning of basal measures is clear: a high level of a given cytokine means an immune response is ongoing which, in the case of asthma or arthritis, could worsen symptoms. With mitogen-stimulated cytokine production, cells are taken from their natural environment and placed in culture with (typically) pharmacologic doses of a mitogen. It is unclear how well these artificial conditions simulate what occurs in a patient during real-life exposure to a pathogen or allergen.

PSYCHOLOGICAL STRESS AND TH1/TH2 CYTOKINES

In earlier decades, stress was believed to exert globally suppressive effects on the immune system including reduced humoral immunity, reduced proliferation of lymphocytes, and reduced functioning (cytotoxicity) of naturally killer cells.[1,17,18] This diminished functioning of the immune system was thought to account for high rates of infectious and neoplastic disease in chronically stressed individuals.[19,20]

The immunosuppression model has been critiqued more recently because it cannot explain why stress exacerbates medical conditions that involve activation of the immune response (e.g., asthma, arthritis, cardiac disease). Also, increasing numbers of studies have illustrated that stress may produce *shifts* in cytokine levels or immunomodulation specifically in regard to Th1 and Th2 cytokines rather than suppression.[4,13,14] Th1 and Th2 cytokines have been shown to shift toward a Th2 response in the presence of certain stressors in healthy individuals,[4,14] that is, psychological stressors may result in suppression of one group of cytokines (Th1) and enhancement of another (Th2). Thus, stress may modulate this axis of cytokines instead of universally suppressing it.

In addition, psychological research has grown increasingly sophisticated in its understanding of stress. While diverse stressors were tested earlier, there is a growing consensus that it is important to distinguish the characteristics of stressors, such as duration, frequency, and severity.[21] Furthermore, not all stressors will affect Th1 and Th2 cytokines in the same way; it is important to understand what types of stressors produce what types of effects on these cytokines. In the sections below, we will define different types of psychological stressors and review empirical studies that describe their impacts on Th1 and Th2 cytokines.

Brief Naturalistic Stressors and Th1/Th2 Cytokines

Acute stressors are negative events that are time-limited in duration, perception, and the responses they elicit.[16] One category of acute stressors is the group of brief naturalistic stressors that occur in the real world (as opposed to acute stressors induced in a laboratory) and are time-limited. Among humans, brief naturalistic stressors are often studied because they provide more ecologically valid stress paradigms that can reveal whether immune changes occur in response to stressors encountered in daily life.[16] Examples include academic stress and brief hospital stays.[4,22]

Overall, the literature illustrates that in healthy individuals, the stress associated with taking academic exams causes a shift toward the Th2 response, as seen by a decrease in Th1 cytokines and a corresponding increase in Th2 cytokines.[4,13,14] In the Marshall et al. study of medical students, taking an exam was associated with a significant increase in IL-10 production and a slight decrease in IFN-γ production.[4] They calculated the IFN-γ :IL-10 ratio before and after the exam period in order to assess shifts across the Th1/Th2 axis, and concluded that the stress of exams resulted in a shift along the axis toward a Th2 response as the IFN-γ :IL-10 ratio decreased. In addition, greater reports of daily hassles were negatively correlated with the IFN-γ: IL-10 ratio, illustrating that psychological self-report measures of stress also are associated with the Th1/Th2 shift toward a Th2 response.

Other studies using the exam stress paradigm reported decreased IFN-γ and IL-2 levels during exam periods, illustrating that Th1 cytokines decrease as a result of exam stress.[14,23] In the Paik et al.[23] and Kang and Fox[14] studies, blood samples were obtained from subjects on the day of or during the week of exams; samples used in the Marshall et al.[4] study were obtained several days after the exam period. These differences in timing may explain why Marshall[4] found small but non-significant differences in Th1 cytokines and Paik [23] and Kang and Fox[14] found significant decreases in Th1 cytokines.

A recent review of the stress and immunity literature concluded, after meta-analyses of over 300 studies, that brief naturalistic stressors exert a reliable effect on cytokine production that involves a shift away from Th1 (cellular) immunity, as shown by a decrease in Th1 cytokines, and toward Th2 (humoral) immunity, as shown by an increase in Th2 cytokines.[5]

The consequences of this shift away from a Th1 cytokine response during brief naturalistic stressors may be harmful based on the potential susceptibility to viruses or bacteria to which the Th1 or cellular arm of the immune system responds. If an individual experiences this type of naturalistic stressor and is exposed to a pathogen, it could be more difficult for his or her immune system to resist these pathogens if the cytokines that help coordinate the response are diminished.

Segerstom and Miller[5] also found in their meta-analysis that functional (as opposed to numerical) measures of the immune response such as natural killer cell cytotoxicity and T cell proliferative responses were decreased in the presence of brief naturalistic stress. Th1 cytokines play a vital role in mediating these responses, which aid in the defense and eradication of viruses and other pathogens. This illustrates additional evidence for a link between stress and a Th1/Th2 cytokine shift. In addition, the shift *toward* Th2 cytokines in the presence of brief naturalistic stressors is interesting to consider in regard to inflammatory diseases such as rheumatoid arthritis and asthma, which have altered cytokine levels that shift toward Th1 and Th2 cytokine profiles, respectively. A shift toward an enhanced humoral response to allergens during a brief naturalistic stressor could promote airway inflammation and obstruction that may affect individuals with asthma. We will discuss these implications later in this chapter.

CHRONIC STRESS AND TH1/TH2 CYTOKINES

In contrast to brief naturalistic stressors, chronic stressors take place over an extended period of time, often with unclear endpoints, and elicit prolonged psychological and biological responses.[5] Chronic stressors in humans are typically studied in naturalistic settings and include stressors such as caring for a chronically ill family member.[16] The literature has shown that chronic unrelenting stress is associated with declines in Th1 and Th2 responses as well as declines in other immune parameters such as natural and specific immune responses.[5] For example, the chronic stressor of serving as a caregiver or having a mother with breast cancer was associated with decreased production of Th1 cytokines including IL-2, IFN-g, and IL-12[17,24,25] as well as decreased production of Th2 cytokines such as IL-4.[26] Thus, chronic stress appears to fit the traditional immunosuppressive theory.

However, not all studies are consistent with this pattern. For example, Glaser et al.[24] found that caregivers expressed greater percentages of IL-10+/CD8+ peripheral blood leukocytes compared to control subjects not experiencing chronic stress. This suggests a shift toward a Th2 cytokine response under chronic stress. They did not find differences in Th1 cytokine expression between caregivers and controls.

Studies investigating the effects of chronic stress have more often examined Th1 rather than Th2 cytokines, and overall reveal a reliable effect of chronic stress decreasing Th1 responses.[5] In contrast, effects on Th2 cytokines may be more uncertain, although a recent meta-analysis concluded that chronic stress reliably decreases Th2 responses when one includes measures of humoral immunity other than cytokine production (e.g., antibodies to vaccination).[5] These types of immunosuppressive effects have important implications for disease susceptibility, including potentially increased risk for infectious and neoplastic diseases under chronic stress.[19,20] At the same time, however, they suggest that diseases characterized by exacerbated inflammatory responses would benefit from the immunosuppressive effects of chronic stress, but this result has not been observed clinically. This suggests that the relationship between chronic stress and Th1/Th2 cytokines in humans is not as straightforward as might initially appear. To help explain associations among chronic stress and inflammatory diseases, we next consider the role of glucocorticoids.

GLUCOCORTICOIDS, TH1/TH2 CYTOKINES, AND PSYCHOLOGICAL STRESS

GLUCOCORTICOIDS AND TH1/TH2 CYTOKINES

Stress hormones, specifically glucocorticoids, influence the polarization of naïve Th0 cells into Th1 and Th2 cells. Glucocorticoids (which take the form of cortisol in humans) are hormones secreted by the hypothalamic–pituitary–adrenal (HPA) axis, often after exposure to stressors. Glucocorticoids exert inhibitory effects on Th1 cytokines and enhancing effects on Th2 cytokines.[9,11,27,28] The relationship between glucocorticoids and Th1/Th2 cytokine production and differentiation adds an important layer to the relationships of psychological stress and cytokines.

The literature illustrates that cortisol levels increase when an individual experiences stressful situations where his or her coping resources are not able to counteract the demands of the environment.[28,29] However, another body of literature finds decreased cortisol levels and blunted cortisol responsiveness when individuals experience chronic stressors.[30-32]

The role of glucocorticoids in stress is complex. This section will review the relationship of stress to hyper- versus hypo-cortisolism profiles and discuss reasons for some discrepancies in previous research. We will also discuss biological evidence regarding stress hormones and the shift toward Th2 cytokines and studies illustrating a preliminary link of glucocorticoids, Th1/Th2 cytokines, and human psychological stress. Finally, we will discuss the notion of glucocorticoid resistance in chronic stress and its implications for shifts or dysregulation along the Th1/Th2 axis.

GLUCOCORTICOIDS AND TH1/TH2 CYTOKINES: BIOLOGICAL LINK

Basic immunology research in the areas of stress hormones and Th1/Th2 cytokines reveals that glucocorticoids act on lymphocytes in order to induce the production of Th2 cytokines and decrease the production of Th1 cytokine precursors and consequently Th1 cytokines.[3,9,11,27,33-35] Specifically, glucocorticoids work by suppressing the production of IL-12 by antigen-presenting cells (recall that IL-12 is necessary for Th1 cell development), and by down-regulating IL-12 receptor expression on T-cells and NK cells — cells that help produce IFN-γ when stimulated by IL-12.[11,36,37]

Glucocorticoids work by directly suppressing IL-12 production, preventing the presence of the cytokines necessary for Th1 development and reducing the ability of IL-12 to stimulate the production of other Th1 cytokines such as IFN-γ. In addition, glucocorticoids induce both IL-4 and IL-10 production.[3,9] Thus, in physiological concentrations, glucocorticoids may cause a shift from a Th1 immune response pattern to Th2 via alteration of cytokine production. Agarwal and Marshall[38] empirically demonstrated the ability of glucocorticoids to shift cytokine levels across the Th1/Th2 axis toward a Th2 response by using dexamethasone, a synthetic glucocorticoid, to model cortisol stress responses. They added exogenous dexamethasone (to mimic the release of hormones during the stress response) to human peripheral blood mononuclear cells (PBMCs) and assessed the alterations in Th1/Th2 cytokine levels (specifically IL-12, IFN-γ, IL-10, and IL-4). They found that dexamethasone decreased Th1 cytokines and increased Th2 cytokines, demonstrating a shift toward Th2 cytokines in response to glucocorticoids.

We next discuss the link among stressors, glucocorticoids, and Th1/Th2 cytokines in ecologically valid human stress paradigms.

Brief Naturalistic Stressors, Glucocorticoids, and Th1/Th2 Cytokines

Preliminary Links

As mentioned above, the literature regarding brief naturalistic stress and the Th1/Th2 axis of cytokines supports a shift toward Th2 cytokines. This stressor–cytokine shift is well established, but the role of glucocorticoids in this shift has not been adequately explored. The literature demonstrates that acute laboratory stressors reliably produce increases in cortisol levels.[39] The greatest effects were found with stressors that relate to social evaluation. In addition, numerous other acute stressors such as academic examinations,[40] public speaking,[41] parachute jumping,[42] hostage imprisonment, and public speaking combined with mental arithmetic in a laboratory[45] have been found to stimulate the HPA axis and produce increases in cortisol.

Few human studies have measured glucocorticoids (cortisol) together with Th1/Th2 cytokines in response to stress. Marshall et al. found no difference in plasma cortisol when comparing 2-day post-exam levels to pre-exam (3 weeks preceding exam) levels.[4] However, they found a shift toward Th2 (IL-10) cytokines and a decrease in Th1 (IFN-γ) cytokines resulting in a decreased IFN-γ:IL-10 ratio as a result of the exam stress. A study by Liu et al.[46] focusing on children with asthma also found no increase in cortisol levels during a school examination, although they found increases in IL-5 levels and decreases in IFN-γ levels.

It appears surprising that no increases in cortisol levels were noted in these two studies because cortisol would be expected to facilitate a Th1-to-Th2 shift. However, the timing of cortisol measures in both studies may explain why no changes were detected. Previous studies illustrated that cortisol reaches it peak in circulation 20 to 40 minutes after the onset of an acute laboratory stressor.[29] In basic biological studies, simply culturing naïve (Th0) cells with glucocorticoids can drive Th1/Th2 cell and cytokine differentiation.[27] When using brief naturalistic stressors, however, the optimal time to measure cortisol responses to stress is more ambiguous because the durations and intensities of naturalistic stressors vary. In the studies cited, temporary changes in cortisol may not have been captured based on the timing of assessments. For example, the studies measured cortisol several days after exams started and assessed cortisol concurrently with cytokines.[4,46] Changes in cortisol may have been more apparent if measures of cortisol were taken during or immediately after the exam. In addition, collecting cortisol measures prior to measuring Th1/Th2 cytokines would have allowed researchers to better assess whether cortisol drives the Th1/Th2 shift.

Other stress hormones such as catecholamines have been shown to cause a shift toward Th2 cytokines at the levels of both antigen-presenting cells and Th1 cells.[3] These hormones may be more responsive during times of brief naturalistic stress and consequently may help drive the shift along the Th1/Th2 axis.

Ultimately, the few studies of brief naturalistic stressors, glucocorticoids, and Th1/Th2 cytokines suggest that additional investigations involving repeated measures to clarify the timing of cortisol responses to naturalistic stressors are important. They will allow researchers to correlate changes in cortisol levels with changes in Th1 and Th2 cytokines in the context of psychological stress paradigms.

CHRONIC STRESS, GLUCOCORTICOIDS, AND TH1/TH2 CYTOKINES

Preliminary Links

The literature regarding chronic stress, glucocorticoids and the Th1/Th2 axis of cytokines is also in its preliminary stages. An increasing body of literature reports that in the face of chronic stress, individuals exhibit decreased or blunted cortisol levels.[31,32,47] However, some researchers found increased cortisol levels in the face of chronic stress.[17,32,48] With respect to cortisol and Th1/Th2 cytokines, Cohen et al.[17] found that cortisol levels were negatively associated with IL-2 levels among individuals whose mothers had breast cancer. This study illustrates a direct relationship between increased glucocorticoids and decreased Th1 cytokine levels under conditions of chronic stress.

Some researchers proposed that chronic stress alters the ability of cortisol to regulate the immune system. For example, Miller et al.[47] found that among adults experiencing chronic stress, immune cells exposed to dexamethasone (a synthetic cortisol) produced higher levels of IL-6 (an integral cytokine in pro-inflammatory responses) compared to the cells of adults not facing chronic stressors. They proposed a model of *glucocorticoid resistance* to explain this finding. Specifically, the model argues that increased cortisol secretion in the presence of chronic unrelenting stress forces the immune system to adapt by down-regulating its glucocorticoid receptors, thus leading to an inability of immune cells to respond effectively to glucocorticoid signals. This results in an inability to shut down certain immune responses that in turn elevates levels of cytokines such as IL-6.[47]

The glucocorticoid resistance model may help explain some of the inconsistent patterns found for cortisol levels and chronic stress. The core idea of glucocorticoid resistance is that the presence of chronic stress results in elevated cortisol levels. Cells then down-regulate their receptors for glucocorticoids to accommodate the elevated levels of cortisol. It is not central to the concept of glucocorticoid resistance that the cortisol levels remain elevated *continuously*, but rather that they remain elevated long enough to alter receptor expression. Indeed, research has shown that sometimes cortisol levels rebound below normal to recover from prolonged periods of elevation.[31] Thus, in humans experiencing chronic stress, elevated cortisol levels may result in glucocorticoid resistance; however, over time, cortisol levels may rebound below normal, resulting in a hypoactive stress system. Thus the different patterns of cortisol with respect to chronic stress may stem in part from differences in the timing of cortisol collection relative to the duration of the chronic stressor.

Consistent with this notion, Bauer et al.[49] found that chronic caregiver stress was associated with decreased lymphocyte sensitivity to glucocorticoids as well as increased salivary cortisol levels. Although this study does not directly support the biological link between increased glucocorticoids and decreased sensitivity to glucocorticoids, it does imply the potential for dysfunction along the Th1/Th2 axis related to cortisol. This idea that altered stress hormones may cause Th1 or Th2 cytokines to remain unregulated may have important implications for inflammatory diseases defined by Th1 or Th2 cytokine predominance — the topic for our next section.

INFLAMMATORY DISEASE AND TH1/TH2 CYTOKINES

Stress has been shown to exacerbate inflammatory diseases such as asthma and rheumatoid arthritis, resulting in increased inflammation and symptomology.[53] However, the mechanism by which stress results in the general worsening of these two conditions is challenging to understand. As noted, asthma is marked by a predominance of a Th2 cytokine profile and RA is marked by a Th1 cytokine profile.[3,12-14] Both diseases are exacerbated by stress. This suggests that a single uniform model of stress, cytokines, and inflammatory disease may not explain both types of diseases.

This section covers the complexities of the interactions of stress and these diseases. We will begin with a discussion of asthma, including cytokine profiles associated with the disease and the impact of stress on immune indicators and clinical symptoms. We will then discuss RA and the role of Th1/Th2 cytokines. The role of altered glucocorticoid functioning in this disease and its implications for Th1/Th2 cytokine expression will also be discussed.

ASTHMA AND TH1/TH2 CYTOKINES

Asthma is an immune-mediated inflammatory disease characterized by (1) airway obstruction, (2) airway inflammation, and (3) increased responsiveness of the airway to stimuli.[54] Researchers have hypothesized that certain cytokines are important for the orchestration of cellular events related to airway inflammation and hyperresponsiveness.[55] For example, Th2 helper cells secrete cytokines (e.g., IL-4, IL-5, and IL-13) that recruit inflammatory cells and release mediators that result in allergic inflammation, smooth muscle contraction, and mucus production.[3,13,14,54-56] Specifically, Th2 cell secretion of IL-4 and IL-13 induces B cells to switch to producing IgE antibodies.[57]

IgE is responsible for allergic responses and the up-regulation of eosinophil adhesion molecules, leading to obstructed airways and mucus production.[58] The longer lasting inflammatory response involves recruitment of eosinophils to the airways, which also promotes airway inflammation and obstruction. Eosinophil count, in turn, has been associated with symptoms and severity levels of asthma.[59,60] Th2 cell secretion of the IL-5 cytokine has been found to increase eosinophil production. Some researchers have argued that the inflammatory response in asthma involves a Th2 mechanism (IL-4, IL-5, and IL-13 cytokines).[55,61,62]

Research has demonstrated that patients with asthma differ from healthy individuals in their cytokine profiles. Asthma patients have cells that produce higher levels of cytokines such as IL-4 and IL-5 compared to healthy individuals[63,65] and greater expression of mRNA for IL-4 and IL-5.[66-68] Following allergen challenge, levels of IL-4 and IL-13 cytokines increase in patients with asthma.[69]

Stress and Asthma

The psychological role of stress in asthma was cited long before scientists uncovered the biological and immunological pathways linking stress and the disease. In the 19th century, asthma was believed to be a "neurotic affection" instigated solely by psychological stress.[54] Research in the past decades reveals a more sophisticated approach to explaining how psychosocial stress "gets inside" the body to impact the expression of asthma symptoms. As reviewed earlier, certain types of psychological stress are related to the suppression of cellular (Th1) immunity and heightened humoral (Th2) immunity in healthy people.[5] If stress is also related among individuals with asthma to this type of shift in Th1/Th2 cytokine profiles, it may indicate one pathway to worsening clinical symptomatology in asthma.[70]

Acute Stress and Asthma

Studies have shown links between brief naturalistic stressors and asthma. For example, in a study by Sandberg and colleagues,[71] children between 6 and 13 years of age recorded asthma symptoms and life stressors over an 18-month period using daily diary and interview assessments. Experiencing an acute life stressor was related to increased risk of asthma exacerbations 4 to 6 weeks after the occurrence of the event.[70,71] In daily diary studies of patients with asthma, acute life stressors were associated with same-day lower peak flow rates and greater self-reports of asthma symptoms.[72] The number of asthma exacerbations induced by colds was found to be higher in asthmatic adults who had high numbers of negative life events and low social support.[73] Finally, an intervention involving disclosure of stressful life experiences improved pulmonary function months later in a sample of patients with asthma.[74]

Studies of the impacts of brief naturalistic stressors in patients with asthma revealed altered immune profiles during times of stress. In a study of the responses of 20 college students with asthma to antigen challenges during times of low stress (mid-semester) and high stress (final exam period), results revealed that during high stress, students' eosinophil and IL-5 production increased, consistent with a Th1/Th2 cytokine shift.[46] In another sample of patients with asthma, taking a school exam was associated with greater stimulated Th2 cytokine (IL-5) production in adolescents with asthma compared to healthy control adolescents.[75] IL-5 levels in adolescents with asthma remained elevated even 2 to 3 weeks after examinations compared to control adolescents.[75]

Kang and colleagues[70] reported that the impact of exam stress on immunity was reduced when students reported having high social support. More specifically, students with asthma who had high social support when they were under stress showed smaller reductions in natural killer cell cytotoxicity compared to students with asthma who lacked social support.

On a neuroendocrine level, in individuals with inflammatory diseases such as asthma, the HPA axis is thought to be dysregulated. Subjects with asthma have been described as having hypocortisolistic profiles or blunted HPA axes.[6] Stress may also contribute to this blunted cortisol profile. For example, in response to an acute laboratory stressor (public speaking), children with asthma displayed lower cortisol responses compared to healthy children.[76] The same patterns were found for children with similar inflammatory conditions (atopic dermatitis).[77]

Chronic Stress and Asthma

With respect to chronic stress, studies of children with asthma revealed that chronic stress alters the clinical profile of asthma. For example, among children with asthma who were experiencing chronic stress, an acute life event produced an increased risk

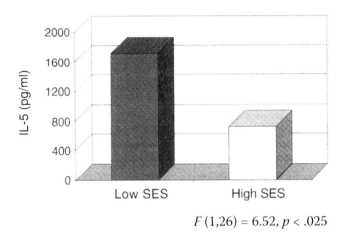

$$F(1,26) = 6.52, p < .025$$

FIGURE 3.1 Asthmatic adolescents from low socioeconomic status neighborhoods had higher stimulated production of the IL-5 Th2 cytokine compared to asthmatic adolescents from high socioeconomic status neighborhoods. (From Chen E et al. (2003). *Psychom. Med.* 65: 984–992. With permission.)

of an asthma attack more quickly (within 2 weeks) compared to children with asthma who did not experience chronic stress.[78] With respect to links to immune measures, adolescents with asthma who came from low socio-economic status (SES) backgrounds had higher levels of stimulated Th2 cytokine IL-5 compared to high SES adolescents with asthma.[79] In addition, chronic stress was found to mediate the relationship between living in a low SES neighborhood and heightened production of IL-5 among adolescents with asthma (see Figure 3.1).

In a study of infants 6 to 18 months old, high levels of chronic stress among caregivers were associated with altered IgE and cytokine expression in their infants, consistent with the patterns of Th2 immunity found in people with asthma.[80] The infants of caregivers who reported greater psychological stress as measured by the Perceived Stress Scale had higher levels of allergen and mitogen-stimulated TNF-α and lower levels of IFN-γ than infants from low-stress households. The number of IgE antibodies was also greater in children whose caregivers reported higher levels of psychological stress. These findings suggest that stress experienced in early life alters Th1/Th2 cytokine profiles toward a dominant Th2 immune response, which in turn may predispose these children to developing chronic inflammatory diseases such as asthma later in life.

Earlier we reviewed evidence documenting that chronic stress had immunosuppressive effects. However, these studies were all conducted in physically healthy individuals undergoing chronic stressor (e.g., serving as a caregiver for a chronically ill family member). In contrast, among individuals with asthma who already have dysregulated immune profiles, it is possible that chronic stress pushes the immune system further toward a Th2 cytokine imbalance, elevating risk for exacerbations of asthma.

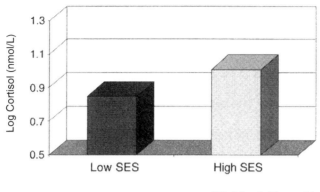

$F(1,26) = 3.03, p < .10$

FIGURE 3.2 Asthmatic adolescents from low socioeconomic status neighborhoods had marginally lower morning cortisol levels than asthmatic adolescents who came from higher socioeconomic status neighborhoods. (From Chen E et al. (2003). *Psychom. Med.* 65: 984–992. With permission.)

On the neuroendocrine level, chronic stress also contributes to a blunted cortisol profile. For example, among women with asthma, low serum cortisol concentrations were found in those who had high levels of life stress and low levels of social coping resources.[81] Adolescents with asthma who came from low SES neighborhoods (conceptualized as high stress) had marginally lower morning cortisol values than adolescents with asthma who came from high SES neighborhoods[79] (see Figure 3.2). These blunted cortisol profiles under high chronic stress may allow inflammatory processes to flourish unchecked, resulting in exacerbations of asthma. Overall, both acute and chronic stressors have been associated with heightened production of Th2 cytokines and blunted cortisol profiles in patients with asthma. This suggests that real-life acute and chronic stressors may shift the Th1/Th2 axis of cytokines and glucocorticoid production in a manner that could lead to heightened and unchecked production of Th2 cytokines in the face of exposure to an antigen, resulting in increased airway obstruction and inflammation for patients with asthma.

RHEUMATOID ARTHRITIS AND TH1/TH2 CYTOKINES

Rheumatoid arthritis (RA) is a chronic inflammatory disorder of unknown etiology.[82] The tissues around one or more joints trigger an inflammatory response that affects joint mobility and can cause increased pain and difficulty in daily life. It is well established in the literature that the balance of Th1/Th2 cytokines is skewed toward a Th1 response in patients with RA.[3,12,34,83] Specifically, RA involves excesses of IL-12 and TNF-α, but IL-10 production is deficient.[34] Psychological stress has been associated with exacerbations of RA.[84] Daily diary studies revealed that weeks of high stress were associated with more clinician-rated disease activity than weeks of low stress among patients with RA.[85] Increases in the number of stressors experienced from week to week were associated with increases in disease activity.[86] Finally, when patients with RA reported high levels of social support and coping behaviors during times of chronic stress or major life events, RA symptoms did not change, suggesting that while stress can exacerbate disease severity, coping and social support may mitigate its effects on RA outcomes.[87]

Research on the effects of stress on Th1/Th2 cytokines in patients with RA is limited. Some studies have shown that subgroups of patients with RA who experience significant increases in interpersonal stress also show increases in certain immune measures such as soluble IL-2 receptor levels.[53,85] Other studies reported blunting of Th2 stress responses and Th1 in RA patients, that is, healthy subjects showed increases in both Th2 (IL-10) and Th1 (IFN-g) cytokine production in response to acute laboratory stressors, while these changes were not evident in patients with RA.[88]

Some research relates to cortisol and RA. One study investigated the effects of an acute laboratory stressor on cortisol in RA patients[12] who exhibited significantly smaller cortisol responses to acute laboratory stressors when compared to healthy control subjects without RA.[12] This study illustrated that individuals with RA have decreased cortisol responses to acute stress, and is consistent with previous literature that describes a hypoactive stress system in terms of basal cortisol profiles in patients with RA.[3,6] However, it should be noted that one study found that RA and healthy patients showed similar cortisol responses to experiences of daily stress events.[89]

The literature on stress and RA in humans does not provide much direct evidence about the implications of a hypoactive stress system in RA on the Th1/Th2 axis of cytokines. However, it is possible that the low levels of glucocorticoids found in RA patients may mean a compromised ability to shift the Th1/Th2 axis toward a Th2 profile under stress (the typical effect of glucocorticoids). This could explain why stress has typically been associated with a worsening of symptoms in RA patients rather than the improvement that would be expected if stress shifted the Th1/Th2 axis toward a Th2 profile.

Some studies involved the use of exogenous glucocorticoids such as dexamethasone to challenge the immune response and act as a biological model for stress.[82,83] DeAntonio et al.[83] performed a glucocorticoid sensitivity assay with PBMCs from RA patients to determine the responsiveness of cytokines to glucocorticoids. They found that IFN-γ and TNF-α levels of RA patients remained elevated after administration of dexamethasone when compared to healthy controls. In addition, higher levels of dexamethasone were needed to inhibit TNF-α cytokines in the RA patients. These findings allude to the decreased ability of RA patients to respond to glucocorticoids. Other studies also reported decreased expression of glucocorticoid receptors in cells of RA patients and consequent reduced sensitivity to circulating glucocorticoids.[11,89,90]

Immune systems of RA patients seem to lack responsiveness to glucocorticoids, and as a result it may be difficult for the immune systems of RA patients to downregulate Th1 cytokines. Thus, when the immune systems in RA patients are challenged by stress, there is a blunted cortisol response as well as glucocorticoid resistance on the part of immune cells, both of which could result in an inability to shift away from the disease Th1 cytokine profile toward a Th2 cytokine response during stress.

Some evidence indicates that psychological stress in RA is characterized by blunted glucocorticoid reactivity. In addition, the decreased glucocorticoid receptor expression and glucocorticoid sensitivity in RA may explain the inability to induce Th2 cytokine production and suppress the damaging elevation in Th1 cytokines when stressors are present. The discussion of Th1/Th2 cytokines and stress in RA is very preliminary, although the links between RA and glucocorticoid expression and functioning set the stage for speculation regarding RA and Th1/Th2 cytokines during stress. Future studies that focus on stress-related alterations in both Th1 and Th2 cytokines in the face of glucocorticoid resistance in RA patients are necessary to achieve a better understanding of the mechanisms involved in exacerbations of RA.

CONCLUSIONS AND FUTURE DIRECTIONS

In the past decade, clinical research on the role of psychological stress on the expression of Th1/Th2 cytokines has moved from conceptualizing the effects of stress as immunosuppressive to considering the immunomodulatory effects of stress. Th1 and Th2 cytokines orchestrate different immune pathways to fight pathogens: Th1 cytokines coordinate cellular immune responses and Th2 cytokines coordinate humoral immune responses. Under stress, one type of immunity may be enhanced and another suppressed, resulting in immunomodulatory (rather than globally immunosuppressive) effects.

The effects of stress on Th1/Th2 cytokines depend on the type of stressor investigated. Psychological stress can be characterized according to the duration and resolution of the stressful event. Brief naturalistic stressors occur during daily life and are time-limited stressors (e.g., academic examinations). Studies have shown that this type of psychological stress elicits predominantly Th2 immune responses. In contrast, chronic stress (e.g., caring for a loved one with dementia) is a prolonged experience often with an unclear endpoint. Studies have shown that this type of stress suppresses both Th1 and Th2 responses.

Glucocorticoids, hormones released during times of psychological stress, inhibit the polarization of Th1 cytokines and enhance Th2 cytokine production. Cortisol levels are affected by stress; however the relationship among stress, hormones, and cytokines is complex and differs by the type of stressor measured. Under conditions of acute stress, glucocorticoids increase, perhaps causing a shift toward Th2 immunity. Studies of chronic stress sometimes reported increases and at other times decreases in cortisol. It is possible that glucocorticoid levels depend on time since onset of a chronic stressor; for example, glucocorticoid levels may be high at the beginning of a chronic stressor, but may then rebound below normal levels as the stressor becomes prolonged. This dysregulation of stress hormones may then impair the cross-regulatory functioning of the Th1/Th2 axis, with implications for inflammatory diseases.

Cytokine profiles specific to asthma and rheumatoid arthritis were considered in this chapter as representative of dominant Th2- and Th1-mediated diseases, respectively. Among patients with asthma, stress has been associated with clinical exacerbations of the disease and as also associated with elevations in Th2 cytokines and low levels of cortisol, suggesting immune and neuroendocrine pathways from stress to asthma. Among patients with rheumatoid arthritis, levels of Th1 cytokines were elevated, although these elevations were not definitively linked to stress.

Patients with RA were also found to have blunted cortisol responses to stress and decreased sensitivity to glucocorticoids, suggesting that alterations to the HPA axis may be partially responsible for elevated Th1 cytokines in RA.

A number of recommendations should be considered in determining future directions for research on the relationship of stress, Th1/Th2 cytokines, and inflammatory diseases. First, it is important to understand the timing of when stressors affect both cytokines and cortisol. Future studies should involve repeated assessments after the onset of a stressor to determine when cytokines peak (or shifts occur) and determine when cortisol profiles become altered. Understanding these temporal patterns may help reconcile inconsistencies in previous research studies that used different timing parameters for assessing cytokines and cortisol. These types of assessments are important for both brief naturalistic stressors and chronic stressors. With respect to chronic stressors, it is also important to assess the effects of the duration of the stressor on cytokine and cortisol profiles. Because stressors persist over time, cell receptors may become up-regulated or down-regulated in response to low or high levels of certain cytokines and cortisol. This may in turn shift cytokine and cortisol profiles over the long term. It is also important for future studies to address the interrelationships of Th1/Th2 cytokines and cortisol in studies of psychological stress in humans. Understanding the effects of cortisol on Th1 and Th2 cytokines in response to both brief naturalistic and chronic stressors will help researchers develop a more accurate overall model of how cortisol regulates the Th1/Th2 axis in the faces of different types of stressors.

Additional studies of patient populations are needed to clarify the biological pathways between stress and disease exacerbation. Few studies of patients with RA focus on how different types of stressors affect Th1 versus Th2 cytokines. In addition, few studies of asthma patients target the role of glucocorticoid resistance in the relationship between stress and Th1/Th2 cytokines. Finally, studies that investigate the links from stress to cytokine and cortisol profiles and from cytokine and cortisol profiles to clinical indicators of disease in patients with inflammatory conditions such as asthma and RA are needed.

Intriguing evidence concerns potential pathways from stress to inflammatory diseases operating through Th1/Th2 cytokines and cortisol. Future research directly addressing these issues in patient populations will help researchers develop biologically plausible alternatives to the immunosuppression model to reveal how psychological stress affects inflammatory conditions.

ACKNOWLEDGMENTS

This research was supported by the Canadian Institutes for Health Research and the Human Early Learning Partnership. The authors would like to thank Gregory Miller for helpful comments on this chapter.

REFERENCES

1. Herbert TB and Cohen S (1993). Stress and immunity in humans: a meta-analytic review. *Psychosom. Med.* 55: 364–379.
2. Seyle H (1975). *The Stress of Life*. McGraw Hill, New York.

3. Elenkov IJ and Chrousos GP (2002). Stress hormones, proinflammatory and anti-inflammatory cytokines and autoimmunity. *Ann. NY Acad. Sci.* 966: 290–303.
4. Marshall GD, Agarwal SK, Lloyd C, Cohen L, Henniger EM, and Morris GJ (1998). Cytokine dysregulation associated with exam stress in healthy medical students. *Brain Behav. Immun.* 12: 297–307.
5. Segerstrom SC and Miller GE (2004). Psychological stress and the immune system in humans: a meta-analytic review of 30 years of inquiry. *Psychol. Bull.* 130: 601–630.
6. Sternberg EM (2001). Neuroendocrine regulation of autoimmune/inflammatory disease. *J. Endocrinol.* 169: 429–435.
7. Romagnani S (2004). T cell subsets (Th1 vs. Th2). *Ann. Allergy Asthma Immunol.* 85: 9–18.
8. Shinkai K, Mohrs M, and Locksley RM (2002). Helper T cells regulate type 2 innate immunity *in vivo. Nature* 420: 825–829.
9. Spellberg B and Edwards JE (2001). Type 1/Type 2 immunity in infectious diseases. *Clin. Infect. Dis.* 21: 76–102.
10. Wills-Karp M (2001). IL-12/IL-13 axis in allergic asthma. *J. Allergy Clin. Immunol.*107: 9–18.
11. Chrousos GP (2000). Stress, chronic inflammation, and emotional and physical well-being: concurrent effects and chronic sequelae. *J. Allergy Clin. Immunol.* 106: 275–291.
12. Dekkers JC, Geenen R, Godaert G, Glaudemans K, Lafeber F, van Doornen L, and Bijlsma J (2001). Experimentally challenged reactivity of the hypothalamic pituitary adrenal axis in patients with recently diagnosed rheumatoid arthritis. *J. Rheumatol.* 28: 1504.
13. Kang D, Coe CL, McCarthy DO, Jarjour NN, Kelly EA, Rodriguez RR, and Busse WW (1997). Cytokine profiles of stimulated blood lymphocytes in asthmatic and healthy adolescents across the school year. *J. Interferon Cytokine Res.* 17: 481–487.
14. Kang D and Fox C (2001). Th1 and Th2 cytokine responses to academic stress. *Res. Nurs. Health* 24: 245–257.
15. Schulze-Koops H and Kalden JR (2001). The balance of Th1/Th2 cytokines in rheumatoid arthritis. *Best Pract. Res. Clin. Rheumatol.* 15: 677–691.
16. Stetler CA, Murali R, Chen E, and Miller GE (2005). Stress, immunity, and disease, in *Handbook of Stress Medicine*, Cooper CL, Ed., Taylor & Francis, London.
17. Cohen E, Klein E, Fried G, Zinder O, and Pollack S (2002). Increased emotional distress in daughters of breast cancer patients is associated with decreased natural cytotoxic activity, elevated levels of stress hormones and decreased secretion of Th1 cytokines. *Int. J. Cancer* 100: 347–354.
18. Kiecolt-Glaser JK, Marucha PT, and Malarkey WB (1995). Slowing of wound healing by psychological stress. *Lancet* 346: 1194–1196.
19. Andersen BL, Keicolt-Glaser JK, and Glaser R (1994). A biobehavioral model of cancer stress and disease course. *Am. Psychol.* 49: 389–404.
20. Cohen S and Williamson GM (1991). Stress and infectious disease in humans. *Psychol. Bull.* 109: 5–24.
21. Cohen S, Kessler RC, and Gordon LU (1997). *Measuring Stress: A Guide for Health and Social Scientists,* Oxford University Press, London.
22. Elliot GR and Eisdorfer C (1982). *Stress and Human Health: An Analysis and Implications of Research*, Springer, New York.
23. Paik I, Toh K, Lee C, Kim J, and Lee S (2000). Psychological stress may induce increased humoral and decreased cellular immunity. *Behav. Med.* 26: 139–141.

24. Glaser R, Keicolt-Glaser JK, Janice K, Malarkey WB, and William B (1998). The influence of psychological stress on the immune response to vaccines, in *Neuromodulation: Molecular Aspects, Integrative Systems, and Clinical Advances*, McCann SM and Lipton JM, Eds., New York Academy of Sciences, New York, pp. 649–644.

25. Vedhara K, Fox JD, and Wang ECY (1999). The measurement of stress-related immune dysfunction in psychoneuroimmunology. *Neurosci. Behav. Rev.* 23: 699–715.

26. Nakano Y, Nakamura S, Hirata M, Harada K, Ando K, Tabuchi T, et al. (1998). Immune function and lifestyle of taxi drivers in Japan. *Ind. Health* 36: 32–39.

27. Rook GAW (1999). Glucocorticoids and immune function. *Ballière Clin. Endocrinol. Metabol.* 13: 567–581.

28. Sapolsky R (1998). *Why Zebras Don't Get Ulcers*. W.H. Freeman, New York.

29. Kirschbaum C and Hellhammer DH (1989). Salivary cortisol in psychobiological research: an overview. *Neuropsychobiology* 22: 150–169.

30. Caplan RD, Cobb S, and French JRP, Jr (1979). White collar work load and cortisol: disruption of a circadian rhythm by job stress? *J. Psychosom. Res.* 23: 181–192.

31. Heim C, Ehlert U, and Hellhammer D (2000). The potential role of hypocortisolism in the pathophysiology of stress-related bodily disorders. *Psychoneuroendocrinology* 25: 1–35.

32. Pruessner JC, Hellhammer DH, and Kirschbaum C (1999). Burnout, perceived stress, and cortisol responses to awakening. *Psychosom. Med.* 61: 197–204.

33. Blotta MH, Umetsu DT, and DeKruyff R.H. (1997). Corticosteroids inhibit IL-12 production in human monocytes and enhance their capacity to induce IL-4 synthesis in CD4+ lymphocytes. *J. Immunol.* 158: 5589–5595.

34. Elenkov IJ, Chrousos GP, and Wilder RL (2000). Neuroendocrine regulation of IL-12 and TNF/IL-10 balance: clinical implications. *Ann. NY Acad. Sci.* 917: 94–105.

35. Wilcken T and De Rijk R (1997). Glucocorticoids and immune function: unknown dimensions and new frontiers. *Immunol. Today* 18: 418–424.

36. Chung FK (2001). Anti-inflammatory cytokines in asthma and allergy: interleukin-10, interleukin-12, and interferon-gamma. *Med. Inflamm.* 10: 51–59.

37. Elenkov IJ (2004). Glucocorticoids and the Th1/Th2 balance. *Ann. NY Acad. Sci.* 1024: 138–146.

38. Agarwal SK and Marshall GDJ (1998). Glucocorticoid-induced type1/type2 cytokine alterations in humans: a model for stress-related immune dysfunction. *J. Interferon Cytokine Res.* 18: 1059–1068.

39. Dickerson SS and Kemeny ME (2004). Acute stressors and cortisol responses: a theoretical integration and synthesis of laboratory research. *Psychol. Bull.* 130: 355–391.

40. Kahn JP, Michaud C, de Talance N, Lazenaire M, Mejean L, and Burlet C (1992). Applications of salivary cortisol determinations to psychiatric and stress research: stress responses in students during academic examinations, in *Assessment of Hormones and Drugs in Saliva in Behavioral Research*, Kirschbaum C, Read GF, and Hellhammer D. Eds., Hogrefe & Huber, Seattle, pp. 111–127.

41. Bassett JR, Marshall PM, and Spillane R (1987). The physiological measurement of acute stress (public speaking).in bank employees. *Int. J. Psychophysiol.* 5: 265–273.

42. Deinzer R, Kirschbaum C, Gresele C, and Hellhammer D (1997). Adrenocortical responses to repeated parachute jumping and subsequent h-CRH challenge in inexperienced healthy subjects. *Physiol. Behav.* 61: 507–511.

43. Cook NJ, Read GF, Walker RF, Harris B, and Riad-Fahmy D (1992). Salivary cortisol and testosterone as markers of stress in normal subjects in abnormal situations, in *Assessment of Hormones and Drugs in Saliva in Behavioral Research*, Kirschbaum C, Read GF, and Hellhammer D, Eds., Hogrefe & Huber, Seattle, pp. 147–162.

44. Rahe RH, Karson S, Howard NS, Jr, Rubin RT, and Poland RE (1990). Psychological and physiological assessments of American hostages freed from captivity in Iran. *Psychosom. Med.* 52: 1–16.

45. Kirschbaum C, Pirke KM, and Hellhammer D (1993). The Trier Social Stress Test: a tool for investigating psychobiological stress responses in a laboratory setting. *Neuropsychobiology* 1–2: 76–81.

46. Liu LY, Coe CL, Swenson CA, Kelly EA, Kita H, and Busse WW (2002). School examinations enhance airway inflammation to antigen challenge. *Am. J. Resp. Crit. Care Med.* 165: 1062–1067.

47. Miller G, Cohen S, and Ritchey A (2002). Chronic psychological stress and the regulation of pro-inflammatory cytokines: a glucocorticoid-resistance model. *Health Psychol.* 21: 531–541.

48. Matthews KA, Gump BB, and Owens JF (2001). Chronic stress influences cardio-vascular and neuroendocrine responses during acute stress and recovery, especially in men. *Health Psychol.* 20: 403–410.

49. Bauer ME, Shanks N, Lightman SL, Wilcock GK, Perks P, and Vedhara K (2000). Chronic stress in caregivers of dementia patients is associated with reduced lympho-cyte sensitivity to glucocorticoids. *J. Neuroimmunol.* 103: 84–92.

50. Miller BD and Wood BL (1994). Psychophysiologic reactivity in asthmatic children: a cholinergically mediated confluence of pathways. *J. Am. Acad. Child Adolesc. Psychiatr.* 33: 1236–1244.

51. Miller BD and Wood BL (1997). Influence of specific emotional states on autonomic reactivity and pulmonary function in asthmatic children. *J. Am. Acad. Child Acolesc. Psychiatr.* 36: 669–677.

52. Thomason B, Brantley P, Jones G, Dyer H, and Morris J (1992). The relation between stress and disease activity in rheumatoid arthritis. *J. Behav. Med.* 15: 215–220.

53. Zautra AJ, Hoffman JM, and Matt KS (1998). An examination of individual differ-ences in the relationship between interpersonal stress and disease activity among women with rheumatoid arthritis. *Arthritis Care Res.* 11: 271–279.

54. Wright RJ, Rodriques M, and Cohen S (1998). Review of psychosocial stress and asthma: an integrated biopsychosocial approach. *Thorax* 53: 1066–1074.

55. Chung FK, Barnes PJ (1999). Cytokines in asthma. *Thorax* 54: 825–857.

56. Marshall GD and Agarwal SK (2000). Stress, immune regulation, and immunity: applications for asthma. *Allergy Asthma Proc.* 21: 241–246.

57. Bacharier LB and Geha RS (2000). Molecular mechanisms of IgE regulation. *J. Allergy. Clin. Immunol.* 105: S547–S548.

58. Marshall GD and Agarwal SK (2000). Stress, immune regulation, and immunity: applications for asthma. *Allergy Asthma Proc.* 21: 241–246.

59. Kamfar HZ, Koshak EE, and Milaat WA (1999). Is there a role for automated eosinophil count in asthma severity assessment? *J. Asthma* 36: 153–158.

60. Ying S, Humbert M, Barkans J, Corrigan CJ, Pfister R, Menz G, Larché M, Robinson DS, Durham SR, and Kay AB (1997). Expression of IL-4 and IL-5 mRNA and protein product by CD4+ and CD8+ T cells, eosinophils, and mast cells in bronchial biopsies obtained from atopic and nonatopic (intrinsic) asthmatics. *J. Immunol.* 158: 3539–3544.

61. Barnes PJ (1994). Cytokines as mediators of chronic asthma. *Am. J. Respir. Crit. Care Med.* 150: S42–S49.

62. Marshall GD and Agarwal SK (2000). Stress, immune regulation, and immunity: applications for asthma. *Allergy Asthma Proc.* 21: 241–246.

63. Walker W, Bode E, Boer L, Hansel TT, Blaser K, and Virchow J (1992). Allergic and nonallergic asthmatics have distinct patterns of T cell activation and cytokine production in peripheral blood and bronchoalveolar lavage. *Am. Rev. Respir. Dis.* 146: 109–115.

64. Ackerman V, Marini M, Vittori E, Bellini A, Vassali G, and Mattoli S (1994). Detection of cytokines and their cell sources in bronchial biopsy specimens from asthmatic patients: relationship to atopic status, symptoms, and level of airway hyperresponsiveness. *Chest* 105: 687–696.

65. Robinson DS, Hamid Q, Ying S, Tsicopoulos A, Barkans J, Bentley AM, Corrigan C, Durham SR, and Kay AB (1992). Predominant Th2-like bronchoalveolar T-lymphocyte population in atopic asthma. *New Engl. J. Med.* 326: 298–304.

66. Corrigan CJ, Hamid Q, North J, Barkans J, Moqbel R, Durham S, Gemou-Engesæth V, and Kay AB (1995). Peripheral blood CD4 but not CD8 T-lymphocytes in patients with exacerbation of asthma transcribe and translate messenger RNA encoding cytokines which prolong eosinophil survival in the context of Th2-type pattern: effect of glucocorticoid therapy. *Am. J. Resp. Cell Mol. Biol.* 12: 567–578.

67. Hamid Q, Azzawi M, Ying S, Moqbel R, Wardlaw AJ, Corrigan CJ, Bradley B, Durham SR, Collins JV, and Jeffery PK (1991). Expression of mRNA for interleukin-5 in mucosal bronchial biopsies from asthma. *J. Clin. Invest.* 87: 1541–1546.

68. Ying S, Durham SR, Corrigan CJ, Hamid Q, and Kay AB (1995) Phenotype of cells expressing messenger RNA for Th2-type (interleukin-4 and interleukin-5) and Th1-type (interleukin-2 and interferon-gamma) cytokines in bronchoalveolar lavage and bronchial biopsies from atopic asthmatic and normal control subjects. *Am. J. Resp. Cell Mol. Biol.* 12: 477–487.

69. Kroegel C, Julius P, Matthys H, Virchow JC, Jr, and Luttmann W (1996). Endobronchial secretion of interleukin-13 following local allergen challenge in atopic asthma: relationship to interleukin-4 and eosinophil counts. *Eur. Respir. J.* 9: 899–904.

70. Kang D, Coe CL, Karaszewski J, and McCarthy DO (1998). Relationship of social support to stress responses and immune function in healthy and asthmatic adolescents. *Res. Nurs. Health* 21: 117–128.

71. Sandberg S, Paton JY, Ahola S, McCann D, McGuinness D, Hillary CR, and Oja H (2000). The role of acute and chronic stress in asthma attacks in children. *Lancet* 356: 982–987.

72. Smyth JM, Soefer MH, Hurewitz A, Kliment A, and Stone AA (1999). Daily psychosocial factors predict levels and diurnal cycles of asthma symptomatology and peak flow. *J. Behav. Med.* 22: 179–193.

73. Smith A and Nicholson K (2001). Psychological factors, respiratory viruses and exacerbation of asthma. *Psychoneuroendocrinology* 26: 411–420.

74. Smyth JM, Stone AA, Hurewitz A, and Kaell A (1999). Effects of writing about stressful experiences on symptom reduction in patients with asthma or rheumatoid arthritis: a randomized trial. *JAMA* 281: 1304–1309.

75. Kang D, Coe C, McCarthy DO, Jarjour NN, Kelly EA, Rodriguez RR, and Busse WW (1997). Cytokine profiles of stimulated blood lymphocytes in asthmatic and healthy adolescents across the school year. *J. Interferon Cytokine Res.* 17: 481–487.

76. Buske-Kirschbaum A, van Auer K, Krieger S, Weis S, Rauh W, and Hellhammer D (2003). Blunted cortisol responses to psychosocial stress in asthmatic children: a general feature of atopic disease? *Psychosom. Med.* 65: 806–810.

77. Buske-Kirschbaum A, Jobst S, Psych D, Wustmans A, Kirschbaum C, Rauh W, and Hellhammer D (1997). Attenuated free cortisol response to psychosocial stress in children with atopic dermatitis. *Psychosom. Med.* 59: 419–426.

78. Sandberg S, Paton JY, Ahola S, McCann DC, McGuinness D, and Hillary CR (2000). The role of acute and chronic stress in asthma attacks in children. *Lancet* 356: 982–987.
79. Chen E, Fisher EB, Bacharier LB, and Strunk RC (2003). Socioeconomic status, stress, and immune markers in adolescents with asthma. *Psychosom. Med.* 65: 984–992.
80. Wright RJ, Finn P, Contreras JP, Cohen S, Wright RO, et al. (2004). Chronic caregiver stress and IgE expression, allergen-induced proliferation, and cytokine profiles in a birth cohort predisposed to atopy. *J. Allergy Clin. Immunol.* 113: 1051–1057.
81. Laube BL, Curbow BA, Costello RW, and Fitzgerald ST (2002). A pilot study examining the relationship between stress and serum cortisol concentrations in women with asthma. *Resp. Med.* 96: 823–828.
82. Demir H, Kelëtimur F, Tunç M, Kirnap M, and Özügül Y (1999). Hypothalamus–pituitary–adrenal axis and growth hormone axis in patients with rheumatoid arthritis. *Scand. J. Rheumatol.* 28: 41–46.
83. DeAntonio SR, Blotta HM, Mamoni PL, Bertolo MB, Foss NT, Moreira AC, and Castro M (2002). Effects of dexamethasone on lymphocyte proliferation and cytokine production in RA. *J. Rheumatol.* 29:46–51.
84. Keefe FJ, Smith SJ, Buffington ALH, Gibson J, Studts JL, and Caldwell DS (2002). Recent advances and future directions in the biopsychosocial assessment and treatment of arthritis. *J. Consult. Clin. Psychol.* 70: 640–655.
85. Zautra AJ, Hamilton NA, Potter P, and Smith B (1999). Field research on the relationship between stress and disease activity in rheumatoid arthritis, in *Neuroendocrine Immune Basis of the Rheumatic Diseases*, Cutolo M et al., Eds., New York Academy of Sciences, New York, pp. 397–412.
86. Zautra AJ, Hoffman JM, Potter P, Matt KS, Yocum D, and Castro L (1997). Examination of changes in interpersonal stress as a factor in disease exacerbations among women with rheumatoid arthritis. *Ann. Behav. Med.* 19: 279–286.
87. Evers AWM, Kraaimaat FW, Geenen R, Jacobs JWG, and Bijlsma JWJ (2003). Stress vulnerability factors as long-term predictors of disease activity in early rheumatoid arthritis. *J. Psychosom. Res.* 55: 293–302.
88. Jacobs R, Pawlak CR, Mikeska E, Meyer-Olson D, Martin M, Heijnen CJ, et al. (2001). Systemic lupus erythematosus and rheumatoid arthritis patients differ from healthy controls in their cytokine pattern after stress exposure. *Rheumatology* 40: 868–875.
89. Catley D, Kaell AT, Kirschbaum C, and Stone AA (2000). A naturalistic evaluation of cortisol secretion in persons with fibromyalgia and rheumatoid arthritis. *Am. Coll. Rheumatol.* 13: 51–61.
90. Schlaghecke R, Kornley E, Wollenhaupt J, and Specker C (1992). Glucocorticoid receptors in rheumatoid arthritis. *Arthritis Rheumatol.* 35: 740–744.

4 Role of Cytokines in Depression

Ghanshyam N. Pandey and Yogesh Dwivedi

CONTENTS

ABSTRACT

A relationship between altered immune function and depression has been suggested. Changes in immune function are followed by the release of cytokines, which cause various behavioral changes, called "sickness behavior," which appears to be very similar to depression. That cytokines may play an important role in the pathophysiology of depression is inferred from many observations: (1) levels of several cytokines, both proinflammatory and anti-inflammatory, have been found to be increased in the serum of patients with depression; (2) administration of cytokines, for example, IFN-α, to cancer patients or to patients with hepatitis C, produced depression in some patients, as diagnosed by DSM criteria; and (3) indirect evidence suggesting a role of cytokines in depression is the observation that stress, which is a major risk factor for depressive illness, alters not only the immune system but also the levels of several cytokines. The mechanism by which cytokines cause depression is not clear at this time, but it is believed that they may do so by interacting and interfering with the serotonin (5HT), the noreprinephrine (NE) systems, and the hypothalamic–pituitary–adrenal (HPA) axis. All of these mechanisms have been implicated in the pathophysiology of depression. For example, some studies suggest that administration of cytokines shifts the metabolism of tryptophan, a precursor in the synthesis of 5HT, to the kynurenine pathway, thus decreasing its availability for the synthesis of 5HT. Cytokines have also been found to interfere with 5HT uptake. Although cytokines have been shown to affect both NE and dopaminergic function by stimulating the release of these amines, the interaction of cytokines with NE is less clear. Cytokine administration has also been found to alter the HPA system specifically in patients receiving IFN-α therapy. In this chapter, we review the evidence, as stated above, suggesting a role of cytokines in the pathophysiology of depression and the mechanisms by which the cytokines may be causing depressive-like symptoms in these patients.

The evidence for the involvement of cytokine in depressive illness is primarily based on observations that the levels of cytokines are altered in the plasma and/or serum of depressed patients. However, there are practically no studies examining the role of cytokines in the CNS of depressed patients. The presence of cytokines in the CNS has been demonstrated by many studies. It is therefore important that future studies also focus on determining the levels of cytokines, either proteins or mRNA, in the postmortem brain obtained from depressed patients or suicidal patients with depression.

INTRODUCTION

There are many interactions of the neural, immune, and neuroendocrine systems, and this has led the question whether the immune system may also be involved in some of the brain-related disorders, such as depression.[1–4] In recent years it has been suggested that depression — one of the major psychiatric disorders known to be related to changes in the neuroendocrine system — may also be related to or caused by changes in the immune system.

According to this hypothesis, peripheral activation of the immune system, followed by the release of pro-inflammatory cytokines, causes various behavioral changes that result in depression, possibly due to the effects of the cytokines on neurochemical and neuroendocrine changes that have been hypothesized to be associated with depression. Although several lines of evidence support an immune hypothesis of depression, the two major ones are derived from the observations that several cytokines have been found to be abnormal in patients with depression[5–31] and that administration of cytokines, particularly interferon (IFN)-α, to patients such as those suffering from hepatitis or cancer induces a syndrome similar to depression.[4,22–33]

Several observations suggest that altered immune states may be present in patients suffering from depressive disorders. For example, Kronfol et al.[34] measured lymphocyte responses to mitogens in patients diagnosed with melancholic depression, and these patients were found to have decreased lymphocyte responses as compared with controls. These findings of lower lymphocyte responsiveness have been replicated by several studies.[34–38] Several investigators also observed that natural killer cell activity was decreased in patients with depression as compared with normal controls.[34,37,39-41] The other immune function studied in depressed patients, neutrophil activity, was found to be lower among depressed patients than control subjects. These studies indicate that the immune process may be reduced in patients with depression (for review, see Weisse[20]).

Cytokines, generally known as chemical messengers between immune cells, comprise a heterogeneous group of messenger molecules produced by immunocompetent cells such as lymphocytes and macrophages. They regulate the immune responses and interact with the central nervous system (CNS).[1-3,20] Because of the suggested relationship between altered immune functions in depression and because cytokines are mediators of immune function and interact with the CNS, the role of cytokines in the pathophysiology of depressive illness has been investigated.

Cytokines are a diverse group of proteins that can be considered the hormones of the immune system. These small molecules are secreted by various cells and act as signals among cells to regulate immune responses to injury and infection. The responses of cytokines are mediated through cytokine receptors. Similar to other receptors, they respond to the presence of specific cytokines and thus produce certain physiological responses. Cytokine receptors are present in soluble forms as well as being associated with cell membranes.

Their classification and nomenclature are complex. The cytokines have been classified into families of interleukins (ILs), tumor necrosis factors (TNFs), interferons (IFNs), chemokines, hematoproteins, and colony stimulating factors. In terms of biological activity, the cytokines have been classified as pro-inflammatory or anti-inflammatory. The pro-inflammatory cytokines involved in the inflammatory process include IL-1, IL-6, IFN-α and TNF-α. The anti-inflammatory cytokines include IL-4, IL-10, and IL-13. Cytokines have been shown to regulate growth, differentiation, and functioning of many cell types. Several cytokines are present in more than one form, and they are termed as α, β, or γ.

One of the two major lines of evidence suggesting that cytokines play an important role in the pathophysiology of depression is derived from the observation that administration of some cytokines such as IFN-α to patients with hepatitis and cancer patients with melanoma produced a symptom known as "sickness behavior," which is very similar to depression.[21-32] The other major evidence for a role of cytokines in the pathophysiology of depression is derived from the observations that the levels of pro- and/or anti-inflammatory cytokines are altered in the serum[15-20] or the cerebrospinal fluid (CSF) of depressed patients.[42,43] Other indirect evidence suggesting a role for cytokines in depression is the observation that stress, which is a major risk factor for depressive illness, alters not only the immune system but also the levels of several cytokines.[44-49]

Cytokines have also been shown to interact with components of the neuroendocrine system such as the hypothalamic–pituitary–adrenal (HPA) axis[50,51] as well as some of the neurotransmitter systems such as serotonin (5HT)[29,52,53] and norepinephrine (NE).[54,55] Abnormalities of the HPA axis,[56] 5HT,[57] and NE[58] have been implicated in the pathophysiology of depression.

In this chapter we will briefly review these studies related to (1) cytokines in depressed patients, (2) cytokine-induced depression in patients, and (3) interaction of cytokines with the HPA axis, with the 5HT and NE systems, and with stress.

STUDIES OF CYTOKINES IN DEPRESSION

Because of the suggested relationship between abnormal immune function and depression and because of the observation that reductions in mitogen-stimulated lymphocyte proliferation and reduced natural killer cell activity have been observed in depressed patients,[5,39-41] the levels of cytokines that are the major mediators of immune function have been determined primarily in the sera of depressed patients and normal control subjects. A significant number of studies in this area have been conducted by Maes and colleagues.

In an initial study, Maes et al.[6] determined the levels of soluble IL-6 receptor (sIL-6R), sIL-2R, and transferrin receptors (TfRs) in the plasma of subjects with major depression. They found that the plasma concentrations of IL-6, sIL-6R, sIL-2R, and TfR were significantly higher in major depressed patients as compared with normal control subjects. They also found a positive correlation between the plasma concentrations of IL-6 and sIL-6R, IL-6 and sIL-2R, IL-6 and TfR, and between sIL-2R and TfR. In addition, they observed that chronic treatment with antidepressant drugs did not cause significant changes in these cytokines. In a subsequent study, Sluzewska et al.[9] studied the plasma concentrations of IL-6, sIL-6R, sIL-2R, TfR, C-reactive protein (CPR), and α_1-acid glycoprotein (AGP) in the plasma of 49 subjects with major depression during an acute phase of the illness and compared the concentrations with those of 15 normal control subjects. They found that the plasma concentrations of IL-6, sIL-6R, sIL-2R, TfR, CRP, and AGP were significantly higher in patients with major depression as compared with normal control subjects, thus replicating their previous finding in another group of patients in Poland.

Maes et al.[7] also determined the levels of the IL-1 receptor antagonist (IL-1-rA) in 68 depressed subjects and 22 normal control subjects and found that the serum levels of IL-1-rA were significantly higher in depressed patients as compared with normal healthy control subjects. They also found a significant and positive relationship between serum IL-1-rA and severity of illness in 44% of the depressed patients. However, they did not find any significant relationship between serum IL-1-rA concentration and HPA axis activity in these subjects (determined by measuring 24-hour urinary cortisol and post-dexamethasone cortisol levels).

In another study, Maes et al.[8] determined the levels of some cytokines in treatment-resistant depressed patients before and after subchronic treatment with antidepressants. They found that the serum levels of IL-6 and IL-1-rA were significantly higher in patients with major depression as compared with normal control subjects. They also found that subchronic treatment with antidepressants had no significant effect on the serum levels of IL-6, IL-1-rA, or IL-6R.

Several other groups have also studied the plasma levels of cytokines in depressed patients and normal control subjects. Berk et al.[10] found that levels of IL-6 when detected were significantly higher in depressed patients as compared with normal controls. They also found that they could not detect IL-6 in 51% of depressed patients and 58% of normal control subjects. However, whenever they could detect IL-6, they found that its levels were significantly increased in the sera of depressed patients as compared with normal control subjects.

In another study, the Maes group[12] found that the serum levels of IL-6, IL-10, and IL-1-rA were significantly higher in patients with major depression as compared with normal control subjects, although these were not statistically significant. The group also found no significant effect of antidepressant treatment on the serum levels of these cytokines.

Another group of investigators who have done significant work on the role of cytokines in depression are Anisman and Merali in Canada. In one study, they determined both the levels of cytokines and also the HPA axis functions in these patients.[11] They sought to determine whether the alterations in cytokines observed in depression are related to the neurovegetative symptom profile or to the chronicity of the illness. They found that the levels of IL-1β were increased in dysthymic patients and were highly correlated with age of onset and duration of illness. They also found that IL-2 production was decreased in all the depressed groups, which included the depression, atypical depression, dysthymic depression, and atypical dysthymic patients. Kim et al.[13] determined the plasma levels of IL-12 in 102 psychiatric patients (34 with major depression, 25 bipolar patients, and 43 schizophrenia patients) and 85 normal control. They found that the levels of IL-12 in patients with major depression were significantly higher than levels of the control group, whereas no differences were found in the bipolar or schizophrenia groups as compared with normal control subjects. Eight weeks of treatment caused significant decreases in the levels of IL-12 in these patients.

TNF-α has important effects on behavioral, endocrine, and immune parameters in rats[44,59,60] and levels of TNF-α have also been determined in the sera of depressed patients. In a recent study, Tuglu et al.[14] determined the levels of TNF-α and CRP in the sera of 26 patients with major depressive disorders (MDDs) and 17 normal control subjects. They found that the levels of TNF-α were significantly higher in MDD patients compared to normal control subjects. When these patients were treated with antidepressants, their levels of TNF-α decreased and were almost similar to levels observed in normal control subjects. These results provide strong evidence that not only are the levels of the cytokine TNF-α decreased in depressed patients but also that treatment with antidepressants normalizes the levels of TNF-α.

Plasma levels of cytokines have also been determined in late-life depression and elderly depressed patients. Thomas et al.[18] found that the levels of plasma IL-1β were significantly higher in elderly depressed patients when compared with normal control subjects, and that the higher levels correlated with current depression severity. Trzonkowski et al.[61] studied pro-inflammatory cytokines in depressed elderly subjects and found elevated levels of TNF-α, IL-6, and cortisol, decreases in the levels of ACTH, and insufficient production of IL-10 in depressed patients as compared with normal control subjects.

Although most of these studies were performed in the plasma of depressed patients, Carpenter et al.[43] determined the levels of cytokines in the CSF of depressed patients and elderly control subjects and the levels of IL-6 in the CSF of 18 subjects with major depression and 26 normal control subjects, but did not find any significant differences.

In summary, these studies strongly suggest that in general, the levels of several cytokines including IL-2, IL-6, and IL-12 and of their soluble receptors were increased in the plasma of depressed patients as compared with normal control subjects.

Another observation was that mitogen-elicited production of the pro-inflammatory cytokines IL-1β, IL-6, and TNF-α was increased in the sera of depressed patients.

The other question was whether the increased levels of cytokines observed in depressed patients were normalized by treatment with antidepressants. As described earlier, several studies determined the levels of cytokines before and after treatment with antidepressant drugs. While it was found that levels of IL-1β and IL-6 normalized after treatment with antidepressant medication,[62,63] treatment with antidepressants did not cause changes in the increased production of soluble IL-2 receptors, IL-6, or IL-6 receptors in major depression.[6] It has also been reported that levels of IL-6, the IL-10 anti-inflammatory cytokine, and IL-1-rA were also moderately increased in depressed patients as compared with normal controls. However, the increased levels of these cytokines were not affected by treatment with antidepressants.

Although studies of cytokines are limited, most suggest increases in the levels of cytokines in the sera of depressed patients. One study that compared cytokines in the CSF of depressed patients and normal control subjects did not find any differences between them, and hence it is unclear whether brain levels of the cytokines are different in depressed patients and normal control subjects. Studies should be carried out in postmortem brains from depressed or depressed suicide subjects to further examine and clarify the role of cytokines in depression.

CYTOKINE-INDUCED DEPRESSION

Cytokine therapy is used in the treatment of several disorders. Cytokines have been found effective in treating various forms of cancer such as renal cell cancer, chronic myelogenous leukemia, several other malignancies, viral infections (e.g., hepatitis C virus), multiple sclerosis, and several skin conditions.[22] The cytokines used for treatment for these purposes include IFN-α, IFN-β and IL-2.[22] The other evidence that cytokines are involved in the pathophysiology of depression is derived from studies of the effects of interferons and other cytokines in inducing depression in these patients.

The administration of cytokines such as IFN-α causes the production of pro-inflammatory cytokines such as IFN-γ, IL-6, and TNF-α. IFN-α also augments the cytotoxic activities of natural killer cells by enhancing IL-2-dependent growth, cytokine production, and antibody-dependent cellular toxicity.[36] Administration of IFN-α and other cytokines also causes changes in serotonergic[29,52,53] and adrenergic[54,55] mechanisms that have been considered as the means by which cytokine administration causes depression in these patients. These mechanisms will be described in detail in the following pages. Several lines of evidence suggest that interferon administration may cause depression-like symptoms such as fatigue, increased sleepiness, difficulty sleeping, irritability, loss of appetite, weight loss, and low mood.[21,25,27] Several of these symptoms together have been termed "sickness behavior." The other psychiatric symptoms produced by IFN-α administration are cognitive changes that involve verbal memory, cognitive speed, and executive function.[64,65]

Because of these effects of interferon, several investigators have systematically examined whether the administration of interferon and IFN-α caused depression in these patients and whether treatment with antidepressants would be beneficial. Systematic studies of the development of depression in patients undergoing IFN-α therapy suggest that 30% to 40% of patients receiving this therapy develop some form of depression as diagnosed by DSM-III-R and assessed by either the Hamilton Depression Rating Scale (HAM-D) or the Montgomery Asberg Depression Rating Scale (MADRS) and DSM-IV criteria (for review, see Loftis and Hauser[22]). For example, Otsubo et al.[66] found that 37% of patients who were treated with IFN-α developed major depressive episodes at least once during TNF-α therapy. Bonaccorso et al.[28–30] found that 40% of patients who received IFN-α therapy developed major depressive disorders as diagnosed by DSM-IV criteria. The symptoms they developed included expressed and unexpressed sadness, irritability, insomnia, loss of appetite, and asthenia. In cancer patients treated with IFN-α, several studies found that these subjects developed some form of depression. Full-blown depressive symptoms were reported in up to 36% of patients on treatment with IFN-α.[31] Because of the reported relationship between IFN-α therapy and the development of depression, several studies systematically and specifically examined the rates of depressive and cognitive symptoms during IFN-α therapy using standard instruments for measuring these affective and cognitive changes. Almost all studies found increases in depressive symptoms during IFN-α therapy.[23,24,26,28–30,32]

IL-2 therapy has also been used to treat cancer patients. The side effects of IL-2 therapy include loss of energy, fatigue, and decreased food intake. Although few studies examine the effects of IL-2 therapy on psychiatric and/or cognitive aspects, Denicoff et al.[67] studied 44 patients with metastatic cancer who had been treated with IL-2 alone or with IL-2 followed by treatment with other lymphokine-activated killer cells. Of the 44 patients, 15 showed severe behavioral changes such as agitation and combative behavior.

Antidepressant Treatment of IFN-α-induced Depression

Because treatment with IFN-α causes a set of symptoms known as "sickness behavior," several of which are similar to those of depression, a systematic effort has been made to examine whether in fact these symptoms meet the diagnostic criteria for depressive illness and whether treatment with antidepressant drugs produces beneficial effects in these patients. Capuron et al.[68] determined the association between immune activation and depressive symptoms in cancer patients on IL-2 therapy.

Musselman and co-investigators[69] examined the effects of antidepressant treatment, specifically paroxetine, on the prevention of depressive symptoms induced by IFN-α treatment. They found that 12 weeks of interferon treatment of 40 patients with malignant melanoma caused some symptoms consistent with the diagnosis of major depression and that in patients pretreated with paroxetine, there appeared to be a decrease in depression induced by IFN-α.[70] Thirty-six patients with malignant melanoma were treated in a double-blind fashion, either with placebo or paroxetine.

Several other studies have also shown that pretreatment with antidepressant drugs can reduce the risk for the development of depression in cancer patients who undergo IFN-α therapy.[69–71] Capuron et al.[70] administered IFN-α therapy to a group of malignant melanoma patients assigned to receive either paroxetine or placebo in a double-blind design. They found that several symptoms of depression such as anxiety, cognitive dysfunction, and pain were more responsive to pretreatment with paroxetine than placebo treatment. However, symptoms of fatigue and anorexia were less responsive to pretreatment with paroxetine. In a similar study, Musselman, et al.[69] found that pre-treatment with paroxetine was beneficial in reducing depressive symptoms in a group of malignant melanoma patients undergoing IFN-α therapy. This kind of approach also provided evidence that cytokine-induced depression is responsive to pretreatment with antidepressant drugs.

IFN-α-INDUCED CHANGES IN CYTOKINE LEVELS IN PATIENTS UNDERGOING IFN-α THERAPY

Because IFN-α treatment causes symptoms of depression in cancer patients and because alterations in cytokine levels have been related to depression, some investigators attempted to determine whether IFN-α therapy will also cause changes in the levels of cytokines. Capuron et al.[68] determined the development of depressive symptoms and the levels of several cytokines in 33 cancer patients undergoing cytokine therapy who were treated with either IL-2 alone or in association with IFN-α. They found that patients treated with IL-2 or IL-2 plus IFN-α displayed depressive symptoms as determined by MADRS, but they also found increased levels of cytokines IL-6, sIL-2R, and IL-10 in these patients.[68]

In summary, the studies of the behavioral and biochemical effects of cytokine therapy in cancer patients indicate it causes behavioral symptoms in some patients which, when assessed by rating and diagnostic instruments, appear to be depression. The pretreatment of these patients with antidepressants before the initiation of cytokine therapy reduces the risk for developing depression. Another finding is that IFN-α treatment causes increases in levels of some cytokines. These observations thus raise a question as to the mechanism by which IFN-α therapy causes the development of depression in these patients.

MECHANISM OF CYTOKINE-INDUCED DEPRESSION

The original amine hypothesis of depressive illness states that there is abnormal function of monoamines such as 5HT and NE in depression. Several studies over the years have provided support for this hypothesis. Another consistent observation in depressive illness is a dysregulation of the HPA axis. It is therefore not surprising that the mechanism by which cytokines cause symptoms of depression in patients undergoing cytokine therapy has been related to their effects on 5HT, NE, and the HPA axis. In the next section we discuss the evidence and the mechanisms by which cytokines alter the 5HT, NE, and the HPA axis systems, which are also interlinked.

INTERACTIONS OF CYTOKINES WITH MONOAMINE SYSTEMS AND HPA

CYTOKINES AND THE 5HT SYSTEM

Effects of Cytokines on Indolamine 2,3-Dioxygenase (IDO)

In its simplest form, according to the serotonin hypothesis of depression, depression may be related either to a decreased availability of 5HT, decreased release or reuptake, alterations in the pre- and postsynaptic receptors for 5HT, or to the 5HT receptor-linked signaling system. Serotonin is synthesized in the brain by conversion of its precursor, an amino acid tryptophan, by tryptophan-hydroxylase and by decarboxylation to 5HT. Tryptophan is largely available in the brain, and the rate-limiting factor in the synthesis of 5HT is tryptophan-hydroxylase.

Another pathway of tryptophan metabolism is related to its metabolism to kynurenine, which is mediated by the IDO enzyme. Kynurenine is further metabolized to several other products including 3-hydroxy-kynurenine and anthranilic acid. Treatment with cytokines may affect the serotonergic system in several ways. First, cytokines may induce a depletion of tryptophan by reducing food intake.[72]

The other major hypothesis of the effect of cytokines on the serotonergic system is related to their enhancement of the activity of IDO, the first enzyme in the kynurenine pathway. As stated above, IDO converts tryptophan to kynurenine. In addition to IFN-α, several other cytokines induce the activity of IDO. Because IFN-α therapy also causes an increase in other cytokines, it is quite possible that induction of the IDO enzyme may be shunting the metabolism of tryptophan more to the kynurenine pathway as opposed to the tryptophan hydroxylase or 5HT pathway. Thus, as a result of the induction of IDO, the synthesis of 5HT, because of the lack of availability of tryptophan, is decreased, and the decrease in 5HT levels and its function may be related to the development of depressive symptoms.[73,74]

That, in fact, cytokine therapy may be causing this shift of tryptophan metabolism toward the kynurenine pathway has been recently demonstrated by the studies of Capuron et al.[75] They treated 26 patients with malignant melanoma with IFN-α and determined the levels of kynurenine, tryptophan, and neopterin in the plasma of these patients. They found that antidepressant-free patients who developed major depression exhibited significantly greater increases in kynurenine and neopterin concentrations and decreases in tryptophan concentration when compared with non-depressed antidepressant-free subjects. In the depressed patients, they also found that tryptophan correlated negatively with depressive, anxious, and cognitive symptoms. These studies thus provide further support to the hypothesis that cytokine treatment shifts the metabolism of tryptophan towards the kynurenine pathway, thus decreasing the biosynthesis of 5HT in the brain of these patients.

Although the major hypothesis of the interaction of cytokines with 5HT relates to its effect on stimulating the IDO enzyme and shunting the metabolism of tryptophan toward the kynurenine pathway, thus decreasing the availability of tryptophan for 5HT biosynthesis, some theories suggest that the effects of cytokines on the serotonergic pathway and depression may be related to both the decreased synthesis of 5HT and the increased production of kynurenine metabolites. These metabolites have been shown to be toxic, and the resultant side effects may also be related to the depression-like symptomatology.[53,76,77]

Other Effects of Cytokines on the 5HT System

In addition to their stimulation of the IDO enzyme, cytokines exert several other effects on the serotonergic system. IL-1, IFN-α, IFN-γ, and TNF-α have been shown to up-regulate the 5HT transporter, thus reducing 5HT concentration in the synapse.[52,78] On the other hand, the IL-4 anti-inflammatory cytokine has been shown to induce a reduction of 5HT uptake.

Cytokines and the NE System

Cytokines have been shown to affect both noradrenergic and dopaminergic functions. For example, IL-1 has been shown to stimulate the release of catecholamines in the periphery and in the CNS. IL-2 has also been shown to stimulate dopaminergic neurotransmission. IL-1 has also been shown to stimulate hypothalamic and pre-optic noradrenergic neurotransmission in rats.[54] Zalcman et al.[55] observed that IL-1-induced increases in the MHPG:NE ratio in the prefrontal cortex (PFC) and hippocampus in mice. Although TNF-α has been shown to cause changes in the adrenergic system, the clinical evidence to support the interaction of cytokines with NE is scarce.

Cytokines and the HPA Axis

Abnormality in the HPA axis has been implicated in the pathophysiology of depression. Abnormal levels of cortisol and non-suppression to dexamethasone administration have been reported widely in patients with depressive illness. Because cytokines can also affect the HPA axis, it is not surprising that the mechanism of cytokine-induced depression in cancer patients has been related to their effects on the HPA axis. Capuron et al.[51] determined HPA axis responsivity in patients undergoing cytokine therapy. They found that ACTH and cortisol responses (but not IL-6 responses) to the initial administration of IFN-α were significantly greater in seven patients who subsequently developed symptoms of major depression as compared with those who did not develop depression. Because of the small number of subjects, it is unclear whether the depression caused by IFN-α in the cancer patients was related to a disturbance in the HPA axis.

FUNCTIONAL ROLES OF IL-2, IL-6, TNF-α, AND IFN IN DEPRESSIVE ILLNESS

As noted earlier, some of the cytokines that have been found to be increased either in sera or CSF of depressed patients include the IL-2, IL-6, sIL-6R, and TNF-α cytokines. Among these, the pro-inflammatory IL-6 and TNF-α cytokines may not only have crucial functions in the CNS but may also be of particular importance in the pathophysiology of depression.

Most of the work carried out by Maes and colleagues suggests that IL-6 and sIL-6-R are increased in patients suffering from major depressive disorders. There appears to be a parallel increase of IL-6 and sIL-6-R in these patients. Because IL-6 and sIL-6-R form a complex and this complex enhances the biological activity of IL-6,[6] and because of the correlation between increased IL-6 levels and cortisol in the plasma of these depressed patients, the suggestion is that IL-6 may play a crucial role in depressive disorders. There also appears to be a correlation between IL-6 and tryptophan levels in depressed patients. The synthesis of 5HT in the CNS is partly dependent on the availability of tryptophan in the blood; this suggests that IL-6 may be crucial in depressive disorders.

The other pro-inflammatory cytokine that may play a crucial role in both the CNS and also in the pathophysiology of depression is TNF-α. One of the most consistent observations in studies of the neurobiology of depressive disorders is the observation of structural abnormalities in the brains of depressed patients.[79-87] These structural abnormalities include decreased hippocampal volume,[88] changes in the PFC, and decreased density of neurons in the PFC and in the anterior cingular cortex.[79-81] Decreases in non-pyramidal neurons have also been found in the post-mortem brains of suicide victims.[82]

The structural abnormalities observed in depressed patients have been related, at least in part, to altered apoptotic processes or to changes in the levels of apoptotic proteins. TNF-α and some of the other cytokines such as IL-1β play an important role in the apoptotic pathways. Two of the three pathways of apoptosis include the death receptor or the extrinsic pathway and the inflammatory or caspase-1-mediated pathway.[89] The extrinsic pathway involves the binding of the death receptor to a specific ligand, and one of these ligands is TNF-α.[90,91] The third pathway, also known as the inflammatory pathway, involves the formation of inflamasomes and consists of caspase-1, caspase-5, and the APAF-1 protein that then converts the pro-IL-1β inflammatory cytokine into its biologically activated form, IL-1β. The TNF-α and IL-1β cytokines are thus involved in the process of apoptosis, and their involvement in the pathophysiology of depressive illness has been suggested. The other evidence that TNF-α may be involved in depression is its playing of an important role in the cognitive impairment and psychic disturbances occurring during HIV infection. Increased TNF-α has also been found in the CSF of HIV patients, and expression of TNF-α mRNA is increased in the brains of AIDS patients. It has been shown recently that TNF-α is not only present in the brain, but may play an important role in synaptic plasticity and modulating responses to neuronal injury.[92]

SUMMARY AND FUTURE STUDIES

In this chapter, we have reviewed the role of cytokines in depression. Several lines of evidence implicate cytokines in the pathophysiology of depression. The evidence appears quite strong. For example, several studies indicate that cytokine therapy of cancer or hepatitis patients causes a syndrome termed "sickness behavior" that is very similar to depression, and that pretreatment with antidepressants in most cases prevents the appearance of these depressive-like symptoms in patients who are being treated with IFN-α.

There appears to be a relationship between cytokine-induced depression and some of the serotonergic and neuroendocrine markers associated with depressive illness. For example, administration of cytokines appears to alter the metabolism of tryptophan by inducing the IDO enzyme and shifting the metabolism of tryptophan to the kynurenine pathway, thus reducing the availability of tryptophan for the biosynthesis of 5HT and possibly producing toxic substances like kynurenine metabolites. Cytokines also appear to interact with the HPA axis and other neurotransmitter systems, i.e., NE, associated with depressive illness. In addition, the levels of cytokines, specifically pro-inflammatory cytokines, have been found to be increased in the sera and, in some cases, in the CSF of depressed patients.

There is still no strong evidence, but some studies suggest that pretreatment with antidepressants prevents the development of depressive symptoms in patients receiving

IFN-α therapy. The failure of antidepressant treatment to normalize cytokine levels in depressed patients may suggest that the alteration of these cytokines in depression is a trait rather than a state marker. Taken together, the evidence strongly points to the involvement of cytokines in depressive illness. Most studies of cytokines in IFN-α-induced depressive illness or in depressed patients have been performed on sera. The functional role of cytokines in the CNS and the changes in the cytokines in the central nervous systems of depressed patients have not been studied. It is therefore not clear whether depressive illness is associated with changes in the levels of cytokines or their receptors in the brain.

Cytokines can be synthesized and are present in the brain.[93] IL-1 was localized in human hypothalamus.[94] Receptors for IL-1 and TNF-α have been shown to be localized with high densities in hippocampus and hypothalamus of the rodent brain.[95] Messenger RNA for IL-1 receptor was found in the mouse brain[96] and IL-1-rA in the rat brain.[97] It has been shown that TNF-α is present in the brain and may play an important role in synaptic plasticity and modulating response to neuronal injury.[92] It is therefore important to study cytokines in the human brain.

Future studies must be directed to measuring the levels of cytokines and their receptors in postmortem brain samples from patients with depression or suicide victims. In recent years, postmortem brain samples from depressed patients and from suicide victims with depression have been studied with regard to the neurotransmitter receptors and the signaling pathways. Studies of cytokines in postmortem brain samples are therefore important to further elucidate the role of cytokines in the pathophysiology of depression.

REFERENCES

1. Müller, N. and Ackenheil, M., Psychoneuroimmunology and the cytokine action in the CNS: implications for psychiatric disorders, *Prog. Neuropsychopharmacol. Biol. Psychiatr.*, 22, 1, 1998.
2. Hopkins, S.J. and Rothwell, N.J., Cytokines and the nervous system. I: expression and recognition, *Trends Neurosci.*, 18, 83, 1995.
3. Kronfol, Z. and Remick, D.G., Cytokines and the brain: implications of clinical psychiatry, *Am. J. Psychiatr.*, 157, 683, 2000.
4. Anisman, H., Kokkinidis, L., and Merali, Z., Further evidence for the depressive effects of cytokines: anhedonia and neurochemical changes, *Brain. Behav. Immunol.*, 16, 544, 2002.
5. Maes, M., Evidence for an immune response in major depression: a review and hypothesis, *Prog. Neuropsychopharmacol. Biol. Psychiatr.*, 19, 11, 1995.
6. Maes, M. et al., Increased plasma concentrations of interleukin-6, soluble interleukin-6, soluble interleukin-2 and transferrin receptor in major depression, *J. Affect. Disord.*, 34, 301, 1995.
7. Maes, M. et al., Increased serum interleukin-1 receptor antagonist concentrations in major depression, *J. Affect. Disord.*, 36, 29, 1995.
8. Maes, M. et al., Increased serum IL-6 and IL-1 receptor antagonist concentrations in major depression and treatment resistant depression, *Cytokine*, 9, 853, 1997.
9. Sluzewska, A. et al., Indicators of immune activation in major depression, *Psychiatr. Res.*, 64, 161, 1996.

10. Berk, M. et al., Acute phase proteins in major depression, *J. Psychosom. Res.*, 43, 529, 1997.
11. Anisman, H. et al., Endocrine and cytokine correlates of major depression and dysthymia with typical or atypical features, *Mol. Psychiatr.*, 4, 182, 1999.
12. Kubera, M. et al., Plasma levels of interleukin-6, interleukin-10, and interleukin-1 receptor antagonist in depression: comparison between the acute state and after remission, *Pol. J. Pharmacol.*, 52, 237, 2000.
13. Kim, Y-K. et al., The plasma levels of interleukin-12 in schizophrenia, major depression, and bipolar mania: effects of psychotropic drugs, *Mol. Psychiatr.*, 7, 1107, 2002.
14. Tuglu, C. et al., Increased serum tumore necrosis factor-α levels and treatment response in major depressive disorder, *Psychopharmacology*, 170, 429, 2003.
15. Musselman, D.L. et al., Higher than normal plasma interleukin-6 concentrations in cancer patients with depression: preliminary findings, *Am. J. Psychiatr.*, 158, 1252, 2001.
16. Nassberger, L. and Traskman-Bendz, L., Increased soluble interleukin-2 receptor concentrations in suicide attempters, *Acta Psychiatr. Scand.*, 88, 48, 1993.
17. Song, C., Dinan, T., and Leonard, B.E., Changes in immunoglobulin, complement and acute phase protein levels in depressed patients and normal controls, *J. Affect. Disord.*, 30, 283, 1994.
18. Thomas, A.J. et al., Increase in interleukin-1-β in late life depression, *Am. J. Psychiatr.*, 162, 175, 2005.
19. O'Brien, S.M., Scott, L.V., and Dinan, T.G., Cytokines: abnormalities in major depression and implications for pharmacological treatment, *Human Psychopharmacol. Clin. Exp.*, 19, 397, 2004.
20. Weisse, C.S., Depression and immunocompetence: a review of the literature, *Psychol. Bull.*, 111, 475, 1992.
21. Yirmiya, R. et al., Cytokines, "depression due to a general medical condition," and antidepressant drugs, *Adv. Exp. Med. Biol.*, 461, 283, 1999.
22. Loftis, J.M. and Hauser, P., The phenomenology and treatment of interferon-induced depression, *J. Affect. Disord.*, 82, 175, 2004.
23. Pavol, M.A. et al., Pattern of neurobehavioral deficits associated with interferon alfa therapy for leukemia, *Neurology*, 45, 947, 1995.
24. Pariante, C.M. et al., Treatment with interferon-alpha in patients with chronic hepatitis and mood or anxiety disorders, *Lancet*, 354, 131, 1999.
25. Renault, P.F. et al., Psychiatric complications of long-term interferon alfa therapy, *Arch. Intern. Med.*, 147, 1577, 1987.
26. Hunt, C.M. et al., Effect of interferon-alpha treatment of chronic hepatitis C on health-related quality of life, *Dig. Dis. Sci.*, 42, 2482, 1997.
27. Valentine, A.D. et al., Mood and cognitive side effects of interferon-alpha therapy, *Semin. Oncol.*, 25, 39, 1998.
28. Bonaccorso, S. et al., Immunotherapy with interferon-α in patients affected by chronic hepatitis C induces an intercorrelated stimulation of the cytokine network and an increase in depressive and anxiety symptoms, *Psychiatr. Res.*, 105, 45, 2001.
29. Bonaccorso, S. et al., Increased depressive ratings in patients with hepatitis C receiving interferon-α-based immunotherapy are related to interferon-α-induced changes in the serotonergic system, *J. Clin. Psychopharmacol.*, 22, 86, 2002.
30. Bonaccorso, S. Depression induced by treatment with interferon-α in patients affected by hepatitis C virus, *J. Affect. Disord.*, 72, 237, 2002.
31. Collier, J. and Chapman, R., Combination therapy with interferon-alpha and ribavirin for hepatitis C: practical treatment issues, *BioDrugs*, 15, 225, 2001.

32. Malaguarnera, M. et al., Interferon alpha-induced depression in chronic hepatitis C patients: comparison between different types of interferon alpha, *Neuropsychobiology*, 37, 93, 1998.

33. Anisman, H. and Merali, Z., Anhedonic and anxiogenic effects of cytokine exposure, *Adv. Exp. Med. Biol.*, 461, 199, 1999.

34. Kronfol, Z. et al., Impaired lymphocyte function in depressive illness, *Life Sci.*, 33, 241, 1983.

35. Calabrese, J.R. et al., Depression, immunocompetence, and prostaglandins of the E series, *Psychiatr. Res.*, 17, 41, 1986.

36. Herberman, R.B., Effect of alpha-interferons on immune function, *Semin. Oncol.*, 24, S9, 1997.

37. Irwin, M. and Gillin, J.C., Impaired natural killer cell activity among depressed patients, *Psychiatr. Res.*, 20, 181, 1987.

38. Maes, M. et al., Depression-related disturbances in mitogen-induced lymphocyte responses and interleukin-1β and soluble interleukin-2 receptor production, *Acta Psychiatr. Scand.*, 84, 379, 1991.

39. Herbert, T.B. and Cohen, S., Depression and immunity: a meta-analytic review, *Psychol. Bull.*, 113, 472, 1993.

40. Irwin, M., Immune correlates of depression, *Adv. Exp. Med. Biol.*, 461, 1, 1999.

41. Maes, M., Major depression and activation of the inflammatory response system, *Adv. Exp. Med. Biol.*, 461, 25, 1999.

42. Levin, J. et al., Cerebrospinal cytokine levels in patients with acute depression, *Neuropsychobiology*, 40, 171, 1999.

43. Carpenter, L.L. et al., Cerebrospinal fluid interleukin (IL)-6 in unipolar major depression, *J. Affect. Disord.*, 79, 285, 2004.

44. Minami, M. et al., Immobilization stress induces interleukin-1b mRNA in rat hypothalamus, *Neurosci. Lett.*, 123, 254, 1991.

45. Merali, Z., Lacosta, S., and Anisman, H., Effect of interleukin-1-β and mild stress on alterations of norepinephrine, dopamine and serotonin neurotransmission: a regional microdialysis study, *Brain Res.*, 761, 225, 1997.

46. Connor, T.J. and Leonard, B.E., Depression, stress and immunological activation: the role of cytokines in depressive disorders, *Life Sci.*, 62, 583, 1998.

47. Leonard, B.E. and Song, C., Stress, depression, and the role of cytokines, *Adv. Exp. Med. Biol.*, 461, 251, 1999.

48. Tilders, F.J.H. and Schmidt, E.D., Cross sensitization between immune and nonimmune stressors, *Adv. Exp. Med. Biol.*, 461, 179, 1999.

49. Anisman, H. and Merali, Z., Cytokines, stress, and depressive illness, *Brain. Behav. Immunol.*, 16, 513, 2002.

50. Maes, M. et al., Relationships between interleukin-6 activity, acute phase proteins and function of the hypothalamic–pituitary–adrenal axis in severe depression, *Psychiatr. Res.*, 49, 11, 1993.

51. Capuron, L. et al., Association of exaggerated HPA axis response to the initial injection of interferon-alpha with development of depression during interferon-alpha therapy, *Am. J. Psychiatr.*, 160, 1342, 2003.

52. Morikawa, O. et al., Effects of interferon-alpha, interferon-gamma and cAMP on the transcriptional regulation of the serotonin transporter, *Eur. J. Pharmacol.*, 349, 317, 1998.

53. Myint, A.M. and Kim, Y.K., Cytokine-serotonin interaction through IDO: a neurodegeneration hypothesis of depression, *Med. Hypoth.*, 61, 519, 2003.

54. Kabiersch, A. et al., Interleukin-1 induces changes in norepinephrine metabolism in the rat brain, *Brain Behav. Immunol.*, 2, 267, 1988.

55. Zalcman, S. et al., Cytokine-specific central monoamine alterations induced by inter-leukin-1, -2 and -6, *Brain Res.*, 643, 40, 1994.
56. Carrol, B.J., The dexamethasone suppression test for melancholia, *Br. J. Psychiatr.*, 140, 292, 1982.
57. Maes, M. and Meltzer, H.Y., The serotonin hypothesis of major depression, in *Psychopharmacology: The Fourth Generation of Progress*, Bloom, F.E. and Kupfer, D.J., Eds., Raven Press, Raven Press, New York, 1995, p. 933.
58. Schatzberger, A.F. and Schildkraut, J.J., Recent studies on norepinephrine systems in mood disorders, in *Psychopharmacology: The Fourth Generation of Progress*, Bloom, F.E. and Kupfer, D.J., Eds., Raven Press, New York, 1995, p. 911.
59. Connor, T.J. et al., An assessment of the effects of central interleukin-1-beta, -2, -6, and tumor necrosis factor-alpha administration on some behavioural, neurochemical, endocrine and immune parameters in the rat, *Neuroscience*, 84, 923, 1998.
60. Yirmiya, R., Endotoxin produces a depressive-like episode in rats, *Brain Res.*, 711, 163, 1996.
61. Trzonkowski, P. et al., Immune consequences of the spontaneous pro-inflammatory status in depressed elderly patients, *Brain Behav. Immunol.*, 18, 135, 2004.
62. Frommberger, U.H. et al., Interleukin-6 (IL-6) plasma levels in depression and schizo-phrenia: comparison between the acute state and after remission, *Eur. Arch. Psychiatr. Clin. Neurosci.*, 247, 228, 1997.
63. Sluzewska, A. et al., Interleukin-6 serum levels in depressed patients before and after treatment with fluoxetine, *Ann. NY Acad. Sci.*, 762, 474, 1995.
64. Meyers, C.A. and Abbruzzese, J.L., Cognitive functioning in cancer patients: effect of previous treatment, *Neurology*, 42, 434, 1992.
65. Meyers, C.A., Mood and cognitive disorders in cancer patients receiving cytokine therapy, *Adv. Exp. Med. Biol.*, 461, 75, 1999.
66. Otsubo, T., et al., Depression during interferon therapy in chronic hepatitis C patients: a prospective study, *Seish. Shink. Zasshi*, 99, 101, 1997.
67. Denicoff, K.D. et al., The neuropsychiatric effects of treatment with interleukin-2 and lymphokine-activated killer cells, *Ann. Intern. Med.*, 107, 293, 1987.
68. Capuron, L. et al., Association between immune activation and early depressive symptoms in cancer patients treated with interleukin-2-based therapy, *Psychoendo-crinology*, 26, 797, 2001.
69. Musselman, D.L. et al., Paroxetine for the prevention of depression induced by high-dose interferon alfa, *New Engl. J. Med.*, 344, 961, 2001.
70. Capuron, L. et al., Neurobehavioral effects of interferon-alpha in cancer patients: phenomenology and paroxetine responsiveness of symptom dimensions, *Neuropsy-chopharmacology*, 26, 643, 2002.
71. Maddock, C., et al., Psychopharmacological treatment of depression, anxiety, irrita-bility and insomnia in patients receiving interferon-α: a prospective case series and a discussion of biological mechanism, *Psychopharmacology*, 18, 41, 2004.
72. Plata-Salaman, C.R., Cytokine-induced anorexia. Behavioral, cellular, and molecular mechanisms, *Ann. NY Acad. Sci.*, 856, 160, 1998.
73. Maes, M., et al., Relationships between lower plasma L-tryptophan levels and immune-inflammatory variables in depression, *Psychiatr. Res.*, 49, 151, 1993.
74. Maes, M., et al., Increased neopterin and interferon-gamma secretion and lower availability of L-tryptophan in major depression: further evidence for an immune response, *Psychiatr. Res.*, 54, 143, 1994.
75. Capuron, L. et al., Interferon-alpha-induced changes in tryptophan metabolism. rela-tionship to depression and paroxetine treatment, *Biol. Psychiatr.*, 54, 906, 2003.

76. Meyers, C.A. et al., Reversible neurotoxicity of interleukin-2 and tumor necrosis factor: correlation of SPECT with neuropsychological testing, *J. Neuropsychiatr. Clin. Neurosci.*, 6, 285, 1994.

77. Wichers, M.C. and Maes, M., The role of indoleamine 2,3-dioxygenase (IDO) in the pathophysiology of interferon-α-induced depression, *J. Psychiatr. Neurosci.*, 29, 11, 2004.

78. Wichers, M. and Maes, M., The psychoneuroimmuno-pathophysiology of cytokine-induced depression in humans, *Int. J. Neuropsychopharmacol.*, 5, 375, 2002.

79. Rajkowska, G., et al., Morphometric evidence for neuronal and glial prefrontal cell pathology in major depression, *Biol. Psychiatr.*, 45, 1085, 1999.

80. Rajkowska, G., Postmortem studies in mood disorders indicate altered numbers of neurons and glial cells, *Biol. Psychiatr.*, 48, 766, 2000.

81. Cotter, D. et al., Reduced neuronal size and glial cell density in area 9 of the dorsolateral prefrontal cortex in subjects with major depressive disorder, *Cereb. Cortex*, 12, 386, 2002.

82. Benes, F.M. et al., A reduction of nonpyramidal cells in sector CA2 of schizophrenics and manic depressives, *Biol. Psychiatr.*, 44, 88, 1998.

83. Benes, F.M., Vincent, S.L., and Todtenkopf, M., The density of pyramidal and non-pyramidal neurons in anterior cingulate cortex of schizophrenic and bipolar subjects, *Biol. Psychiatr.*, 50, 395, 2001.

84. Rossi, A. et al., Temporal lobe structure by magnetic resonance in bipolar affective disorders and schizophrenia, *J. Affect. Disord.*, 21, 19, 1991.

85. Baumann, B. and Bogerts, B., The pathomorphology of schizophrenia and mood disorders: similarities and differences, *Schizophr. Res.*, 39, 141, 1999.

86. Benes, F.M., Davidson, J., and Bird, E.D., Quantitative cytoarchitectural studies of the cerebral cortex of schizophrenics, *Arch. Gen. Psychiatr.*, 43, 31, 1986.

87. Benes, F.M. et al., Deficits in small interneurons in prefrontal and cingulate cortices of schizophrenic and schizoaffective patients, *Arch. Gen. Psychiatr.*, 48, 996, 1991.

88. Sheline, Y.I. et al., Hippocampal atrophy in recurrent major depression, *Proc. Natl. Acad. Sci. USA*, 93, 3908, 1996.

89. Adams, J.M. and Cory, S., Apoptosomes: engines for caspase activation, *Curr. Opin. Cell Biol.*, 14, 715, 2002.

90. Boatright, K.M. and Salvesen, G.S., Mechanisms of caspase activation, *Curr. Opin. Cell. Biol.*, 15, 725, 2003.

91. Ashkenazi, A. and Dixit, V.M., Death receptors: signaling and modulation, *Science*, 281, 1305, 1998.

92. Beattie, E.C. et al., Control of synaptic strength by glial TNF-α, *Science*, 295, 2282, 2002.

93. Licinio, J. and Wong, M.L., The role of inflammatory mediators in the biology of major depression: central nervous system cytokines modulate the biological substrate of depressive symptoms, regulate stress-responsive systems, and contribute to neurotoxicity and neuroprotection, *Mol. Psychiatr.*, 4, 317, 1999.

94. Breder, C.D., Dinarello, C.A., and Saper, C.B., Interleukin-1 immunoreactive innervation of the human hypothalamus, *Science*, 240, 321, 1988.

95. Schobitz, B. et al., Cellular localization of interleukin 6 mRNA and interleukin 6 receptor mRNA in rat brain, *Eur. J. Neurosci.*, 5, 1426, 1993.

96. Cunningham, E.T. Jr. et al., In situ histochemical localization of type I interleukin-1 receptor messenger RNA in the central nervous system, pituitary, and adrenal gland of the mouse, *J. Neurosci.*, 12, 1101, 1992.

97. Licinio, J., Wong, M.L., and Gold, P.W., Localization of interleukin-1 receptor antagonist mRNA in rat brain, *Endocrinology*, 29, 562, 1991.

5 Loneliness, Dysphoria, Stress, and Immunity: A Role for Cytokines

Louise C. Hawkley, Jos A. Bosch, Christopher G. Engeland, Phillip T. Marucha, and John T. Cacioppo

CONTENTS

WHY STUDY IMMUNITY AND CYTOKINES IN LONELINESS?

Human existence is founded on social bedrock, so it is not surprising that the most stressful experiences people endure are typically those that strain or break social connections. The oft-reported health benefits of social integration and, conversely, the health risks of social isolation (House et al.[1,2]) are not limited to the presence or absence of social ties but include satisfaction with social relationships. When personal relationships are perceived to be inadequate to meet intimate and social needs, loneliness may ensue. Although social isolation contributes to loneliness by depriving individuals of opportunities to have their social needs met,[3–5] lonely individuals can feel as though they live isolated existences even when they are with others.[6,7] For this reason, loneliness is characterized as *feelings* of social isolation, absence of companionship, and rejection by peer groups,[8,9] with feelings of an isolated life in a social world forming the dominant experience.[10,11]

Negative and dissatisfying personal relationships have been shown to be powerful modulators of immune processes,[12,13] and loneliness is no exception. For instance, loneliness has been associated with lower natural killer (NK) cell activity, poorer blastogenic response to PHA, and higher levels of circulating EBV antibodies.[14–16] The important question for the purpose of this chapter, however, is, "Why study immunity in loneliness?"

One answer to this question follows on the well-known relationship between social isolation and health outcomes.[1] Objective social isolation is not linked to any one disease pathway but is a risk factor for a broad array of illnesses and causes of death including cancer, cardiovascular disease, and diabetes. An understanding of the processes that link social isolation with broad-based morbidity and mortality will therefore benefit from greater specificity in identifying intervening factors to help explain how social isolation contributes to diverse disease states. Research at the psychological level of analysis, namely the study of loneliness, may help bridge the gap between the epidemiological (i.e., objective social isolation) and biological (i.e., disease) levels of analysis.

The United States is experiencing rapidly growing numbers of older individuals who are also increasingly likely to find themselves living alone and possibly lonely in their old age. The aging of America is occurring at a stunning rate: in 1950, adults over the age of 65 comprised 8% of the United States population; in 2000 they represented 12%; and by 2030 they are projected to represent 20% of the population.[17,18] Moreover, among the more than 27 million people who live alone, a full 36% are over the age of 65,[19] and this proportion is projected to increase in the future.[20] Objective social isolation carries the risk of engendering loneliness, and this risk is particularly high in older individuals. Indeed, although loneliness is relatively constant throughout adult life, older individuals (over 75) report significantly higher levels of loneliness than do younger adults.[21]

Notably, an increasingly large number of elderly individuals are finding themselves socially isolated at the same time that their immune functioning is exhibiting signs of decline. It is widely known that older individuals are more vulnerable to immune challenges than are young adults. Prime examples of their vulnerability include their heightened susceptibility to bacterial (e.g., pneumonia) and viral (e.g., influenza) diseases.[22] Social isolation and loneliness could serve to further compromise immune functioning of already immune-compromised older adults.[23,24] In fact, because younger adults possess a resilient physiology, loneliness may not exert a demonstrable influence on immune functioning until older age. Elucidation of the pathways by which immunity is influenced by loneliness could be informative in the search for appropriate treatment targets in a growing population of older and isolated adults.

A final reason to study immunity in loneliness derives from the dual facts that the effects of social relationships on health outcomes seem to unfold over long periods of time (years) and that loneliness tends to be self-perpetuating.[25] Lonely individuals tend to be more anxious, pessimistic, and fearful of negative evaluation than nonlonely individuals, and consequently, they are more likely to act and relate to others in an anxious, self-protective fashion. Moreover, lonely individuals perceive that they have little control over their ability to fulfill their social needs.[26] Not only are lonely individuals less accepting of nonlonely others than are nonlonely individuals,[27] but lonely people are also recognized as lonely by others and are viewed more negatively than are nonlonely people.[27,28] Once others form the impression that a person is lonely, their behaviors toward that individual can reinforce the lonely individual's negative social expectancies[29,30] and sustain his or her isolated existence. The continual social deficit felt by lonely individuals and the caustic nature of their social cognition provide a neural basis for the chronic activation of physiological pathways that, over time, could have deleterious effects on health.

STRESS, DYSPHORIA, AND LONELINESS

One set of physiological pathways potentially linking loneliness to health consequences involves the stress-responsive hypothalamic–pituitary–adrenocortical (HPA) and sympathetic–adrenomedullary (SAM) endocrine systems, and the sympathetic (SNS) and parasympathetic (PNS) nervous systems. Lonely and nonlonely individuals may differ in stress exposure, stress reactivity, stress buffering, and restorative processes that enhance stress resistance. Each of these factors may independently or synergistically contribute to loneliness-related differences in physiological activity.[31]

For instance, to the extent lonely individuals experience more frequent and/or more intense stress than do nonlonely individuals, they may exhibit more frequent, more prolonged, and/or greater activation of the HPA and SAM systems. Consistent with increased HPA and SAM activation, loneliness has been linked with a greater post-awakening rise in cortisol[32] and increased urinary excretion of cortisol and epinephrine.[15,33] The immunosuppressive effects of HPA and SAM activation may place lonely individuals at an immune disadvantage relative to more socially connected individuals.

Loneliness is itself a stressor that produces negative affects (e.g., anxiety, depression), negative reactivity (e.g., irritability, hostility, mistrust), and lowered feelings of self-worth (see review by Ernst et al.[34]). Indeed, loneliness and dysphoria exhibit considerable experiential overlap, and this is reflected in significant correlations ($r > .4$) between scores on the R-UCLA Loneliness Scale[10] and the Beck Depression Inventory (BDI)[35] or the Center for Epidemiologic Studies Depression (CESD) Scale.[36] However, results of factor analyses of items from this loneliness scale and either depression scale support the notion that loneliness and depressed affect are distinct constructs on theoretical and statistical grounds.[37] Moreover, loneliness appears to have stronger effects on depressive symptomatology than depression has on loneliness. For instance, loneliness was a stronger predictor of depression in older men than women despite greater susceptibility to and higher levels of depression in women.[38]

On the other hand, depression and dysphoria may, at least in some instances, account for the effects of loneliness on physiological functioning. Depression, for instance, has been associated with alterations of the HPA system,[39] down-regulation of the cellular immune response,[40] and stimulation of the production of pro-inflammatory cytokines associated with cardiovascular disease, diabetes, and other age-related chronic conditions.[41,42] Indeed, the cytokine hypothesis of depression is based on the assumption that a chronic stressor (e.g., as might be produced by loneliness) can lead to increased cytokine levels which, in turn, elicit depressed affect.[43]

Stress and dysphoria have also been directly related to plasma markers of inflammation (e.g., IL-6, C-reactive protein, gp130). Examination stress, for example, has been associated with local increases in IL-1β levels in crevicular exudate (the plasma fluid between the gums and the teeth) after accumulation of oral bacteria.[44] Glaser et al.[45] found that influenza vaccination increased plasma IL-6 levels in elderly individuals who reported high numbers of depressive symptoms. Cohen et al.[46] found that higher levels of perceived stress were positively associated with nasal IL-6 secretion (in conjunction with more severe clinical symptoms) in adults infected with influenza. Even without obvious sources of antigenic stimulation, consistent associations can be found between depressive and stress-related symptoms and elevated plasma markers of inflammation.[47-50] Thus, psychological distress appears to have an intrinsic capacity to activate various components of the immune system.

ACUTE STRESS, IMMUNITY, AND CYTOKINES

The study of physiological stress responses has benefited from a distinction between acute (short-lasting) and chronic stress, and the same distinction may be useful when considering the means by which loneliness may affect physiological functioning. Loneliness is not only a source of chronic stress, but has also been associated with greater acute stress. For example, in our comprehensive study of undergraduate students,[6] lonely individuals reported more daily "hassles" (in both frequency and severity) and fewer and less intense "uplifts" than did nonlonely individuals. In addition, the routine activities in which these students engaged every day were rated as more stressful by lonely than by nonlonely individuals.[51] We next consider the differential impacts of acute and chronic stress on immunological functioning to introduce mechanisms by which stress experienced by lonely individuals may influence health.

The immune effects of acute stress have been well documented in animal studies. Placing a rodent in an unfamiliar open field causes a rise in both core body temperature (CBT) and circulating levels of IL-6.[52] Other acute stressors such as foot shock and restraint have been shown to cause fever and increase quantities of circulating leukocytes, acute phase proteins (APPs), and IL-6; these effects may last for days (reviewed by Maier et al.[53]). In addition, very intense stressors (e.g., inescapable tail shocks) produce the same set of sickness behaviors induced by LPS (increases in sleep; decreases in food and water intake, activity, and social interactions). Thus, stress appears able to make animals genuinely sick, even without antigenic stimulation.

Many of the immune alterations induced by acute stress also occur during systemic inflammation. These include increases in both circulating leukocytes and plasma levels of IL-6, and activation of the acute phase response that causes increases of APPs such as protease inhibitors and haptoglobin.[54,55] Importantly, activation of these immune components alone does not necessarily cause sickness or inflammation. Rather, when induced by acute stress, these changes serve largely to limit pathogen growth, buffer inflammation and minimize damage to the organism in the event of infection. For instance, APPs function to remove cellular debris, inhibit pathogen growth, promote bacterial destruction by the activation of complement, and stimulate IL-1ra synthesis.[56,57] In addition, protease inhibitors (e.g., C reactive protein, serum amyloid A) limit the tissue damage that occurs from excess inflammation.[56] Enzymatic activity in blood is also shifted to a state that is less conducive for bacterial growth/replication.[58] Lastly, the systemic actions of IL-6 during infection appear to be largely anti-inflammatory in nature (see section titled "IL-6: Pro-Inflammatory or Anti-Inflammatory?"). The statement that acute stress causes immune activation (or suppresses immune activity) is misleading. Rather, acute stress seems to prime the immune system, placing it into a state of readiness to combat potential injury and infection. This is logical from an evolutionary standpoint: in a fight-or-flight situation, an organism might be injured and would then have to deal with subsequent inflammation, tissue repair, and infection. Placing the immune system in a state of readiness prior to such an injury will conceivably increase survival rate.

In support of this idea of priming the immune response, Dhabhar[59] has repeatedly shown that acute stress (2-hour physical restraint) in mice enhances delayed type hypersensitivity (DTH) reactions that represent cell-mediated immune responses, and this effect is reversed by adrenalectomy indicating HPA involvement. This enhancement is likely due to a mobilization of leukocytes from blood to skin, which is induced by stress and is hypothesized to increase immune surveillance in the skin.[60] This enhancement also occurs due to increased migration of skin dendritic cells mediated via norepinephrine, which results in greater priming of CD8(+) T cells in draining lymph nodes and increases the recruitment of these effector cells to the skin upon challenge.[61] Thus, stress appears to prime the DTH response by inducing the migration of immune cells prior to antigen challenge.

Using a model of oral wound healing in humans, we recently observed that individuals with higher anticipatory stress (of the wounding procedure) healed significantly faster than individuals who were less stressed at the time of wounding. This appeared related to higher circulating levels of glucocorticoids (GCs) at the time of wounding and decreased inflammation in the wound tissue 24 hours post-wounding.[62] Other studies have shown that animals previously stressed with inescapable tail shocks and then challenged with LPS displayed enhanced induction of pro-inflammatory cytokines,[63] and an augmentation of both fever and sickness behaviors.[64] Similar stressors also activate the acute phase response[65] and enhance recovery from bacterial challenge.[66] Moreover, macrophages from stressed rats exhibited increased production of nitrite (in vitro) when challenged with keyhole limpet hemocyanin (KLH). However, in the absence of KLH, macrophage nitrite production was similar in stressed and nonstressed animals. Thus, stress primed but did not activate nitrite production.[67] Taken together, these findings indicate that acute stress can both prime and increase the effectiveness of the immune response against antigenic challenge and injury.

How stress is able to influence cytokine levels and sickness may stem back to basic energy production in the body. GCs catalyze the conversion of glycogen to glucose and muscle protein to amino acids, antagonize the actions of insulin (resulting in decreased uptake of glucose to fat and muscle), and liberate fatty acids from fat reserves. The overall effect is that GCs liberate stored energy by increasing glucose availability to the peripheral tissues, muscles, and brain. The immune system requires vast amounts of energy for tissue repair, increased metabolism, and fever maintenance. Evidence suggests that the immune system has made use of GCs as an energy production system from a very early time point in evolution and, indeed, even primitive organisms such as mollusks exhibit activation of such a system upon immune challenge (see Maier et al.[53] for review).

In vertebrates, peripheral immune activation (e.g., infection) leads to the release of pro-inflammatory cytokines (e.g., IL-1β, TNF-α) that signal the brain through a variety of mechanisms. This, in turn, induces the release of a variety of substances centrally (e.g., IL-1β, prostaglandins) that signal the hypothalamus, raising the set point for core body temperature and activating the HPA axis. This results in GC release, which liberates energy for immune activation such as fever. Fever is an adaptive response to infection as it bolsters the immune system and inhibits bacterial growth and reproduction.[58] Thus, one of the original purposes of GC release may have been to liberate stored energy for fever maintenance and tissue repair.

During a fight-or-flight situation (a situation of acute stress requiring complex, integrated responses), energy demands are high and immediate, and are largely met by GC release. However, the fight-or-flight response is evolutionarily younger than the immune system (very primitive creatures incapable of fight-or-flight responses possess immune mechanisms for dealing with infection). Based on this, Maier and Watkins[54] proposed that as organisms evolved, GC release — which was already used for quick energy production by the immune system — also became utilized when a fight-or-flight response was needed. As a result, the stress response began to stimulate the same circuitry stimulated following infection. In fact, stress appears to activate the same cascade of events as LPS does (central activation causing fever and HPA activation), although this stems from a neural pathway rather than from peripheral cytokine release.[53] Figure 5.1 illustrates this circuitry.

Tail shock and social isolation both cause central increases in brain IL-1β; immobilization stress increases brain IL-1β mRNA; and IL-1ra (icv) blocks endocrine and behavioral responses to some stressors.[53] Furthermore, following intense stress (e.g., tail shock), the central release of IL-1β is related to increases in plasma cytokine levels (e.g., IL-1β, IL-6) and sickness behaviors,[68] all of which can be blocked by the pre-administration of IL-1β antagonists (e.g., IL-1ra, α-MSH) centrally but not peripherally.[53] These findings suggest that central increases in IL-1β influence peripheral inflammatory responses that occur following psychological stress.

In summary, acute stress activates many peripheral components of innate and even some components of acquired (e.g., DTH) immunity which, in turn, are protective in nature or serve to prime the immune system for antigenic challenge. However, IL-1β may also be released centrally, and under intense stress this can lead to peripheral IL-1β and IL-6 release, along with increased inflammation, fever, and sickness behaviors. These data suggest that the repeated and more intense bouts of acute stress experienced by lonely compared to nonlonely individuals represent one mechanism by which loneliness may have a negative impact on immune activity and health.

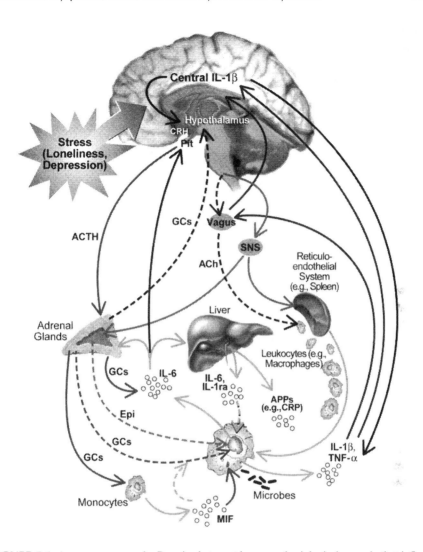

FIGURE 5.1 Acute stress cascade. Perceived stress triggers a physiological cascade that influences inflammatory processes. Activation of the SNS primes the immune system by mobilizing leukocytes from the spleen (as well as lungs, marginal pools, and bone marrow pools) into the blood. Stress-induced vagal withdrawal results in reduced ACh release and permits inflammatory activity of tissue macrophages in the vagally innervated reticulendothelial system (liver, heart, spleen, GI tract). Acute psychological stressors also stimulate the release of IL-1β in the brain and initiate direct activation of the HPA axis, which culminates in the secretion of GCs (e.g., cortisol). Under severe stress, brain IL-1β appears capable of causing signs of low-grade peripheral inflammation (e.g., fever, elevated plasma cytokine levels). Circulating GCs reduce/contain this inflammation by inhibiting the release of these cytokines. GCs also stimulate IL-6 production which in turn induces hepatic APPs (e.g., CRP) that help minimize cellular damage. However, GCs induce macrophages to release MIF, which reduces immune cell sensitivity to the anti-inflammatory actions of GCs and promotes TNF-α release. This may help sustain low-grade inflammation during conditions of chronic stress (see Figure 5.2). Solid arrows represent stimulatory effects and dashed arrows represent inhibitory effects. (Illustration by Karen Dirr, M.A.M.S., University of Chicago.)

Proper HPA functioning largely prevents the peripheral release of pro-inflammatory cytokines following acute stress.[69] Chronic stress, however, involves a lasting dysregulation of the HPA axis, and also a resistance to the immunosuppressant effects of GCs.[70,71] The higher degrees of peripheral inflammation and sickness reported in chronically stressed individuals may stem from decreased ability to prevent peripheral inflammation following the stress-induced release of IL-1β centrally.

CHRONIC STRESS, DYSPHORIA, GLUCOCORTICOID SENSITIVITY, AND MACROPHAGE MIGRATORY INHIBITORY FACTOR

Loneliness is aversive, and when social needs go unmet for extended periods of time, the stress of perceived isolation may pervade every other aspect of life. The chronic stress of loneliness is further exacerbated by the repeated and intense bouts of acute stress that are common to lonely individuals. Indeed, stress responses to even relatively minor recurring daily stressors can accumulate and have long-term consequences on health.[72] Chronic stress therefore represents a second mechanism that may lead to greater peripheral inflammation and sickness in lonely rather than nonlonely individuals. Moreover, loneliness has been shown to be a strong predictor of depressive symptomatology,[37,38] and depression offers another venue for loneliness to make inroads on immune functioning and health. GCs play a key role in determining the physiological consequences of chronic stress and depression and thus provide a useful avenue to examine how loneliness may affect health.

The observation that chronic stress can potentiate inflammatory processes appears at odds with the potent anti-inflammatory effects of GCs and other stress hormones. One possible explanation for this discrepancy, discussed earlier, is that the systemic signs of inflammation may have been misinterpreted, and actually reflect a response that helps to contain inflammatory processes (cf. reference 73). Thus, as inflammation is primarily a localized event, many of the systemic "pro-inflammatory" mediators that are elevated in distressed individuals may function in conjunction with GCs to keep this process localized.

An additional possibility is that protracted stress diminishes the immune system's sensitivity to GCs that normally control the inflammatory cascade. Strong support for this hypothesis comes from the work of Sheridan et al., who employed social disruption (SDR) as a stress model in animals.[74–76] In this experimental model, male mice are housed in groups of five until a stable hierarchy develops. An aggressive intruder is introduced, after which excessive fighting re-establishes the social hierarchy. In a series of studies, it was found that SDR stress induces a strong HPA activation in the defeated animals,[76,77] and simultaneously leads to glucocorticoid resistance in splenocytes activated with LPS.[77] It is relevant to add that chronic restraint stress does not result in glucocorticoid resistance, and may even increase sensitivity to GCs, despite the fact that this stressor induces similar HPA activation to that of SDR.[76,78,79] Hence, the induction of glucocorticoid sensitivity appears stressor-specific. Consistent with the glucocorticoid sensitivity hypothesis, the SDR-induced reduction in glucocorticoid sensitivity results in greater proneness to hyperinflammation, leading to increased mortality from experimental influenza infection and septic shock.[76,78]

Studies in humans confirmed and extended the results of animal experiments. In human studies, glucocorticoid sensitivity is often measured *ex vivo*. Immune cells are incubated with a bacterial endotoxin (e.g., LPS) or a mitogen (e.g., PHA) in combination with varying concentrations of GCs (e.g., dexamethasone). Using this approach, studies have found a reduced glucocorticoid sensitivity of immune cells (e.g., greater *in vitro* production of IL-6 and TNF-α in the presence of dexamethasone) in spousal caregivers of dementia patients,[80] in parents of children undergoing cancer treatment,[81] and in stress-related syndromes such as vital exhaustion and depression.[82–84]

Thus, both animal and human studies provide good support for the hypothesis that psychological stressors can down-regulate the GC sensitivity of immune cells. As shown in Figure 5.2, this can result in an increased release of pro-inflammatory cytokines (e.g., IL-1β, TNF-α), and suggests that the consequences of GC resistance may include elevated pro-inflammatory cytokine responses to inflammatory stimuli. Although it is still unclear how stress-induced GC resistance is mediated, macrophage migratory inhibitory factor (MIF) is one candidate. In two studies described below, we explored whether MIF is up-regulated by psychological stress.

MIF is one of the earliest identified cytokines, discovered nearly 40 years ago, although its exact functions remained elusive for many years.[85] Studies using pure recombinant MIF and specific neutralizing antibodies have shown MIF to be a potent pro-inflammatory cytokine and a key modulator of immune and inflammatory processes.[86,87] In the early 1990s, it was discovered that MIF overrides the anti-inflammatory actions of GCs, and restores macrophage cytokine production and T cell activation during treatment with immunosuppressive levels of GCs.[88,89] Subsequent studies demonstrated a critical role of MIF in various inflammatory processes and syndromes, including atherosclerosis, wound repair, rheumatoid arthritis, inflammatory lung diseases, and sepsis, whereas MIF-neutralizing antibodies reduced disease severity and mortality in models of arthritis, glomerular nephritis, and sepsis.[86,89–105]

Monocytes/macrophages and T cells are probably the main immune cells to produce MIF.[87] Interestingly, MIF secretion by leukocytes is induced rather than suppressed by low concentrations of synthetic GCs.[88,93] Animal studies have revealed other remarkable associations between MIF and HPA axis activities.[106] MIF is a significant pituitary protein (0.05% of total protein. As a comparison, ACTH forms 0.2% and prolactin 0.08% of pituitary protein[101]) secreted by the same cells of the anterior pituitary that secrete ACTH. Pituitary MIF partly derives from ACTH-containing secretory granules.[89,107,108] Moreover, *in vitro* studies showed that CRH is a potent MIF secretagogue, although the signaling pathway appears distinct from that controlling ACTH release.[108,109] MIF is also expressed in the adrenals,[110,111] and adrenal MIF protein expression is reduced in animals that have their pituitaries surgically removed, indicating that adrenal MIF production is dependent on stimulation by pituitary hormones.[110] Animal studies further show that plasma levels of MIF increase in response to various HPA-activating signals, including endotoxin and handling stress.[88] The latter finding provided the first indication that psychological stressors may up-regulate plasma MIF levels.

Although the regulation of MIF was extensively studied in rodents, data on humans is somewhat sparser. In healthy human subjects, MIF is at relatively high

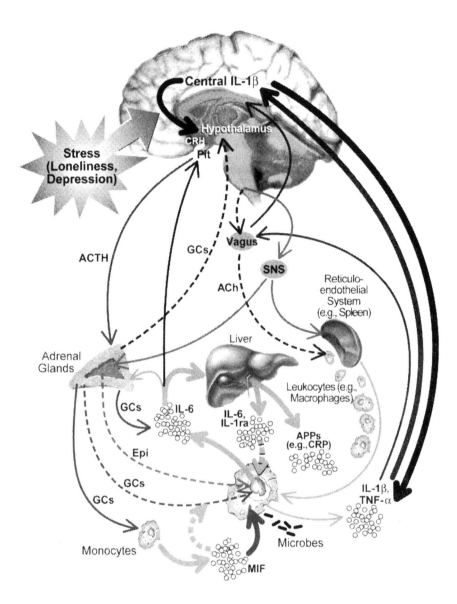

FIGURE 5.2 Impact of chronic stress. Despite higher circulating levels of GCs under conditions of chronic stress, the anti-inflammatory effects of GCs appear substantially lessened. This is due to the formation of GC insensitivity by many immune cells, and may be mediated by MIF production. The end result is that susceptibility to inflammation and its associated morbidities (e.g., sickness, disease) may be greater in chronically stressed (e.g., lonely, depressed) individuals. Solid arrows represent stimulatory effects and dashed arrows represent inhibitory effects. Thicker arrows represent effects made stronger due to chronic stress. (Illustration by Karen Dirr, M.A.M.S., University of Chicago.)

plasma concentrations (2 to 8 ng/ml), and much higher concentrations are found in inflammatory disease and sepsis.[97,101,112,113] Consistent with the MIF–HPA association in animals, MIF shows a circadian cycle that parallels that of cortisol.[114] In contrast with the findings of animal studies, however, plasma levels of MIF are not affected by various HPA stimulants or inhibitors, including injections of CRH or ACTH, the insulin tolerance test, and the dexamethasone suppression test.[113] Likewise, we did not observe an effect of acute stress (public speaking) on plasma MIF levels, in spite of the fact that this laboratory stressor had a strong effect on plasma ACTH and cortisol levels.[48]

Our data did indicate, however, that protracted forms of distress can affect MIF levels in both humans and animals. For our human studies, we selected undergraduate students (mean age 20.4) who scored in the upper or lower quintile of their peer group on the BDI.[48] The BDI is one of the most frequently used self-report questionnaires for assessing depression and dysphoria, and high scores on this questionnaire are predictive of the presence of clinical depression.[115] Approximately 4 to 6 weeks after initial screening, subjects were invited to the laboratory where they underwent a 15-minute public speaking task (i.e., giving a presentation in front of a camera and an audience). Participants who at the time of this laboratory visit had BDI scores indicative of mild to moderate depression (13) were denoted dysphoric ($N = 36$); subjects with BDI scores 5 were denoted nondysphoric ($N = 39$). Although the 15-minute speaking stressor had no effect on plasma MIF levels, the participants in the dysphoric group had higher average levels of MIF. Dysphoria was also associated with marginally increased numbers of peripheral blood lymphocytes ($p < .05$). Subsequent analyses to detect potential confounders showed that the two groups did not differ in gender or ethnic composition, age, body mass index, smoking, alcohol consumption, or average hours of exercise or sleep, and the use of these variables as covariates in the analyses did not attenuate the observed group differences.[48]

We also investigated MIF expression in the SDR animal model (described above). This model has shown that glucocorticoid resistance does not develop until after 4 to 5 days of SDR. Quantitative polymerase chain reaction (PCR) tests of the spleens and pituitaries of mice exposed to 6 days of SDR showed a 50% increase in MIF gene expression in both tissues (J.F. Sheridan, personal communication). Additional experiments in which spleens were removed after 1, 3, or 6 days of SDR demonstrated that MIF expression did not significantly increase until day 6. Hence, MIF expression shows a pattern that appears to parallel the kinetics of the development of glucocorticoid resistance (J.F. Sheridan, personal communication).

To conclude, both animal and human studies show that chronic stress is associated with reduced immune cell sensitivity to the anti-inflammatory actions of GCs, and stress-induced elevations in MIF may be potential mediators of this effect. However, correlation is not causation, and additional experiments are clearly needed to confirm a role of MIF in stress-related glucocorticoid resistance. For the SDR paradigm, further experiments with MIF knock-out animals appear the most obvious ways to proceed. Correlational studies in humans could examine statistical associations of MIF expression, glucocorticoid sensitivity, and indices of distress. Such research might help explain the link between stress and inflammatory conditions such as atherosclerosis, autoimmunity, and allergic diseases, and also help to solve the paradox of how stressors can act as both immunosuppressants and immunostimulants.

IL-6: PRO-INFLAMMATORY OR ANTI-INFLAMMATORY?

A hallmark of immune activation in major depression is increased production of IL-6.[116] Indeed, many studies have linked IL-6 with immune activation during aging, stress and disease[50,117] and cite this cytokine as an important marker for inflammatory events. Taken a step further, the most common interpretation is that IL-6 release is pro-inflammatory, although most studies that relate increased inflammation or fever to elevated levels of IL-6 are correlational in nature. Is IL-6 truly a pro-inflammatory cytokine? For instance, of the pro-inflammatory cytokines released during infection, IL-6 correlates most closely with fever and HPA activation (both temporally and quantitatively).[118-120] It has been clearly shown that IL-6 rises in concordance with both IL-1β and TNF-α, as each stimulates the synthesis and release of IL-6.[121] We propose that a misinterpretation exists in the literature, as many of the reports that IL-6 acts in a pro-inflammatory manner during systemic infection have been largely inferred on the basis of its stronger correlation with fever, HPA activity, and other indices of inflammation more than either IL-1β or TNF-α.

IL-6 certainly has pro-inflammatory qualities during infection; it acts as a strong progenitor of myeloid cell differentiation (e.g., macrophages, neutrophils) and is involved in cell maturation and maintenance (e.g., NK cells, CD8(+) T cells). However, IL-6 also has many anti-inflammatory properties during infection. For instance, it is released in response to rising levels of IL-1 and TNF-α,[121] and dampens the inflammation caused by these pro-inflammatory cytokines through a variety of mechanisms: (1) once released, IL-6 directly inhibits the further synthesis of both IL-1β and TNF-α,[122,123] (2) the administration of IL-6 in humans causes the induction of the soluble receptors IL-1ra and p55[57] that inhibit IL-1β and TNF-α activity, respectively, and (3) IL-6 acts at both the pituitary gland and the adrenals to activate the HPA axis and is the main modulator of the release of GCs during immune

Although IL-6 is routinely mentioned in the literature in the same context as the IL-1β and TNF-α cytokines, it should be noted that the biological effects of IL-6 are very different from those of the two pro-inflammatory cytokines. Although systemic administration of IL-1β and TNF-α causes high fever and even septic shock at relatively low doses, fairly high doses of IL-6 are tolerated and do not cause shock in mice, dogs, or primates.[56]

Furthermore, unlike IL-1β and TNF-α, IL-6 does not cause (1) the up-regulation of major inflammatory mediators (e.g., chemokines, prostaglandins, nitric oxide, matrix metalloproteinases), (2) the induction of cyclooxygenase activity, (3) tissue damage by proteases, or (4) the synthesis of adhesion molecules (e.g., intracellular adhesion molecule, ICAM-1).[56,57,122] Rather, IL-6 is a chief mediator of the acute phase response[125] that serves to limit pathogen growth, inflammation, and tissue damage. T-cell mediated inflammation such as delayed type hypersensitivity and adjuvant arthritis or triggered by superantigen is inhibited by IL-6.[56,123]

Finally, in a murine model of toxic shock, it has been shown that IL-6 pretreatment decreases mortality rates in a dose-dependent fashion and treatment with IL-6 antibodies increases mortality rates, likely due to the inhibitory effect IL-6 has on TNF-α release.[123] Similarly, treatment with IL-6 antibodies increases mortality in a septic shock model.[126] Thus, although IL-6 is one of the main cytokines released during bacterial infection and inflammation, its principal systemic actions may be anti-inflammatory. In summary, the authors encourage readers to allow for this possibility when interpreting results that involve correlations between immune activation or disease severity and levels of IL-6.

CONCLUSION

Sociodemographic changes in the United States are finding increasing numbers of people living alone, and a growing percentage of these isolated individuals are elderly. Given the risk for morbidity and mortality associated with social isolation and loneliness, one challenge for researchers is to identify mechanisms by which social factors take a toll on physiological functioning and health. Relatively recent developments in the field of immunology have introduced cytokines as potential players in the physiological processes that link psychosocial factors with increased risk for disease.

Investigations of the numerous actions of cytokines involved in psycho-neuro-immune interactions are ongoing, and examinations of the role of cytokines in the pathways that lead from loneliness to morbidity and mortality have only begun. Because cytokine research is in its infancy, special care must be taken to ensure that empirical evidence supports inferences regarding the role of cytokines in physiological and health outcomes. A role for IL-6 is a case in point. Although typically referred to as a pro-inflammatory cytokine, an anti-inflammatory interpretation of IL-6 actions is consistent with data from many studies. For example, although greater age-related increases in IL-6 among current and former caregivers (relative to controls) may mark inflammatory processes,[127] IL-6 increases may reflect an attempt to contain inflammation. Indeed, decreases in IL-6 under conditions of chronic stress may signal failure in self-regulation of the inflammatory process.

The recently discovered role of MIF in immune processes is another reminder that much has yet to be learned regarding the interplay among psychological, endocrine (i.e., HPA), and immune systems. The pro-inflammatory actions of MIF are particularly interesting in their potential to explain the development of glucocorticoid resistance, an especially troubling consequence of chronic stress and depression. Because loneliness may operate through distress and dysphoria to affect health, MIF may play an important role in increasing the risks for morbidity and mortality in lonely individuals.

It appears obvious that loneliness can contribute to disease processes through its influence on acute and chronic stress. Figure 5.1 illustrates the main cascade of physiological changes that occur following acute stress. Figure 5.2 illustrates how chronic stress impacts this same cascade of events and how it promotes peripheral inflammation to a greater extent than does acute stress. Overall, acute stress typically elicits an adaptive response, as it primes the immune system, placing it into a state of readiness to combat potential injury and infection. Conversely, chronic stress, an overshoot of this response, is generally maladaptive to the organism. Observation of Figure 5.2 indicates that a chronic stressor such as loneliness can cause low-grade peripheral inflammation which, in turn, has been linked to inflammatory diseases such as diabetes, cardiovascular disease (e.g., atherosclerosis), and autoimmune disorders (e.g., rheumatoid arthritis, lupus). Whether chronic stress works causally or synergistically with underlying disease mechanisms remains unresolved. Nevertheless, the outcomes of these processes can be influenced by the stress and depression associated with loneliness. Indeed, the known centrality of social relationships to well-being implies that loneliness may extract a great cost on human health, the mechanisms for which have only begun to be explored.

ACKNOWLEDGMENT

This research was supported by National Institute on Aging Program Grants PO1 AG-18911 and P01 AG-16321, and National Institutes of Health Grant P50 DE-13749.

REFERENCES

1. House, J.S., Landis, K.R., and Umberson, D., Social relationships and health, *Science*, 241, 540, 1988.
2. Seeman, T.E., Health promoting effects of friends and family on health outcomes in older adults, *Am. J. Hlth. Promot.*, 14, 362, 2000.
3. de Jong-Gierveld, J., Developing and testing a model of loneliness, *J. Pers. Soc. Psychol.*, 53, 119, 1987.
4. Fees, B.S., Martin, P., and Poon, L.W., A model of loneliness in older adults, *J. Gerontol. Psychol. Sci.*, 54, P231, 1999.
5. Henderson, A.S., Scott, R., and Kay, D.W., The elderly who live alone: their mental health and social relationships, *Austr. NZ J. Psychiatr.*, 20, 202, 1986.
6. Cacioppo, J.T. et al., Lonely traits and concomitant physiological processes: the MacArthur Social Neuroscience Studies, *Int. J. Psychophys.*, 35, 143, 2000.
7. van Baarsen, B. et al., Lonely but not alone: emotional isolation and social isolation as two distinct dimensions of loneliness in older people, *Educat. Psychol. Measur.*, 61, 119, 2001.
8. Austin, B.A., Factorial structure of the UCLA Loneliness Scale, *Psychol. Rep.*, 53, 883, 1983.
9. Hawkley, L.C., Browne, M.W., and Cacioppo, J.T., How can I connect with thee? Let me count the ways, *Psychol. Sci.*, 16, 798, 2005.
10. Russell, D., Peplau, L.A., and Cutrona, C.E., The revised UCLA Loneliness Scale: concurrent and discriminant validity evidence, *J. Pers. Soc. Psychol.*, 39, 472, 1980.
11. Hays, R.D. and DiMatteo, M.R., A short-form measure of loneliness, *J. Person. Assess.*, 51, 69, 1987.
12. Kiecolt-Glaser, J.K., Stress, personal relationships, and immune function: health implications, *Brain Behav. Immun.*, 13, 61, 1999.
13. Uchino, B.N., Cacioppo, J.T., and Kiecolt-Glaser, J.K., The relationship between social support and physiological processes: a review with emphasis on underlying mechanisms and implications for health, *Psychol. Bull.*, 119, 488, 1996.
14. Glaser, R. et al., Stress, loneliness, and changes in herpes virus latency, *J. Beh. Med.*, 8, 249, 1985.

15. Kiecolt-Glaser, J.K. et al., Urinary cortisol levels, cellular immunocompetency, and loneliness in psychiatric inpatients, *Psychosom. Med.*, 46, 15, 1984.

16. Kiecolt-Glaser, J.K. et al., Stress and the transformation of lymphocytes by Epstein–Barr virus, *J. Beh. Med.*, 7, 1, 1984.

17. Meyer, J., Age: 2000, in *Census 2000 Brief*, U.S. Census Bureau, Government Printing Office, Washington, D.C., 2001.

18. U.S. Census Bureau, *Projections of the Total Resident Population by 5-year Age Groups, and Sex with Special Age Categories, Middle Series*, 2025-2045 (NP-T3-F), Population Projections Program, Government Printing Office, Washington, D.C., 2000.

19. Hobbs, F. and Stoops, N., *Demographic Trends in the 20th Century*, Census 2000 Special Reports Series CENSR-4, U.S. Census Bureau, Government Printing Office, Washington, D.C., 2002.

20. U.S. Census Bureau, *Projections of the Number of Persons Living Alone by Age and Sex: 1995 to 2010*, Series 1, 2, and 3, Population Projections Program, Government Printing Office, Washington, D.C., 1996.

21. Andersson, L., Loneliness research and interventions: a review of the literature, *Aging Ment. Hlth.*, 2, 264, 1998.

22. Yoshikawa, T.T., Clinical relevance of age-related immune dysfunction, *Clin. Infect. Dis.*, 31, 578, 2000.

23. Hawkley, L.C. and Cacioppo, J.T., Stress and the aging immune system, *Brain Behav. Immun.*, 18, 114, 2004.

24. Kiecolt-Glaser, J.K. and Glaser, R., Stress and immunity: Age enhances the risks, *Curr. Dir. Psychol. Sci.*, 10, 18, 2001.

25. Cacioppo, J.T. and Hawkley, L.C., People thinking about people: the vicious cycle of being a social outcast in one's own mind, in *The Social Outcast: Ostracism, Social Exclusion, Rejection, and Bullying*, Williams K.D., Forgas J.P., and von Hippel W., Eds., Psychology Press, New York, 2005, p. 91.

26. Solano, C.H., Loneliness and perceptions of control: general traits versus specific attributions, *J. Soc. Beh. Pers.*, 2, 201, 1987.

27. Rotenberg, K.J. and Kamill, J., Perception of lonely and non-lonely persons as a function of individual differences in loneliness, *J. Soc. Pers. Relat.*, 9, 325, 1992.

28. Lau, S. and Gruen, G.E., The social stigma of loneliness: effect of target person's and perceiver's sex, *Pers. Soc. Psychol. Bull.*, 18, 182, 1992.

29. Rotenberg, K., Loneliness and interpersonal trust, *J. Soc. Clin. Psychol.*, 13, 152, 1994.

30. Rotenberg, K.J., Gruman, J.A., and Ariganello, M., Behavioral confirmation of the loneliness stereotype, *Basic Appl. Soc. Psychol.*, 24, 81, 2002.

31. Hawkley, L.C. and Cacioppo, J.T., Loneliness and pathways to disease, *Brain Behav. Immun.*, 17, S98, 2003.

32. Steptoe, A. et al., Loneliness and neuroendocrine, cardiovascular, and inflammatory stress responses in middle-aged men and women, *Psychoneuroendocrinology*, 29, 593, 2004.

33. Hawkley, L.C., Masi, C.M., Berry, J.D., and Cacioppo, J.T., Loneliness is a unique predictor of age-related differences in systolic blood pressure, *Psychol. Aging*, 21, 152, 2006.

34. Ernst, J.M. and Cacioppo, J.T., Lonely hearts: psychological perspectives on loneliness, *Appl. Prev. Psychol.*, 8, 1, 1999.

35. Beck, A.T. and Beck, R.W., Screening depressed patients in a family practice: a rapid technique, *Postgrad. Med.*, 52, 81, 1972.

36. Radloff, L.S., The CES-D Scale: a self-report depression scale for research in the general population, *Appl. Psychol. Measur.*, 1, 385, 1977.

37. Cacioppo, J.T. et al., Loneliness within a nomological net: is social connectedness central? Under review, 2004.

38. Cacioppo, J.T. et al., Loneliness and depressive symptoms, self-rated health, and chronic health conditions: evidence from two population-based studies, under review, 2004.

39. Tsigos, C. and Chrousos, G.P., Hypothalamic–pituitary–adrenal axis, neuroendocrine factors and stress, *J. Psychosom. Res.*, 53, 865, 2002.

40. Miller, A.H., Neuroendocrine and immune system interactions in stress and depression, *Psychiat. Clin. N. Am.*, 21, 443, 1998.

41. Dantzer, R. et al., Cytokines and depression: fortuitous or causative association? *Molec. Psych.*, 4, 328, 1999.

42. Kiecolt-Glaser, J.K. and Glaser, R., Depression and immune function: central pathways to morbidity and mortality, *J. Psychosom. Res.*, 53, 873, 2002.

43. Leonard, B.E. and Song, C., Stress, depression, and the role of cytokines, in *Cytokines, Stress, and Depression*, Dantzer R., Wollman E.E., and Yirmiya R., Eds., Kluwer Academic Publishers, New York, 1999, p. 251.

44. Deinzer, R. et al., Acute stress effects on local IL-1β responses to pathogens in a human *in vivo* model, *Brain Behav. Immun.*, 18, 458, 2004.

45. Glaser, R. et al., Mild depressive symptoms are associated with amplified and prolonged inflammatory responses after influenza virus vaccination in older adults, *Arch. Gen. Psychiatr.*, 60, 1009, 2003.

46. Cohen, S., Doyle, W.J., and Skoner, D.P., Psychological stress, cytokine production, and severity of upper respiratory illness, *Psychosom. Med.*, 61, 175, 1999.

47. Miller, G.E. et al., Clinical depression and inflammatory risk markers for coronary heart disease, *Am. J. Cardiol.*, 90, 1279, 2002.

48. Bosch, J.A. et al., Elevated macrophage migration inhibitory factor in dysphoric young adults, in preparation.

49. Penninx, B.W. et al., Inflammatory markers and depressed mood in older persons: results from the Health, Aging and Body Composition Study, *Biol. Psychiatry*, 54, 566, 2003.

50. Kiecolt-Glaser, J.K. et al., Chronic stress and age-related increases in the proinflammatory cytokine IL-6, *Proc. Natl. Acad. Sci. USA*, 100, 9090, 2003.

51. Hawkley, L.C. et al., Loneliness in everyday life: cardiovascular activity, psychosocial context, and health behaviors, *J. Pers. Soc. Psychol.*, 85, 105, 2003.

52. LeMay, L.G., Vander, A.J., and Kluger, M.J., The effects of psychological stress on plasma interleukin-6 activity in rats, *Physiol. Behav.*, 47, 957, 1990.

53. Maier, S.F., Bi-directional immune-brain communication: implications for understanding stress, pain, and cognition, *Brain Behav. Immun.*, 17, 69, 2003.

54. Maier, S.F. and Watkins, L.R., Bidirectional communication between the brain and the immune system: implications for behaviour, *Animal Behav.*, 57, 741, 1999.

55. Yeager, M.P., Guyre, P.M., and Munck, A.U., Glucocorticoid regulation of the inflammatory response to injury, *Acta Anaesthiol. Scand.*, 48, 799, 2004.

56. Barton, B., The biological effects of interleukin 6, *Med. Res. Rev.*, 16, 87, 1996.

57. Tilg, H., Dinarello, C., and Mier, J., IL-6 and APPs: Anti-inflammatory and immunosuppressive mediators, *Immunol. Today*, 18, 428, 1997.

58. Hart, B.L., Biological basis of the behavior of sick animals, *Neurosci. Biobehav. Rev.*, 12, 123, 1988.

59. Dhabhar, F.S., Stress-induced augmentation of immune function: the role of stress hormones, leukocyte trafficking, and cytokines, *Brain Behav. Immun.*, 16, 785, 2002.

60. Dhabhar, F.S. and McEwen, B.S., Stress-induced enhancement of antigen-specific cell-mediated immunity, *J. Immunol.*, 156, 2608, 1996.

61. Saint-Mezard P. et al., Psychological stress exerts an adjuvant effect on skin dendritic cell functions *in vivo*, *J. Immunol.*, 171, 4073, 2003.
62. Engeland, C.G., Cacioppo, J.T., and Marucha, P.T., Stress hormones modulate the healing rates of oral wounds, in preparation.
63. Johnson, J.D. et al., Prior stressor exposure sensitizes LPS-induced cytokine production, *Brain Behav. Immun.*, 16, 461, 2002.
64. Johnson, J.D. et al., Effects of prior stress on LPS-induced cytokine and sickness responses, *Am. J. Physiol.*, 284, R422, 2003.
65. Deak, T. et al., Evidence that brief stress may induce the acute phase response in rats, *Am. J. Physiol.*, 273, R1998, 1997.
66. Deak, T. et al., Acute stress may facilitate recovery from a subcutaneous bacterial challenge, *Neuroimmunomodulation*, 6, 344, 1999.
67. Fleshner, M. et al., Acute stressor exposure both suppresses acquired immunity and potentiates innate immunity, *Am. J. Physiol.*, 275, R870, 1998.
68. Johnson, J.D. et al., The role of IL-1-beta in stress-induced sensitization of proinflammatory cytokine and corticosterone responses, *Neuroscience*, 127, 569, 2004.
69. Nguyen, K.T. et al., Time course and corticosterone sensitivity of the brain, pituitary, and serum interleukin-1-beta protein response to acute stress, *Brain Res.*, 859, 193, 2000.
70. Avitsur, R., Stark, J.L., and Sheridan, J.F., Social stress induces glucocorticoid resistance in subordinate animals, *Horm. Behav.*, 39, 247, 2001.
71. O'Connor, K.A. et al., Inescapable shock induces resistance to the effects of dexamethasone, *Psychoneuroendocrinology*, 28, 481, 2003.
72. McEwen, B.S., Protective and damaging effects of stress mediators, *New Engl. J. Med.*, 338, 171, 1998.
73. Tracey, K.J., The inflammatory reflex, *Nature*, 420, 853, 2002.
74. Bailey, M.T. et al., Physical defeat reduces the sensitivity of murine splenocytes to the suppressive effects of corticosterone, *Brain Behav. Immun.*, 18, 416, 2004.
75. Engler, H. et al., Effects of repeated social stress on leukocyte distribution in bone marrow, peripheral blood and spleen, *J. Neuroimmunol.*, 148, 106, 2004.
76. Padgett, D.A. et al., Social stress and the reactivation of latent herpes simplex virus type 1, *Proc. Natl. Acad. Sci. USA*, 95, 7231, 1998.
77. Stark, J.L. et al., Social stress induces glucocorticoid resistance in macrophages, *Am. J. Physiol. Regul. Integr. Comp. Physiol.*, 280, R1799, 2001.
78. Quan, N. et al., Social stress increases the susceptibility to endotoxic shock, *J. Neuroimmunol.*, 115, 36, 2001.
79. Bauer, M.E. et al., Restraint stress is associated with changes in glucocorticoid immunoregulation, *Physiol. Behav.*, 73, 525, 2001.
80. Bauer, M.E. et al., Chronic stress in caregivers of dementia patients is associated with reduced lymphocyte sensitivity to glucocorticoids, *J. Neuroimmunol.*, 103, 84, 2000.
81. Miller, G.E., Cohen, S., and Ritchey, A.K., Chronic psychological stress and the regulation of pro-inflammatory cytokines: a glucocorticoid-resistance model, *Hlth. Psychol.*, 21, 531, 2002.
82. Miller, A.H., Pariante, C.M., and Pearce, B.D., Effects of cytokines on glucocorticoid receptor expression and function: glucocorticoid resistance and relevance to depression, *Adv. Exp. Med. Biol.*, 461, 107, 1999.
83. Wirtz, P.H. et al., Reduced glucocorticoid sensitivity of monocyte interleukin-6 production in male industrial employees who are vitally exhausted, *Psychosom. Med.*, 65, 672, 2003.
84. Bauer, M.E. et al., Altered glucocorticoid immunoregulation in treatment resistant depression, *Psychoneuroendocrinology*, 28, 49, 2003.

85. Bucala, R., Neuroimmunomodulation by macrophage migration inhibitory factor (MIF), *Ann. NY Acad. Sci.*, 840, 74, 1998.

86. Donn, R.P. and Ray, D.W., Macrophage migration inhibitory factor: molecular, cellular and genetic aspects of a key neuroendocrine molecule, *J. Endocrinol.*, 182, 1, 2004.

87. Calandra, T. and Roger, T., Macrophage migration inhibitory factor: a regulator of innate immunity, *Nat. Rev. Immunol.*, 3, 791, 2003.

88. Calandra, T. et al., MIF as a glucocorticoid-induced modulator of cytokine production, *Nature*, 377, 68, 1995.

89. Bernhagen, J. et al., MIF is a pituitary-derived cytokine that potentiates lethal endotoxaemia, *Nature*, 365, 756, 1993.

90. Bernhagen, J. et al., An essential role for macrophage migration inhibitory factor in the tuberculin delayed-type hypersensitivity reaction, *J. Exp. Med.*, 183, 277, 1996.

91. Nishihira, J., Novel pathophysiological aspects of macrophage migration inhibitory factor (review), *Int. J. Mol. Med.*, 2, 17, 1998.

92. Rossi, A.G. et al., Human circulating eosinophils secrete macrophage migration inhibitory factor (MIF): potential role in asthma, *J. Clin. Invest.*, 101, 2869, 1998.

93. Leech, M. et al., Macrophage migration inhibitory factor in rheumatoid arthritis: evidence of proinflammatory function and regulation by glucocorticoids, *Arthritis Rheum.*, 42, 1601, 1999.

94. Calandra, T. et al., Protection from septic shock by neutralization of macrophage migration inhibitory factor, *Nat. Med.*, 6, 164, 2000.

95. Leech, M. et al., Regulation of macrophage migration inhibitory factor by endogenous glucocorticoids in rat adjuvant-induced arthritis, *Arthritis Rheum.*, 43, 827, 2000.

96. Abe, R. et al., Regulation of the CTL response by macrophage migration inhibitory factor, *J. Immunol.*, 166, 747, 2001.

97. Beishuizen, A. et al., Macrophage migration inhibitory factor and hypothalamo–pituitary–adrenal function during critical illness, *J. Clin. Endocrinol. Metab.*, 86, 2811, 2001.

98. Lehmann, L.E. et al., Plasma levels of macrophage migration inhibitory factor are elevated in patients with severe sepsis, *Intensive Care Med.*, 27, 1412, 2001.

99. Burger-Kentischer, A. et al., Expression of macrophage migration inhibitory factor in different stages of human atherosclerosis, *Circulation*, 105, 1561, 2002.

100. Ashcroft, G.S. et al., Estrogen modulates cutaneous wound healing by downregulating macrophage migration inhibitory factor, *J. Clin. Invest.*, 111, 1309, 2003.

101. Baugh, J.A. and Donnelly, S.C., Macrophage migration inhibitory factor: a neuroendocrine modulator of chronic inflammation, *J. Endocrinol.*, 179, 15, 2003.

102. Lai, K.N. et al., Role for macrophage migration inhibitory factor in acute respiratory distress syndrome, *J. Pathol.*, 199, 496, 2003.

103. Chen, Z. et al., Evidence for a role of macrophage migration inhibitory factor in vascular disease, *Arterioscler. Thromb. Vasc. Biol.*, 24, 709, 2004.

104. Ichiyama, H. et al., Inhibition of joint inflammation and destruction induced by anti-type II collagen antibody/lipopolysaccharide (LPS)-induced arthritis in mice due to deletion of macrophage migration inhibitory factor (MIF), *Cytokine*, 26, 187, 2004.

105. Nakamaru, Y. et al., Macrophage migration inhibitory factor in allergic rhinitis: its identification in eosinophils at the site of inflammation, *Ann. Otol. Rhinol. Laryngol.*, 113, 205, 2004.

106. Petrovsky, N. and Bucala, R., Macrophage migration inhibitory factor (MIF): a critical neurohumoral mediator, *Ann. NY Acad. Sci.*, 917, 665, 2000.

107. Nishino, T. et al., Localization of macrophage migration inhibitory factor (MIF) to secretory granules within the corticotrophic and thyrotrophic cells of the pituitary gland, *Mol. Med.*, 1, 781, 1995.

108. Waeber, G. et al., Transcriptional activation of the macrophage migration-inhibitory factor gene by the corticotropin-releasing factor is mediated by the cyclic adenosine 3',5'-monophosphate responsive element-binding protein CREB in pituitary cells, *Mol. Endocrinol.*, 12, 698, 1998.

109. Tierney, T. et al., Macrophage migration inhibitory factor is released from pituitary folliculo-stellate-like cells by endotoxin and dexamethasone and attenuates the steroid-induced inhibition of interleukin 6 release, *Endocrinology*, in press, 2004.

110. Fingerle-Rowson, G. et al., Regulation of macrophage migration inhibitory factor expression by glucocorticoids *in vivo*, *Am. J. Pathol.*, 162, 47, 2003.

111. Imamura, K. et al., Identification and immunohistochemical localization of macrophage migration inhibitory factor in human kidney, *Biochem. Mol. Biol. Int.*, 40, 1233, 1996.

112. Fingerle-Rowson, G.R. and Bucala, R., Neuroendocrine properties of macrophage migration inhibitory factor (MIF), *Immunol. Cell Biol.*, 79, 368, 2001.

113. Isidori, A.M. et al., Response of serum macrophage migration inhibitory factor levels to stimulation or suppression of the hypothalamo–pituitary–adrenal axis in normal subjects and patients with Cushing's disease, *J. Clin. Endocrinol. Metab.*, 87, 1834, 2002.

114. Petrovsky, N. et al., Macrophage migration inhibitory factor exhibits a pronounced circadian rhythm relevant to its role as a glucocorticoid counter-regulator, *Immunol. Cell Biol.*, 81, 137, 2003.

115. Beck, A.T., Steer, R.A., and Garbin, M.G., Psychometric properties of the Beck Depression Inventory: twenty-five years of evaluation, *Clin. Psychol. Rev.*, 8, 77, 1988.

116. van West, D. and Maes, M., Activation of the inflammatory response system: a new look at the etiopathogenesis of major depression, *Neuroendocrinol. Lett.*, 20, 11, 1999.

117. Yudkin, J.S. et al., Inflammation, obesity, stress and coronary heart disease: is interleukin-6 the link?, *Atherosclerosis*, 148, 209, 2000.

118. Engel, A. et al., Kinetics and correlation with body temperature of circulating interleukin-6, interleukin-8, tumor necrosis factor alpha and interleukin-1 beta in patients with fever and neutropenia, *Infection*, 22, 160, 1994.

119. Lenczowski, M. et al., Individual variation in hypothalamus-pituitary-adrenal responsiveness of rats to endotoxin and interleukin-1b, *Ann. NY Acad. Sci.*, 856, 139, 1998.

120. Roth, J. et al., Kinetics of systemic and intrahypothalamic IL-6 and tumor necrosis factor during endotoxin fever in guinea pigs, *Am. J. Physiol.*, 265, R653, 1993.

121. Luheshi, G.N. et al., Febrile response to tissue inflammation involves both peripheral and brain IL-1 and TNF-a in the rat, *Am. J. Physiol.*, 272, R862, 1997.

122. Barton, B., IL-6: Insights into novel biological activities, *Clin. Immunol. Immunopathol.*, 85, 16, 1997.

123. Barton, B., Shortall, J., and Jackson, J., Interleukins 6 and 11 protect mice from mortality in a staphylococcal enterotoxin-induced toxic shock model, *Infect. Immun.*, 64, 714, 1996.

124. Bethin, K., Vogt, S., and Muglia, L., Interleukin-6 is an essential, corticotropin-releasing hormone-independent stimulator of the adrenal axis during immune system activation, *Proc. Natl. Acad. Sci. USA*, 97, 9317, 2000.

125. Streetz, K.L. et al., Mediators of inflammation and acute phase response in the liver, *Cell. Mol. Biol.*, 47, 661, 2001.

126. Barton, B.E. and Jackson, J.V., Protective role of interleukin 6 in the lipopolysaccharide-galactosamine septic shock model, *Infect. Immun.*, 61, 1496, 1993.

127. Steptoe, A. et al., Inflammatory cytokines, socioeconomic status, and acute stress responsivity, *Brain Behav. Immun.*, 16, 774, 2002.

6 Stress, Cytokines, and Peripheral Analgesia

Peter John Cabot

CONTENTS

INTRODUCTION

Stress has been well documented to induce cytokine expression and evoke the release of cytokines and corticotropin releasing factor (CRF). Moreover, both stressful stimuli and cytokine release have a direct link to pain pathways and involvement in analgesia. The involvement in pain pathways exists in regions within the brain as well as peripheral tissues. Envisaged as a component of survival response, stress can evoke a potent analgesic effect, albeit short lived. Stress-induced analgesia (SIA) has in many models demonstrated an immediate and potent effect as well as roles for both opioid and non-opioid mediated mechanisms.[1,2] The basis for a non-opioid or opioid mechanism can be differentiated by the ability for antagonism by the opiate antagonist naloxone or sympathetic control.

This chapter describes the link between analgesia and stress, with particular emphasis on the involvement of the immune system in the analgesia associated with stress and cytokines. A number of excellent reviews cover parts only touched on in this review, such as central processes in stress-induced analgesia and non-opioid mechanisms in stress-evoked analgesia.[3,4]

STRESS EVENTS AND LINK TO ANALGESIA

In general, animals exposed to some forms of natural or manifested threatening stimuli will encounter reduced reactions to painful stimuli. These threatening stimuli vary widely and across many different strains and the reactions can be varied and complex.[5,6] In addition, SIA may differ between animals of the same species simply on the basis of its breeding source.[6] This provides some insight into the complexity of the interpretation of the experiments on stress evoked analgesia.

CENTRAL ROLE FOR STRESS-INDUCED ANALGESIA

A large body of work addresses the roles of receptor classes and central mechanisms involved in stress-induced analgesia. In general, the responses through the nervous and endocrine systems trigger signals to the hypothalamus that activate the autonomic nervous system,[3] leading to increased CRF and increases in the secretion of adrenocorticotropic hormone (ACTH) and endogenous opioids within the central nervous system (CNS).[4] Changes have been seen in analgesic effects with numerous stress initiators under many agonist- and antagonist-controlled studies. Gaba-ergic,[7] serotinergic,[8] and NMDA[5,9,10] pathways are certainly involved in both opioid- and non-opioid-related analgesia associated with stress. Antagonist-dependent effects have been documented and studies have postulated that stress is an indicator of the central link between pain pathways and thermoregulatory pathways.[11]

Regions throughout the brain have been also demonstrated to have differential involvement in analgesia resulting from stress. The rostral ventromedial medulla was shown to have altered effects in stressed as opposed to non-stressed animals in terms of tonic pain perception and responses to morphine.[12] Potent analgesia may be produced by electrical stimulation of medial brainstem sites which was cross-tolerant with opioid-dependent mechanisms produced by foot shock stress.[13] This did not occur with non-opioid elicitation of responses, albeit that non-opioid-induced analgesia was induced by electrical stimulation in the same medial brainstem sites. These findings were similar to an early study by the same group, showing that the opioid and non-opioid SIA emanated from the same brain centers.[14,15]

MODELS OF STRESS-INDUCED ANALGESIA

One of the most abundantly utilized stimuli for evoking SIA is forced swim stress. This method has variable outcomes based on swim duration, water depth, and water temperature.[16] The complexity of the response is due mostly to a mixture of the fear associated with the depth (or inability to stand) and the temperature of the pool. Lapo et al. (2003) demonstrated that the forced swim-evoked SIA is more predicted by a combination of the fear as well as the hypothermia than by either stimulus alone.[16] This was highlighted by comparison of repeated swims by freely swimming mice versus naive mice in shallow cold water, and allowing the mice to stand without fear associated to depth. The complexity in the cold forced swim stimuli is exposed in the responses to temperature as well.

The physical nature of SIA has been shown to vary with temperature of elicitation at the extremes of hot and cold for the stress event. For example, studies at 32°C have shown decreases in formalin (a noxious pain-producing agent) responses indicative of changes in tonic pain and evidence of analgesia.[17] Swim temperatures of 2°C showed a delay in onset of pain in response to formalin injection, but no change in response threshold.[9] With similar cold swim stress models, albeit different inflammatory pain induction, compounds such as Freund's complete adjuvant (FCA) and carrageenan resulted in pronounced analgesia. Indeed, rats with FCA-induced inflammation showed potent but short-lived opioid-dependent analgesic responses.[18,19] Analgesia from swim stress (0°C to 4°C) has shown distinct peripheral mechanisms of opioid peptide release and action at peripheral opioid receptors.[20] A number of studies described this result.[18,20,21] These researchers rationalize that the SIA is due in part to the accumulation of opioid-containing immune cells within inflamed tissue as the major source for opioid peptide within the inflamed tissue.[18,20,21] The release and subsequent analgesia associated with opioid-containing immune cells will be discussed in more detail below.

Foot shock-evoked analgesia has similarly shown strain dependence among other parameters in eliciting SIA. Charles River SD rats showed predominance of non-naloxone-antagonized SIA as compared to Long Evans and Holtzman SD rats that both had SIA antagonized by naloxone; all were inhibited by naltrexone, an alternative opioid receptor antagonist to naloxone.[6] This finding highlighted the opioid-dependent pathways as having a major role in SIA, but identified unusual differences in reactivity to the specific opioid antagonists.[22] It is commonly assumed that stimulation of non-opioid or opioid analgesia or both is associated with shock parameters, region of the body shocked, age, and strain. These were significant as they highlight a problem in utilizing one antagonist in defining opioid action in SIA, which is the usual scenario for defining an opioid or non-opioid role in SIA.

Another paradigm for the induction of SIA is a forced walk. Similar to cold water swim stress and foot shock-evoked SIA, there is a degree of controversy related to the bases of opioid or non-opioid SIA. Moreover, forced walk SIA opioid or non-opioid nature appears to be dependent on the duration of the walk as well as the antagonist utilized for defining the mechanism.[23] Interestingly, age was also shown to be a confounding factor, with mice at 4, 24, and 48 weeks differing in SIA.[10] Many other methods for producing SIA, for example, food restriction,[24] predator threat,[6] and auditory stimulus,[25] have shown varying degrees of opioid and non-opioid involvement in SIA.

It is plausible that both opioid and non-opioid mechanisms as defined by antagonists are in fact at times related but independent of each other under certain experimental conditions. For instance, NMDA receptor action is know to affect the outcome of opioid action, heavily documented in studies on reward and dependence but also evident in pain.[26] It is clear that there must be separate mechanisms in some forms of evoked SIA, as cross tolerance has been shown to not exist between the opioid and non-opioid forms.[27]

OPIOIDS IN INFLAMMATION IN THE PERIPHERY: ROLE FOR IMMUNE SYSTEM

A large amount of evidence has been accumulated for the local action of opioids within inflamed tissue. Evidence demonstrates the presence of precursor genes and subsequent peptides of all three classes of endogenous opioid peptides in immune cells that reside in inflamed tissue. Through this mechanism, these events have a powerful influence over opioid action within peripheral tissues. These infiltrating immune cells provide endogenous opioid peptides that act at local receptors to reduce pain.[28]

Knockout mice have provided additional insight into the roles of opioids in SIA. Mice that lack the prodynorphin gene did not show SIA as a result of potentiation of cocaine placement preference. This was confirmed by blockade by the nor-BNI kappa opioid antagonist in wild-type mice.[29] Similarly, delta opioid receptor action in SIA has been isolated by both specific antagonism by selective antagonists such as naltrindole and confirmation in receptor knockout models.[30] The next section will focus on the role of the immune system through directed infiltration into sites of inflammation and the subsequent release of opioids from these immune cells under stress and in the presence of cytokines.

INFLAMMATION AND IMMUNE CELL RECRUITMENT

A major component of the reaction to inflammatory challenge is the increased expression and accumulation of cytokines in inflamed tissue. Cytokines have an integral role in all aspects of initiation, cell adhesion, and repair in inflammatory challenge. This section will briefly describe the cell infiltration process with an emphasis on lymphocyte migration. A major source for cytokines within inflamed tissue is from infiltrating immune cells in addition to the endothelium. Infiltrating immune cells accumulate in inflamed or injured tissue as a part of the host defense mechanism and circulate through collecting ducts to localized lymph nodes that drain from the tissue.

Leukocyte homing in general is a multi-step process involving the sequential activation of various adhesion molecules located on immune cells and on the vascular endothelium.[31,32] The homing patterns of lymphocyte subsets differ and can be explained by their reaction to distinct combinations of molecular signals that are mediated by active mechanisms of lymphocyte — endothelial cell recognition via cell adhesion molecules.[31,32]

Endothelial cells express immune cell-adhesion molecules (CAMs) that play a direct role in lymphocyte migration.[31,32] Circulating immune cells express CAMs either constitutively or in response to local concentrations of cytokines produced during an inflammatory response. An immune cell in its transition from a naive status may undergo many changes in CAM expression on the path to a recirculating memory-type cell.

Adhesion and extravasation of lymphocytes occur through several sequential steps: (1) rolling, (2) activation by chemoattractant stimulus, (3) arrest and adhesion, and (4) transendothelial migration.[32,33] During an inflammatory response, cytokines and other mediators act upon the local endothelium, inducing the expression of selectins and other chemoattractants. Immune cells attach loosely to the endothelium by a low affinity selectin — carbohydrate interaction, for example, P- and E-selectin molecules on the endothelium bind to cutaneous lymphocyte-associated antigen (CLA) or mucin-like CAMs on lymphocytes.[32,34] This primary adhesion tethers the lymphocyte briefly, thus allowing sufficient time for it to sample the vessel for soluble or endothelial surface pro-adhesive factors required for the latter steps.[34]

The immune cell slows and rolls along the endothelial membrane; it can be activated by cytokines such as interleukin-1 (IL-1) or tumor necrosis factor-alpha (TNF-alpha) that are expressed intrinsically in the endothelium or are secreted locally by other inflammatory cells.[35] Binding of these cytokines to G-protein-coupled receptors on the lymphocyte leads to activation of integrins such as LFA-1 on the membrane. Activation leads to a conformational change in integrin molecules such as ICAM-1, resulting in a strong adhesion to the endothelium. In fact, it has been shown that infiltrating immune cells may avoid the selectin migration step and are slowed and tethered through integrins alone.[33]

The molecular mechanisms involved in the final step, transendothelial migration, are poorly understood. The same integrins involved in lymphocyte arrest on endothelium are also involved in this final process.[35] Hence, lymphocyte extravasation depends on the surface charges of the interacting cells, the hemodynamic shear force in the vascular bed, and the expression of complementary sets of adhesion molecules on both the lymphocytes and the endothelium. These factors serve to bring different migratory behaviors to different subsets of lymphocytes.

PERIPHERAL OPIOID ACTION AND STRESS-INDUCED ANALGESIA IN INFLAMMATION

Stress has been shown to alter the prodynorphin, proenkephalin, and pro-opiomelanocortin (POMC) expression,[36-39] the resultant peptides (dynorphins, enkephalins, and endorphins), and the three classes of opioid receptors at which they act (mu, delta, and kappa).[40-42] Ultimately, a stress event will increase opioid peptide production and release both in the central and peripheral nervous systems. The role of both central and peripheral opioid mechanisms cannot be easily dissociated by the use of typical antagonists such as naloxone or naltrexone.[16] These antagonists will block both central and peripheral mechanisms at systemic doses. The differentiation has been achieved more readily with quaternary antagonists such as naloxone methiodide. These are utilized to describe peripheral effects due to their limited ability to cross the blood–brain barrier as they are ionized at physiological pH.

A clear peripheral role for opioids in inflammatory pain has been demonstrated through immune-derived opioid action. Immune-derived release of endogenous opioid peptides has been shown to evoke potent analgesic responses in rats with FCA-induced inflammation of the hind paw. Local inflammatory factors such as CRF, IL-1, TNF-alpha,[43] and IL-6[43] when injected into the inflamed paw produced potent analgesia.[19] This CRF- and IL-1-induced analgesic response was produced only when injected by the intraplantar route; when equivalent doses were given by the intravenous route, there was no evidence of an analgesic effect.[21] The analgesic effect appeared to be mediated by both cytokine and CRF receptors within the tissue as selective antagonists blocked the analgesia completely. Furthermore, this cytokine- and CRF-evoked analgesia was inhibited by a locally applied specific antibodies to beta-endorphin (END), methionine enkephalin (MET), dynorphin-A (DYN),[21,44] and by specific and selective antagonists to the three major classes of opioid receptors. This strongly suggests that opioids mediate this analgesic response directly within the inflamed tissue and the effects are directly coupled to local inflammatory mediators present within inflamed tissue.

In addition to peripheral analgesia evoked by intraplantar CRF and IL-1, cold water swim stress can also evoke potent peripheral analgesia in the inflamed paws of FCA-treated rats.[21,44,45] This stress-induced analgesic effect is also blocked by specific CRF antibodies, selective CRF antagonists, and antisense oligodeoxynucle-otides for CRF.[19,21,44,46,47] Analgesic effects were not evident within non-inflamed paws and not affected by CRF blockade. These findings clearly identify opioid peptides as potent local analgesic compounds released by activation of CRF receptors in inflamed tissue.

OPIOID PRESENCE IN IMMUNE CELLS

Opioids are expressed and released from immune cells within inflamed tissue.[48] Substantial evidence has been gathered for the presence of opioid peptides within immune cells.[44,49-51] Even though END derived from POMC has been shown to be expressed in the highest quantity in immune cells, peptides from proenkephalin such as MET and prodynorphin-producing DYN have also been identified in immune cells.[52] Our studies have shown that both END and mRNA encoding its POMC precursor are present in immune cells.[44] Many researchers have reported truncated and full length mRNA transcripts for POMC in activated immunocytes[53-55] as well as the resultant peptides. The role of truncated precursor proteins has yet to be determined, but is speculated to still produce active peptides, albeit there may be some differences in expression of the peptides.[56-58]

Consistent with an alteration in pain responses in disease, opioid peptide precursor proteins and mRNA are increased in circulating immune cells. Lymphocytes of rats that had FCA-induced inflammation of the hind paw had pronounced increases in POMC mRNA.[44] Moreover, lymphocytes that had not migrated through inflamed tissue had increases in END content and were identified to be predominantly memory type T-cells.[44,59] Numerous immune cells express and contain opioid peptides. Early stages of inflammation have been characterized as predominantly opioid-containing granulocytes with monocytes and macrophages predominating later in the disease cascade.[60] Numbers of infiltrating immune cells showed a direct correlation with analgesia due to cold water swim stress.

Production of opioid peptides in immunocytes is inherently linked to the activation of immune cells, for instance, incubation of lymphocytes with the T-cell mitogen known as concanavalin-A activates T-cells, thereby inducing an increase in the production of opioid peptides and their precursor messages.[54,61] The regulation of expression is bidirectional for opioids and cytokines. Not only does the regulation of opioid precursor message occur in immunocytes, but opioids also regulate cytokine expression. Increased expression of IL-1-beta and TNF-alpha was shown to correlate with proenkephalin expression in leukocytes in inflammation.[62] A direct action has also been shown for IL-4 and IL-10 on human PBMC for proenkephalin expression.[63]

Opioid receptors also exist on these immune cells,[64,65] although their role in peripheral analgesia is as yet undiscovered.[66] However, they may have indirect effects because they regulate expression of cytokines and modulate immune cell function.[67,68] Immunosuppression may even be an outcome of acute dosing as opposed to chronic opioid use.[69]

RELEASE OF IMMUNE-DERIVED OPIOIDS

The release of END from immunocytes by local inflammatory factors such as CRF, adrenergics,[70] and cytokines have been extensively studied.[18,19,21,71,72] Recent studies have shown that lymphocytes collected from rats with inflamed paws exhibit dose-dependent release of END evoked by CRF and IL-1. This effect was dose dependently antagonized by specific antagonists, alpha-helical CRF, and IL-1 receptor antagonist, respectively. END release was higher from the non-inflamed lymph nodes (LNs), which correlated with higher content of END in the non-inflamed LNs. Circulating lymphocytes did not release significant amounts of END. This is consistent with the finding that only a small portion of these cells contain END. Importantly, CRF and IL-1 release of END from immune cells was calcium-dependent and was evoked by increasing potassium concentrations. These findings strongly suggested that END is released from vesicles, similar to vesicular release of END from nerve terminals[44] (see Figure 6.1).

The release of END from lymphocytes was mirrored for MET and DYN in subsequent studies. These opioid peptides revealed a unique difference in release profiles. MET was released through a dose-dependent mechanism by the cytokine IL-1 which was antagonized by IL-ra. However, MET was not released from lymphocytes by CRF.[52] In contrast, IL-1 did not release DYN, but was dose dependently released by CRF. This was different from END and demonstrated a differential role for cytokines and inflammatory factors in mediating pain responses. Importantly, these findings correlated directly with pain responses. Antibodies to MET had no effect on CRF-induced analgesia yet blocked IL-1, while antibodies against DYN blocked CRF induced analgesia but not IL-1.[21,52]

LYMPHOCYTE TRAFFICKING AND ITS ROLE IN PERIPHERAL ANALGESIA

It is clear from studies that lymphocyte trafficking plays an important role not only in the augmentation of inflammation but as the limiting factor in initiation of peripheral analgesia via this mechanism. Activated lymphocytes have increased expression of opioid peptides and home preferentially to the injured tissue where they secrete opioids to reduce pain.[48,73–75] However, the mechanisms underlying the migration of opioid-containing immunocytes to inflamed tissue have only recently begun to be investigated.

The blockade of selectins with fucoidin, a glycoprotein found in some seaweeds, has been demonstrated to inhibit lymphocyte adhesion to endothelium. Reduced adhesion results in a marked reduction in lymphocyte infiltration and a significant

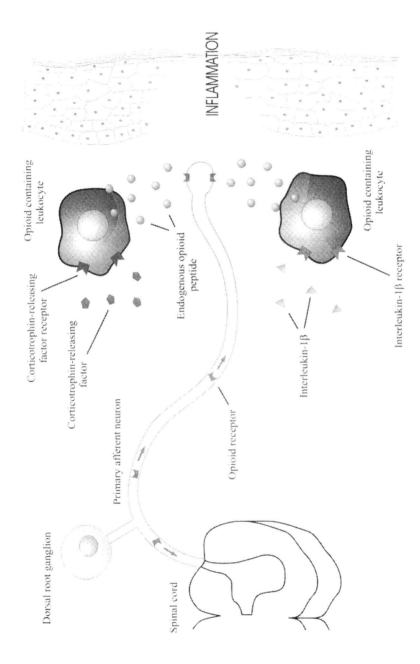

FIGURE 6.1 Immune infiltration in localized inflammation, followed by stress and cytokine-evoked release of opioid peptides close to peripheral sensory nerve fibres. (Illustration by Daniel Kapitzke.)

decrease in the presence of END-containing lymphocytes within inflamed paw tissue.[75] Consistent with this change in END-containing lymphocyte numbers in inflamed tissue, CRF- and stress-induced analgesia was also significantly lowered as was the amount of END available for producing an analgesic response.[75] More recently, this group has shown a link to specific adhesion molecules blocked by fucoidin, and demonstrated co-expression of opioid peptides with adhesion molecules L-selectin and P-selectin on immune cells.[74] It seems to be selective to only a limited group of adhesion molecules which has implications for immunoregulatory and antiinflammatory therapy.[73]

Opioids themselves have an immunosuppressive or immune cell modulating capability. Mu-opioid receptors have been shown to be inherently involved in lymphocyte apoptosis as a consequence of psychological stress.[76] Restraint stress over 12 days showed marked inhibition of lymphocyte proliferation, IL-2, and IFN-gamma production which was not evident in MOR knockout mice. This is consistent with numerous reports of reduced lymphocyte proliferation in patients on opioid therapy[69] and the direct involvement for opioid receptors on immune cells acting as immune modulators.[77] However, there may be some desensitization of these effects because these factors are not evident in long-term users of opioids.[69] Opioid addicts had similar numbers of immune cell populations but, importantly, showed reduced cytokine production, which had an impact on activation-induced apoptosis of the lymphocytes.[78] Similarly, morphine and ketarolac reduced IL-6 blood levels after 2 days of treament[79] and reduced IL-6 within wounds directly after surgery.[80]

IMMUNOSUPPRESSION, STRESS, AND IMMUNE-DERIVED ANALGESIA

The greatest body of work in this area concentrates on the immunosuppressive actions of opioids. Acute opioid therapy has been repeatedly demonstrated to result in reduce cell proliferation and suppression of immune cell responses.[69] Moreover, stress has been well associated through opioid induced mechanisms to induce an immunosuppressive response that can be blocked by opioid antagonists such as naltrexone.[81,82] Swim stress has been shown to reduce IL-1 and TNF-alpha,[83] which would account for reduced immune cell activity and a reduction in opioid-releasing ability from immune cells in response to stress, yet to be proven.

In addition to an opioid role in stress-induced immunosuppression, reports suggest that immunocompromised patients experience increased pain associated with disease or injury.[84] An association has been made between increased sensitivity to pain and disease status. This is emphasized in patients suffering from either AIDS or cancer.[85-88] In these reviews of treatment paradigms, under-treatment of pain was commonly identified.[87,89] A more direct link between immune system function and pain in patient groups was seen with increased pain due to poly-neuropathy as correlated to a reduction in CD4+ cell numbers in AIDS patients.[90] Similarly, HIV/AIDS patients suffering increased stress also suffered increased pain scores. Whether this corresponds to inflammatory pain was not investigated.[91]

Consistent with these findings, reductions in lymphocyte numbers resulting from cyclosporin-A-induced immunosuppression produced complete inhibition of IL-1, CRF-induced, and stress-induced analgesia in studies on rats.[21,44] More recently, our studies have shown an increase in baseline nociceptive thresholds with cyclosporin-A-induced immunosuppression.[66] This has been combined with low levels of END in inflamed tissue and reduced infiltration as a result of reduced immunocyte function. Importantly, this was reversed with a single bolus injection of donor concanavalin-A-stimulated lymphocytes. These findings clearly demonstrate the importance of the immune system in pain and highlight the need for further research.

REFERENCES

1. Lewis, J.W., J.T. Cannon, and J.C. Liebeskind, Opioid and nonopioid mechanisms of stress analgesia. *Science*, 1980. 208: 623–625.
2. Lewis, J.W., et al., Opioid and non-opioid mechanisms of foot shock-induced analgesia: role of the spinal dorsolateral funiculus. *Brain Res*, 1983. 267(1): 139–144.
3. Yamada, K. and T. Nabeshima, Stress-induced behavioral responses and multiple opioid systems in the brain. *Behav Brain Res*, 1995. 67(2): 133–145.
4. Amit, Z. and Z.H. Galina, Stress-induced analgesia plays an adaptive role in the organization of behavioral responding. *Brain Res Bull*, 1988. 21(6): 955–958.
5. Vendruscolo, L.F., F.A. Pamplona, and R.N. Takahashi, Strain and sex differences in the expression of nociceptive behavior and stress-induced analgesia in rats. *Brain Res*, 2004. 1030(2): 277–283.
6. Helmstetter, F.J. and M.S. Fanselow, Strain differences in reversal of conditional analgesia by opioid antagonists. *Behav Neurosci*, 1987. 101(5): 735–737.
7. Tokuyama, S., M. Takahashi, and H. Kaneto, Participation of GABAergic systems in the production of antinociception by various stresses in mice. *Jpn J Pharmacol*, 1992. 60(2): 105–110.
8. Tokuyama, S., M. Takahashi, and H. Kaneto, Involvement of serotonergic receptor subtypes in the production of antinociception by psychological stress in mice. *Jpn J Pharmacol*, 1993. 61(3): 237–242.
9. Fuchs, N., B. Kerr, and R. Melzack, Delayed nociceptive response following cold-water swim in the formalin test: possible mechanisms of action. *Exp Neurol*, 1996. 139(2): 291–298.
10. Onodera, K., et al., Age-related differences in forced walking stress-induced analgesia in mice. *Drugs Exp Clin Res*, 2001. 27: 193–198.
11. Benedek, G. and M. Szikszay, Sensitization or tolerance to morphine effects after repeated stresses. *Prog Neuropsychopharmacol Biol Psychiatr*, 1985. 9(4): 369–380.
12. Mitchell, J.M., D. Lowe, and H.L. Fields, The contribution of the rostral ventromedial medulla to the antinociceptive effects of systemic morphine in restrained and unre-strained rats. *Neuroscience*, 1998. 87(1): 123–133.
13. Terman, G.W., E.R. Penner, and J.C. Liebeskind, Stimulation-produced and stress-induced analgesia: cross-tolerance between opioid forms. *Brain Res*, 1985. 360: 374–378.
14. Cannon, J.T., et al., Evidence for opioid and non-opioid forms of stimulation-pro-duced analgesia in the rat. *Brain Res*, 1982. 243(2): 315–321.
15. Cannon, J.T. and J.C. Liebeskind, Analgesic effects of electrical brain stimulation and stress: brain stem mechanisms. *Pain Headache*, 1987. 9: 283–294.

16. Lapo, I.B., M. Konarzewski, and B. Sadowski, Analgesia induced by swim stress: interaction between analgesic and thermoregulatory mechanisms. *Pflugers Arch*, 2003. 446(4): 463–469.

17. Vaccarino, A.L., P. Marek, and J.C. Liebeskind, Stress-induced analgesia prevents the development of the tonic, late phase of pain produced by subcutaneous formalin. *Brain Res*, 1992. 572: 250–252.

18. Binder, W., et al., Sympathetic activation triggers endogenous opioid release and analgesia within peripheral inflamed tissue. *Eur J Neurosci*, 2004. 20: 92–100.

19. Schafer, M., et al., Expression of corticotropin-releasing factor in inflamed tissue is required for intrinsic peripheral opioid analgesia. *Proc Natl Acad Sci USA*, 1996. 93: 6096–6100.

20. Stein, C., et al., Opioids from immunocytes interact with receptors on sensory nerves to inhibit nociception in inflammation. *Proc Natl Acad Sci USA*, 1990. 87(1): 5935–5939.

21. Schafer, M., L. Carter, and C. Stein, Interleukin-1-beta and corticotropin-releasing factor inhibit pain by releasing opioids from immune cells in inflamed tissue. *Proc Natl Acad Sci USA*, 1994. 91(10): 4219–4223.

22. Urca, G., S. Segev, and Y. Sarne, Stress induced analgesia: its opioid nature depends on the strain of rat but not on the mode of induction. *Brain Res*, 1985. 343(2): 216–222.

23. Onodera, K., et al., Differential involvement of opioid receptors in stress-induced antinociception caused by repeated exposure to forced walking stress in mice. *Pharmacology*, 2000. 61(2): 96–100.

24. Wideman, C.H., H.M. Murphy, and S.B. McCartney, Interactions between vasopressin and food restriction on stress-induced analgesia. *Peptides*, 1996. 17(1): 63–66.

25. Helmstetter, F.J. and S. Bellgowan, Hypoalgesia in response to sensitization during acute noise stress. *Behav Neurosci*, 1994. 108(1): 177–185.

26. Lee, H.J., et al., Intracisternal NMDA produces analgesia in the orofacial formalin test of freely moving rats. *Prog Neuropsychopharmacol Biol Psychiatry*, 2004. 28(3): 497–503.

27. Terman, G.W., J.W. Lewis, and J.C. Liebeskind, Opioid and non-opioid mechanisms of stress analgesia: lack of cross-tolerance between stressors. *Brain Res*, 1983. 260(1): 147–150.

28. Janson, W. and C. Stein, Peripheral opioid analgesia. *Curr Pharm Biotechnol*, 2003. 4(4): 270–274.

29. McLaughlin, J., M. Marton-Popovici, and C. Chavkin, Kappa opioid receptor antagonism and prodynorphin gene disruption block stress-induced behavioral responses. *J Neurosci*, 2003. 23(13): 5674–5683.

30. LaBuda, C.J., et al., Stress-induced analgesia in mu-opioid receptor knockout mice reveals normal function of the delta-opioid receptor system. *Brain Res*, 2000. 869: 1–5.

31. Hunt, S.W., 3rd, et al., T-lymphocyte interactions with endothelium and extracellular matrix. *Crit Rev Oral Biol Med*, 1996. 7(1): 59–86.

32. Mackay, C.R. and B.A. Imhof, Cell adhesion in the immune system. *Immunol Today*, 1993. 14(3): 99–102.

33. Mackay, C., Lymphocyte migration: a new spin on lymphocyte homing. *Curr Biol*, 1995. 5(7): 733–736.

34. Santamaria, L.F., et al., Allergen specificity and endothelial transmigration of T cells in allergic contact dermatitis and atopic dermatitis are associated with the cutaneous lymphocyte antigen. *Int Arch Allergy Immunol*, 1995. 107: 359–362.

35. Mackay, C.R. and U.H. von Andrian, Immunology. Memory T cells: local heroes in the struggle for immunity. *Science*, 2001. 291: 2323–2324.

36. Watanabe, Y., N.G. Weiland, and B.S. McEwen, Effects of adrenal steroid manipulations and repeated restraint stress on dynorphin mRNA levels and excitatory amino acid receptor binding in hippocampus. *Brain Res*, 1995. 680: 217–225.

37. Harbuz, M., et al., Rapid changes in the content of proenkephalin A and corticotrophin releasing hormone mRNAs in the paraventricular nucleus during morphine withdrawal in urethane-anaesthetized rats. *Brain Res Mol Brain Res*, 1991. 9(4): 285–291.

38. Zhou, Y., et al., Hypothalamic–pituitary–adrenal activity and pro-opiomelanocortin mRNA levels in the hypothalamus and pituitary of the rat are differentially modulated by acute intermittent morphine with or without water restriction stress. *J Endocrinol*, 1999. 163(2): 261–267.

39. Wiedenmayer, C., et al., Stress-induced preproenkephalin mRNA expression in the amygdala changes during early ontogeny in the rat. *Neuroscience*, 2002. 114(1): 7–11.

40. Nikulina, E.M., et al., Social defeat stress increases expression of mu-opioid receptor mRNA in rat ventral tegmental area. *Neuroreport*, 1999. 10(14): 3015–3019.

41. Mantione, K., et al., Effects of cold stress on morphine-induced nitric oxide production and mu-opiate receptor gene expression in *Mytilus edulis* pedal ganglia. *Neuroendocrinol Lett*, 2003. 24: 68–72.

42. Cadet, J. et al., Cold stress alters *Mytilus edulis* pedal ganglia expression of mu opiate receptor transcripts determined by real-time RT-PCR and morphine levels. *Brain Res Mol Brain Res*, 2002. 99(1): 26–33.

43. Czlonkowski, A., C. Stein, and A. Herz, Peripheral mechanisms of opioid antinociception in inflammation: involvement of cytokines. *Eur J Pharmacol*, 1993. 242(3): 229–235.

44. Cabot, J., et al., Immune cell-derived beta-endorphin: production, release, and control of inflammatory pain in rats. *J Clin Invest*, 1997. 100(1): 142–148.

45. Mousa, S.A., et al., Involvement of corticotropin-releasing hormone receptor subtypes 1 and 2 in peripheral opioid-mediated inhibition of inflammatory pain. *Pain*, 2003. 106(3): 297–307.

46. Schafer, M., S.A. Mousa, and C. Stein, Corticotropin-releasing factor in antinociception and inflammation. *Eur J Pharmacol*, 1997. 323(1): 1–10.

47. Mousa, S.A., et al., Local upregulation of corticotropin-releasing hormone and interleukin-1 receptors in rats with painful hindlimb inflammation. *Eur J Pharmacol*, 1996. 311: 221–231.

48. Mousa, S.A., Morphological correlates of immune-mediated peripheral opioid analgesia. *Adv Exp Med Biol*, 2003. 521: 77–87.

49. Likar, R., et al., Increased numbers of opioid expressing inflammatory cells do not affect intra-articular morphine analgesia. *Br J Anaesth*, 2004. 93(3): 375–380.

50. Mousa, S.A., et al., Subcellular pathways of beta-endorphin synthesis, processing, and release from immunocytes in inflammatory pain. *Endocrinology*, 2004. 145(3): 1331–1341.

51. Przewlocki, R., et al., Gene expression and localization of opioid peptides in immune cells of inflamed tissue: functional role in antinociception. *Neuroscience*, 1992. 48(2): 491–500.

52. Cabot, J., et al., Methionine, enkephalin, and dynorphin A-release from immune cells and control of inflammatory pain. *Pain*, 2001. 93(3): 207–212.

53. Wajs, E., E. Kutoh, and D. Gupta, Melatonin affects pro-opiomelanocortin gene expression in the immune organs of the rat. *Eur J Endocrinol*, 1995. 133(6): 754–760.

54. Linner, K.M., H.E. Quist, and B.M. Sharp, Expression and function of proenkephalin A messenger ribonucleic acid in murine fetal thymocytes. *Endocrinology*, 1996. 137(3): 857–863.

55. Sharp, B. and K. Linner, What do we know about the expression of proopiomelanocortin transcripts and related peptides in lymphoid tissue? *Endocrinology*, 1993. 133(5): 1921A–1921B.

56. Lyons, D. and J.E. Blalock, Pro-opiomelanocortin gene expression and protein processing in rat mononuclear leukocytes. *J Neuroimmunol*, 1997. 78: 47–56.

57. Blalock, J.E., Proopiomelanocortin and the immune-neuroendocrine connection. *Ann NY Acad Sci*, 1999. 885: 161–172.

58. Blalock, J.E., Natural painkillers. *Nat Med*, 1997. 3(12): 1302.

59. Mousa, S.A., et al., Beta-endorphin-containing memory cells and mu-opioid receptors undergo transport to peripheral inflamed tissue. *J Neuroimmunol*, 2001. 115: 71–78.

60. Rittner, H.L., et al., Opioid peptide-expressing leukocytes: identification, recruitment, and simultaneously increasing inhibition of inflammatory pain. *Anesthesiology*, 2001. 95(2): 500–508.

61. Manfredi, B., et al., Age-related changes in mitogen-induced beta-endorphin release from human peripheral blood mononuclear cells. *Peptides*, 1995. 16(4): 699–706.

62. Chadzinska, M., et al., Expression of proenkephalin (PENK) mRNA in inflammatory leukocytes during experimental peritonitis in Swiss mice. *Pol J Pharmacol*, 2001. 53(6): 715–718.

63. Kamphuis, S., et al., Role of endogenous pro-enkephalin A-derived peptides in human T cell proliferation and monocyte IL-6 production. *J Neuroimmunol*, 1998. 84(1): 53–60.

64. Carr, D.J., et al., Opioid receptors on cells of the immune system: evidence for delta- and kappa-classes. *J Endocrinol*, 1989. 122(1): 161–168.

65. Carr, D.J., et al., Anti-opioid receptor antibody recognition of a binding site on brain and leukocyte opioid receptors. *Neuroendocrinology*, 1990. 51(5): 552–560.

66. Hermanussen, S., M. Do, and J. Cabot, Reduction of beta-endorphin-containing immune cells in inflamed paw tissue corresponds with a reduction in immune-derived antinociception: reversible by donor activated lymphocytes. *Anesth Analg*, 2004. 98(3): 723–729.

67. Shavit, Y., et al., Effects of a single administration of morphine or foot shock stress on natural killer cell cytotoxicity. *Brain Behav Immun*, 1987. 1(4): 318–328.

68. Carr, D.J., et al., Opioid modulation of immunoglobulin production by lymphocytes isolated from Peyer's patches and spleen. *Ann NY Acad Sci*, 1992. 650: 125–127.

69. Vallejo, R., O. de Leon-Casasola, and R. Benyamin, Opioid therapy and immunosuppression: a review. *Am J Ther*, 2004. 11(5): 354–365.

70. Kavelaars, A., R.E. Ballieux, and C.J. Heijnen, *In vitro* beta-adrenergic stimulation of lymphocytes induces the release of immunoreactive beta-endorphin. *Endocrinology*, 1990. 126(6): 3028–3032.

71. Stein, C., Opioid receptors on peripheral sensory neurons. *Adv Exp Med Biol*, 2003. 521: 69–76.

72. Cabot, J., Immune-derived opioids and peripheral antinociception. *Clin Exp Pharmacol Physiol*, 2001. 28(3): 230–232.

73. Machelska, H., et al., Selectins and integrins but not platelet-endothelial cell adhesion molecule-1 regulate opioid inhibition of inflammatory pain. *Br J Pharmacol*, 2004. 142(4): 772–780.

74. Mousa, S.A., et al., Co-expression of beta-endorphin with adhesion molecules in a model of inflammatory pain. *J Neuroimmunol*, 2000. 108: 160–170.

75. Machelska, H., et al., Pain control in inflammation governed by selectins. *Nat Med*, 1998. 4(12): 1425–1428.

76. Wang, J., et al., Mu-opioid receptor mediates chronic restraint stress-induced lymphocyte apoptosis. *J Immunol*, 2002. 169(7): 3630–3636.

77. Sharp, B.M., Opioid receptor expression and intracellular signaling by cells involved in host defense and immunity. *Adv Exp Med Biol*, 2003. 521: 98–105.

78. Sibiryak, S.V., et al., The immune status and lymphocyte apoptosis in opioid addicts. *Russ J Immunol*, 2001. 6(3): 281–290.

79. Kim, M.H. and T.S. Hahm, Plasma levels of interleukin-6 and interleukin-10 are affected by ketorolac as an adjunct to patient-controlled morphine after abdominal hysterectomy. *Clin J Pain*, 2001. 17(1): 72–77.

80. Eriksson-Mjoberg, M., et al., Infiltration of morphine into an abnormal wound; effects on pain relief and endocrine/immune response. *Pain*, 1997. 73(3): 355–360.

81. Shavit, Y., et al., Endogenous opioids may mediate the effects of stress on tumor growth and immune function. *Proc West Pharmacol Soc*, 1983. 26: 53–56.

82. Terman, G.W., et al., Intrinsic mechanisms of pain inhibition: activation by stress. *Science*, 1984. 226: 1270–1277.

83. Connor, T.J., et al., Acute stress suppresses pro-inflammatory cytokines TNF-alpha and IL-1beta independent of a catecholamine-driven increase in IL-10 production. *J Neuroimmunol*, 2005. 159: 119–128.

84. Merine, D.S., et al., Right lower quadrant pain in the immunocompromised patient: CT findings in 10 cases. *Am J Roentgenol*, 1987. 149(6): 1177–1179.

85. Brady, A., et al., Pain management guidelines: implications for managed care: a roundtable discussion. *Med Interface*, 1997. Suppl: 10–32.

86. Lefkowitz, M., Pain management for the AIDS patient. *J Fla Med Assoc*, 1996. 83(10): 701–704.

87. Lebovits, A.H., et al., Pain in hospitalized patients with AIDS: analgesic and psychotropic medications. *Clin J Pain*, 1994. 10(2): 156–161.

88. Wyatt, S.H. and E.K. Fishman, The acute abdomen in individuals with AIDS. *Radiol Clin North Am*, 1994. 32(5): 1023–1043.

89. Breitbart, W., et al., Patient-related barriers to pain management in ambulatory AIDS patients. *Pain*, 1998. 76: 9–16.

90. Hewitt, D.J., et al., Pain syndromes and etiologies in ambulatory AIDS patients. *Pain*, 1997. 70: 117–123.

91. Smith, M.Y., et al., The impact of PTSD on pain experience in persons with HIV/AIDS. *Pain*, 2002. 98: 9–17.

7 Alexithymia, Stress, and Immunity

Olivier Guilbaud, Maurice Corcos, and Philippe Jeammet

CONTENTS

INTRODUCTION

The goal of this chapter is to appreciate the relationships between a specific cognitive emotional processing style characterized by an intellectual inability to identify and verbalize emotional feelings (alexithymia) and its impact on immunity. The impact of stress on immunity has obviously been detailed, but little is known about this specific impaired emotional regulation style and its impact on immune response.

Considering the relationship between negative emotions and immunity, we will then provide a description of alexithymia. After a brief review of the literature on alexithymia and stress and immunity, we will present a psychoneuroendocrinoimmunological pathway linking alexithymia and the characteristics of the immune response of chronic stressors.

EMOTIONAL PROCESSING AND IMMUNE RESPONSE

Several studies have related psychological characteristics, behaviors, and emotions to onset and progression of diseases including allergies, asthma, peptic ulcers, autoimmune diseases, and so-called psychosomatic disorders. However, the biological mechanisms mediating these changes remain poorly understood and the links between emotional states and the onset of organic disease are still controversial.

What is best known is the effect of stress on immunity. It is well known that psychological stress can down-regulate various aspects of the cellular immune response. Recent evidence indicates that acute stress and chronic stress inhibit the type 1 pro-inflammatory cytokines and stimulate the production of type 2 anti-inflammatory cytokines. Through this mechanism, endogenous catecholamines may systematically cause a selective suppression of Th1 responses and a Th2 shift toward dominance of humoral immunity. This could constitute a feedback loop mechanism protecting the organism from an "overshoot" of pro-inflammatory cytokines and other products of activated macrophages with tissue-damaging potential. However, the results of these studies are sometimes contradictory. The results vary with the nature of stressor, stressor duration, interpersonal events, uncontrollability of the stressor, and ways of coping with emotions.[1] Indeed, under certain conditions, acute stress boosts Th1 responses through induction of pro-inflammatory cytokines and inhibits Th2 responses. Integrating certain psychological traits and various aspects of stress-induced reactivity could help us to untangle the discrepancies among studies.

For instance, negative emotions that are associated with the inability to cope with them contribute indirectly to immune dysregulation. The way to cope with negative affect or personality disorder associated with impaired emotional regulation has been an interesting field for exploring the relationships and mechanisms linking affect regulation and immune function. For example, specific coping styles such as denial and repression were associated with altered immunity. Subjects classified as repressors of negative affect exhibited lower immune responses than other groups of subjects.[2] Some studies found significant associations between immunological parameters reflective of HIV progression and psychopathological characteristics such as denial and distress.[3] Marsland et al.[4] found lower antibody responses during the standard course of hepatitis B vaccinations in healthy graduate participants with high trait negative affects. It has also been shown that activated personality temperament with specific cognitive processing (speaking and thinking quickly) was protective under stress conditions in terms of T and B lymphocyte counts.[5]

WHAT IS ALEXITHYMIA?

Particular attention has been paid to specific cognitive–affective disturbances such as alexithymia. The term was coined by Sifneos[6] in 1972 from the Greek for lack (a), word (lexis), and emotion (thymos) to mean "no words for feelings." Alexithymia is a clinical dimension defined by a set of cognitive–affective deficits characterized by inaccuracy in identifying and describing emotions, difficulty in distinguishing between feelings and bodily sensations, paucity of daydreaming, limited fantasies and introspection, and thought characterized by pragmatic content with a highly descriptive mode of expression.

In other words, people with alexithymic features have difficulties in verbally identifying and expressing emotional stress. Alexithymia is a difficult concept to operationalize and only a few instruments to do so are sufficiently reliable and valid. Several scales are used to measure alexithymia, but only the Toronto Alexithymia Scale (TAS)[7] can be regarded as having sufficient psychometric properties. This dimension was first studied in classical somatic disorders as asthma, multiple sclerosis, ulcerative colitis, essential hypertension, irritable bowel syndrome, and rheumatoid arthritis. Alexithymic characteristics were suggested to occur more frequently in individuals with so-called psychosomatic disorders. This is still a matter of controversy because alexithymia has been found in patients suffering from psychiatric conditions such as mood disorders, anxiety, phobias, post-traumatic stress disorders, and addictive behaviors[8,9] without so-called psychosomatic disorders. Freyberger[10] distinguished primary alexithymia from secondary alexithymia. The former has been attributed to an organic substratum (neurophysiological and neuroanatomical) while the latter has been related to consequences of the distress observed in the psychiatric disorder.

ALEXITHYMIA AND STRESS

NEUROENDOCRINE AND IMMUNE PATHWAYS OF STRESS

The influence of the autonomic nervous system on immune function is exerted primarily through the sympathetic fibers that innervate the lymphoid organs and through circulating catecholamines. It is especially involved during acute stress. The immunoregulatory actions of the catecholamines are mediated mainly by β2–adrenoreceptors that are expressed on splenocytes and peripheral blood cells. *In vivo*, chemical sympathectomy suppresses cell-mediated (T-helper-1) responses and may enhance antibody (T-helper-2) responses.[11] The sympathetic nervous system (SNS) has been linked to increased natural killer cell activity (NKCA) with enhancement of cellular (Th1) immune response.

A major endocrine response to stress, especially during chronic stress, consists of the activation of the hypothalamo–pituitary–adrenal (HPA) axis, leading to the secretion of ACTH from the pituitary and corticoids from the adrenal and subsequent immunosuppression. The paraventricular nucleus (PVN) of the hypothalamus contains neurons that manufacture the neuropeptide corticotropin-releasing factor (CRF) that generates the changes in ACTH and glucocorticoid profiles that characterize the HPA axis stress response. It has been shown that acute stress heightens cardiac sympathetic activation and plasma catecholamine concentrations, whereas chronic stress (such as caregivers dealing with progressive dementia) results in elevated blood pressure and plasma levels of ACTH and decreased cellular immune response with lower levels of interleukin-1b.[12] Those subjects who had elevated plasma levels of ACTH exhibited the greatest diminutions in cellular immune response.

In addition, recent studies suggest that acute stress induces cell-mediated immunity (Th1 immune responses) while chronic stress induces humoral (Th2) immune responses.[13–16] Larson et al.[17] found an association between acute stress in healthy volunteers and increases in the cell-mediated (Th1 immune) response, with elevated rates of interferon-c produced by peripheral blood mononuclear cells (PBMCs) and increased NKCA that may be connected to the sympathetic pathway. For example, acute activation of the SNS in healthy subjects after acute physical and psychological stress led to leukocytosis with increased levels of lymphocytes, monocytes, and granulocytes and elevated *in vitro* production of interleukin-6 by PBMCs.[18] During chronic stress, catecholamines potently inhibited type 1 cytokines (IL-2 and IL-12) and stimulated type 2 cytokines (IL-10).[14] It has also been shown[2] that subjects classified as repressors of negative affect have lower immune responses than other groups of subjects.

ASSOCIATION OF ALEXITHYMIA WITH SYMPATHETIC OVER-REACTIVITY

A rapidly increasing body of evidence[19-23] suggests that alexithymic characteristics are related to sympathetic over-reactivity. Alexithymics exhibited higher heart rates[19,24] higher electrodermal activity,[25,26] and lower oxygen consumption. Papciak et al.[24] found that alexithymia was related to a higher baseline heart rate. Friedlander et al.[25] found a higher tonic skin conductance level. Martin et al.[22] observed that alexithymic subjects had altered tryptophan metabolisms while Rabavilas[23] reported greater skin conductance responses. Moreover, during acute stress, sympathetic responsiveness is unchanged or lower in alexithymics compared to nonalexithymics.[24,25,27]

Nemiah et al.[29] observed a smaller increase in oxygen consumption during a mental stress test while Newton and Contrada[27] found a smaller heart rate increase in alexithymics giving personally relevant speeches. Wehmer et al.[28] described smaller skin conductance reactivity during exposure to stressors such as viewing emotional scenes. Although results of studies of tonic and reactive autonomic functioning are relatively consistent for resting periods, the results are still controversial for conditions of acute stress. Alexithymia is associated with higher tonic levels of sympathetic activity at baseline and lower sympathetic reactivity during acute stress. The constant hyperactivity of autonomic functioning at baseline suggests that alexithymic subjects may have the same physiological arousal observed under chronic stress conditions, while distress remains emotionally unnoticed.

ALEXITHYMIA, IMMUNITY, AND ENDOCRINE PATHWAYS

Some empirical studies have found impaired immune responses in alexithymic subjects. Todarello et al.[30,31] found that alexithymic women had lower counts of almost all lymphocytic subsets compared to non-alexithymic women. Dewaraja et al.[32] observed decreased cytotoxic lymphocyte counts (for the natural killer subset CD57–CD16 + cells and killer-effective T cell CD8 + CD11a + cells) in highly alexithymic men compared to non-alexithymics. In previous research,[33] we found a significant positive correlation between alexithymic features, notably the first dimension (difficulty in identifying feelings), and serum levels of IL-4. IL-4 is a modulator of key cytokines known to regulate the type 1–type 2 cytokine balance.

We recently found decreased production of interleukin-1β, interleukin-2, and interleukin-4 by stimulated peripheral mononuclear blood cells with lower CD4/CD8 ratios in alexithymic subjects. We also observed a reduced ratio of Th1/Th2 (IL-2/IL-10) in the alexithymics.[34] Lindholm et al.[35] observed that alexithymia was associated with higher cortisol levels following dexamethasone administration, even after controlling for depression. It is known that increased production of glucocorticoid can promote type 2 cytokine production.[13] This may be one possible neuroendocrine pathway associated with immune perturbation in alexithymic subjects.

TOWARD A
PSYCHONEUROENDOCRINOIMMUNOLOGICAL
APPROACH TO ALEXITHYMIA

In many ways, the neuroendocrine and immune response of alexithymics seems to follow the same pattern observed in subjects afflicted with chronic stress. Alexithymia and stress have been connected on a theoretical basis[36] with a sympathetic over-reactivity in both cases (Figure 7.1).

Alexithymic features may be connected with aberrant means of handling psychosocial stress. Due to their inability to identify and verbalize their emotions, alexithymics may present an exceptional stress reaction with poorly developed channels for proper emotional discharge. These subjects present a dissociation between subjective and physiological stress responses. In this kind of specific emotional expressive style, there are reduced or unnoticed reports of stress coupled with high autonomic, somatic, and behavioral responsivity. The decoupling response between the feeling state and physiological arousal at baseline may increase alexithymic individuals' risks for stress-related illness.[24,37]

Because affect differentiation is impaired and emotional stress is unnoticed, the arousal remains active, thereby disturbing the autonomic and pituitary–adrenal axis and the immune system. Thus alexithymics may suffer from an over-reactivity of the SNS and an overdrive of the HPA axis with glucocorticoid resistance. The sympathetic nervous system would primarily exert its action on immune response through the stimulation of the β2-adrenoreceptor–cAMP-protein kinase A pathway by catecholamines. Through their actions on β2-adrenoreceptor, norepinephrine and epinephrine inhibit the type 1 cytokines, such as interleukin-2 and interferon-gamma by antigen-presenting cells and T helper (Th) 1 cells, and stimulate the production of type 2 cytokines such as interleukin (IL)-4 and -10.

The hyperactivity of the HPA axis results in the secretion of glucocorticoids favoring humoral immunity while suppressing cell-mediated immunity due to a shift in cytokine balance toward a type 2 cytokine response. Glucocorticoids also act through their classic cytoplasmic nuclear receptors on antigen-presenting cells to suppress the production of the main inducer of Th1 responses of IL-12.[38] They also down-regulate the expression of IL-12 receptors on T and natural killer cells.

Endogenous catecholamines and glucocorticoids systematically may cause selective suppression of Th1 responses and cellular immunity and a Th2 shift toward dominance of humoral immunity as observed in subjects afflicted with chronic stress. Glaser et al.[15] observed that a chronic stressor such as caregiving was associated with a shift from Th1 to Th2 cytokine response.

During the resting period, alexithymic subjects may exhibit decreased cellular immune responses mediated by profound changes in cytokine secretions with a shift toward a type 2 cytokine pattern favoring humoral immunity responses. The enhanced production of type 2 cytokines and decreased production of type 1 cytokines may generate a vulnerability to infectious and allergic diseases.[39] Nevertheless, in a precedent study,[34] we found a global decrease of most of the cytokines (IL-1, IL-2, IL-4) produced by stimulated PBMCs in alexithymic subjects. However, there was a decreased ratio of IL-2/IL-10 in favor of a more pronounced reduction of

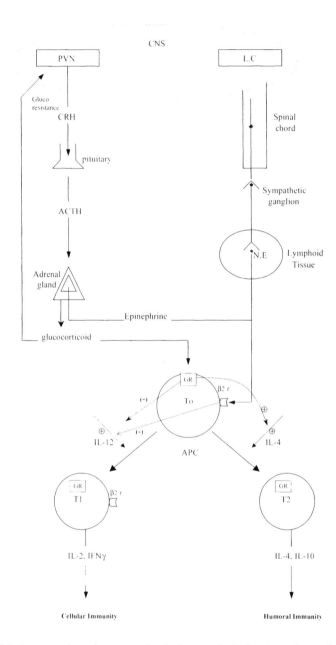

FIGURE 7.1 A proposed psychoneuroendocrinoimmunological pathway for alexithymia. Ihibition of the Th1 response and preservation of Th2 response due to over-reactivity of the HPA axis and the SAS in alexithymics. (Abbreviations: HPA, hypothalamic-pituitary-adrenal axis; SAS, sympathetic adrenomedullary system; CNS, central nervous system; PVN, paraventricular nuclei; LC, locus coeruleus; CRH, corticotropin-releasing hormone; ACTH, adrenocorticotropin hormone; APC, antigen presenting cell; N.E, norepinephrin; GR, glucocorticoid receptor; β2 r, beta 2 adrenoreceptor; IL, interleukin; To, TO lymphocytes; T1, T1 lymphocytes; T2, T2 lymphocytes.)

Th1 cytokines. Whether alexithymia is associated with a specific shift toward Th2 cytokine response[33] or whether it is associated with a global impaired immune response touching all Th1 and Th2 cytokine responses is still unknown.[34]

Alexithymic subjects may be prone to stress-related disorders due to chronically increased levels of sympathetic and HPA activation prior to stress with lower responses of these neuroendocrine systems during a stress-related activation associated with impaired immune response.

Further studies should assess several endocrine and immune parameters (adrenoreceptor, dexamethasone test and HPA axis, T and B lymphocyte numbers and subsets, spontaneous production of Th1 and Th2 cytokines and after mitogen stimulation of PBMCs, lymphoproliferative response IgE antibody production, and eosinophil count) at rest and after acute stress.

REFERENCES

1. Peters ML, Godaert GL, Ballieux RE, Brosschot JF, Sweep FCG, Swinkels LMJ,Van Vliet M, and Heijnen CJ. Immune responses to experimental stress: effects of mental effort and uncontrollability. *Psychosom Med* 1999; 61: 513–524.
2. Shea JD, Burton R, and Girgis A. Negative affect, absorption, and immunity. *Physiol Behav* 1993; 53: 449–457.
3. Ironson G, Friedman A, Klimas N, et al. Distress, denial and low adherence to behavioural interventions predict faster disease progression in gay men infected with human immunodeficiency virus. *Int J Behav Med* 1994; 1: 90–105.
4. Marsland AL, Cohen S, Rabin BS, and Manuck SB. Associations between stress, trait negative affect, acute immune reactivity and antibody to hepatitis injection in healthy young adults. *Health Psychol* 2001; 20(1): 4–11.
5. Gruzelier J, Smith F, Nagy A, and Henderson D. Cellular and humoral immunity, mood and exam stress: the influence of self-hypnosis and personality predictors. *Int J Psychophysiol* 2001; 42(1): 55–71.
6. Sifneos PE. The prevalence of 'alexithymic' characteristics in psychosomatic patients. *Psychother Psychosom* 1973; 22: 255.
7. Bagby R, Parker JDA, and Taylor GJ. The 20-item Toronto Alexithymia Scale. I. Item selection and cross-validation of the factor structure. II. Convergent, discriminant, and concurrent validity. *J Psychosom Res* 1994; 38(1): 33–40.
8. Haviland MG, Hendryx MS, Shaw DG, and Henry JP. Alexithymia in women and men hospitalized for psychoactive substance dependence. *Compr Psychiatr* 1994; 35(2): 124–128.
9. Loas G, Fremaux D, Otmani O, Lecercle C, and Jouvent R. Relationships between the emotional and cognitive components of alexithymia and dependency in alcoholics. *Psychiatr Res* 2000; 96: 63–74.
10. Freyberger H. Supportive psychotherapeutic techniques in primary and secondary alexithymia. *Psychother Psychosom* 1977; 28: 337–342.
11. Madden KS, Sanders VM, and Felten DL. Catecholamine influences and sympathetic neural modulation of immune responsiveness. *Pharmacol Toxicol* 1995; 35: 417.
12. Caioppo JT, Berntson GC, Malarkey WB, Kiecolt-Glaser JK, Sheridan JF, Poehlmann KM, Burleson MH, Ernst JM, Hawkley LC, and Glaser R. Autonomic, neuroendocrine, and immune responses to psychological stress: the reactivity hypothesis. *Ann NY AcadSci* 1998; 840: 664–673.

13. Agarwal SK and Marshall Jr. GD. Dexamethasone promotes type 2 cytokine production primarily through inhibition of type 1 cytokines. *J Interferon Cytokine Res* 2001; 21: 147–155.

14. Elenkov IJ, Papanicolaou DA.Wilder RL, and Chrousos GP. Modulatory effects of glucocorticoids and catecholamines on human interleukin-12 and interleukin-10 production: clinical implications. *Proc Assoc Am Phys* 1996; 108: 374–381.

15. Glaser R, MacCallum RC, Laskowski BF, Malarkey WB, Sheridan JF, and Kiecolt-Glaser JK. Evidence for a shift in the Th-1 to Th-2 cytokine response associated with chronic stress and aging. *J Gerontol A Biol Sci Med Sci* 2001; 56: M477–482.

16. Marshall GD. Agarwall SK, Lloyd C, Cohen L, Henninger EM, and Morris GJ. Cytokine dysregulation associated with exam stress in healthy medical students. *Brain Behav Immun* 1998; 12: 297–307.

17. Larson MR, Ader R, and Moynihan JA. Heart rate, neuroendocrine, and immunological reactivity in response to an acute laboratory stressor. *Psychosom Med* 2001; 63: 493.

18. Goebels MU, Mills PJ, Irwin MR, and Ziegler MG. Interleukin-6 and tumor necrosis factor-α production after acute psychological stress, exercise, and infused isoproterenol: differential effects and pathways. *Psychosom Med* 2000; 62: 591–598.

19. Fukunishi I, Sei H, Morita Y, Rahe RH. Sympathetic activity in alexithymics with mother's low care. *J Psychosom Res* 1999; 46: 579–589.

20. Gundel H, Greiner A, Ceballos-Baumann AO, Von Rad M, Forstl H, and Jahn T. Increased level of tonic sympathetic arousal in high versus low alexithymic cervical dystonia patients. *Psychother Psychosom* 2002; 52: 461–468.

21. Infrasca R. Alexithymia, neurovegetative arousal and neuroticism: an experimental study. *Psychother Psychosom* 1997; 66(5): 276–280.

22. Martin JB and Pihl RO. Influence of alexithymic characteristics on physiological and subjective stress responses in normal individuals. *Psychother Psychosom* 1986; 45: 66–67.

23. Rabavilas AD. Electrodermal activity in low and high alexithymia neurotic patients. *Psychother Psychosom* 1987; 47: 101–104.

24. Papciak AS, Feuerstein M, and Spiegel JA. Stress reactivity in alexithymia: decoupling of physiological and cognitive responses. *J Hum Stress* 1985; 11(3): 135–142.

25. Friedlander L, Lumley MA, Farchione T, and Doyal G. Testing the alexithymia hypothesis: physiological and subjective responses during relaxation and stress. *J Nerv Ment Dis* 1997; 185(4): 233–239.

26. Stone LA and Nielson KA. Intact physiological response to arousal with impaired emotional recognition in alexithymia. *Psychother Psychosom* 2001; 70(2): 92–102.

27. Newton TL and Contrada RJ. Repressive coping and verbal-autonomic response dissociation: the influence of social context. *J Pers Soc Psychol* 1992; 62: 159–167.

28. Wehmer F, Brejnak C, Lumley M, and Stettner L. Alexithymia and physiological reactivity to emotion-provoking visual scenes. *J Nerv Ment Dis* 1995; 183: 351–357.

29. Nemiah JC, Sifneos PE, and Apfel-Savitz R. A comparison of oxygen consumption of normal and alexithymic subjects in response to affect-provoking thoughts. *Psychother Psychosom* 1977; 28: 167–171.

30. Todarello O, Casamassima A, Marinaccio M, La Pesa MW, Caradonna L, Valentino L, and Marinaccio L. Alexithymia, immunity and cervical intraepithelial neoplasia: a pilot study. *Psychother Psychosom* 1994; 61: 199–204.

31. Todarello O, Casamassima A, Daniele S, Marinaccio M, Fanciullo F, Valentino L, Tedesco N, Wiesel S, Simone G, and Marinaccio L. Alexithymia, immunity and cervical intraepithelial neoplasia: replication. *Psychother Psychosom* 1997; 66: 208–213.

32. Dewaraja R, Tanigawa T, Araki S, Nakata A, Kawamura N, Ago Y, and Sasaki Y. Decreased cytotoxic lymphocyte counts in alexithymia. *Psychother Psychosom* 1997; 66: 83–86.

33. Corcos M, Guilbaud O, Paterniti S, Curt F, Hjalmarsson L, Moussa M, Chambry J, Loas G, Chaouat G, and Jeammet P. Correlation between serum levels of interleukin-4 and alexithymia scores in healthy female subjects: preliminary findings. *Psychoneuroendocrinology* 2003, in press.

34. Guilbaud O, Chaouat G, Curt F, Berthoz S, Touitou C, Strebler M, Dugré-Le Bigre C, Loas G, Jeammet P, and Corcos M. Impaired immune and automatic response in alexithymic women, manuscript submitted.

35. Lindholm T, Lehtinen V, Hyyppa MT, and Puukka P. Alexithymic features in relation to the dexamethasone suppression test in a Finnish population sample. *Am J Psychiatry* 1990;147: 1216–1219.

36. Martin, JB and Pihl, RO. Influence of alexithymia hypothesis: theoretical and empirical considerations. *Psychother Psychosom* 1985; 43(4): 169–176.

37. Lumley MA, Stettner L, and Wehmer F. How are alexithymia and physical illness linked? A review and critique of pathways. *J Psychosom Res* 1996; 41(6): 505–518.

38. Elenkov IJ, Wilder RL, Chrousos GP, and Vizi ES. The sympathetic nerve: an integrative interface between two supersystems: the brain and the immune system. *Pharmacol Rev* 2000; 52: 595–638.

39. Iwakabe K, Shimada M, Ohta A, Yahata T, Ohmi Y, Habu S, and Nishimura T. The restraint stress drives a shift in Th1/Th2 balance toward Th2-dominant immunity in mice. *Immunol Lett* 1998; 62: 39–43.

8 Roles of Mu-Opioid Receptor and Endogenous Opiates in Stress-Induced Immunosuppression

Jennifer Kelschenbach, Horace H. Loh, and Sabita Roy

CONTENTS

INTRODUCTION

Clinical and anecdotal evidence provides support for the idea that stressful life experiences may result in impaired immune function, and therefore may render an individual more susceptible to infections. Stress in all of its many forms is considered a huge risk factor for disease. Therefore, it is paramount to understanding the immunological consequences of stress and the mechanisms by which immunosuppression is manifested. The work of many groups has documented the fact that stress significantly alters many aspects of the immune system, at both the adaptive and innate levels. In addition, in recent years it has been debated whether morphine has a direct mode of action or whether it indirectly activates the neuroendocrine and sympathetic systems.

Therefore, it is the goal of this chapter to review the contribution of the mu-opioid receptor (MOR) and the endogenous opiates to stress-induced immunosuppression.

EFFECTS OF PSYCHOLOGICAL AND PHYSICAL STRESSORS ON IMMUNE FUNCTIONING

Psychological and physical stressors have both been demonstrated to alter parameters of both the innate and adaptive immune systems. One of the first realizations that stress alters the body's immune system was suggested by anecdotal evidence that demonstrated that emotional stress resulted in increased susceptibility to illness. Since these first observations, several studies have demonstrated that stress — physical and mental — renders the immune system vulnerable to infection. Numerous elements and immune cell responses have been examined following application of a stressor, and in most cases stress diminished the capabilities of the tested parameter.

Normally, a stressor elicits physiological changes that allow an individual to cope with a particular stressor. These physiological alterations include activation of the hypothalamic–pituitary–adrenal (HPA) axis, resulting in the release of glucocorticoids, stimulation of the sympathetic system resulting in epinephrine and norepinephrine release, and the mobilization of endogenous opioid peptides. Chronic activation of these stress responses is believed to cause dysfunction in many systems including the immune system.[1]

A variety of stress models have been used to address the question of how stress affects the functioning of the immune system. Schedlowski et al. examined immune parameters of first-time parachutists and found that the functional capacity of natural killer (NK) cells increased immediately after jumping, followed by a significant decrease 1 hour later. These results suggest that quick mobilization of NK cells may be one of the initial adaptive mechanisms to cope with stress.[2] However, this increased functionality was not maintained, and it can therefore be speculated that during chronic stressful experiences, NK cell mobilization and increased activity may not be an efficient defense strategy.

This process of NK cell activity was further investigated utilizing a stress model in which infant squirrel monkeys were separated from their mothers for various time periods, followed by assessment of NK cell cytolytic activity. The first day of separation resulted in a significant decrease in the lytic responses against target cells, but this deficit returned to baseline by the conclusion of the study.

To determine the mechanism by which this defect occurred, investigators administered RU-486, a glucocorticoid receptor blocker, and naltrexone, an opioid antagonist. Interestingly, administration of these compounds did not alter the observed decrement in lytic responses, suggesting that stress augments a number of pathways to bring about decreased functioning. The authors commented that the recovery of the response within 1 week of the initiation of the stressor demonstrated the resiliency of the immune system. However, it is important to note that the recovery in responding paralleled behavioral adaptations made by the infants in response to the stress, and that similar recovery may not occur with persistent stress.[3] Other studies examined the effects of surgical stress on monocyte and polymorphonuclear cell functioning. They demonstrated that the stress associated with surgery resulted in depressed monocyte performance as measured by phagocytotic activity, and it was further noted that this decrement correlated significantly with increased cortisol levels.

It is important to add that postoperative recovery was not compromised, which suggests that immune decrements recovered and did not impede recuperation.[4] This study along with the others presented introduces the possibility that acute and chronic stress periods may have differential effects on immune functioning.

This idea was explored by subjecting rats to either acute or chronic social stress using a confrontation model in which male rats were introduced to male–female groups for either 2 (acute) or 48 (chronic) hours. The study demonstrated that 2 hours of confrontation resulted in decreased lymphocyte numbers and decreased T cell proliferative responses to concanavalin-A (Con-A). Chronic stress (48 hours of confrontation) resulted in similar findings of cell numbers and proliferative responses but at a lower magnitude, thus suggesting that acute and chronic stresses may not result in similar immune deficits. This difference should be considered when examining stress-induced dysfunctions.[5]

These studies clearly demonstrate that stress does impact the immune system, but the studies focused on NK cells and monocytes — two cell types that act early in an immune response. Numerous reports have also demonstrated the effects of stress on cell-mediated and humoral responses, processes that occur at a later phase in the immune response. Karp et al. used a restraint stress model to evaluate the effects of psychological stress on antibody production in mice. Stressed mice exhibited higher serum levels of IgM and IgG anti-KLH (keyhole limpet hemocyanin) antibodies.

Additionally, administration of cyclophosphamide to stressed animals significantly increased anti-KLH IgG titers compared to saline treated non-stressed controls. These data indicate that stress can modulate a humoral-mediated immune response, and that low dose administration of immunomodulatory drugs makes a subject more reactive to particular stressors.[6]

Numerous studies have examined the effects of examination and other academic-related stresses on immune functioning. It has been demonstrated that salivary IgA levels are reduced for as long as 2 weeks following a major academic exam.[7] In addition, in a study that investigated the effects of stress associated with an oral academic examination of graduate students, plasma cortisol levels were significantly elevated 1 hour prior to the exam, but not 6 to 8 weeks preceding it. Conversely, mitogen-induced lymphocyte proliferation was reduced 6 to 8 weeks prior to the exam, suggesting that lengthy anticipatory periods before an expected stressor modulates immune function.

Stressed students reported more feelings of malaise including headaches, sore throats, and fatigue. Finally, this study also suggested that cortisol release is associated with immediate stressors, whereas immune alterations are sensitive to distant stressful experiences.[8]

Academic stress has also been demonstrated to affect T helper cell differentiation. Marshall et al. measured type 1 cytokine (IFN-γ) and type 2 cytokine (IL-10) levels released from peripheral blood mononuclear cells (PBMCs) of students experiencing exam-related stress, and found that stress resulted in decreased IFN-γ:IL-10 ratios. These results suggest that psychological stresses associated with academic exams can shift the type 1–type 2 cytokine balance toward type 2, thus resulting in immune dysregulation.[9] The studies cited concentrated on the effects that chronic stress has on immune functioning. However, it has been demonstrated that acute mental stress can also affect certain immune parameters. Participants subjected to a brief experimental stressor (a frustrating 21-minute laboratory task) showed significant decreases in phytohemagglutinin (PHA)-stimulated T cell mitogenesis, reduced T helper:T suppressor cell ratios, and increases in NK cell number, all indicating that acute mental stressors can negatively impact immune functioning.[10] Interestingly, some studies also implied that the way in which an individual copes with stressful experiences may predict decrements in immune operation.

Futterman et al. evaluated the impact of a bone marrow transplant on the immunological and psychological status of the patient's spouse or partner, and found that the greatest alterations in immune parameters occurred during the waiting period before the transplant procedure. The decrement in immune variables also correlated with declined psychological status, and it was determined that less escape–avoidance coping predicted better immune functioning.[11]

WITHDRAWAL STRESS AND IMMUNE DYSFUNCTION

The studies and investigations described above focused mainly on the consequences to the immune system resulting from exposure to "common" stressors such as academic stress, surgical stress, restraint stress, and the stress associated with mental anguish. However, an area of study that has received considerably less attention and is of particular interest to our laboratory is the stress associated with drug withdrawal. This type of stress contains both psychological and physical elements; therefore, a careful examination of this process and the consequences it imparts on the immune system is warranted.

One study examining the effects of cocaine withdrawal on immune functioning found that proliferative responses of peripheral blood lymphocytes to Con A were significantly reduced from 2 hours and up to 6 days during cocaine withdrawal. Plasma corticosterone concentrations were significantly elevated up to 24 hours after cocaine cessation, but returned to baseline levels at 2 days of withdrawal. Additionally, the suppressive effects of withdrawal were abolished in animals undergoing adrenalectomies or those administered the RU-486 glucocorticoid antagonist, indicating that the effects of withdrawal on cellular immunity were mediated by a glucocorticoid pathway.[12] However, it is important to note that deficits in lymphocyte proliferation were seen up to 6 days of withdrawal despite the return of corticosterone to basal levels. This may suggest that the stress associated with drug withdrawal may activate additional pathways that affect immune function.

Two reports from Rahim et al. examined the effects of morphine withdrawal on immune functioning in mice. Their first study compared the consequences to immune function of both abrupt and precipitated morphine withdrawal. Examining the ability of murine splenocytes to mount an *in vitro* antibody response to sheep red blood cells was used to assess immune deficits. The findings demonstrated that initiation of withdrawal in dependent animals by either method resulted in significant immunosuppression between 24 and 48 hours post-withdrawal. However, the period of onset and recovery differed between the two modes of withdrawal, with abrupt withdrawal resulting in an early decline followed by a protracted deficit (144 hours), whereas precipitated withdrawal produced an initial potentiation (3 hours) followed by a decline that recovered within 72 hours.[13]

These findings are interesting because they suggest that the mode of withdrawal also has an effect on the observed immune deficits. This group of authors went on to determine the causes of the observed deficit in the plaque-forming cell (PFC) response following morphine withdrawal. They stated that the observed dysfunction was a result of impaired macrophage function, as evidenced by the findings that macrophages obtained from withdrawn spleens displayed reduced expression of the co-stimulatory molecule B7.2 and had depressed cytokine production.

Also, the addition of either normal unfractionated spleen cells, macrophage enriched spleen cells, or purified CD11b+ cells was able to restore the PFC response.[14] This report adds new understanding but does not explain other observed deficits following morphine withdrawal, such as impaired cytotoxic T cell activities[15] and decreased T cell proliferative responses to PHA.[16] Other reports demonstrated no significant alterations to macrophage function as measured by proliferation and TNF-α production.[15]

Our laboratory recently demonstrated that morphine withdrawal contributes to T helper cell differentiation by biasing cells toward the Th2 lineage,[17] and the contribution of the innate immune system, particularly the role of macrophages, is currently under investigation. In summary, this section demonstrates that various stressors impart severe decrements to immune functioning (summarized in Table 8.1). The following sections will examine the contributions of morphine, endogenous opiates, and the mu-opioid receptor to stress-induced immunosuppression.

ROLE OF MU-OPIOID RECEPTOR IN STRESS-INDUCED IMMUNOSUPPRESSION

MU-OPIOID RECEPTOR EXPRESSION ON IMMUNE CELLS

The fields of opiate pharmacology and immunology connected after the observations that opioid administration significantly impaired an individual's immune system and produced vulnerability to infection by pathogenic agents. One of the first questions addressed was whether opioid drugs acted indirectly on the central nervous system to activate neuroendocrine and sympathetic systems, which subsequently mediated the immune system, or whether the opiates potentially had direct effects on cells of the immune system. To achieve a direct mode of action, researchers speculated that immune cells would have to express receptors for the opioids, and this speculation compelled a significant number of groups to examine this possibility.

The earliest efforts used pharmacological and ligand binding studies to provide support for the existence of opioid receptors on the cells of the immune system. The advent of genetic cloning and polymerase chain reaction (PCR) techniques added valuable tools for addressing the existence of opioid receptors on cells of the immune system. These techniques demonstrated the expression of all three opioid receptors on several immune cells including CD4 + T helper cells (reviewed in reference 18).

TABLE 8.1
Stress and Immune Dysfunction

Stressor	Type of Stressor	Immune Cells Involved	Immune Parameters	Reference
Infant removal from mother	Psychological	NK cells	↓ lytic response	Coe. C.L. et al. [3]
Surgical stress	Psychological	Monocytes; PMNs	↓ phagocytic activity	Dahanukar, S.A. et al. [4]
Social stress/ confrontation	Psychological	Th cells	↓ proliferative responses	Stefanski, V. et al. [5]
Restraint stress	Psychological	B cells	↑ levels of IgM and IgG	Karp. J.D. et al. [6]
Academic stress	Psychological	B cells	↓ salivary IgA levels	Deinzer. R. et al. [7]
		Th cells	↓ proliferative responses	Lacey. K. et al. [8]
		PBMCs	Th1 → Th2 shift	Marshall, G.D. Jr. et al. [9]
Cocaine withdrawal	Psychological and physical	Lymphocytes	↓ proliferative responses	Avila, A.H. et al. [12]
Morphine withdrawal	Psychological and physical	Splenocytes	↓ PFC response	Rahim, R.T. et al. [13]
		Macrophages	↓ expression of B7.2 and cytokine production	Rahim, R.T. et al. [14]
		Tc cells	↓ cytotoxic activity	Bhargava, H. et al. [15]
		Th cells	↓ proliferative responses	Govitrapong, P. et al. [16]
		Th cells	Th1 → Th2 shift	Kelschenbach, J. et al. [17]

Specifically, utilizing the reverse transcriptase polymerase chain reaction (RT-PCR), cDNA clones of the mu-,[19] delta-, and kappa-[20] opioid receptors were obtained from several immune cells.

Chuang et al. demonstrated the expression of the mu-opioid receptor gene in various cell types including, the human hybrid B and T cell CEM line, the Ragi line (human B cells), human CD4+ cells, human monocytes and macrophages, and various others.[19] Our laboratory, using similar techniques, demonstrated the existence of delta- and kappa-opioid cDNA transcripts in MOLT-4 and CEM T cell lines and in human peripheral blood lymphocytes.[20] Additionally, mu-opioid receptor transcripts have been demonstrated to be expressed in rat peritoneal macrophages.[21]

Our group was also one of the first to report on the expression of a full-length cDNA encoding the delta-opioid receptor in unactivated mouse thymocytes.[22] In all cases, the transcripts obtained from the immune cells were nearly identical to opioid receptor cDNAs isolated from neuronal sources. These observations suggest that

TABLE 8.2
Opioid Receptor Expression on Immune Cells

Opioid Receptor	Immune Cell	Identifying Technique	Reference
μ	CEM line (hybrid B and T cell line) Ragi line (human B cells) CD4+ cells Monocytes and macrophages	RT-PCR	Chuang, T.K. et al. [19]
δ	MOLT-4 T cells CEM T cells Lymphocytes Murine thymocytes	RT-PCR	Wick, M.J. et al. [20] Sedqi, M., et al. [22]
κ	MOLT-4 T cells CEM T cells Lymphocytes	RT-PCR	Wick, M.J. et al. [20]
Opioid 'orphan' receptor	Lymphocytes	cDNA library screen	Wick, M.J. et al. [23]

opiate drugs may directly mediate their diverse array of effects by binding to receptors expressed on cells of the immune system. It is also important to note that the cDNA clone, AT7-5EU, was isolated after a screen of an activated human lymphocyte cDNA library in search for homology to brain opioid receptors. This clone was demonstrated to encode for the opioid "orphan" receptor, and the protein coding region shared complete homology with a reported opioid orphan receptor cloned from human brain.

Another interesting finding is that this receptor has not been shown to bind opioids.[23] There have also been reports that implicate the existence of novel, non-classical opioid receptors and binding sites on immune cells that are selective for morphine.[18] The importance of all of these findings (summarized in Table 8.2) relates to the idea that opioids, both endogenous and exogenous, may exert their myriad effects on the immune system in a direct manner.

MU-OPIOID RECEPTOR SIGNALING

Prior to discussing the involvement of the mu-opioid receptor in stress-induced immunosuppression, a brief overview of opioid receptor signaling and the effects that morphine, the prototypical mu-opioid receptor alkaloid agonist, has on immune functioning is warranted. First, there is sufficient evidence from both selective ligand binding studies and molecular cloning to demonstrate the existence of three classes of opioid receptors: mu, kappa, and delta. As described above, several cells of the immune system express most if not all of these receptors.

Cloning of these receptors confirmed that they belong to the G-protein-coupled superfamily of seven transmembrane receptors, and transduce their signals directly or through the involvement of second messengers that stimulate multiple effector systems. It was well known, even prior to cloning, that all three receptors couple to adenylyl cyclase, K^+ and Ca^+ channels, and phosphatidyl inositol turnover via the pertussis toxin-sensitive G_i/G_o G proteins. Through these interactions opioids are able to mediate adenylyl cyclase and Ca^+ channel inhibition and activate inwardly rectifying K^+ channels (reviewed in Reference 24). Opiates may exert their myriad effects on the immune system through these receptors and their downstream partners.

EFFECT OF MORPHINE ON IMMUNE FUNCTION

Before discussing the role that the mu-opioid receptor plays in stress-induced immunosuppression, a brief commentary on the influence of morphine on immune functioning is necessary because morphine may act directly on cells of the immune system via these receptors. It was demonstrated in rhesus monkeys that daily low doses of morphine suppressed PBMC and NK cell activity, as well as reducing the number of CD8 + and CD4 + T cells.[25] Acute exposure to morphine has also been demonstrated to inhibit phagocytosis of murine macrophages, and chronic exposure results in an apparent desensitization.[26]

Morphine and heroin treatments *in vitro* have been shown to significantly increase the production of IL-1β, IL-2, TNF-α, and IFN-γ from mouse splenocyte cultures, as well as stimulate the production of anti-inflammatory cytokines TGF-β1 and IL-10.[27] Our laboratory demonstrated that *in vitro* morphine treatment of PBMCs or splenocytes results in T helper cell differentiation toward the Th2 lineage.[28] We demonstrated that morphine treatment impairs mitogen-stimulated lymphocyte proliferation by interfering with transcriptional activation of the IL-2 gene,[29] and showed that morphine modulates IFN-γ promoter activity through two distinct cAMP dependent pathways, specifically the NF-κβ and AP-1/NFAT pathways.[30] This brief discussion of the work of our lab and several others (summarized in Table 8.3) clearly demonstrates that morphine has a profound effect on immune functioning, at both the innate and adaptive levels.

The next logical question posed by investigators and based on morphine's effects and the findings that immune cells express opioid receptors, is whether morphine exerts these effects directly by acting on cells of the immune system via opioid receptors. One of the crucial tools utilized to address this question is the mu-opioid receptor knock-out (MORKO) mouse. These mice were generated by replacing the major coding region of the MOR gene (exon 2 and exon 3) with the Neo[r] coding sequence. This strategy results in a complete loss of mu-opioid receptors because the coding sequences for six of the seven transmembrane domains are deleted.

Specifically, a double-selection targeting vector was generated by replacing an *XhoI/XbaI* fragment that spans the entire exon 2 and 3 region with a Neo[r] cassette followed by ligation of a thymidine kinase expression cassette to the 3' end of this segment. The targeting vector was introduced into HM1 ES cells derived from the 129/Ola mouse strain by electroporation, and MOR-targeted ES clones were injected into blastocysts derived from C57/BL6 mice. Finally, heterozygotes and homozygotes

TABLE 8.3
Effect of Morphine on Immune Functioning

Cell Type	Effect	Reference
PBMCs	Suppressed activity	Carr, D.J. et al. [25]
	Th1 → Th2 shift	Roy, S. et al. [28]
NK cells	Suppressed activity	Carr, D.J. et al. [25]
T cells	↓ number	Carr, D.J. et al. [25]
	Modulated IFN-γ promoter activity via cAMP	Wang, J. et al. [30]
Murine macrophages	↓ phagocytosis	Tomei, E.Z. et al. [26]
Murine splenocytes	↑ IL-1β, IL-2, TNF-α, IFN-γ, TGF-β1, IL-10 production	Pacifici, R. et al. [27]
	Th1 → Th2 shift	Roy, S. et al. [28]
Murine thymocytes	↓ activation of IL-2 gene	Roy, S. et al. [29]

of MOR-targeted mice were obtained by a standard breeding program.[31] These mice have been utilized extensively by our group to address the contribution of the mu-opioid receptor to both morphine- and stress-mediated immune deficits.

We first demonstrated that morphine modulation of several immune functions is attributable to the mu-opioid receptor, including macrophage phagocytosis and secretion of TNF-α, which was not abolished in morphine-treated MORKO mice.[32] Subsequently, we demonstrated that low dose morphine treatment of lymph node-derived T lymphocytes results in impaired Con-A-induced proliferation and IL-2 and IFN-γ production. This decrement was accompanied by an increase in apoptosis, and these effects were lost in MORKO mice. Conversely, high doses of morphine were associated with an increase in inducible nitric oxide (NO) synthase mRNA expression. These results suggest that low dose morphine through its effects on lymphocyte mu-opioid receptors results in apoptosis, whereas higher doses trigger NO release.[33]

Other researchers have also investigated the role of the mu-opioid receptor in morphine-induced immunosuppression, and noted that morphine-induced lymphoid organ atrophy and diminished NK cell activity are lost in MORKO mice. However, it is important to note that the MOR gene in the mice used in this study was generated by an insertion strategy, as opposed to the method described above.[34] Finally, these studies have demonstrated that the mu-opioid receptor plays a crucial role in morphine-mediated immune deficits, but there is still the question of how the mu-opioid receptor mediates stress-induced immunosuppression.

As mentioned previously, the immunosuppressive effects of morphine and the endogenous opiates may be indirect actions of glucocorticoid release. This idea has been suggested by the work of Bryant et al., who administered morphine to both adrenalectomized and sham animals and found that morphine implantation, significantly increased corticosterone in sham animals. In addition, morphine-pelleted animals displayed splenic and thymic atrophy as well as impaired lymphocyte proliferative responses; these morphine-induced effects were absent in adrenalecto-mized mice, implicating the rise in corticosterone as a mediator of these effects.[35]

These findings again pose the question whether morphine acts directly or indi-rectly to bring about immune changes. Our laboratory addressed this question in several publications that examined the contribution of the HPA axis. It was demon-strated that morphine mediated elevations in corticosterone levels were mediated by the mu-opioid receptor, as evidenced by a loss in corticosterone increases in MORKO mice.[36] Subsequent studies utilizing MORKO mice demonstrated that morphine-induced immunosuppression is mediated by the mu-opioid receptor, and that only a few deficits are amplified in the presence of corticosterone. Specifically, inhibition of IFN-γ synthesis and activation of macrophage cytokine production are corticosterone-independent events.[37]

Researchers in our laboratory also examined the effects of stress on immune processes using a restraint stress model. It was demonstrated that stressed WT mice had decreased splenocyte numbers accompanied by increased apoptosis. This effect was lost in MORKO mice, despite the finding that corticosterone concentrations were similar for both WT and MORKO animals. These results therefore indicate that the mu-opioid receptor is involved in stress-induced immunosuppression, and that this effect is not entirely mediated by a glucocorticoid pathway.[38] In summary, the question of whether morphine imparts a direct effect on immune functioning by acting on opiate receptors on immune cells, or whether it acts indirectly by activating receptors in the central nervous system (CNS) to release catecholamines and/or steroids that then indirectly affect immune parameters is an area that requires further examination.

ROLE OF ENDOGENOUS OPIOIDS IN STRESS-INDUCED IMMUNOSUPPRESSION

The endogenous opioids are peptides that are known to be components of the stress response and are divided into four families: the enkephalins, the endorphins, the dynorphins, and the endomorphins. The enkephalins are small, 5-amino acid peptides that exist in two forms: leucine enkephalin and methionine enkephalin. The endor-phins (predominantly beta-endorphin) are 31-amino acid peptides that contain the met-enkephalin sequence, but are synthesized separately by a different precursor.

This precursor, pro-opiomelanocortin (POMC), is also cleaved to form melano-cyte stimulating hormone (MSH) and adrenocorticotropic hormone (ACTH). The endorphins and enkephalins act primarily on mu- and delta-opioid receptors to exert their inhibitory effects. The dynorphins exist in several forms that range from 10 to 17 amino acids in length, and they exert their effects primarily on kappa receptors. Finally, the endomorphins exist in two different forms, both 4 amino acids in length, and interestingly do not share homology with classical opiates.[39]

The role of the endogenous opioids in the CNS is fairly well established, but the existence of these peptides in the immune system has only recently been acknowl-edged. Therefore, the activity of these compounds in immune functioning is under profound investigation. Beta-endorphin (BE) and its POMC precursor are found in PBMCs. BE is constitutively synthesized. Concentrations are independent of opioid plasma concentration and can be elevated in response to certain stimuli such as stress.

Pharmacological studies examining BE concentration modulations revealed that dopamine and gamma-aminobutyric acid (GABA) provide inhibitory control, whereas serotonin imparts stimulatory regulation.[40] In addition, BE is also found in lymphocytes and is thought to be involved in the control of inflammatory pain. Cabot et al. demonstrated that BE-producing lymphocytes home to inflamed tissue where they secrete BE to control pain; following the release of peptide, the lymphocytes migrate to regional lymph nodes.[41]

The existence of endogenous opioids in the cells of the immune system suggests that they serve a relevant function. The work of many groups has been designed to reveal possible functions of the endogenous opioids in immune operation.

A significant amount of work has been done to try to establish a role for the opioids in immune functioning. It has been demonstrated that *in vitro* treatments of CD4+ T cells with endorphins results in increased IL-2, IL-4, and IFN-γ cytokine production.[42] On the other hand it has also been demonstrated that BE treatment of splenocytes results in inhibition of PHA-stimulated proliferation.[43] Enhanced neutrophil activity, as assessed by the expression of complement receptors and superoxide anion generation, was demonstrated after treatment of neutrophils with BE and met-enkephalin.[44]

Many of the functions of the endogenous opioids have been implicated due to the observation that opiate antagonist administration blocks many of the effects. For example, rats subjected to inescapable foot shocks exhibited elevated tumor growth, and this effect was abolished by treatment with naltrexone, an opiate antagonist, suggesting a role for the endogenous opioids.[45] Mice exposed to odors produced by foot shock-stressed donor mice demonstrated enhanced antibody responses and increases in IL-4 production that were eliminated following naltrexone treatment, once again suggesting a role for the endogenous opioids in mediating stress-induced immune alterations.[46]

Sacerdote et al. demonstrated that treatment of splenocytes with the antagonist naloxone resulted in an increase in IL-2 and IFN-γ production accompanied by a decrease in IL-4 and IgG antibody titers. These results suggest that naloxone treatment polarizes T helper cells toward a Th1 effector population, and imply that naloxone may be removing the regulatory effects of endogenous opioids that may shift the balance toward Th2.[47] Interestingly, administration of met-enkephalin before restraint stress abolished stress-induced immune alterations including elevations of glucocorticoids.

However, met-enkephalin administration alone exerted effects on the immune system similar to those seen following stress, including decreased NK activity and a deficit in PFC response.[48] In summary, the work described in this section clearly points to a role for endogenous opioids in the modulation of the immune system, and like stress and exogenous opiates (morphine), it appears that these compounds have an inhibitory mode of action.

CONCLUSION

This chapter has hopefully outlined the current understanding of the roles of the mu-opioid receptor and the endogenous opioids in stress-induced immunosuppression. The opening sections described work directed to understanding the mechanisms by which stress brings about immune dysfunction. Several different and versatile models of stress clearly demonstrate that it has a profound impact on immune system function. The chapter also describes the impact of morphine on the immune system and, like stress, morphine imparts severe immunosuppression.

Finally, the closing sections described the role of the mu-opioid receptor and the endogenous opioid system. A fair amount of work has been done, but there remain huge gaps of knowledge that must be investigated. Uncovering the mechanisms by which stress brings about immunosuppression is a worthwhile endeavor given the vast number of situations and means by which countless people deal with stress.

REFERENCES

1. Padgett, D.A. and Glaser, R. How stress influences the immune response. *Trends Immunol* 24(8), 444, 2003.
2. Schedlowski, M., Jacobs, R., Stratmann, G., Richter, S., Hadicke, A., Tewes, U., Wagner, T.O., and Schmidt, R.E. Changes of natural killer cells during acute psychological stress. *J Clin Immunol* 13(2), 119, 1993.
3. Coe, C.L. and Erickson, C.M. Stress decreases lymphocyte cytolytic activity in the young monkey even after blockade of steroid and opiate hormone receptors. *Dev Psychobiol* 30, 1, 1997.
4. Dahanukar, S.A., Thatte, U.M., Deshmukh, U.D., Kulkarni, M.K., and Bapat, R.D. The influence of surgical stress on the psychoneuro–endocrine–immune axis. *J Postgrad Med* 42(1), 12, 1996.
5. Stefanski, V. and Engler, H. Effects of acute and chronic social stress on blood cellular immunity in rats. *Phys Behav* 64(5), 733, 1998.
6. Karp, J.D., Smith, J., and Hawk, K. Restraint stress augments antibody production in cyclophosphamide-treated mice. *Phys Behav* 70, 271, 2000.
7. Deinzer, R., Kleineidam, C., Stiller-Winkler, R., Idel, H., and Bach, D. Prolonged reduction of salivary immunoglobulin A (sIgA) after a major academic exam. *Int J Psychophys* 37, 219, 2000.
8. Lacey, K., Zaharia, M.D., Griffiths, J., Ravindran, A.V., Merali, Z., and Anisman, H. A prospective study of neuroendocrine immune alterations associated with the stress of an oral academic examination among graduate students. *Psychoneuroendocrinology* 25, 339, 2000.
9. Marshall Jr., G.D., Agarwal, S.K., Lloyd, C., Cohen, L., Henninger, E.M., and Morris, G.J. Cytokine dysregulation associated with exam stress in healthy medical students. *Brain Behav Immun* 12, 297, 1998.
10. Bachen, E.A., Manuck, S.B., Marsland, A.L., Cohen, S., Malkoff, S.B., Muldoon, M.F., and Rabin, B.S. Lymphocyte subset and cellular immune response to a brief experimental stressor. *Psychosom Med* 54(6), 673, 1992.
11. Futterman, A.D., Wellisch, D.K., Zighelboim, J., Luna-Raines, M., and Weiner, H. Psychological and immunological reactions of family members to patients undergoing bone marrow transplantation. *Psychosom Med* 58(5), 472, 1996.
12. Avila, A.H., Morgan, C.A., and Bayer, B.M. Stress-induced suppression of the immune system after withdrawal form chronic cocaine. *JPET* 305(1), 290, 2003.
13. Rahim, R.T., Adler, M.W., Meissler Jr., J.J., Cowan, A., Rogers, T.J., Geller, E.B., and Eisenstein, T.K. Abrupt or precipitated withdrawal from morphine induces immunosuppression. *J Neuroimmunol* 127, 88, 2002.

14. Rahim, R.T., Meissler Jr., J.J., Zhang, L., Adler, M.W., Rogers, T.J., and Eisenstein, T.K. Withdrawal from morphine in mice suppresses splenic macrophage function, cytokine production, and costimulatory molecules. *J Neuroimmunol* 144, 16, 2003.

15. Bhargava, H.N., Thomas, P.T., Thorat, S., and House, R.V. Effects of morphine tolerance and abstinence on cellular immune function. *Brain Res* 642, 1, 1994.

16. Govitrapong, P., Suttitum, T., Kotchabhakdi, N., and Uneklabh, T. Alterations of immune functions in heroin addicts and heroin withdrawal subjects. *JPET* 286, 883, 1998.

17. Kelschenbach, J., Barke, R.A., and Roy, S. Morphine withdrawal contributes to Th cell differentiation by biasing cells toward the Th2 lineage. *J Immunol* 175(4), 2655, 2005.

18. Sharp, B.M., Roy, S., and Bidlack, J.M. Evidence for opioid receptors on cells involved in host defense and the immune system. *J Neuroimmunol* 83, 45, 1998.

19. Chuang, T.K., Killam Jr., K.F., Chuang, L.F., Kung, H.F., Sheng, W.S., Chao, C.C., Yu, L., and Chuang, R.Y. Mu opioid receptor gene expression in immune cells. *Biochem Biophys Res Comm* 216(3), 922, 1995.

20. Wick, M.J., Minnerath, S.R., Roy, S., Ramakrishnan, S., and Loh, H.H. Differential expression of opioid receptors in human lymphoid cell lines and peripheral blood lymphocytes. *J Neuroimmunol* 64(1), 29, 1996.

21. Sedqi, M., Roy, S., Ramakrishnan, S., Elde, R., and Loh. H.H. Complementary DNA cloning of a mu-opioid receptor from rat peritoneal macrophages. *Biochem Biophys Res Comm* 209(2), 563, 1996.

22. Sedqi, M., Roy, S., Ramakrishnan, S., and Loh, H.H. Expression cloning of a full-length cDNA encoding delta opioid receptor form mouse thymocytes. *J Neuroimmunol* 65(2), 167, 1996.

23. Wick, M.J., Minnerath, S.R., Roy, S., Ramakrishnan, S., and Loh, H.H. Expression of alternate forms of brain opioid 'orphan' receptor mRNA in activated human peripheral blood lymphocytes and lymphocytic cell lines. *Brain Res Mol Brain Res* 32(2), 342, 1995.

24. Piros, E.T., Hales, T.G., and Evans, C.J. Functional analysis of cloned opioid receptors in transfected cell lines. *Neurochem Res*. 11, 1277, 1996.

25. Carr, D.J. and France, C.P. Immune alterations in morphine treated rhesus monkeys. *JPET* 267(1), 9, 1993.

26. Tomei, E.Z. and Renaud, F.L. Effect of morphine on Fc-mediated phagocytosis by murine macrophages *in vitro*. *J Neuroimmunol* 74, 111, 1997.

27. Pacifici, R., di Carlo, S., Bacosi, A., Pichini, S., and Zuccaro, P. Pharmacokinetics and cytokine production in heroin and morphine treated mice. *Int J Immunopharm* 22, 603, 2000.

28. Roy, S. Balasubramanian, S., Sumandeep, S., Charboneau, R., Wang, J., Melnyk, D., Beilman, G.J., Vatassery, R., and Barke, R.A. Morphine directs T cells toward Th2 differentiation. *Surgery* 130, 304, 2001.

29. Roy, S., Chapin, R.B., Cain, K.J., Charboneau, R.G., Ramakrishnan, S., and Barke, R.A. Morphine inhibits transcriptional activation of IL-2 in mouse thymocytes. *Cellular Immunol* 179, 1, 1997.

30. Wang, J., Barke, R.A., Charboneau, R., Loh, H.H., and Roy, S. Morphine negatively regulates interferon-γ promoter activity in activated murine T cells through two distinct cyclic AMP dependent pathways. *J Biol Chem* 278(39), 37622, 2003.

31. Loh, H.H., Liu, H., Cavalli, A., Yang, W., Chen, Y., and Wei, L. Mu opioid receptor knockout in mice: effects on ligand-induced analgesia and morphine lethality. *Molec Brain Res* 54, 321, 1998.

32. Roy, S., Barke, R.A., and Loh, H.H. Mu-opioid receptor knockout mice: role of mu-opioid receptor in morphine-mediated immune functions. *Molec Brain Res* 61, 190, 1998.

33. Wang, J., Charboneau, R., Balasubramanian, S., Barke, R.A., Loh, H.H., and Roy, S. Morphine modulates lymph node derived T-lymphocyte function: role of caspase-3,-8, and nitric oxide. *J Leuk Biol* 70, 527, 2001.

34. Gaveriaux-Ruff, C., Matthes, H.W.D., Peluso, J., and Kieffer, B. Abolition of morphine immunosuppression in mice lacking the μ-opioid receptor gene. *Proc Natl Acad Sci USA* 95, 6326, 1998.

35. Bryant, H.U., Bernton, E.W., Kenner, J.R., and Holaday, J.W. Role of adrenal cortical activation in the immunosuppressive effects of chronic morphine treatment. *Endocrinology* 128(6), 3253, 1991.

36. Roy, S., Wang, J., Balasubramanian, S., Sumandeep, Charboneau, R. Barke, R., and Loh, H.H. Role of hypothalamic-pituitary axis in morphine-induced alteration in thymic cell distribution using mu-opioid receptor knockout mice. *J Neuroimmunol* 116, 147, 2001.

37. Wang, J., Charboneau, R., Balasubramanian, S., Barke, R. A., Loh, H. H., and Roy, S. The immunosuppressive effects of chronic morphine treatment are partially dependent on corticosterone and mediated by the mu-opioid receptor. *J Leuk Biol* 71, 782, 2002.

38. Wang, J. Charboneau, R. Barke, R.A., Loh, H.H., and Roy, S. Mu-opioid receptor mediates chronic restraint stress-induced lymphocyte apoptosis. *J Immunol* 169, 3630, 2002.

39. www.archway.ac.uk

40. Panerai, A.E. and Sacerdote, P. Beta-endorphin in the immune system: a role at last? *Trends Immunol Today* 18(7), 317, 1997

41. Cabot, P.J., Carter, L., Gaiddon, C., Zhang, Q., Schafer, M., Loeffler, J.P., and Stein, C. Immune cell derived beta-endorphin. *J Clin Invest* 100(1), 142, 1997.

42. van der Bergh, P., Dobber, R., Ramlal, S., Rozing, J., and Nagelkerken, L. Role of opioid peptides in the regulation of cytokine production by murine CD4+ T cells. *Cell Immunol* 154(1), 109, 1994.

43. Panerai, A.E., Manfredi, B., Granucci, F., and Sacerdote, P. The beta-endorphin inhibition of mitogen-induced splenocytes proliferation is mediated by central and peripheral paracrine/autocrine effects of the opioid. *J Neuroimmunol* 58, 71, 1995.

44. Menzebach, A., Hirsch, J., Hempelmann, G., and Welters, I.D. Effects of endogenous and synthetic opioid peptides on neutrophil function *in vitro*. *Brit J Anaesthesia* 91(4), 546, 2003.

45. Lewis, J.W., Shavit, Y., Terman, G.W., Nelson, L.R., Gale, R.P., and Liebeskind, J.C. Apparent involvement of opioid peptides in stress-induced enhancement of tumor growth. *Peptides* 4(5), 635, 1983.

46. Moynihan, J.A., Karp, J.D., Cohen, N., and Ader, R. Immune deviation following stress odor exposure: role of endogenous opioids. *J Neuroimmunol* 102, 145, 2000.

47. Sacerdote, P., Manfredi, B., Gaspani, L., and Panerai, A.E. The opioid antagonist naloxone induces a shift from type 2 to type1 cytokine pattern in BALB/cJ mice. *Blood* 95(6), 2031, 2000.

48. Morotti, G., Gabrilovac, J., Rabatic, S., Smejkal-Jagar, L., Rocic, B., and Haberstock, H. Met-enkephalin modulates stress-induced alterations of the immune response in mice. *Pharmacol Biochem Behav* 54(1), 277, 1996.

9 Stress, Opioid Peptides, and Immune Response

Javier Puente, Marion E. Wolf, M. Antonieta Valenzuela, and Aron D. Mosnaim

CONTENTS

INTRODUCTION

Endorphins, enkephalins, and dynorphins, and endogenous peptides synthesized by a wide variety of cell types, are involved in the regulation of multiple biological processes in the animal kingdom. During the course of evolution, these chemical mediators have been conserved in vertebrate and invertebrate organisms, emphasizing the vital importance of their actions. One of their roles is the immunomodulatory function over both the innate and specific immune responses.

Opioid peptides and cytokines share many properties; they are both low molecular weight peptides characterized by the redundancy and pleiotropy of their effects.[1,2] Their actions can be felt at paracrine and autocrine levels, and in some situations such as stress, also systemically. The demonstration in the early 1980s of communications among the three main regulatory systems (nervous, endocrine, and immunological) in vertebrate organisms led to the realization that chemical signals or mediators originating from any one of these systems may influence the other two.[3]

Recognition of a role for the opioid peptides in the modulation of the immune response is of particular importance. These substances act directly upon specific opioid receptors present in practically all cellular types implicated in the immune response, including lymphocytes B and T, natural killer (NK) cells, monocytes, macrophages, and neutrophils.[4] Lymphocytes may also synthesize these peptides, allowing for the action of these substances at different levels because they are present in circulation and may migrate toward areas of need.[5] In fact, this peptide–immune cell interaction appears to engage wide participation of the innate and specific immune responses and may be critical in conditions as diverse as stress, inflammation, and pain

The hypothalamus–hypophysis–effector (adrenal) gland and the sympathetic system–adrenal medulla axis are two of the principal pathways involved in stress modulation of the immune response since immunocompetent cells also express receptors for neuroendocrine system-related substances such as catecholamines and cortisol. Some of the stress-related molecules (biointegrators), such as epinephrine and pro-opiomelanocortin (POMC), have the role of coordinating the whole organism to produce an adequate response to this condition. Regulated hydrolysis of the POMC polyprotein can generate various regulatory peptides such as melanocyte-stimulating hormones (α, β, and γ-MSH), adrenocorticotropin (ACTH), β-lipotropin hormones, β-endorphin, dynorphins, and enkephalins.

Most of the more than 20 endogenous opioid peptides identified in mammals derive from one of three protein precursor families: POMC, proenkephalins, and proendorphins. This review analyzes the effects of these peptides upon immuno-competent cells. It will also discuss the capacities of these cells to produce some of these same peptides, both under physiological conditions and in response to certain pathological circumstances such as stress, inflammation, and pain.

ENDOGENOUS OPIOID PEPTIDES AND THEIR RECEPTORS

ENDOGENOUS OPIOID PEPTIDES

Morphine received its name from Morpheus, the Greek god of sleep. It and other exogenous opioid-like substances with alkaloid chemical structures produce anal-gesia through interaction with specific mu-type (μ) opioid receptors.[6] Since the isolation of the enkephalins from pig brain in the early 1970s,[7] three main families of endogenous opioid peptides (enkephalins, endorphins, and dynorphins) have been described as having multiple physiological functions and pharmacological effects. Two enkephalins, methionine-enkephalin [H-Tyr-Gly-Gly-Phe-Met-OH (MET)] and leucine-enkephalin [H-Tyr-Gly-Gly-Phe-Leu-OH (LEU)], best characterized by their analgesic properties, show greater specificity for delta (δ) than for μ receptors.

These pentapeptides derive from three precursor proteins: POMC, preproenkephalin (proenkephalin A), and preprodynorphin (proenkephalin B). The POMC molecule encodes the MET and LEU sequences as well as those of other non-opioid fragments including β-lipotropin, ACTH, and MSH. While proenkephalin A contains six copies of MET and one of LEU, proenkephalin B produces dynorphin A and B peptides that contain the LEU sequence. Precursors for peptides such as endomorphin 1 and 2 that share many identified opioid peptide actions (e.g., μ agonists with analgesic properties) are still unknown. All these peptides are present in the central nervous system (CNS) and released in response to various stimuli such as stress and pain. Enkephalins are also produced in the adrenal gland and, along with endorphins, in the leukocytes. The effects of dynorphin A are rather conflictive and, paradoxically, have been shown to produce hyperalgesia. Recently a new 17-amino acid endogenous opioid peptide designated nociceptin or orphanin FQ has been reported.[8,9] This peptide, derived from higher molecular weight precursors, acts upon the newly designated opioid-like receptor 1 (ORL-1) that has approximately a 50% homology with the classic opioid receptors.[10]

OPIOID RECEPTORS

Endogenous opioid peptides act upon specific receptors, namely μ,κ (ketocyclazocine), and δ, and their effects are blocked by specific antagonists, the most representative being naloxone and naltrexone (Table 9.1).[11-13] Molecular cloning techniques have shown the presence of these receptors in components of the immune system.[14-16] All three of them are part of the receptor family coupled to protein G (GPCR), formed by one peptidic chain with seven transmembrane regions.[17] The transductor protein Gi, a heterotrimer structure formed by the α, β, and γ subunits, participates in signal transduction and regulation of receptor expression.[17] A fourth member of this GPCR family known as ORL-1 is considered an example of so-called reverse pharmacology because it was discovered before its nociceptin ligand.[18]

TABLE 9.1
Leukocytes: Opioid Peptides and Receptors

Opioid Agonists	Binding Affinity	Precursor	Leukocyte Receptors
β-endorphin	μ > δ	Pro-opiomelanocortin	T lymphocytes, NK cells, monocytes/ macrophages, polymorphonuclear cells
Enkephalins	δ > μ	Pro-enkephalin	T lymphocytes, NK cells, monocytes/ macrophages, polymorphonuclear cells
Dynorphin	κ > μ	Pro-dynorphin	T lymphocytes, monocytes/macrophages
Nociceptin/orphanin FQ	—	Nociceptin/orphanin FQ precursor	T lymphocytes

The presence of all of these receptors has been demonstrated in components of the immune system e.g., lymphocytes T and B, monocytes/macrophages, and neutrophils. Their transcripts have been detected in immunocompetent cells, initially using radioligand and fluorescence assays and later by RT-PCR techniques.[19,20] Low receptor levels in lymphocytes are increased by cell activation. Thus, *in vivo* administration (animal models) of the staphylococcal enterotoxin B (SEB) exotoxin known to interact with lymphocytes T TCR, stimulated delta opioid receptor (DOR) expression in these cells.[21] *In vitro* studies, using vegetal lectine phytohemagglutinin (PHA) to stimulate lymphocytes produce increased DOR, T CD4, and CD8 expression; PHA also elicited increased anti-CD3 expression in murine splenocytes.[22]

ORL-1 is also present in lymphocytes, and its nociceptin ligand stimulates T lymphocyte activation and proliferation.[23] It is not therefore unexpected that opioid peptides, having specific receptors in both the nervous and immune systems, are considered immunomodulators, thus allowing for a close relationship of both systems.

Signal transduction mechanisms mediated by opioid receptors are diverse and complex. The presence in the CNS of different receptor subtypes (μ_{1-3}, δ_{1-2}, and κ_{1-3}) is further complicated as they may, in turn, associate to protein G from various Gi or Go structures. Activation of these different protein G molecules may stimulate or inhibit adenylate cyclase, resulting in alterations in cyclic AMP levels.[17] Although signal transduction mechanisms involving immunocompetent cell opioid peptide receptors are not yet well characterized, μ and δ receptor activation stimulated MAPkinases, which in turn activated transcriptional factors such as ATF-2 via phosphorylation.[19,22]

STRESS AND EFFECTS OF OPIOID PEPTIDES ON THE IMMUNE SYSTEM

OPIOID PEPTIDES AND IMMUNE RESPONSE

The pioneering research of Joseph Wybran in the mid-1970s[24] demonstrating the presence of opioid receptors in immunocompetent cells marked the beginning of a large ongoing research effort to elucidate the response of the immune system to substances with opioid-like pharmacological properties. Although this work produced a substantial amount of data, a number of factors rendered this information rather difficult to interpret:

1. The presence of opioid and non-opioid effects described in various systems, particularly in the CNS[25] as a general characteristic after a challenge with opioid peptides. One example is the demonstration of specific β-endorphin non-opioid receptors in rat lymphocytes.[26]
2. The difficulty of determining the "possible" effects of opioid peptide fragments on opioid receptors. Complicating the issue even further, depending on the tissue or fluid studied, proteolysis of a given peptide may give rise to a qualitatively and/or quantitatively different mix of parent compound fragments,

e.g., human tissue and plasmatic MET and LEU metabolism.[27–31] We can only speculate about the relative contribution of the parent compound and its various fragments to a particular overall immune response: MET and β- endorphin metabolites have been shown to stimulate NK cell activity.[27,32–35]

3. The effects of opioid peptides on the CNS or the immune system are complex and results of similar *in vitro* and *in vivo* experiments do not always coincide. Additionally, the mechanisms responsible for regulating circulating opioid peptide levels are not yet well understood, although the levels are important because they may influence the magnitude and direction of elicited immune responses.

Circulating opioid peptide levels may change significantly in patients suffering from pain-associated medical conditions. Thus, the basal plasma MET and LEU levels are significantly higher in migraineurs during acute migraine episodes than levels measured when the same individuals are migraine pain-free.[29] In inflammation-associated pain, leukocyte migration is responsible for the delivery of endogenous opioids to the irritated area.[4,5,36–38] Both of these examples indicate a relationship between the occurrence of pain and the response by the opioid system. Plasma MET and LEU levels are tightly regulated at various stages of their synthesis, release, and degradation. This latter process, carried out almost completely by plasmatic aminopeptidase,[28,30] can be inhibited by a number of currently used drugs — a fact worth considering when devising rational approaches to the pharmacological modulation of the endogenous opioid system.[39–42]

STRESS, INFLAMMATION, AND PAIN

Although the influence of physical and psychological stress on the immune system was suspected for a long time, the first scientific reports describing this influence appeared only in the middle of last century. Results from a large number of studies on a variety of experimental models consistently showed that, depending on the type and duration of the applied paradigm, stress may stimulate or reduce immune system response. It is generally accepted that models of acute stress elicit stimulation and those of chronic stress produce reduction of this response.[43,44] Alterations in homeostasis induced by conditions such as stress, inflammation, and infection test the integrity and strength of the interconnection of the nervous, endocrine, and immunological systems, including alterations caused by the many implicated mediators including hormones, neuropeptides, neurotransmitters, and cytokines.[45–47] The hypothalamic–pituitary–adrenal (HPA) axis is critical in maintaining physiological homeostasis; opioid peptides are known to play an important role in this process.[48]

STRESS AND THE HPA AXIS

The response of the HPA axis to stress caused by inflammatory, psychological, and environmental factors is complex and largely depends on hypothalamic control, magnitude, duration of the stress-producing stimulus, and the dynamics of secretion

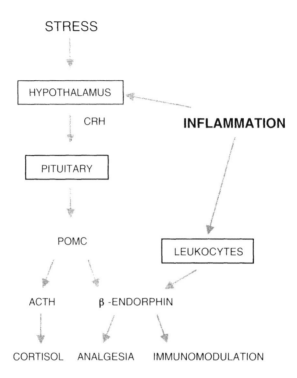

FIGURE 9.1 Generation of CRH and/or ACTH after HPA axis activation by stress and inflammation. Resultant substances such as cortisol and β-endorphin are immunomodulators of the innate and specific immune responses. Inflammation also stimulates leukocyte synthesis and release of opioid peptides.

and actions of the implicated chemical mediators (Figure 9.1). Hypothalamic stimulation results in hypothalamic paraventricular nuclei secretion of corticotrophin-releasing hormone (CRH) toward the hypophysis where it induces POMC expression and release.[49,50] POMC then undergoes specific post-translational processing, generating ACTH, β-lipoprotein, and β-endorphin. ACTH secreted into the circulation, in turn, induces adrenal gland expression and release of glucocorticoids.[49,51] Substances involved in the regulation of a wide variety of genes implicated in the control of the immune response inhibit the expression of select pro-inflammatory cytokines and leukocyte adhesion molecules and stimulate the expression of anti-inflammatory cytokines and lymphocyte apoptosis.[52-55]

Many central (hypothalamic, hyphophysiary) and peripheral factors can stimulate biochemical pathways leading to the synthesis and release of POMC and ACTH. Thus, POMC expression is stimulated by CRH, vasopressin, catecholamines, and cytokines, and inhibited by glucocorticoids. The role of cytokines, particularly those with pro-inflammatory properties is most relevant. POMC stimulation results in increased cortisol formation, thus antagonizing their own pro-inflammatory actions in a process seen as an important physiological control mechanism.[56-59] The hypothalamus and hyphophysis express cytokines and their receptors. There is evidence for the autocrine and paracrine effects of cytokines, in particular those of the gp130 family [IL-6, IL-11, leukemia inhibitory factor (LIF), oncostatin M, ciliary neurotrophic factor (CNF), and cardiotropin 1].[49,60]

This type of mechanism was demonstrated in genetically defective (knockout) mice for the gene CRF (CRFKO). In this model, lipopolyssacharide (LPS) challenge stimulated the synthesis of pro-inflammatory cytokines, indicating that these mice can still have viable biochemical pathways to synthesize ACTH in response to inflammation, emphasizing the complexity of mechanisms regulating ACTH production.[59]

In addition to the local synthesis of cytokines, there is also the probability that peripherally produced cytokines may exert their effects at the level of the hypothalamus or hypophysis.[61,62] Whether peripheral pro-inflammatory cytokines enter the brain is still a controversial subject, but it is generally accepted that a great number of cytokines are expressed constitutively in the brain, including the hypothalamus, and that their synthesis is induced during inflammation.[63]

OPIOID AGONISTS μ AND δ, MORPHINE, β-ENDORPHIN, AND ENKEPHALINS

The most important *in vivo* effects of β-endorphin, a μ and δ opioid receptor agonist, on the immune system relate to its immunosuppressant properties. Its administration directly to the brain or intravenously decreases various immunological functions, e.g., mitogen-induced lymphocyte proliferation and NK cell cytotoxicity, an effect antagonized by naloxone and naltrexone.[64-66] Furthermore, β-endorphin induces a T helper 2 type (TH2) effect, whereas naloxone acting as an immune response enhancer elicits a T helper 1 type (TH1) effect.[66,67] However, opioid receptor δ synthetic nonpeptidic agonists such as SNC80 enhance the immune response, again emphasizing the complexity of opioid actions.[68-69]

In general, opioid peptides act as immunosuppressants *in vivo*. Among the most notable effects of the chronic use of morphine, a powerful immunosuppresor acting upon μ receptors, are the decrease of bone marrow cellular proliferation and lymphocyte apoptosis, as manifested in mice thymus and spleen hypoplasia.[70-75] These serious effects are even more severe in immature T lymphocytes.[74,75] Similar observations, e.g., characteristic lymphopenia, have been reported to accompany chronic stress and in surgical patients and individuals subjected to psychological stress.[76-81]

In animal restriction models, naloxone treatment previous to stressor application blocked the development of apoptosis, emphasizing the role of opioid-like substances in this process.[82] Mechanisms believed to be involved in this type of stress-induced lymphocyte apoptosis include Fas receptor induction in lymphocytes, thus favoring Fas–FasL interaction with the resulting caspase enzyme activation as the cause of apoptosis.[72-83,84] HPA axis-released glucocorticoids also contribute to lymphocyte apoptosis, thus potentiating this process.[51]

Sepsis or septic shock, manifested in infection as well as in inflammatory and immunological alterations, is another example of severe pathological stress in which endogenous and exogenous opioids may produce immunosuppressant effects via mechanisms involving opioid receptors.[85-88] Recent animal studies have shown that naltrexone administration previous to LPS sepsis induction provides protection from some of the deleterious effects of this condition and prevents the mortality commonly associated with its occurrence.[89] Current evidence shows naltrexone as inhibiting *in vivo* LPS-induced macrophage tumor necrosis factor-α (TNF-α) generation, a process thought to happen through a mechanism independent of the macrophage, perhaps occurring at the CNS level, as this opioid receptor antagonist does not inhibit *in vitro* macrophage TNF-α secretion.[89] The immune responses in other animal models of septic shock not based on TNF-α generation, e.g., lymphocyte stimulation by superantigens or via Fas activation, were not influenced by naltrexone, emphasizing the selectivity of the opioid-mediated effects.[88,89]

Further affirmation of the role of opioids in inflammatory processes via the μ opioid receptor (MOR) comes from finding that administration of μ receptor agonists such as (D-Arg2,Lys4)dermorphin-(1,4)-amide (DALDA) and (D-Ala2,N-Me-Phe4,Gly5-ol)-enkephalin (DAMGO or DAGO) inhibit colon inflammation.[90] Both substances block release in the colon of pro-inflammatory cytokines such as TNF-α and interferon-γ (IFN-γ), an effect antagonized by naloxone. The fact that neither DALDA nor DAMGO significantly crosses the blood–brain barrier indicates that the protector effect is mediated by peripheral mechanisms.[90]

There is ample evidence showing that the circulating level of MET and LEU, pentapeptides synthesized and released in the adrenal gland, hypothalamus, and lymphocytes, are increased in response to stress, inflammation, and pain.[29,91-94] Depending on experimental conditions, particularly the doses used, the enkephalins may stimulate or inhibit various immune functions *in vivo*.[2,95] Thus, these peptides increase the humoral and cellular immune responses,[96] for example, phagocytosis,[97] NK cell cytotoxicity,[98] IFN-γ secretion, and lymphocyte proliferation.[99] This led some investigators to consider their use as coadjuvant therapies for conditions characterized by decreased immune system activity such as AIDS and various carcinomas.[99] Enkephalins may also act as immunosuppressants, and in some cases their actions are dependent on animal gender.[95,100] As with other opioids, the effects of enkephalin may result from a direct action upon opioid receptors in immune cells or indirectly via interaction with CNS-located receptors. The actual mechanisms of most enkephalin effects are unknown and probably include a mixture of both types of actions. Considering their multiple biological effects, the enkephalins are currently considered cytokines by most authors.[1,2-101]

Results obtained mostly from *in vitro* studies indicate that substances with opioid-like activities, particularly enkephalins and endorphins, may stimulate or inhibit various immunological functions such as PHA mitogenic action, effect of pokeweed mitogen (PWM) on lymphocyte T and B proliferation, cytokine secretion, NK cell cytotoxicity, and macrophage and neutrophil phagocytic activity in health and disease.[102-108] The immune response is dependent on factors as diverse as the opioid dose tested and the initial status of the sample's immune system (above, below, or within normal control range). Furthermore, effects observed *in vitro* do not always coincide with those obtained *in vivo*, and not all opioid peptide effects are inhibited by their classic antagonists.

The magnitude and direction of the *in vitro* effect of MET and/or β-endorphin on NK cell cytotoxicity of PBMC preparations obtained from different patient populations appear to be dependent on the particular disease condition of the group studied. Thus, MET challenge significantly decreased NK cell activity in PBMC samples obtained from a group of post-traumatic stress disorder patients.[103] Similar results were recorded after the addition of opioid peptide to PBMC preparations from migraineurs obtained during acute migraine episodes.[109,110] Although the mechanisms involved in these opioid peptide–PBMC–NK cell interaction are yet to be elucidated, it has been suggested that they may result from quantitative and/or qualitative changes in NK cell subpopulations associated with various disease conditions. Little is known regarding changes in lymphocyte subpopulations that may be associated with stress-related pain, but preliminary results indicate significant increases in the relative levels of circulating CD3+, CD16+, and CD56+ cells in migraine patients.[111] Furthermore, increases in CD56+ cells and in NK cell activity were observed in an acute human pain model.[112]

OPIOID PEPTIDES AND LEUKOCYTES

Immunocompetent cells such as T and B lymphocytes, neutrophils, eosinophils, monocytes, and macrophages can synthesize opioid peptides from POMC, a process stimulated by CRH and a few cytokines such as IL-1β.[4,36–38,92] Lymphocyte migration, in response to tissue inflammation, is followed by the release of stored peptides which may help to restore the structures and functions of affected areas. Inflammation is considered part of a host complex and beneficial response in reply to an external challenge or tissue damage. It involves the active participation of the vascular endothelium, the innate and in some cases also the specific immune response.[5] The innate response initiates this process, generating warning signals guiding the ensuing participation of components of the specific immune response.

Blood leukocyte migration toward the inflammation site takes place in various stages: (1) endothelial cell activation, (2) circulating leukocyte activation, and (3) leukocyte chemoattraction. Inflammation-activated leukocytes, particularly T lymphocytes, express higher levels of POMC mRNA and opioid peptides which, upon release at the inflammation site, may interact with sensitive opioid receptors producing analgesia.[5,38] In fact, this characteristic "inflammation-derived analgesic effect" is blocked by specific opioid antagonists and by specific anti-opioid peptide-specific antibodies. Thus, immunological cells with the potential to express higher opioid peptide levels, particularly MET and β-endorphin, in response to inflammation, have the ability to migrate and release these substances to injured tissue and lymphatic ganglia.[113] Polymorphonuclear leukocyte-like neutrophils that constitute the host's first line of defense against inflammation also contain opioids, further emphasizing the importance of this response in analgesia. Opioid-mediated analgesia may also be induced in animal models of stress (cold-water swimming) and post-surgery in humans.[37,114-117]

COMPLEX REGULATION OF OPIOID RECEPTORS

Immune cellular response to opioid receptor agonists is subject to multiple regulatory mechanisms. These include (1) control of agonist synthesis and metabolism, e.g., rapid and complete human *in vivo* and *in vitro* aminopeptidase degradation of MET and LEU, (2) regulation of the level of opioid receptor expression at the cellular level, and (3) receptor desensitization, a rapid development resulting in decreased or no receptor response. The latter process, occurring after opioid binding and receptor activation, may be completed after receptor internalization and down-regulation. The two types of desensitization described are homologous and heterologous.

HOMOLOGOUS DESENSITIZATION

The opioid agonist is responsible for receptor-G protein decoupling in a process involving receptor phosphorylation by a specific G protein-coupled receptor kinase (GRK) followed by the association of the β-arrestin protein to the receptor.[118,119] GRK phosphorylation of opioid receptor serine/threonine residues facilitates its interaction with β-arrestin. These events alter GPCR-mediated signal transduction, leading to receptor-protein G decoupling and its subsequent endocytosis.[120,121] It is well established that the various opioid receptor agonists studied differ in their relative abilities to produce receptor desensitization, with morphine, for example, being much less effective than the endogenous opioid peptides and a number of other agonists tested.[121-124] Homologous desensitization allows the explanation of complex biological phenomenon such as opioid dependence and tolerance.

HETEROLOGOUS DESENSITIZATION

A heterologous bidirectional regulation exerted by chemokines and opioid peptides over the expression of their receptors has been described. This effect corresponds to heterologous receptor desensitization.[125-126] Based on the positions of conserved cysteine amino acids, chemokines have been grouped into four families (C, CC, CXC, and CXCR) that interact with Gi protein coupled GPCR-type receptors designated CR1, CCR1-11, CXCR1-5, and CX3CR, respectively[127] The most important biological function of the chemokines is chemotaxis, a property of particular relevance in inflammation-associated leukocyte recruitment and migration. Through their actions upon μ, κ, and δ receptor opioid peptides, they also chemorecruit T lymphocytes, monocytes/macrophages, and neutrophils.[128-130]

These findings made it relatively easy to establish a heterologous regulation for these mediators. Thus, experiments based on pretreatment with MET and morphine inhibited neutrophil chemotactic response to IL-8 (CXCL8), an agonist of CXCR1 and CXCR2 receptors.[130] MET pretreatment blocked the effects of RANTES (CCL5) agonists CCR1, CCR3 and CCR5 on Jurkat cells.[126] As could be expected from a bidirectional receptor regulation, chemokines inhibited the chemotactic response to opioid agonists. In fact, pretreatment with RANTES inhibited leukocyte chemotactic response to the DAMGO μ-selective agonist.[126]

In conditions associated with overexpression of chemokines and opioid peptides, such as inflammation or stress, regulation of the final immune system response will reflect the balance of mediator effects. The findings that CCR5 and CXCR4 receptors are also co-receptors of the HIV-1 virus responsible for AIDS have increased the interest in this type of interaction. *In vitro* experiments using PHA (which stimulates DOR expression) challenged PBMC showed that the addition of the delta receptor agonist SNC-80 decreased expression of the HIV-1 virus in CD4+ T lymphocytes. This inhibitory effect on virus replication was inhibited by naltrindole.[131] Heterologous desensitization studies in monocytes/macrophages using opioid μ and δ receptor agonists produced a decrease in HIV-1 virus infectivity, an effect associated with desensitization of the CCR5 receptor.[132] Explanation for these findings could include a diminished cellular surface receptor expression and/or alterations in signal transduction mechanisms. Mu receptor phosphorylation as a result of chemokine treatment apparently prevents the action of opioid agonists, thus providing a possible explanation for the mechanism of desensitization.[133]

The study of animal models genetically deficient in the expression of opioid receptors has provided important information regarding the *in vivo* role of opioid ligands. Thus, recognized morphine immunosuppressant effects were lacking in μ receptor knockout mice, validating the critical importance of such receptors for morphine actions.[134] It should be noted that a number of *in vivo* and *in vitro* studies determined immunological parameters in these animals; numbers and lymphocyte distribution were similar to those of normal controls.[135,136] Although preliminary experiments showed increases in the numbers of splenocytes and in the overall humoral immune responses of κ opioid receptor knockout (KORKO) mice,[137] significant changes in the immune systems of δ opioid receptor knockout (DORKO) mice have been yet to be observed.[138] These studies are mostly of a preliminary nature but hold great future promise for a better understanding the functional roles of opioid receptors, which may hopefully lead to the rational design of pharmacological treatments of conditions as diverse as pain, inflammation, obesity, and a host of neuropsychiatric diseases.

ACKNOWLEDGMENTS

This research was supported by Proyectos FONDECYT-CHILE# 1880874 and 1901115, the National Headache Foundation of Chicago, Illinois, and Asthmatic Children's Aid, Skokie, Illinois.

REFERENCES

1. Peterson, P., Molitor, T., and Chao, Ch., The opioid-cytokine connection, J. Neuroimmunol., 83, 63, 1998.
2. Plotnikoff, N. et al., Methionine enkephalin, a new cytokine: human studies, Clin. Immunol. Immunopathol., 82, 93, 1997.
3. Haddad, J., Saade, N., and Safieh-Garabedian, B., Cytokines and neuro–immune–endocrine interactions: a role for the hypothalamic–pituitary–adrenal revolving axis, J. Neuroimmunol., 133, 1, 2002.
4. Smith, E., Opioid peptides in immune cells, Adv. Exp. Med., Biol., 521, 51, 2003.
5. Stein, C., Shäfer, M., and Machelska, H., Attacking pain at its source: new perspectives on opioids, Nature Med., 9, 1003, 2003.
6. Goldstein, H.B. and Akil, H., Opioids analgesics, in Goodman & Gilman's The Pharmacologic Basis of Therapeutics, Hardman, J.G. and Limbird, L.E., Eds., McGraw-Hill, New York, 2001, 569.
7. Hughes, J. et al., Identification of two-related pentapeptides from the brain with potent opiate agonist activity, Nature, 258, 577, 1975.
8. Meunier, J.C. et al., Isolation and structure of the endogenous agonist of opioid receptor-like ORL1 receptor, Nature, 377, 532, 1995.
9. Reinscheid, R.K. et al., Orphanin FQ: a neuropeptide that activates an opioid like G protein coupled receptors, Science, 270, 792, 1995.
10. Zeilhofer, H.U. and Calo, G., Nociceptin/orphanin FQ and its receptor-potential targets for pain therapy, J. Pharmacol. Exp. Ther., 306, 423, 2003.
11. Martin, W.E., Opioid antagonists, Pharmacol. Rev., 19, 464, 1967.
12. Martin, W.R., Pharmacology of opioids, Pharmacol. Rev., 35, 285, 1984.
13. Vaupel, B., Naloxone fails to antagonize the σ effect of PCP and SKF-10047 in the dog, Eur. J. Pharmacol., 92, 1136, 1983.
14. Chang, T.K. et al., Mu opioid receptor gene expression in immune cells, Biochem. Biophys. Res. Commun., 216, 922, 1995.
15. Sharp, B.M. et al., Detection of basal levels and induction of delta opioids receptor mRNA in murine splenocytes, J. Neuroimmunol., 78, 198, 1997.
16. Chuang, L.F. et al., Expression of kappa opioids receptors in human and monkey lymphocytes, Biochem. Biophys. Res. Commun., 209, 1003, 1995.
17. Tso, P.H. and Wong, Y.H., Molecular basis of opioid dependence: Role of signal regulation by G-proteins, Clin. Exp. Pharmacol. Physiol., 30, 307, 2003.
18. Hawes, B., Graziano, M., and Lambert, D.G., Cellular actions of nociceptin: transduction mechanisms, Peptides, 21, 961, 2000.
19. Sharp, B.M., Opioid receptor expression and function, J. Neuroimmunol., 147, 3, 2004.
20. Gaveriaux-Ruff, C. et al., Antibody response and allogeneic mixed lymphocyte reaction in mu, delta and kappa opioid receptor knockout mice, J. Neuroimmunol., 147, 121, 2004.
21. Shahabi, N.A. et al., Expression of delta opioid receptors by splenocytes from SEB-treated mice and effects on phosphorylation of MAPkinase, Cell. Immunol., 205, 84, 2000.
22. Shahabi, NA., McAllen, K. and Sharp, B.M., Phosphorylation of activating transcription factor (ATF-2) in murine splenocytes through delta opioid receptors, Cell. Immunol., 221, 122, 2003.

23. Waits, P. et al., Nociceptin/orphanin FQ modulates human T cell function *in vitro, J. Neuroimmunol.*, 149, 110, 2004.

24. Wybran J. et al., Suggestive evidence for receptors for morphine and methionine-enkephalin on normal human blood, *J. Immunol.*, 123, 1068, 1979.

25. Wolleman, M. and Benyhe, S., Non-opioid action of opioid peptides, *Life Sci.*, 75, 257, 2004.

26. Hazum, E., Chang, K. and Cuatrecasas, P., Specific nonopiate receptors for β-endorphin, *Science*, 205, 1033, 1979.

27. Kowalski, J., Immunological action of Met enkephalin fragments, *Eur. J. Pharmacol.* 347, 95, 1998.

28. Mosnaim, A.D. et al., Studies of the *in vitro* human plasma degradation of methionine-enkephalin, *Biochem.Pharmacol.*, 19, 729, 1988.

29. Mosnaim, A.D. et al., Plasma methionine enkephalin level: a biological marker for migraine? *Headache*, 25, 259, 1985.

30. Venturelli, F. et al., Control mechanisms of peripheral enkephalin hydrolysis in mammalian plasma, *Comp. Biochem. Physiol.*, 83c, 307, 1986.

31. De Wied, D. and van Ree, J., Non-opiate effects of neuropeptides derived from beta-endorphin, *Pol. J. Pharmacol. Pharm.*, 39, 623, 1987.

32. Navolotskaya, E.V. et al., beta-Endorphin-like peptide SLTCLVKGFY is a selective agonist of nonopioid beta-endorphin receptor, *Biochem. Biophys. Res. Commun.*, 292, 799, 2002.

33. Navolotskaya, E.V. et al., Synthetic beta-endorphin-like peptide immunorphin binds to non-opioid receptors for beta-endorphin on T lymphocytes, *Peptides*, 22, 2009, 2001.

34. Owen, D.L. et al., The C-terminal tetrapeptide of beta-endorphin (MPF) enhances lymphocyte proliferative responses, *Neuropeptides*, 32, 131, 1998.

35. Williamson, S.A. et al., Differential effects of beta-endorphin fragments on human natural killing, *Brain Behav. Immun.*, 1, 329, 1987.

36. Stein, C. et al., Opioids from immunocytes interact with receptors on sensory nerves to inhibit nociception in inflammation, *Proc. Natl. Acad. Sci. USA*, 87, 5935, 1990.

37. Rittner, H.L. et al., Opioid peptide-expressing leukocytes: identification, recruitment and simultaneously increasing inhibition of inflammatory pain, *Anesthesiology*, 95, 500, 2001.

38. Schäfer, M., Cytokines and peripheral analgesia, *Adv. Exp. Med. Biol.*, 521, 40, 2003.

39. Mosnaim, A.D. et al., Degradation kinetics of leucine-enkephalin by plasma samples from healthy controls and various patient population: in vitro drug effects, *Am. J. Ther.*, 7, 185, 2000.

40. Mosnaim, A.D. et al., *In vitro* human plasma leucine[5]-enkephalin degradation is inhibited by a select number of drugs with the phenothiazine molecule in their chemical structure, *Pharmacology*, 67, 6, 2003.

41. Mosnaim, A.D. et al., Inhibition of human plasma leucine[5]-enkephalin aminopeptidase hydrolysis by various endogenous peptides and a select number of clinically used drugs, *Am. J. Ther.*, 11, 459, 2004.

42. Mosnaim, et al., Phenothiazine molecule provides the basic chemical structure for various classes of pharmacotherapeutic agents, *Am. J. Ther.*, in press, 2006.

43. Kielcot-Glaser, J. et al., Psychoneuroimmunology and psychosomatic medicine: back to the future, *Psychosom. Med.*, 64, 15, 2002.

44. Ader, R. and Cohen, N., Psychoneuroimmunology: conditioning and stress, *Annu. Rev. Psychol.*, 44, 53, 1993.

45. Wilder, R.L., Neuroendocrine–immune system interactions and autoimmunity, *Annu. Rev. Immunol.*, 13, 307, 1995.

46. Besedovsky, H. and del Ray, A., Immune–neuro–endocrine interactions: facts and hypothesis, *Endocr. Rev.*, 18, 206, 1996.

47. Thurnbull, A.V. and Rivier, C.L., Regulation of the hypothalamic–pituitary–adrenal axis by cytokines: actions and mechanisms of action, *Physiol. Rev.*, 79, 1, 1999.

48. Drolet, G. et al., Role of endogenous opioid system in the regulation of the stress response, *Prog. Neuropsychopharmacol. Biol. Psychiat.*, 25, 729, 2001.

49. Chesnokova, V. and Melmed, S., Neuro–immuno–endocrine modulation of the hypothalamic–pituitary–adrenal (HPA) axis by gp130 signalling molecules, *Endocrinology* 143, 1571, 2002.

50. Melmed, S., The immuno–neuro–endocrine interface, *J. Clin. Invest.*, 108, 1563, 2001.

51. Padgett, D. and Glaser, R., How stress influences the immune response, *Trends Immunol.*, 24, 444, 2003.

52. Barnes, P.J., Anti-inflammatory actions of glucocorticoids: molecular mechanisms, *Clin. Sci. (Lond.)*, 94, 557, 1998.

53. Adcock, I.M. and Ito, K. Molecular mechanisms of corticosteroid actions, *Monaldi Arch. Chest Dis.*, 55, 256, 2000.

54. DeRijk, R. et al., Exercise and circadian rhythm-induced variations in plasma cortisol differentially regulate interleukin 1 beta (IL-1 beta), IL-6 and tumor necrosis factor alpha (TNF alpha) productions in humans: high sensitivity of TNF alpha and resistance of IL-6, *J. Clin. Endocrinol. Metab.*, 82, 2182, 1997.

55. Elenkov, U. and Chrousos, G.P., Stress hormone, Th1/Th2 patterns, pro/anti-inflammatory cytokines and susceptibility to disease. *Trends Endocrinol. Metab.*, 10, 359, 1997.

56. Rivest, S., How circulating trigger the neuronal circuits that control the hypothalamic–pituitary–adrenal axis, *Psychoneuroendocrinology*, 26, 761, 2001.

57. Auernhammer, C.J. and Melmed, S., Leukemia-inhibitory factor-neuroimmune modulator of endocrine function, *Endocr. Rev.*, 21, 313, 2000.

58. Arzt, E., The gp130 cytokine family signalling in the pituitary gland: a paradigm for cytokine-neuroendocrine pathways, *J. Clin. Invest.*, 108, 1729, 2001.

59. Kariagina, A. et al., Hypothalamic–pituitary cytokine network, *Endocrinology*, 145, 104, 2004.

60. Mulla, A. and Buckingham, J.C., Regulation of the hypothalamo–pituitary–adrenal axis by cytokines, *Baillieres Best Pract. Res. Clin. Endocrinol. Metab.*, 13, 503, 1999.

61. Wang, Z., Ren, S.G. and Melmed, S., Hypothalamic and pituitary leukemia inhibitory factor gene expression *in vivo*: a novel endotoxin-inducible neuroendocrine interface, *Endocrinology*, 137, 2947, 1996.

62. Lebel, E., Vallieres, L. and Rivest, S., Selective involvement of interleukin-6 in the transcriptional activation of the suppressor of cytokine signalling-3 in the brain during systemic immune challenges, *Endocrinology*, 141, 3749, 2000.

63. Allan, S. and Rothwell, N., Cytokines and acute neurodegeration, *Nat. Rev. Neurosci.* 2, 734, 2001.

64. Panerai, A.E. et al., The β–endorphin inhibition of mitogen-induced splenocytes proliferation is mediated by central and peripheral paracrine/autocrine effects of the opioid, *J. Neuroimmunol.*, 58, 71, 1995.

65. Schneider, G.M. and Lysle, D.T., Effects of centrally administered opioid agonists on macrophage nitric oxide production and splenic lymphocyte proliferation, *Adv. Exp. Med. Biol.*, 402, 81, 1996.

66. Sacerdote, P., Limiroli, E., and Gaspani, L., Experimental evidence for immunomodulatory effects of opioids, *Adv. Exp. Med. Biol.*, 521, 106, 2003.

67. Manfredi, B. et al., Evidence for an opioid inhibitory effect on T cell proliferation, *J. Neuroimmunol.*, 44, 43, 1993.

68. Nowak, J.E. et al., Rat natural killer cell, T cell and macrophage functions after intracerebroventricular injection of SNC 80, *J. Pharmacol. Exp.Ther.*, 286, 931, 1998.

69. Gómez-Flores, R. et al., Activation of tumor necrosis factor-α and nitric oxide production by rat macrophages following *in vitro* stimulation and intravenous administration of the delta-opioid agonist SNC 80, *Life Sci.*, 68, 2675, 2001.

70. Fuchs, B.A. and Pruett S.B., Morphine induces apoptosis in murine thymocytes *in vivo* but not *in vitro*: involvement of both opiate and glucocorticoid receptors, *J. Pharmacol. Exp. Ther.*, 266, 417, 1993.

71. Sei, Y. et al., Morphine-induced thymic hypoplasia is glucocorticoid dependent, *J. Immunol.*, 146, 194, 1991.

72. Yin, D. et al., Fas-mediated cell death promoted by opioids, *Nature*, 397, 2118, 1999.

73. Roy, S. et al., Chronic morphine treatment selectively suppresses macrophage colony formation in bone marrow, *Eur. J. Pharmacol.*, 195, 359, 1991.

74. Lopez, M. et al., Spleen and thymus cell subsets modified by long-term morphine administration and murine AIDS-II, *Int. J. Immunopharmacol.*, 15, 909, 1993.

75. Roy, S. et al., Role of hypothalamic-pituitary axis in morphine induced alteration in thymic cell distribution using μ-opioid receptor knock-out mice, *J. Neuroimmunol.*, 116, 147, 2001.

76. Pariante, C. et al., Chronic caregiving stress alters peripheral blood immune parameters: role of age and severity of stress, *Psychother. Psychosom.*, 66, 199, 1997.

77. Zorrila, E. et al., The relationship of depression and stressors to immunological assays: a meta-analytical review, *Brain Behav. Immun.*, 15, 199, 2001.

78. Galinowsky, A., Stress and panic: immunologic aspects, *Encephale*, 19, 147, 1993.

79. Kunes, P. and Krejsek, J., CD4 lymphopenia and post-operative immunosuppression in cardiac surgery, *Cas. Lek. Cesk.*, 139, 361, 2000.

80. Capitanio, J. and Lerche, N., Psychosocial factors and disease progression in simian AIDS: a preliminary report, *AIDS* 5, 1103, 1991.

81. Padgett, D., Marucha, P. and Sheridan, J., Restraint stress slows cutaneous wound healing in mice, *Brain Behav. Immun.*, 12, 64, 1998.

82. Yin, D. et al., Chronic restraint stress promotes lymphocyte apoptosis by modulating CD95 expression, *J. Exp. Med.*, 191, 1423, 2000.

83. Maher, S. et al., Activation-induced cell death: the controversial role of Fas and Fas ligand in immune privilege and tumour counterattack, *Immunol. Cell Biol.*, 80, 131, 2002.

84. Ju, S.T. et al., Fas(CD95)/FasL interactions required for programmed cell death after T-cell activation, *Nature*, 373, 444, 1995.

85. Cohen, J., Immunopathogenesis of sepsis, *Nature*, 420, 885, 2002.

86. Karima, R. et al., The molecular pathogenesis of endotoxic shock and organ failure, *Mol. Med. Today*, 5, 123, 1999.

87. Yirmiya, R. et al., Behavioral effects of lipoplysaccharide in rats: involvement of endogenous opioids, *Brain Res.*, 648, 80, 1994.

88. Xu, T., Wang, T., and Han, J., Centrally acting endogenous hypotensive substances in rats subjected to endotoxic shock, *Life Sci.*, 51, 1817, 1992.

89. Greeneltech, K. et al., The opioid antagonist naltrexone blocks acute endotoxic shock by inhibiting tumor necrosis factor-α production, *Brain Behav. Immun.*, 18, 476, 2004.

90. Philippe, D. et al., Anti-inflammatory properties of the μ-opioid receptor supports its use in the treatment of colon inflammation, *J. Clin. Invest.*, 111, 1329, 2003.

91. Silverstein, J. et al., Adrenal neuropeptide mRNA but not preproenkephalin mRNA induction of stress is impaired by ageing in Fisher 344 rats, *Mech. Ageing Dev.*, 101, 233, 1998.

92. Cabot, P.J., Immune-derived opioids and peripheral antinociception, *Clin. Exp. Pharmacol. Physiol.*, 28, 230, 2001.

93. Tisher, A. et al., Enkephalin-like immunoreactivity in human adrenal medullary cultures, *Lab. Invest.*, 48, 13, 1983.

94. Zurawski, G. et al., Activation of mouse T-helper cells induces abundant pre-proenkephalin mRNA synthesis, *Science*, 232, 772, 1986.

95. Gabrilovac, J. and Marotti, T., Gender-related differences in murine T and B lymphocyte proliferative ability in response to *in vivo* Met^5-enkephalin administration, *Eur. J. Pharmacol.*, 392, 101, 2000.

96. Radulovic, J. and Jankovic, B., Opposing activities of brain opioid receptors in the regulation of humoral and cell-mediated immune response in the rat, *Brain Res.*, 661, 189, 1994.

97. Marotti, T. et al., Met-enkephalin modulates stress-induced alterations of the immune response in mice, *Pharmacol. Biochem. Behav.*, 54, 277, 1996.

98. Kowalski, J., Effect of enkephalins and endorphins on cytotoxic activity of natural killer cells and macrophages/monocytes in mice, *Eur. J. Pharmacol.*, 326, 251, 1997.

99. Plotnikoff, N.P. et al., Enkephalins and T-cell enhancement in normal volunteers and cancer patients, *Ann. NY Acad. Sci.*, 496, 608, 1987.

100. Marotti, T., Rabatic, S., and Gabrilovac, J., A characterization of *in vivo* immunomodulation by met-enkephalin in mice, *Int. J. Immunopharmacol.*, 15, 919, 1993.

101. Liu, X.H. et al., A new cytokine: the possible effect pathway of methionine enkephalin, *World J. Gastroenterol.*, 9, 169, 2003.

102. Puente, J. et al., Enhancement of human natural killer cell activity by opioid peptides: similar response to methionine-enkephalin and β-endorphin, *Brain Behav. Immun.*, 6, 32, 1992.

103. Mosnaim, A.D. et al., *In vitro* studies of natural killer cell activity in post traumatic stress disorder patients: response to methionine-enkephalin challenge, *Immunopharmacology*, 25, 107, 1993.

104. Hermick, L.M. and Bidlack, J.M., Beta-endorphin stimulates rat T lymphocyte proliferation, *J. Neuroimmunol.*, 29, 239, 1990.

105. Dulinin, K.V., Zakharova, L.A., and Khegal, J.A., Immunomodulating effect of met-enkephalin on different stages of lymphocyte proliferation induced with concanavalin A *in vitro*, *Immunopharmacol. Immunotoxicol.*, 16, 463, 1994.

106. Prete, P., Levin, E., and Pedram, A., The *in vitro* effects of endogenous opiates on natural killer cells, antigen-specific cytolytic T cells, and T cell subsets, *Exp. Neurol.*, 92, 349, 1986.

107. Sizemore, R.C., Dienglewics, E., and Gorttlieb, A., Modulation of concanavalin-induced, antigen-nonspecific regulatory cell activity by leu-enkephalin and related peptides, *Clin. Immunol. Immunopathol.*, 60, 310, 1991.

108. Dokur, et al., β-endorphin modulation of interferon-γ, perforin and granzyme B levels in splenic NK cells: effects of ethanol, *J. Neuroimmunol.*, 166, 29, 2005.

109. Mosnaim, A.D. et al., *In vitro* studies of natural killer cell activity in migraineurs: changes in response to methionine-enkephalin challenge during an acute migraine episode, *Headache Q.*, 4, 36, 1993.

110. Mosnaim, A.D. et al., *In vitro* studies of natural killer cell activity in migraineurs: changes in response to β-endorphin challenge during an acute migraine episode, *Headache Q.*, 5, 142, 1994.

111. Mosnaim, A.D. et al., Flow cytometric analysis of lymphocyte subsets in migraine patients during and outside of an acute headache attack, *Cephalalgia*, 18, 197, 1998.

112. Greisen, J. et al., Acute pain induces an instant increase in natural killer cell cytotoxicity in human and this response is abolished by local anesthesia, *Br. J. Anaesth.*, 83, 235, 1999.

113. Brack, A. et al., Mobilization of opioid-containing polymorphonuclear cells by hematopoietic growth factors and influence on inflammatory pain, *Anesthesiology*, 100,149, 2004.

114. Shäfer, M., Carter, L., and Stein, C., Interleukin 1 beta and corticotropin–releasing factor inhibit pain by releasing opioids from immune cells in inflamed tissue, *Proc. Natl. Acad. Sci. USA*, 91, 4219, 1994.

115. Shäfer, M. et al., Expression of corticotropin-releasing factor in inflamed tissue is required for intrinsic peripheral opioid analgesia, *Proc. Natl. Acad. Sci. USA*, 93, 6096, 1996.

116. Stein, C. et al., A. Local analgesic effect of endogenous opioid peptides, *Lancet*, 343, 321, 1993.

117. Machelska, H. et al., Pain control in inflammation governed by selectins, *Nat. Med.*, 4, 1425, 1998.

118. Fergusson, S., Evolving concepts in G protein-coupled receptor endocytosis: the role in receptor desensitization and signalling, *Pharmacol. Rev.*, 53, 1, 2001.

119. Zhiyi Zuo., The role of opioid receptor internalization and β-arrestins in the development of opioid tolerance. *Anesth. Analg.*, 101, 728, 2005.

120. Goodman, O. et al., Role of arrestins in G-protein-coupled receptor endocytosis, *Adv. Pharmacol.*, 42, 429, 1998.

121. Ferguson, S. et al., Molecular mechanisms of G protein-coupled receptor desensitization and resensitization, *Life Sci.*, 62, 1561, 1998.

122. Dang, Vu C. and Williams, J.T., Morphine-induced μ-opioid receptor desensitization., *Mol. Pharmacol.*, 68, 1127, 2005.

123. Yu, Y. et al., Mu opioid receptor phosphorylation, desensitization and ligand efficacy, *J. Biol. Chem.*, 272, 28869, 1997.

124. Zhang, J. et al., Role of G protein-coupled receptor kinase in agonist-specific regulation of mu-opioid receptor responsiveness, *Proc. Natl. Acad. Sci. USA.*, 95, 7157, 1998.

125. Steele. A. et al., Interactions between opioid and chemokine receptors: heterologous desensitisation, *Cytokine Growth Factor Rev.*, 13, 209, 2002.

126. Rogers, T.J. et al., Bidirectional heterologous desensitization of opioid and chemokine receptors, *Ann. NY Acad. Sci.*, 917, 19, 2000.

127. Murphy, P.M. et al., International union of pharmacology, XXII. Nomenclature for chemokine receptors, *Pharmacol Rev.*, 52, 145, 2000.

128. Ruff, M.R. et al., Opiate receptor-mediated chemotaxis of human monocytes, *Neuropeptides*, 5, 363, 1985.

129. Van Epps, D. and Saland, L., Beta-endorphin and met-enkephalin stimulate human peripheral blood mononuclear cell chemotaxis, *J. Immunol.*, 132, 3046, 1984.

130. Grimm, M. et al., Opiates transdeactive chemokine receptors: delta and mu opiate receptor-mediated heterologous desensitization, *J. Exp. Med.*, 188, 317, 1998.

131. Sharp, B. et al., Immunofluorescence detection of δ opioid receptors (DOR) on human peripheral blood CD4+ T cells and DOR-dependent suppression of HIV-1 expression, *J. Immunol.*, 167, 1097, 2001.

132. Szabo, I. et al., Selective inactivation of CCR5 and decreased infectivity of R5 HIV-1 strains mediated by opioid-induced heterologous desensitisation, *J. Leukoc. Biol.*, 74, 1074, 2003.

133. Szabo, I. et al., Heterologous desensitization of opioid receptors by chemokines inhibits chemotaxis and enhances the perception of pain, *Proc. Natl. Acad. Sci. USA*, 99, 10276, 2002.

134. Gaveriaux-Ruff, C. et al., Abolition of morphine-immunosuppression in mice lacking the μ-opioid receptor gene, *Proc. Natl. Acad. Sci. USA*, 95, 6326, 1998.

135. Kieffer, B., Opioids: first lessons from knockout mice, *Trends Pharmacol.*, 20, 19, 1999.

136. Gaveriaux-Ruff, C. et al., Antibody response and allogeneic mixed lymphocyte reaction in mu-, delta-, and kappa-opioid receptor knockout mice, *J. Neuroimmunol.*, 147, 121, 2004.

137. Gaveriaux-Ruff, C. et al., Enhanced humoral response in kappa-opioid receptor knockout mice, *J. Neuroimmunol.*, 134, 72, 2003.

138. Gaveriaux-Ruff, C. et al., Immunosuppression by delta-opioid antagonist naltrindole: delta and triple mu/delta/kappa-opioid receptor knockout mice reveal a non-opioid activity, *J. Pharmacol. Exp. Ther.*, 298, 1193, 2001.

10 Met-Enkephalin in Oxidative Stress

Tihomir Balog, Sandra Sobočanec, Višnja Šverko,
Helena Haberstock-Debić, and Tatjana Marotti

CONTENTS

INTRODUCTION

Hugo Besedovsky demonstrated immune system–brain communications more than 35 years ago. His recent findings concern the ability of IL-1 (centrally mediated immune challenge) to induce hypoglycemia (response of immune tissue on periphery). We no longer question whether injection of immune modulators can affect the brain or whether the immune system can interfere with neurotransmitters or the neuroendocrine system. The questions today concern the advantages or disadvantages of such "cooperation" between systems.[1]

In the case of information exchanges, the nervous system (which is stimulated by cognitive stresses) can control the immune system via the hypothalamo–pituitary–adrenal axis. By contrast, the immune system can alert the brain. This interaction involves the actions of small molecules such as neuropeptides and cytokines. The co-localization of such molecules found in the nervous[2] and immune[3] systems further supports the hypothesis that opioid peptides and cytokines are the principal messengers of this bidirectional communication. In 1997, Plotnikoff et al.[4] proposed the methionine-enkephalin (met-enkephalin) opioid peptide as one of the cytokines of the immune system because it is produced by cells of the immune system and influences numbers of immunocompetent and accessory cells and functions engaged in bodily defense.

It is generally assumed that the "brain–immune" axis also exists during stress.[5] Release and/or expression of enkephalins can be regulated by different factors such as stress,[6] exercise,[7] hormones,[8] and cytokines.[9] Thus, there is a tight connection among cytokines, opioid peptides, and stress. Cytokines, as mediators of numerous processes such as tissue repair, hematopoiesis, inflammation, and involvement in specific and non-specific immune responses,[10] share some of these functions[4] with opioid peptides (like met-enkephalin). The effects of stress are mediated via the hypothalamic–pituitary–adrenal axis by the release of steroid hormones, catecholamines, enkephalins, endorphins,[11] and cytokines.[12]

In mediation, modulation, and regulation of stress-induced changes, enkephalins are closely related to steroids, catecholamines, and certain pituitary hormones.[13–15] The widespread distribution of enkephalins throughout the limbic system (including the extended amygdala, cingulate cortex, entorhinal cortex, septum hippocampus, and hypothalamus) is consistent with a direct role in the modulation of stress responses. Taken together, these facts reflect a need for correlation and investigation of a possible relation and/or interference of opioid peptides, stress, and cytokines.

MET-ENKEPHALIN, RESTRAINT STRESS, AND IMMUNITY

There was a striking similarity in the alterations of the immune reactivity induced by stress and met-enkephalin. Met-enkephalin and stress similarly elevated phagocytosis, proliferative capacity of spleen cells, and corticosterone (CS) while natural killer (NK) cell activity was decreased.[13] However, stress- or met-enkephalin-elevated plasma CS concentrations returned to the normal range after combined treatment with stress and met-enkephalin. Also, beta-endorphin under physiological conditions elevated the levels of cortisol in peripheral blood, and suppressed the levels in stressed animals.[16]

The enhancing effect of stress on phagocytic ability of mice spleen cells was attenuated by exposure to met-enkephalin prior to stress.[13] In contrast, the inhibitory effect of stress on the primary antibody response to SRBC was only partially reversed. The inhibitory effect of stress on concanavalin-A (Con-A)-driven proliferative capacities of mice spleen cells was abolished in mice treated with met-enkephalin before stress. Met-enkephalin injected before stress did not alter stress-induced NK inhibition. These data additionally speak in favor of the hypothesis that met-enkephalin and stress share common mechanisms by which immune functions are modulated.

Pretreatment of mice with naloxone, an opioid receptor antagonist (30 mg/kg body weight [bw]), abrogated met-enkephalin-induced alteration of phagocytic activity and T-cell proliferation. However, NK activity and plaque forming cell (PFC) responses remained unchanged.[13] Studying the mechanisms of action of met-enkephalin, we found both glucocorticoid-dependent and glucocorticoid-independent actions.[17] Met-enkephalin effects on T- and B-cell functions were absent in adrenalectomized mice, whereas the suppressive effect on NK cells was still present.

MET-ENKEPHALIN AND OXIDATIVE STRESS

Enkephalins and opioid peptides have been identified as immunomodulators in situations of oxidative stress[18] that occurs when biological systems encounter excess of pro-oxidant and/or have reduced antioxidant capacities. Oxidative stress is the state of imbalance between the physiological production of partly toxic reactive oxygen species (ROS) and the scavenging of ROS with antioxidant enzyme. Experimental studies indicated that reactive oxygen species are primary mediators in the pathogenesis of immune and non-immune injuries. Their intermediates play a critical role in limiting tissue damage and preventing or inhibiting infection, secondary to enhancing inflammation and prolonging immune reaction.

Met-enkephalin and its analogs can modulate release of ROS from different cells.[19] Marotti et al.[20] have shown a donor-dependent up-regulation of superoxide anion release from human neutrophils while Šverko et al.[21] demonstrated met-enkephalin-modulated lipid peroxidation (LPO) in liver and thymus of mice. Recently Lin et al.[22] provided evidence that endomorphins can protect human mononuclear blood cells from oxidative damage.

One of the mechanisms responsible for pathological consequences in the livers of animals exposed to oxidative stress may be the stimulation of LPO. We demonstrated that during restraint stress, met-enkephalin does not affect basal LPO per se. Rather, met-enkephalin and stress are adjunct modulators of LPO in that the high dose of met-enkephalin (10 mg/kg bw) additionally elevated LPO levels in stressed mice. This was noticed only early after the onset of stress (2 hours). This elevation of stress-induced LPO superposed by met-enkephalin was paralleled by a corticosterone increase that followed the same pattern: additional increases in 10 mg/kg met-enkephalin-stressed mice after 2 hours of stress; after 6 hours of stress at the same dose, CS levels were down-regulated.[23] In creating a cellular pro-oxidant state often characterized by increased LPO, stress and met-enkephalin seemed to share similar properties. Both increased LPO, primarily in the livers of pretreated animals. Again, the dose of met-enkephalin seemed to be an important parameter. The higher dose (10 mg/kg bw) increased while the lower dose (2.5 mg/kg body weight) decreased LPO in the livers of mice. At the same time the effect was gender-related — observed only in male mice while both doses were ineffective in female mice (see Figure 10.1).[21]

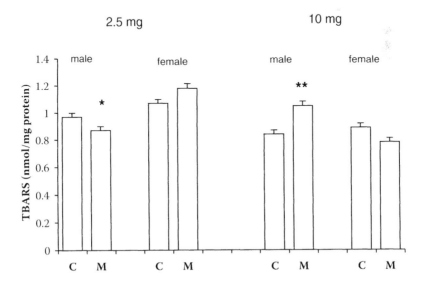

FIGURE 10.1 TBARS (thiobarbituric acid reactive substance) concentrations in the livers of male and female mice injected with 2.5 or 10 mg/kg body weight (bw) met-enkephalin (M) or saline (C). Bars represent mean ± SEM. * p <0.05, ** p <0.01.

MET-ENKEPHALIN AND NITRIC OXIDE

The same ability to switch stimulated functions back to normal and inability to restore suppressed immune functions were observed in other functions of met-enkephalin-treated mice. Marotti et al.[24] demonstrated that met-enkephalin *in vivo* bimodally regulated nitric oxide (NO) release of mouse peritoneal macrophages. The effect was dose-dependent in that low (2.5 mg/kg bw) and high dose (10 mg/kg bw) stimulated NO release and the intermediate dose (5 mg/kg bw) of met-enkephalin suppressed it. The stimulative, but not the suppressive, dose of met-enkephalin was opioid-receptor-mediated as demonstrated by the abolishing effect of naloxone (Figure 10.2).

NO is a pleiotropic mediator that, among other biological effects, causes apoptosis in a variety of cell types including macrophages, lymphocytes, T-cells, and neurons.[25] Balog et al.[26] demonstrated that only 2.5 mg/kg bw of met-enkephalin induced apoptosis visualized by condensed chromatin, nuclei fragmentation, and shrunken cells (Figure 10.3a–c). This was surprising since 10 mg/kg bw also elevated NO release but this increase was not associated with increased apoptosis. The reason for this may lie in the fact that NO is not a universal inducer of apoptosis as stated by Albina et al.[27]

Dynorphine also modulates NO release *in vitro* from the J774 cell line (see Figure 10.4).[28] Functional links between the neuroendocrine and immune systems are often related to the cytokine network, with IL-1 and TNF playing the central role.[29] In fact, IL-1β even suppresses apoptosis by increasing NO production.[30,31]

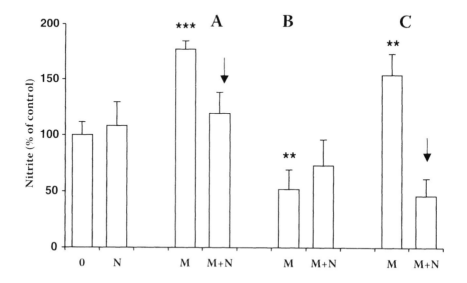

FIGURE 10.2 *In vivo* effect of met-enkephalin (M) on NO release; 2.5 mg/kg bw (A), 5 mg/kg body weight (bw) (B) and 10 mg/kg bw (C) and/or 10 mg/kg bw naloxone (N). Data expressed as mean ± SD percent of control (0) macrophages from saline-treated mice. ** p < 0.01. *** p < 0.001.

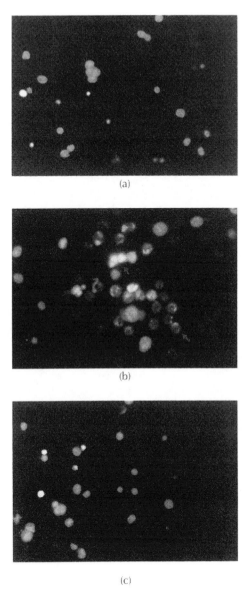

FIGURE 10.3 Detection of apoptotic cell DNA fragmentation (arrows) in macrophages of control mice injected with saline (a), macrophages of mice injected *in vivo* with 2.5 mg/kg body weight (bw) (b), or 10 mg/kg bw met-enkephalin (c).

One of the cytokines responsible for the enhanced NO release may be IFNγ since only IFNγ (in suboptimal concentrations) and met-enkephalin significantly increased NO *in vitro*. However, the main candidate seems to be IL-1, which was induced by met-enkephalin *in vivo* at a concentration of 2.5 mg/kg bw (Figure 10.5) and also induced apoptosis. The effect could be abrogated by anti-IL-1 antibody (Figure 10.6).[24] The higher dose of met-enkephalin (10 mg/kg bw) that does not induce NO release

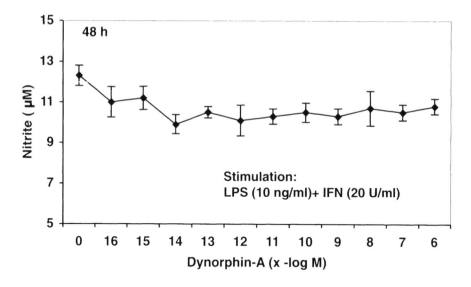

FIGURE 10.4 Effect of dynorphine A on NO release by J774 cells stimulated with LPS plus IFN-γ in the presence of graded concentrations of dynorphine A. Control cells represented by shaded areas were stimulated with LPS plus IFN-γ (without dynorphine). Data expressed as mean ± SD.

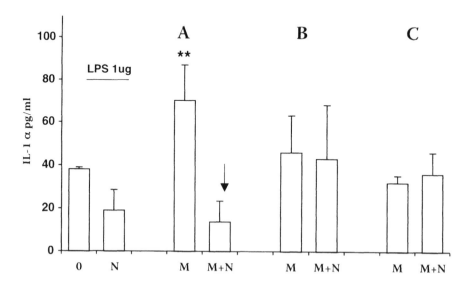

FIGURE 10.5 *In vivo* effect of met-enkephalin (M); 2.5 mg/kg body weight (bw) (A), 5 mg/kg bw (B), and 10 mg/kg bw (C) and/or naloxone (N) on IL-1 secretion of mouse peritoneal macrophages. Control mice received saline (0). Data expressed as mean ± SD. ** p <0.01.

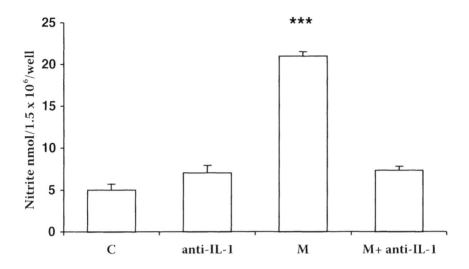

FIGURE 10.6 Blocking effect of anti-IL-1 antibody on NO release from mouse peritoneal macrophages from saline (C) or met-enkephalin (M) (2.5 mg/kg body weight) treated mice. Data expressed as mean ± SD. *** p < 0.001.

also lacks effect on apoptosis. Our study[32] speaks in favor of these assumptions. Mouse peritoneal macrophages co-stimulated with LPS (1 μg) and 10^{-10} M met-enkephalin abrogated TNF activity induced by LPS (Figure 10.7) and at the same time potentiated IL-1 activity compared to LPS alone (data not shown).

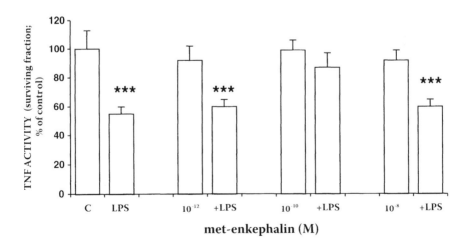

FIGURE 10.7 TNF activity in supernatants of adherent mouse spleen cells cultured with 1 μg LPS and/or met-enkephalin (M) of graded concentration. Data expressed as mean ± SD percentage of TNF activity in the supernatant of control (C) splenocytes cultured in RPMI-1640 (100%). *** p < 0.001.

POSSIBLE PATHWAYS OF EFFECTS EXERTED BY MET-ENKEPHALIN

Additional evidence that the modulatory action of met-enkephalin may be mediated through the up-regulation of cytokines is provided by the fact that the supernatant of the respective cell culture augmented phagocytosis. We recently demonstrated that met-enkephalin can modulate reactive radicals through the level of antioxidant enzymes (Figure 10.8). Surprisingly, the modulatory role of met-enkephalin in the regulation of oxidant/antioxidant processes in the brains of mice seems to follow the same pattern; the stimulatory effect of met-enkephalin on LPO, catalase (CAT), and superoxide dismutase (SOD) activity was efficiently diminished by naloxone, while met-enkephalin-induced suppression of glutathione peroxidase (Gpx) activity was much less affected by naloxone.[33]

It seems that the modulatory effect of opioids, in addition to HPA regulation (via hormones) and cytokine regulation, can be, at least in the case of free radical release, regulated by the activities of enkephalin-degrading enzymes on target cells. Aminopeptidase N (APN, CD13) seems to be the major proteolytic enzyme involved in the degradation of neuropeptides, as demonstrated for the synaptic membranes of the rat brain.[34,35] Such correlation was observed in experiments with human neutrophils, where the release of superoxide anions from human neutrophils from different donors was regulated by the amount of APN on the respective neutrophils (Figure 10.9).[36]

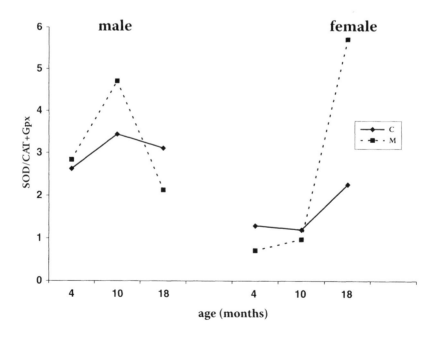

FIGURE 10.8 Effect of met-enkephalin on tSOD/CAT + Gpx ratios of antioxidant enzymes in brains of control (C) and met-enkephalin (M) treated mice of both sexes.

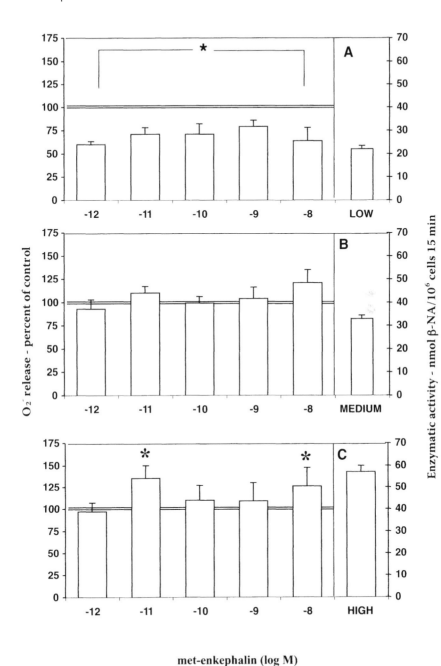

FIGURE 10.9 Superoxide anion release (O_2^-) from human neutrophils preincubated with graded concentrations of met-enkephalin (M) in correlation with the level of aminopeptidase N (APN) activity (β-NA) of the respective cells (low A, medium B, high C). Control neutrophils were incubated with RPMI-1640. Data expressed as mean ± SD. * p < 0.05.

Neutrophils with low APN activity, if preincubated with met-enkephalin, released reduced amounts of superoxide anion. In contrast, neutrophils with high APN activity released increased amounts of superoxide anion after preincubation with met-enkephalin. The paradox that a high concentration of degradative enzyme may preserve the stimulatory effect of met-enkephalin can be explained in light of the published work of Haberstock et al.[37] During the process of hydrolysis of met-enkephalin, low amounts of APN prefer the formation of TGG (Tyr-Gly-Gly), which suppresses superoxide anion release.[37]

MODULATION BY ENKEPHALIN: GENDER MATTERS

Mouse strain differences and gender (and even age) should never be overlooked in studies of stress and interactions of mediators like opioids with the neuroendocrine–immune axis. It was shown recently that *in vivo* administration of met-enkephalin affects the proliferative ability of murine T- and B-lymphocytes in a gender-associated manner.[38] Because of its high oxygen consumption, high lipid concentration, and relatively poor antioxidant defense, the brain is highly vulnerable to oxidative stress[39] and produces more ROS per gram of tissue than any other organ.[40] Enkephalins can modulate release of ROS from different cells as well.[19]

Neurons have a diminished capacity to deal with redox imbalance; this is why even minor cellular stresses have the ability to lead to irreversible injury and contribute to the pathogenesis of neurodegenerative diseases.[41] In the case of oxidative stress (measured by LPO products), our recent study demonstrated that the male brains of mice are less resistant to oxidation than female brains.[33] The difference is mainly due to higher CAT and lower LPO activities in the female brain. Met-enkephalin decreased resistance to stress in the brains of both sexes, but the effect appeared earlier in males (10 months of age) than in females (18 months of age).

The mechanism of diminution of resistance to stress differed in males and females: in males via regulation of oxidative processes and in females via regulation of antioxidative enzyme activity. The gender-related difference in response to peripherally administered met-enkephalin may be a result of differently induced/released cytokines or hormones. According to the results of Borg et al., IL-1 can induce both mRNA expression of antioxidant enzyme and antioxidant enzyme activity.[42] O' Donnell and Lynch[43] showed that IL-1 can trigger LPO. However, in the same study, no differences in plasma concentrations of IL-1 between met-enkephalin-treated and control male and female mice were noticed. One possible reason may be the fact that IL-1 in the plasma may not reflect IL-1 levels in the brain. In favor of the latter suggestion is that in measuring oxidant/antioxidant status in the livers of met-enkephalin pretreated mice, the increased resistance to oxidative stress in old males was paralleled with changes in IL-1 plasma levels.[33] Gonadal steroids may be candidates for such gender-related differences since they play an important role in immunomodulation by opioids.[15,44] Male animals seem to be more susceptible to both peptide and non-peptide opioid effects on immune and antinociceptive responses.[45,46]

Other candidates (especially in case of regulation of oxidant/antioxidant processes) are growth hormone (GH) and prolactin (PRL) because of their influences on immune functions.[47] Opioid peptides have been shown to induce secretion of GH and PRL.[8]

CONCLUSION

Our work and that of others strongly points to a tight connection of cytokines, opioid peptides, and stress (restraint and oxidative). Although stress and met-enkephalin affected several immune functions in the same direction and to similar extent, when combined, they either reversed or attenuated the effect of stress or met-enkephalin per se. The mediation, modulation, and regulation of stress-induced changes were affected by met-enkephalin in both glucocorticoid-dependent and glucocorticoid-independent ways.

Stress-induced increase of lipid peroxidation was superposed by met-enkephalin and paralleled by corticosterone increase. Conversely, met-enkephalin-induced nitric oxide release was regulated by IL-1 release. Met-enkephalin-modulated free radical release via gender and age-regulated antioxidative enzymes seems to involve gonadal hormones and possibly prolactin and growth hormone. The existing data of integrated studies seem to be the fact that among the different immune functions examined, only the stimulatory effect of met-enkephalin, either glucocorticoid-dependent or glucocorticoid-independent, could be abolished by naloxone.

REFERENCES

1. Besedovski, H.O. and del Rey, A., Introduction: immune-neuroendocrine network, *Front. Horm. Res.*, 29, 1, 2002.
2. Hughes, I. et al., Identification of two related pentapeptides from the brain with potent opiate agonist activity, *Nature*, 258, 577, 1975.
3. Weigent, D.A. and Blalock, J.E., Production of peptide hormones and neurotransmitters by the immune system, *Chem. Immunol,*. 69, 1, 1997.
4. Plotnikoff, N.P. et al., Methionine enkephalin: a new cytokine — human studies, *Clin. Immunol. Immunopathol.*, 82, 93, 1997.
5. Dallman, M.F. et al., Stress, feedback and facilitation in the hypothalamo–pituitary–adrenal axis, *J. Neuroendocrin.*, 4, 517, 1991.
6. Yamamoto, M. et al., Effects of single and repeated prolonged stress on mu-opioid receptor mRNA expression in rat gross hypothalamic and midbrain homogenates, *Brain Res.*, 980, 191, 2003.
7. Harbach, H. et al., β-endorphin (1-31) in the plasma of male volunteers undergoing physical exercise, *Psychoneuroendocrinology,* 25, 551, 2000.
8. Fanciulli, G. et al., Prolactin and growth hormone response to intracerebroventricular administration of the food opioid peptide gluten exorphin B5 in rats, *Life Sci.*, 71, 2383, 2002.
9. Low, K.G., Allen, R.G., and Melner, M.H., Differential regulation of proenkephalin expression in astrocytes by cytokines, *Endocrinology,* 131, 1908, 1992.
10. Haddad, J.J., Saade, N.E., and Safieh-Garabedian, B., Cytokines and neuro–immune–endocrine interactions: a role for the hypothalamic–pituitary–adrenal revolving axis, *J. Neuroimmunol.*, 133, 1, 2002.
11. Plotnikoff, N.P. et al., Enkephalins: immunomodulators, *Fed. Proc.*, 44, 118, 1985.

12. Safieh-Garabedian, B. et al., Cytokine-mediated or direct effects of thymulin on the nervous system as assessed by pain-related behavior, *Neuroimmunomodulation,* 6, 39, 1999.

13. Marotti, T. et al., Met-enkephalin modulates stress-induced alterations of the immune response in mice, *Pharmacol. Biochem. Behav.,* 54, 277, 1996.

14. Simerly, R.B., Young, B.J., and Carr, A.M., Co-expression of steroid hormone receptors in opioid peptide-containing neurons correlates with patterns of gene expression during the estrus cycle, *Mol. Brain Res.,* 40, 275, 1996.

15. Hammer, R.P., Zhou, L., and Cheung, S., Gonadal steroid hormones and hypothalamic opioid circuitry, *Horm. Behav.,* 28, 431, 1994.

16. Domanski, E., Romanoviez, K., and Kerdelhue, B., Enhancing effect of intracerebrally infused β-endorphin antiserum on the secretion of cortisol in food-shocked sheep, *Neuroendocrinology,* 57, 127, 1993.

17. Marotti, T., Rabati, S., and Gabrilovac, J., A characterization of the *in vivo* immunomodulation by met-enkephalin in mice, *Int. J. Immunopharmacol.,* 15, 919, 1993.

18. Rebrova, Y.T., The effect of synthetic enkephalins on prostaglandin systems and lipid peroxidation in isolated heart in the activation of free radical processes, *Pathophysiology,* 5, 20, 1998.

19. Kowalski, J., Immunologic action of (Met 5) fragments, *Eur. J. Pharmacol.,* 347, 95, 1998.

20. Marotti, T., Šverko, V., and Hršak, I., Modulation of superoxide anion release from human polymorphonuclear cells by met- and leu-enkephalin, *Brain Behav. Immun.,* 4, 13, 1990.

21. Šverko, V. et al., Met-enkephalin modulates lipid peroxidation and total sialic acid level in CBA mice in age- and sex-dependent manners, *Exp. Gerontol.,* 37, 1413, 2002.

22. Lin, X. et al., Endomorphins, endogenous opioid peptides, provide antioxidant defense in the brain against free radical-induced damage, *Biochim. Biophys. Acta,* 1639, 195, 2003.

23. Šverko, V. et al., Influence of methionine-enkephalin on stress-induced parameters, *Int. J. Immunopharmacol.,* 19, 691, 1997.

24. Marotti, T. et al., The role of cytokines in met-enkephalin-modulated nitric oxide release, *Neuropeptides,* 32, 57, 1998.

25. Pagliaro, P., Differential biological effects of products of nitric oxide (NO) synthase: it is not enough to say NO, *Life Sci.,* 73, 2137, 2003.

26. Balog, T. et al., The effect of methionine-enkephalin on nitric oxide release in mice is age- and gender-related, *Pharmacol. Res.,* 44, 287, 2001.

27. Albina, J.E. et al., Nitric oxide-mediated apoptosis in murine peritoneal macrophages, *J. Immunol.,* 150, 5080, 1993.

28. Gabrilovac, J., Balog, T., and Andreis, A., Dynorphin-A[1-17] decreases nitric oxide release and cytotoxicity induced with lipopolysaccharide plus interferon-γ in murine macrophage cell line J774, *Biomed. Pharmacother.,* 57, 351, 2003.

29. Peterson, P.K., Molitor, T.W., and Chao, C.C., The opioid-cytokine connection, *J. Neuroimmunol.,* 83, 63, 1998.

30. Kim, P.K.M. et al., The regulatory role of nitric oxide in apoptosis, *Int. Immunopharmacol.,* 1, 1421, 2001.

31. Chun, S.Y. et al., Interleukin β-1 suppresses apoptosis in rat ovarian follicles by increasing nitric oxide production, *Endocrinology,* 136, 3120, 1995.

32. Marotti, T. et al., Modulation of lipopolysaccharide-induced production of cytokines by methionine-enkephalin, *Immunol. Lett.,* 40, 43, 1994.

33. Balog, T. et al., Met-enkephalin modulates resistance to oxidative stress in mouse brain, *Neuropeptides*, 38, 298, 2004.

34. Matasas, R. et al., The metabolism of neuropeptides: phase separation of synaptic membrane preparations with Triton X-114 reveals the presence of aminopeptidase N, *Biochem. J.*, 231, 445, 1985.

35. Miller, B.C. et al., Methionine enkephalin is hydrolyzed by aminopeptidase N on CD4+ and CD8+ spleen T cells, *Arch. Biochem. Biophys.*, 317, 174, 1994.

36. Balog, T. et al., The role of aminopeptidase N in Met-enkephalin modulated superoxide anion release, *Immunopharmacology*, 41, 11, 1999.

37. Haberstock, H. and Marotti, T., The relevance of intact enkephalin molecule in predominantly opioid receptor mediated superoxide anion release, *Neuropeptides*, 29, 357, 1995.

38. Gabrilovac, J. and Marotti, T., Gender-related differences in murine T- and B-lymphocyte proliferative ability in response to *in vivo* Met5-enkephalin administration, *Eur. J. Pharmacol.*, 392, 101, 2000.

39. Halliwell, B., Oxidants and the central nervous system: some fundamental questions. Is oxidant damage relevant to Parkinson's disease, Alzheimer's disease, traumatic injury or stroke? *Acta Neurol. Scand. Supp.*, 126, 23, 1989.

40. Reiter, R.J., Oxidative processes and antioxidative defense mechanism in the aging brain, *FASEB J.*, 9, 526, 1995.

41. Perry, G. et al., Is oxidative damage the fundamental pathogenic mechanism of Alzheimer's and other neurodegenerative diseases? *Free Radical Biol. Med.*, 33, 1475, 2002.

42. Borg, L.A. et al., IL-1 increases the activity of superoxide dismutase in rat pancreatic islets, *Endocrinology*, 130, 2851, 1992.

43. O'Donnell, E. and Lynch, M.A., Dietary antioxidant supplementation reverses age-related neuronal changes, *Neurobiol. Aging*, 19, 461, 1998.

44. Zhu, Y-S. et al., Molecular analysis of estrogen induction of preproenkephalin gene expression and its modulation by thyroid hormones, *Mol. Brain Res.*, 91, 23, 2001.

45. Matulka, R.A. et al., Evaluation of strain and sex-dependency of cocaine-induced immunosuppression in B6C3F1 and DBA/2 mice, *J. Pharmacol. Exp. Ther.*, 279, 12, 1996.

46. Cicero, T.J., Nock, B., and Meyer, E.R., Gender-related differences in the antinociceptive properties of morphine, *J. Pharmacol. Exp. Ther.*, 279, 767, 1996.

47. Bolzan, A.D. et al., Relationship between pituitary hormones, antioxidant enzymes, and histopathological changes in the mammary gland of senescent rats, *Exp. Gerontol.*, 32, 297, 1997.

11 Chronic Stress Induces Death of Lymphocytes

Erwei Sun, Lixin Wei, Arthur I. Roberts, Catherine Liu, and Yufang Shi

CONTENTS

ABSTRACT

Alterations in the immune system are recognized as an important contributing factor to the effects of stress on health. While acute stress generally enhances immune responses, chronic stress is associated with immunosuppression. The decrease in mitogen-stimulated lymphocyte proliferation and in lymphocyte numbers has been well established in animals and humans after chronic stress. We show that the reduction in lymphocyte numbers is a result of apoptosis, triggered mainly by the Fas-FasL pathway. Also, we report that stress-induced lymphocyte depletion depends on endogenous opioids, which enhance lymphocyte sensitivity to apoptosis through the up-regulation of Fas expression. Further studies of the cellular and molecular mechanisms will lead to a better understanding of how stress affects the immune system and provide information for the development of strategies to prevent the deleterious effects of chronic stress on the immune system.

INTRODUCTION

The body's response to stress can be defined as adaptive changes to physical, pathological, or psychological stressors. Stress is so common in modern societies that virtually everyone experiences severe stressful events during a lifetime. Although the body generally responds to protect our organ systems from damage, prolonged responses to stress are often detrimental to health. Stress affects almost every system of the body and elicits a whole set of complicated responses.

In contrast to studies of changes in the neural and endocrine systems, immune system alterations during stress have been explored only in the last decade, although they were recognized as early as the 1940s.[1] While the effects of stress on immune responses are complicated by the study model, type, and duration of stress, it is generally accepted that acute stress enhances immune responses whereas chronic stress diminishes immune responses.[2] Stress-induced immunosuppression has been associated with increased susceptibility to and progression of disease, including promotion of infection, acceleration of tumor development, and, paradoxically, increased autoimmunity.[3–10]

For the past several years, we have focused on the impact of chronic stress on the immune system and established that endogenous opioids and the Fas–Fas ligand (FasL) system play crucial roles in the decreased cellularity in immune organs. In this review, we will briefly present our findings that a dramatic loss of lymphocyte cellularity and a significant decrease in lymphocyte proliferation occur in the chronic restraint and hindlimb unloading stress models in mice. We will describe how opioids play a role in mediating these changes in the immune system by promoting the expression of Fas on lymphocytes.[11,12]

CHRONIC STRESS INDUCES LYMPHOCYTE APOPTOSIS

The immune system is highly sensitive to stress, although its effects vary depending on the type and duration of stress and model used.[13–16] It is believed that an acute stressor presenting an immediate threat or intense physical activity usually enhances immune responses, while longer-term chronic stress is down-regulatory.[17] Furthermore, prolonged chronic stress is correlated with various disorders such as autoimmune diseases, tumorigenesis, and infectious diseases.

Chronic Stress Induces Immune Suppression

Chronic stress occurs when a continuous or intermittent stressful situation persists for a prolonged period. In animal experiments, chronic stress is often applied for more than a day. Many experiments show that chronic stress inhibits the immune system. Concanavalin A (Con A)-stimulated proliferation of lymphocytes from either the peripheral blood or lymph nodes is significantly decreased in rats stressed by changes in the light–dark cycle.[18] Another rat emotional stress model that involved randomly giving empty water bottles to rats trained to drink water at set times showed decreases in spleen weight and specific IgG antibody levels in response to ovalbumin immunization.[19]

We believe that stress-induced immunosuppression should render these animals at higher risk of opportunistic infections. In fact, in a mouse wound healing and infection model, restraint stress delayed healing by 30% and dramatically increased opportunistic infections, with a 2- to 5-log increment in bacterial load and a nearly 60% increase in infection rate.[10] This was further verified using anti-orthostatic suspension (hindlimb unloading) of mice infected with *Klebsiella pneumoniae*, which led to dramatically decreased survival compared to controls.[9]

Clinically, caregivers are considered to be subjected to chronic stress and serve as good models to study chronic stress in humans. It has been shown that caregivers have significantly lower numbers of T cells than the general population.[20] They also have poorer antibody and cytokine responses to influenza virus infection,[22] demonstrating that stress reduces the immune response to viral infection. Even long-term professional stress negatively influences the immune system. When a group of nurses was monitored for their immune function, it was discovered that those with higher work-related stress scores showed weaker immune responses compared to those with lower stress scores.[21]

Research has revealed that HIV-infected men with high stress levels progress more rapidly to AIDS as compared to those with lower stress levels.[23] In addition, patients stressed by traumatic injuries show low levels of responses in their immune systems. In spinal cord injury patients, both natural and adaptive immune responses were dramatically decreased 2 weeks after injury, while rehabilitation therapy partially restored normal immune function.[24]

In a study comparing the effects on immunity of laparoscopic operations compared with open surgery, immunosuppression was found to be proportional to the extent of operational trauma, as reduced immune responses were seen only in the open surgery group.[25] Similarly, in athletes, the prolonged physical stress associated with athletic training and competition may dampen their immune functions and make them more vulnerable to negative health outcomes.[26] Therefore, chronic stress has proved to induce immunosuppression both in animal models and in humans.

CHRONIC STRESS INDUCES LYMPHOCYTE APOPTOSIS

Apoptosis is an evolutionarily conserved "cell suicide" program present in all nucleated metazoan cells.[27,28] It is an active cell death process characterized by the activation of proteases, autodestruction of chromatin, nuclear condensation, cellular membrane blebbing, and vesicularization of internal components. Apoptotic cell death can be found in many physiological and pathological processes such as development, differentiation, tumorigenesis, and infection.[29,30] During immune responses, apoptosis is also important for cytotoxic cells that kill their targets[31] in the eradication of pathogen-infected cells, in the elimination of out-of-date immune cells, and in the pathogenesis of autoimmune disorders.[32,33]

One of the best-characterized examples of T cell apoptosis is activation-induced cell death (AICD). We have demonstrated that apoptosis can be induced specifically in immature thymocytes *in vivo* by administration of an antibody against the T cell antigen receptor (TCR).[34,35] Similarly, in both humans and mice, AICD has been proposed to be the main mechanism for elimination of excessive cells following immune responses, which is believed to play a crucial role in the maintenance of immune homeostasis.[33,36] Defects in the apoptotic machinery of lymphocytes lead to their accumulation in lymphoid organs and potentiate autoimmune disorders.

On the other hand, excessive apoptosis results in immunodeficiency, such as is induced by HIV in AIDS.

Lymphopenia is a common phenomenon during stress. It has been observed in surgical patients,[25,37-39] long-term and intensely exercised athletes,[40,41] and persons undergoing various types of physiological stress.[42] Likewise, lymphocyte reduction has also been found in animals subjected to restraint stress.[43] Using the physical restraint mouse model, we investigated the effects of chronic stress on lymphocyte apoptosis.[18] When Balb/c mice were subjected to a 12-hour daily physical restraint regimen for 2 days,[44] they showed 35% to 40% reductions in lymphocyte numbers in the spleen in comparison to control animals.

To investigate whether cell loss was due to apoptosis, the DNA strand breaks typical of apoptosis were detected in splenic histological sections by the terminal deoxyribonucleotidyl transferase-mediated dUTP-digoxigenin nick-end labeling (TUNEL) method. We found a significant increase in TUNEL-positive cells in stressed mice, indicating that the reduction of splenocytes is likely due to the induction of apoptosis in these cells.[45] In another chronic stress model, mice subjected to hindlimb unloading for 2 days also showed increased apoptosis in the spleen.[46]

While the number of lymphocytes decreases in almost every immune organ in response to stress, the sensitivities of different subsets may vary according to the model employed. Thymocytes are affected similarly to splenocytes, as stress causes a marked decrease in thymus weight and thymocyte number and a dramatic increase in thymocyte apoptosis. Interestingly, thymocytes seem to be more sensitive to stress, as apoptotic cells appear in the thymus as early as 6 hours after stress; in contrast, apoptosis in the peripheral lymphoid organs becomes apparent only after 12 hours or more.

Among all thymocyte subpopulations, CD4+CD8+ (double-positive) cells are most sensitive, suggesting that immature thymocytes are more easily affected by stress.[43] One study found that mature T cells are more sensitive than B cells in C57BL/6 mice,[47] while we recently found B cells are more sensitive in Balb/c mice subjected to hindlimb unloading for 2 days (Sun et al., unpublished data). It should be pointed out that a decrease in numbers in one lymphocyte subset may significantly increase the percentage of other cell subsets as detected by flow cytometry, although their absolute numbers may be unchanged. This is a critical issue when one examines cell population changes solely by flow cytometry. For example, we have seen that although the percentage of T cells significantly increases after stress, their absolute number is still significantly decreased (Sun et al., unpublished data).

Clearly, lymphocyte apoptosis is the main mechanism in the reduction of lymphocyte numbers after stress. Although apoptosis can be instigated by various mechanisms, our experiments reveal that the Fas–FasL interaction is most critical.

STRESS-INDUCED LYMPHOCYTE APOPTOSIS BY FAS–FASL MECHANISM

It has long been recognized that the Fas–FasL interaction plays a critical role in homeostasis of the immune system. We have found that chronic restraint stress-induced lymphocyte reduction is related to the increase of Fas expression.[12] Interestingly, stress-induced lymphocyte reduction could be blocked by interfering with the interaction between Fas and FasL by using either Fas fusion protein or antibody against FasL.[12,46] Mice were injected with serum from SCID mice bearing tumors of either 3T3 fibrosarcoma engineered to secrete with Fas–Ig fusion protein[48] or control 3T3 fibrosarcoma. Thus administered, serum containing Fas–Ig prevented stress-induced reductions in splenocyte numbers, while control serum had no effect.

When Fas–Ig-containing serum was adsorbed with protein A Sepharose beads, its protective effect was completely eliminated. In the same experiment, the Fas–Ig serum did not change the number of splenocytes in unstressed mice. We also found that a neutralizing antibody against FasL, MFL3,[49] but not an isotype control, blocked stress-induced lymphopenia. Splenocytes from stressed animals showed dramatically enhanced sensitivity to FasL-mediated apoptosis, as verified by co-culturing them with FasL-transfected L929 cells or control cells. We found that only splenocytes from stressed mice could be induced to undergo apoptosis by the FasL-expressing cells but lymphocytes from unstressed mice could not. In contrast, control L929 cells had no effect on splenocytes from either stressed or unstressed animals. These data indicate the critical role of the ligation between Fas and FasL in mediating stress-induced lymphocyte reduction.

To further elucidate the role of Fas, we utilized mice bearing an autosomal recessive mutation in Fas, C3H.MRL.Fas[lpr], and their appropriate background controls, C3H/HeJ. When these strains of mice were subjected to physical restraint, the typical reduction in lymphocyte numbers was observed only in control C3H/HeJ mice, but not in Fas-deficient C3H.MRL.Fas[lpr] mice. Therefore, the absence of FasL prevented stress-induced lymphocyte reduction in these mice, further supporting the pivotal role of Fas in stress-mediated immunosuppression.

Besides lymphocytes, stress-induced apoptosis has also been found in testicular tubules.[50] Since Sertoli cells in the testes express high levels of FasL,[51] it is possible that testicular tubular apoptosis during stress is mediated through increased Fas expression and the Fas–FasL pathway. The source of FasL in the initiation of lymphocyte apoptosis, however, is elusive. Although there is evidence with human cells that co-culture of post-operative monocytes with T cells increases T cell apoptosis,[52] using our mouse hindlimb unloading model, we found that depletion of macrophages *in vivo* before stress did not prevent lymphocyte losses, suggesting that the requisite FasL does not originate from macrophages (Erwei et al., unpublished data). We are continuing our experiments to determine the identity of the cells that provide the FasL necessary for Fas-mediated lymphocyte apoptosis during stress.

NEUROENDOCRINE FACTORS MEDIATING STRESS-INDUCED LYMPHOCYTE APOPTOSIS

Stress elicits complicated responses in the neural, endocrine, and immune systems. The hypothalamic–pituitary–adrenal (HPA) axis is critical for the release of hormones or transmitters during stress. Among them, three categories have been emphasized: glucocorticoids, catecholamines, and endogenous opioids. Our recent data suggest that during stress, thymocyte apoptosis is likely mediated by glucocorticoids or indirectly by opioids, while apoptosis in peripheral immune organs such as the spleen occurs via a direct effect of endogenous opioids.

GLUCOCORTICOIDS

It is well known that steroid hormones are immunosuppressive and *in vitro* experiments have shown that dexamethasone induces murine splenocyte and thymocyte apoptosis. Ayala et al. reported that during sepsis stress, increased apoptosis was observed in both thymocytes and bone marrow cells, but, unlike in thymocytes, apoptosis in bone marrow cells could not be blocked by the glucocorticoid antagonist, RU486.[43] In a 35-week chronic stress model by alternation of the light–dark (L-D) rhythm in rats, stressed rats were immunosuppressed, but there was no difference in adrenal activity compared to controls, suggesting that glucocorticoids were not involved.[18]

To examine the role of glucocorticoids in restraint-induced lymphocyte reduction, we performed adrenectomy before stress. We found no significant differences in restraint-induced lymphocyte reduction in adrenectomized mice and sham-operated mice.[53] We further verified this observation by experiments in hindlimb unloading stressed mice in which RU486 could block only thymocyte reduction, but not splenocyte reduction.[46]

Freier and Fuchs found that although injection of morphine could reduce thymocyte numbers, culture of thymocytes with morphine could not induce apoptosis, indicating that the effects of morphine on thymocytes are indirect.[54] Since the effect of morphine on thymocytes *in vivo* can be blocked by the opioid antagonist, naltrexone, as well as RU486, the HPA axis must play a critical role in this process. Accumulating data suggest that opioids play a critical role in stress-induced apoptosis of both immature and mature T cells, and the difference is that opioids act indirectly through HPA axis in immature T cells, but directly on mature peripheral T cells.

OPIOIDS

Opioids and Their Receptors

Opiates are an old class of drugs derived from the milky latex of the poppy plant, *Papaver somniferum*, and have been used for centuries as analgesics. Morphine is the primary alkaloid in opium. Opiates have effects on pain perception, consciousness, motor control, mood, and autonomic function, and often induce physical dependence or addiction. In 1975, Hughes et al. discovered the existence of an endogenous morphine-like substance, enkephalin.[55] Thereafter, several endogenous opioid peptides were identified in mammals and humans.[45,56]

These endogenous opioids and exogenous opiates exert their effects through specific surface receptors, all of which are 60-kD proteins and are currently classified into three groups: mu, delta, and kappa.[57,58] The existence of different opioid receptors was predicted mainly by pharmacological approaches and they differ in their affinities for various opioid ligands and in their pharmacological profiles.[59-61] Opioid antagonists such as naloxone or naltrexone specifically block the opioid receptors.[62-64] They have chemical structures similar to opioids and they block the effects of opioids by preventing their binding to receptors by competitive displacement.

Immunosuppression Induced by Chronic Stress Is Mediated by Endogenous Opioids

Opioids have been shown to regulate immune responses in both vertebrates and invertebrates.[65] Although the effect of opioids on immune function is complicated and depends on the study model used, administration of morphine or endogenous opioid is known to inhibit phagocytic activity and lymphocyte function.[66,67] Morphine-initiated inhibition of macrophage activity can be blocked *in vivo* and *in vitro* by the opioid antagonist naltrexone.[68] Similarly, *in vivo* administration of morphine reduced the antibody responses to sheep red cells[69–71] and tetanus toxoid, and the immunosuppression may be due to the decrease of spleen cellularity.[70]

In most studies, morphine-induced immunosuppression can be blocked by naltrexone, indicating the involvement of classical opioid receptors.[70,72] In our studies using the restraint stress model in mice, we found that administration of naltrexone or naloxone completely blocked the reduction in splenocyte numbers in stressed mice; the same treatment had no effect on unstressed mice, however.[12] When spleen tissue was analyzed by the TUNEL assay, we found that both antagonists blocked the appearance of TUNEL-positive cells. The importance of opioids has also been verified in μ-opioid receptor knockout (MORKO) mice.[73] As all three opioid receptors have been identified in lymphocytes, it is predictable that knocking out opioid receptors should block stress-induced lymphocyte death if opioids play a key role. Indeed, when μ-opioid receptor knockout mice were subjected to restraint stress for 12 hours daily for 2 days, there was essentially no apoptosis and no reduction in splenocyte number or in activation-induced cytokine production.

Interestingly, both wild-type and MORKO mice displayed significant elevations of plasma corticosterone.[74] Therefore, opioid-mediated apoptosis of immune cells plays an important role in stress-induced immunosuppression. Our recent studies have further revealed that opioids likely promote apoptosis by boosting the membrane expression of Fas on immune cells, thus enhancing their sensitivity to FasL-induced apoptosis.[11] *In vitro*, morphine enhanced the expression of Fas in a mouse T cell hybridoma cell line (A1.1), primary mouse splenocytes, and human peripheral lymphocytes. Similarly, injection of morphine increased Fas mRNA expression in mouse spleen, heart, and lung. Interestingly, the reduction in splenocyte numbers in mice administered with morphine could be blocked by co-administration of serum containing soluble Fas fusion protein (Fas-Ig), but not control serum.[11] These data clearly show that the level of Fas expression has an important role in opioid-induced lymphocyte apoptosis.

Free Radicals Increase Sensitivity to Fas–FasL-Mediated Apoptosis

Oxidation is essential for cellular energy metabolism, but this process generates numerous pro-oxidants that are highly toxic to the cells, such as free radicals and superoxides. Therefore, many antioxidants exist within cells to neutralize these pro-oxidants. Several studies have shown that stress-induced lymphocyte reduction can be blocked by antioxidants.[53,75–77]

In light of our implication of the Fas-FasL system in stress-induced apoptosis, we hypothesize that over-production of pro-oxidants during stress may increase the sensitivity of cells to Fas–FasL-mediated apoptosis. To this end, we cultured normal splenocytes with peroxide (H_2O_2) and agonistic Fas antibody (Jo2) and then analyzed DNA content as an indicator of apoptosis. We found that while either H_2O_2 or Jo2 alone induced only minimal apoptosis, in combination they dramatically promoted apoptosis.[78] This study implies that oxidants may be involved in the Fas–FasL apoptotic machinery although a detailed mechanism remains elusive.

SUMMARY

It has been established that chronic stress results in immunosuppression that is most likely due to enhancement of lymphocyte apoptosis. Opioids play an important role in promoting lymphocyte apoptosis by enhancing Fas expression in lymphocytes. It is not known how increased Fas expression contributes to the death machinery within cells. Recently, Fas rafting (or clustering) has been recognized as an important step in the transduction of death signals from the cell membrane to intracellular death molecules.[79–82]

It may be possible that increased Fas density in stressed lymphocytes lowers the threshold for rafting and formation of the death-inducing signaling complex (DISC) (Figure 11.1). Free radicals may further increase the sensitivity of cells to FasL-induced apoptosis via an unknown mechanism. Although glucocorticoids are involved in thymocyte apoptosis, their role in peripheral lymphocyte loss seems to be minor. Since a dysregulated immune system may be a major contributor to many diseases such as infection, autoimmunity, or tumors, further studies of the mechanisms and regulators involved in stress-induced lymphocyte apoptosis should provide the insight necessary for the development of novel strategies to prevent and treat these stress-associated disorders.

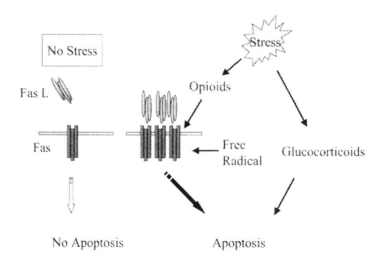

FIGURE 11.1 Mechanisms of lymphocyte apoptosis during chronic stress.

ACKNOWLEDGMENTS

This work was supported by grants from the National Institutes of Health (AI50222 and AI43384) and the National Space Biomedical Research Institute (IIH 00208).

REFERENCES

1. Kiecolt-Glaser J.K., McGuire L., Robles T.F., and Glaser R. (2002). Psychoneuroimmunology and psychosomatic medicine: back to the future. *Psychosom Med* 64, 15.
2. Ader R. and Cohen N. (1993). Psychoneuroimmunology: conditioning and stress. *Annu Rev Psychol* 44, 53.
3. Sklar L.S. and Anisman H. (1979). Stress and coping factors influence tumor growth. *Science* 205, 513.
4. Sklar L.S. and Anisman H. (1981). Stress and cancer. *Psychol Bull* 89, 369.
5. Sklar L.S., Bruto V., and Anisman H. (1981). Adaptation to the tumor-enhancing effects of stress. *Psychosom Med* 43, 331.
6. Sklar L.S. and Anisman H. (1980). Social stress influences tumor growth. *Psychosom Med* 42, 347.
7. Poliak S., Mor F., Conlon P., Wong T., Ling N., Rivier J., Vale W., and Steinman L. (1997). Stress and autoimmunity: the neuropeptides corticotropin-releasing factor and urocortin suppress encephalomyelitis via effects on both the hypothalamic–pituitary–adrenal axis and the immune system. *J Immunol* 158, 5751.
8. Winfield J.B. and Jarjour W.N. (1991). Stress proteins, autoimmunity, and autoimmune disease. *Curr Top Microbiol Immunol* 167, 161.
9. Sonnenfeld G., Aviles H., Belay T., Vance M., and Fountain K. (2002). Stress, suspension and resistance to infection. *J Gravit Physiol* 9, P199.
10. Rojas I.G., Padgett D.A., Sheridan J.F., and Marucha P.T. (2002). Stress-induced susceptibility to bacterial infection during cutaneous wound healing. *Brain Behav Immunol* 16, 74.
11. Yin D., Mufson R.A., Wang R., and Shi Y. (1999). Fas-mediated cell death promoted by opioids. *Nature* 397, 218.
12. Yin D., Tuthill D., Mufson R.A., and Shi Y. (2000). Chronic restraint stress promotes lymphocyte apoptosis by modulating CD95 expression. *J Exp Med* 191, 1423.
13. Bartolomucci A., Sacerdote P., Panerai A.E., Peterzani T., Palanza P., and Parmigiani S. (2003). Chronic psychosocial stress-induced down-regulation of immunity depends upon individual factors. *J Neuroimmunol* 141, 58.
14. Mediratta P.K., Bhatia J., Tewary S., Katyal V., Mahajan P., and Sharma K.K. (2003). Attenuation of the effect of progesterone and 4′-chlordiazepam on stress-induced immune responses by bicuculline. *Ind J Physiol Pharmacol* 47, 288.
15. Hawkley L.C. and Cacioppo J.T. (2004). Stress and the aging immune system. *Brain Behav Immun* 18, 114.
16. Kang D.H., Kim C.J., and Suh Y. (2004). Sex differences in immune responses and immune reactivity to stress in adolescents. *Biol Res Nurs* 5, 243.
17. Campisi J., Leem T.H., and Fleshner M. (2003). Stress-induced extracellular Hsp72 is a functionally significant danger signal to the immune system. *Cell Stress Chaperones* 8, 272.
18. Kort W.J. and Weijma J.M. (1982). Effect of chronic light–dark shift stress on the immune response of the rat. *Physiol Behav* 29, 1083.
19. Shao F., Lin W., Wang W., Washington W.C., Jr., and Zheng L. (2003). The effect of emotional stress on the primary humoral immunity of rats. *J Psychopharmacol* 17, 179.

20. Pariante C.M., Carpiniello B., Orru M.G., Sitzia R., Piras A., Farci A.M., Del Giacco G.S., Piludu G., and Miller A.H. (1997). Chronic caregiving stress alters peripheral blood immune parameters: the role of age and severity of stress. *Psychother Psychosom* 66, 199.

21. De Gucht V., Fischler B., and Demanet C. (1999). Immune dysfunction associated with chronic professional stress in nurses. *Psychiatry Res* 85, 105.

22. Kiecolt-Glaser J.K., Glaser R., Gravenstein S., Malarkey W.B., and Sheridan J. (1996). Chronic stress alters the immune response to influenza virus vaccine in older adults. *Proc Natl Acad Sci USA* 93, 3043.

23. Baier-Bitterlich G., Fuchs D., and Wachter H. (1997). Chronic immune stimulation, oxidative stress, and apoptosis in HIV infection. *Biochem Pharmacol* 53, 755.

24. Cruse J.M., Lewis R.E., Jr., Bishop G.R., Kliesch W.F., Gaitan E., and Britt R. (1993). Decreased immune reactivity and neuroendocrine alterations related to chronic stress in spinal cord injury and stroke patients. *Pathobiology* 61, 183.

25. Mattila-Vuori A., Salo M., Iisalo E., Pajulo O., and Viljanto J. (2000). Local and systemic immune response to surgery under balanced anaesthesia in children. *Paediatr Anaesth* 10, 381.

26. Clow A. and Hucklebridge F. (2001). The impact of psychological stress on immune function in the athletic population. *Exerc Immunol Rev* 7, 5.

27. Chinnaiyan A.M. and Dixit V.M. (1996). The cell-death machine. *Curr Biol* 6, 555.

28. Meier P., Finch A., and Evan G. (2000). Apoptosis in development. *Nature* 407, 796.

29. Kerr J.F., Wyllie A.H., and Currie A.R. (1972). Apoptosis: a basic biological phenomenon with wide-ranging implications in tissue kinetics. *Br J Cancer* 26, 239.

30. Martins L.M. and Earnshaw W.C. (1997). Apoptosis: alive and kicking in 1997. *Trends Cell Biol* 3, 111.

31. Moretta A. (1997). Molecular mechanisms in cell-mediated cytotoxicity. *Cell* 90, 13.

32. Chervonsky A.V., Wang Y., Wong F.S., Visintin I., Flavell R.A., Janeway C.A., Jr., and Matis L.A. (1997). The role of Fas in autoimmune diabetes. *Cell* 89, 17.

33. Lenardo M., Chan K.M., Hornung F., McFarland H., Siegel R., Wang J., and Zheng L. (1999). Mature T lymphocyte apoptosis: immune regulation in a dynamic and unpredictable antigenic environment. *Annu Rev Immunol* 17, 221.

34. Shi Y., Bissonnette R., Parfrey N., Szalay M., Kubo R., and Green D. (1991). *In vivo* administration of monoclonal antibodies to the CD3 T cell receptor complex induces cell death (apoptosis) in immature thymocytes. *J Immunol* 146, 3340.

35. Shi Y.F., Sahai B.M., and Green D.R. (1989). Cyclosporin A inhibits activation-induced cell death in T-cell hybridomas and thymocytes. *Nature* 339, 625.

36. Wesselborg S., Janssen O., and Kabelitz D. (1993). Induction of activation-driven death (apoptosis) in activated but not resting peripheral blood T cells. *J Immunol* 150, 4338.

37. Galinowski A. (1993). Stress and panic: immunologic aspects. *Encephale* 19, 147.

38. Iwagaki H., Morimoto Y., Kodera M., and Tanaka N. (2000). Surgical stress and CARS: involvement of T cell loss due to apoptosis. *Rinsho Byori* 48, 505.

39. Kunes P. and Krejsek J. (2000). CD4 lymphopenia and postoperative immunosuppression in cardiac surgery. *Cas Lek Cesk* 139, 361.

40. Pedersen B.K., Bruunsgaard H., Jensen M., Krzywkowski K., and Ostrowski K. (1999). Exercise and immune function: effect of ageing and nutrition. *Proc Nutr Soc* 58, 733.

41. Pedersen B.K., Bruunsgaard H., Klokker M., Kappel M., MacLean D.A., Nielsen H.B., Rohde T., Ullum H. and Zacho M. (1997). Exercise-induced immunomodulation: possible roles of neuroendocrine and metabolic factors. *Int J Sports Med* 18 Suppl 1, S2.

42. Zakowski S.G., McAllister C.G., Deal M., and Baum A. (1992). Stress, reactivity, and immune function in healthy men. *Health Psychol* 11, 223.

43. Ayala A., Herdon C.D., Lehman D.L., Ayala C.A., and Chaudry I.H. (1996). Differential induction of apoptosis in lymphoid tissues during sepsis: variation in onset, frequency, and the nature of the mediators. *Blood* 87, 4261.

44. Bonneau R.H., Sheridan J.F., Feng N., and Glaser R. (1993). Stress-induced modulation of the primary cellular immune response to herpes simplex virus infection is mediated by both adrenal-dependent and independent mechanisms. *J Neuroimmunol* 42, 167.

45. Kosterlitz H.W. and Hughes J. (1977). Peptides with morphine-like action in the brain. *Br J Psychiatry* 130, 298.

46. Wei L.X., Zhou J.N., Roberts A.I., and Shi Y.F. (2003). Lymphocyte reduction induced by hindlimb unloading: distinct mechanisms in the spleen and thymus. *Cell Res* 13, 465.

47. Dominguez-Gerpe L., and Rey-Mendez M. (2001). Alterations induced by chronic stress in lymphocyte subsets of blood and primary and secondary immune organs of mice. *BMC Immunol* 2, 7.

48. Ju S.T., Panka D.J., Cui H., Ettinger R., el-Khatib M., Sherr D.H., Stanger B.Z., and Marshak-Rothstein A. (1995). Fas(CD95)/FasL interactions required for programmed cell death after T-cell activation. *Nature* 373, 444.

49. Kayagaki N., Yamaguchi N., Nagao F., Matsuo S., Maeda H., Okumura K., and Yagita H. (1997). Polymorphism of murine Fas ligand that affects the biological activity. *Proc Natl Acad Sci USA* 94, 3914.

50. Barnes C.J., Covington B.W., Cameron I.L., and Lee M. (1998). Effect of aging on spontaneous and induced mouse testicular germ cell apoptosis. *Aging (Milano)* 10, 497.

51. Bellgrau D., Gold D., Selawry H., Moore J., Franzusoff A., and Duke R.C. (1995). A role for CD95 ligand in preventing graft rejection. *Nature* 377, 630.

52. Kono K., Takahashi A., Iizuka H., Fujii H., Sekikawa T., and Matsumoto Y. (2001). Effect of oesophagectomy on monocyte-induced apoptosis of peripheral blood T lymphocytes. *Br J Surg* 88, 1110.

53. Venkatraman J.T. and Pendergast D.R. (2002). Effect of dietary intake on immune function in athletes. *Sports Med* 32, 323.

54. Freier D.O. and Fuchs B.A. (1993). Morphine-induced alterations in thymocyte subpopulations of B6C3F1 mice. *J Pharmacol Exp Ther* 265, 81.

55. Hughes J., Smith T.W., Kosterlitz H.W., Fothergill L.A., Morgan B.A., and Morris H.R. (1975). Identification of two related pentapeptides from the brain with potent opiate agonist activity. *Nature* 258, 577.

56. Kosterlitz H.W. and Hughes J. (1977). Opiate receptors and endogenous opioid peptides in tolerance and dependence. *Adv Exp Med Biol* 85B, 141.

57. Grudt T.J. and Williams J.T. (1995). Opioid receptors and the regulation of ion conductances. *Rev Neurosci* 6, 279.

58. Stefano G.B. (1998). Autoimmunovascular regulation: morphine and anandamide and ancondamide stimulated nitric oxide release. *J Neuroimmunol* 83, 70.

59. Connor M. and Christie M.D. (1999). Opioid receptor signalling mechanisms. *Clin Exp Pharmacol Physiol* 26, 493.

60. Narita M., Funada M., and Suzuki T. (2001). Regulations of opioid dependence by opioid receptor types. *Pharmacol Ther* 89, 1.

61. Olley J.E. (1989). Opiate receptors: ligands and methods of study. *Clin Exp Pharmacol Physiol* 16, 535.

62. Crabtree B.L. (1984). Review of naltrexone, a long-acting opiate antagonist. *Clin Pharm* 3, 273.

63. Hameroff S.R. (1983). Opiate receptor pharmacology: mixed agonist/antagonist narcotics. *Contemp Anesth Pract* 7, 27.

64. O'Malley S.S. (1996). Opioid antagonists in the treatment of alcohol dependence: clinical efficacy and prevention of relapse. *Alcohol* Suppl 1, 77.

65. Webster N.R. (1998). Opioids and the immune system. *Br J Anaesth* 81, 835.

66. McCarthy L., Wetzel M., Sliker J.K., Eisenstein T.K., and Rogers T.J. (2001). Opioids, opioid receptors, and the immune response. *Drug Alcohol Depend* 62, 111.

67. Stefano G.B., Salzet B., and Fricchione G.L. (1998). Enkelytin and opioid peptide association in invertebrates and vertebrates: immune activation and pain. *Immunol Today* 19, 265.

68. Rojavin M., Szabo I., Bussiere J.L., Rogers T.J., Adler M.W., and Eisenstein T.K. (1993). Morphine treatment *in vitro* or *in vivo* decreases phagocytic functions of murine macrophages. *Life Sci* 53, 997.

69. Lefkowitz S.S. and Chiang C.Y. (1975). Effects of certain abused drugs on hemolysin forming cells. *Life Sci* 17, 1763.

70. Bussiere J.L., Adler M.W., Rogers T.J., and Eisenstein T.K. (1993). Effects of *in vivo* morphine treatment on antibody responses in C57BL/6 bgJ/bgJ (beige) mice. *Life Sci* 52, PL43.

71. Bhargava H.N., Thomas P.T., Thorat S., and House R.V. (1994). Effects of morphine tolerance and abstinence on cellular immune function. *Brain Res* 642, 1.

72. Bussiere J.L., Adler M.W., Rogers T.J., and Eisenstein T.K. (1992). Differential effects of morphine and naltrexone on the antibody response in various mouse strains. *Immunopharmacol Immunotoxicol* 14, 657.

73. Roy S., Barke R.A., and Loh H.H. (1998). MU-opioid receptor-knockout mice: role of mu-opioid receptor in morphine mediated immune functions. *Brain Res Mol Brain Res* 61, 190.

74. Wang J., Charboneau R., Barke R.A., Loh H.H., and Roy S. (2002). Mu-opioid receptor mediates chronic restraint stress-induced lymphocyte apoptosis. *J Immunol* 169, 3630.

75. Brohee D. and Neve P. (1994). Effect of dietary high doses of vitamin E on lymphocyte subsets in young and old CBA mice. *Mech Ageing Dev* 76, 189.

76. Meerson F.Z., Sukhikh G.T., and Pletsityi K.D. (1985). Prevention of the stress-induced decrease in natural killer activity by using a beta-adrenergic blocker and vitamin E. *Biull Eksp Biol Med* 99, 646.

77. Singh A., Failla M.L., and Deuster P.A. (1994). Exercise-induced changes in immune function: effects of zinc supplementation. *J Appl Physiol* 76, 2298.

78. Shi Y., Devadas S., Greeneltch K.M., Yin D., Allan Mufson R., and Zhou J.N. (2003). Stressed to death: implication of lymphocyte apoptosis for psychoneuroimmunology. *Brain Behav Immun* 17, Suppl 1, S18.

79. Wagenknecht B., Roth W., Gulbins E., Wolburg H., and Weller M. (2001). C2-ceramide signaling in glioma cells: synergistic enhancement of CD95-mediated, caspase-dependent apoptosis. *Cell Death Differ* 8, 595.

80. Grassme H., Cremesti A., Kolesnick R., and Gulbins E. (2003). Ceramide-mediated clustering is required for CD95-DISC formation. *Oncogene* 22, 5457.

81. Grassme H., Jekle A., Riehle A., Schwarz H., Berger J., Sandhoff K., Kolesnick R., and Gulbins E. (2001). CD95 signaling via ceramide-rich membrane rafts. *J Biol Chem* 276, 20589.

82. Cremesti A., Paris F., Grassme H., Holler N., Tschopp J., Fuks Z., Gulbins E., and Kolesnick R. (2001). Ceramide enables fas to cap and kill. *J Biol Chem* 276, 23954.

12 Interleukin-10 and the Hypothalamic–Pituitary–Adrenal Axis

Eric M. Smith, Huolin Tu,
and Thomas K. Hughes, Jr.

CONTENTS

INTRODUCTION

Interleukin-10 (IL-10) was initially reported as a factor produced by T helper-type 2 (Th2) lymphocytes, monocytes/macrophages, and B cells that inhibit Th1 cells.[1–4] IL-10's spectrum of activities quickly expanded from inhibiting production of cytokines by activated Th1 cells, macrophages, and NK cells. Studies have now shown that many immunoregulatory activities can be attributed to IL-10.[2,5–8] Its production and activity are fundamental to our understanding of the change in the cytokine profile with the progression of AIDS from Th1 to Th2 cytokines and the importance of the Th1/Th2 ratio as an indicator of a pro- or anti-inflammatory profile with implications for health. In the 15 years since its discovery,[1] IL-10 has been found to be synthesized by many cell types, including non-immune system cells, and have many diverse activities. One of the most significant of IL-10's "non-immune" activities is on the hypothalamic–pituitary–adrenal (HPA) axis, particularly in regard to the stress pathway.

In response to stressors, the mammalian neuroendocrine system is initiated by the hypothalamus producing corticotropin-releasing hormone (CRF), thereby stimulating the release of corticotrophin (ACTH) by the anterior pituitary gland, which causes the adrenals to produce glucocorticosteroid hormones (GCS). The major glucocorticoid in humans is cortisol (hydrocortisone) and in rodents it is corticosterone. Glucocorticoid production can result in, but is not limited to, increased lipolysis and gluconeogenesis, protein catabolism, effects on musculoskeletal and connective tissue, central nervous system function, and modulation of immune responses (mostly suppression).[9] Research over the past two decades has strongly suggested that the immune and neuroendocrine systems' functions and actions are intimately associated. Neuropeptide hormones can directly affect the immune system, and cytokines can directly affect the neuroendocrine system.[10,11] There are many sites in the stress response pathway where cytokines may act and alter outcomes.

To date, the cytokines most studied in the neuroendocrine system are pro-inflammatory, including IL-1, IL-6, and TNFα. They generally exert positive effects on neuroendocrine responses on all levels of the HPA axis.[12] However, we have found that IL-10, an anti-inflammatory cytokine, affects the HPA axis as well, as it induces the production of CRF and ACTH in hypothalamic and pituitary cells, respectively.[13–15] The clinical relevance of this is emphasized by recent studies showing an association of IL-10 levels, stress, and aging.[16,17] Thus, it appears that both pro-inflammatory and anti-inflammatory cytokines can activate the HPA axis. The literature suggests that changes in the balance of pro-inflammatory and anti-inflammatory cytokines occur with age and an anti-inflammatory phenotype correlates with longevity,[18] which may be mediated in part by the effects of cytokines on the HPA axis.

IL-10 AND THE IMMUNE SYSTEM

BIOLOGIC ACTIVITY

IL-10 is a member of the class 2 α-helical cytokines. The other members include IL-19, IL-20, IL-22, IL-24, IL-26, interferons (IFN-α, -β, -ε, -κ, -δ, -τ, and -γ), and interferon-like molecules (limitin, IL-28A, IL-28B, and IL-29). Mouse IL-10 (mIL-10) exists as a homodimer, with a molecular mass of approximately 35 to 40 kDa. The mIL-10 gene contains five exons encoding the entire mIL-10 mRNA sequence. The first exon is comprised of 5'-untranslated sequences, the signal sequence, and the N terminal 34 amino acids. Exon V contains the C terminal, 30 amino acids, and the entire 3'-untranslated region of the ~1.4 kb mIL-10 mRNA. Human IL-10, which has a molecular weight of about 18 kDa, shares only 73% amino acid homology with mIL-10.[19] In humans, IL-10 is produced by multiple cell types: induced T cell clones stimulated with antisera against CD3 and phorbol myristic acid[20] or by Epstein–Barr virus-infected B cells and by B cell lymphomas.[21] In addition, there are viral IL-10 homologues encoded for by Epstein–Barr virus (BCRF1),[22,23] orf poxvirus (ovIL-10),[24] and cytomegaloviruses (cmvIL-10).[25] Screening EST databases for IL-10 homologues has identified at least three other class

2 cytokines with 20% to 28% identity with IL-10, including IL-19, IL-20, and IL-22[4]; however, these cytokines bind different receptors, are produced by different cells, and seem to mediate different activities

The principal function of IL-10 appears to be limiting the magnitude of an immune response. This occurs through multiple mechanisms, which explains in part the many activities of IL-10. Human IL-10 inhibits the synthesis of various T cell products, including IFN-γ and granulocyte–monocyte colony-stimulating factor (GM-CSF) by activated human peripheral blood mononuclear cells.[1] Murine IL-10 inhibits the synthesis of IL-2, IL-3, TNF, IFN-γ, and GM-CSF by Th1 cells in response to antigen plus antigen-presenting cells. Along with the reduction in cytokine synthesis, there is also reduced expression of class II antigens on the presenting cells.[26] The growth and cytolytic activities of mouse CD8+ cytotoxic T cells are enhanced by murine IL-10.[27] Co-incubation of thymocytes and T cells with IL-7 or IL-2 plus IL-4, mouse or human IL-10, can function as a growth stimulatory co-factor.[3] Also, IL-10 in combination with IL-4 or IL-3 plus IL-4 will stimulate mast cell viability and growth.[28] Therefore, IL-10 is a powerful co-factor in addition to its potent primary functions.

IL-10 was named the cytokine synthesis inhibitory factor due to its ability to inhibit the production of numerous monokines such as IL-1α, IL-1β, IL-6, IL-8, and TNF-α.[5,8] Other monocyte/macrophage activities in the murine and human systems are also affected, such as cellular morphology and adhesion.[29] In the immune system, IL-10 is synthesized not only by Th2 type T cells, but bacterial lipopolysaccharide (LPS) and a variety of other stimulants induce macrophages and monocytes to produce high levels of IL-10 *in vitro*.[29] Furthermore, IL-10 production appears to be under negative feedback in an autoregulatory mechanism because IL-10 mRNA expression in LPS-activated monocytes becomes inhibited.[30]

IL-10 and the Th2 cytokines are associated with enhanced humoral responses and contributing to this is that B cells are stimulated in many ways by IL-10. When highly purified B cells from spleens of naïve/normal mice are treated with IL-10, their viability *in vitro* is enhanced and class II MHC expression is up-regulated.[31] Proliferation of anti-CD40 antibody-activated B cells is enhanced and also their differentiation into antibody-secreting cells. Cell numbers and DNA synthesis are augmented and the differentiation into antibody secreting cells results in large amounts of most immunoglobulin isotypes being produced.[32] IL-10 will function as a co-factor with transforming growth factor β to drive naive B cells into IgA secretion following activation with anti-CD40 antibodies.[33] Further co-factor functions of IL-10 occur through effects on T cell cytokine synthesis and activity. IL-10 enhances the *in vitro* proliferation of murine thymocytes and T cells that have been activated with IL-2 and IL-4; IL-10 seems to modulate T cell development.[3,34]

In vivo studies that manipulate IL-10 in combination with an infectious challenge are particularly revealing about IL-10's fundamental role in the immune system. IL-10's ability to suppress IFN-γ and enhance antibody production suggests it is an important factor during infection. For example, the production of IFN-γ by CD4+ T cells follows infection by a variety of parasites. The subsequent production of IL-10 during the infection is a means by which parasites could escape from IFN-γ's anti-parasitic activities.[8,35] During viral infections such as HIV, IL-10 is thought to play a major role in the shift of Th1 to a Th2 profile that contributes to the progression to AIDS.[36] As mentioned, several viruses produce viral IL-10s such as BCRF1, orfIL-10, and cmvIL-10. These viruses are likely to persist in the host and the viral IL-10 may contribute to the host's inability to control these viruses.[21] Finally, mice deficient in IL-10 demonstrate the critical role of this cytokine in normal maintenance of immune functioning. These animals develop enterocolitis and other symptoms similar to Crohn's disease.[37]

IL-10 RECEPTOR SIGNAL TRANSDUCTION

The IL-10 receptor (IL-10R) as currently understood is a multi-protein complex related to another Class 2 cytokine receptor family member, the interferon gamma receptor complex.[4,38–40] Two gene products, IL-10R1 and IL-10R2, make up the complex as homodimers, i.e., R1:R1 and R2:R2. The genes for R1 and R2 are similar and IL-10 itself binds as a homodimer to activate the cell surface receptors. The presence of IL-10R was initially thought to be limited to hematopoietic cells such as B, T, NK, and monocytic cells. Our lab and others have shown other cells, neurons and neuroendocrine cells in particular, may express IL-10R.[41] Expression of R1 alone is not sufficient to transduce IL-10-mediated signals, and IL-10R2 knockout (KO) mice develop chronic inflammatory bowel disease identical to that of the IL-10 KO mice.[37] Human IL-10R is species-specific, whereas murine IL-10R can bind both murine and human IL-10 with similar affinity.[42]

Like other class 2 cytokine receptors, binding to IL-10R activates JAK/STAT (*Janus* kinase/signal transducers and activators of transcription) intracellular signaling pathways. JAK1 is constitutively bound to IL-10R1, and TYK2 constitutively associates with the IL-10R2 chain.[43–45] IL-10 activates STAT1α and STAT3 in most IL-10R-positive cell types and can result in differential assembly into STAT1 homodimers, STAT3 homodimers, and STAT1:STAT3 heterodimers. The significance of this differential assembly of STAT complexes is not known, but may result in differential binding to STAT binding elements (SBEs) regulating different genes and distinguish IL-10 activation from other STAT-inducing cytokines such as IFN-γ which results in STAT binding to the IFN-γ activating sequence (GAS) and subsequent IFN-γ-related activities.[46] There also appears to be differential activation of STATs by IL-10 in T cells and monocytes,[43] which could also account for the different effects of IL-10. STAT3 activation is critical, as IL-10 does not inhibit LPS-induced cytokine production in STAT3 KO mice but will inhibit synthesis in STAT1α KO macrophages.[47]

There appear to be at least two mechanisms for IL-10 inhibition of cytokine synthesis. Among the genes activated by STAT1 and STAT3 are possible effector proteins, the suppressors of cytokine signaling 1 and 3 (SOCS-1/3) which suppress cytokine synthesis.[38] The other mechanism is based on evidence that IL-10 inhibits NF-κB activity in monocytic cells.[48,49] In addition, it was recently shown that IL-10 inhibits IL-6 production in microglia through prevention of NF-κ B activation.[50] NF-κ B is a key transcription factor regulating cytokine synthesis and many cell surface proteins involved in immune responses, and thus could serve as a critical target to inhibit cytokine synthesis. The controversy over which is the primary if not sole intracellular signaling pathway for IL-10 has not been solved. It suggests multiple pathways that may be affected by IL-10, depending upon the target cells and/or co-factors and makes it important to determine which pathways are utilized by neuroendocrine cells.

IL-10 AND IMMUNE RESPONSES IN THE CENTRAL NERVOUS SYSTEM (CNS)

The first reports of IL-10 in the brain were in association with neuroinflammation diseases such as multiple sclerosis (MS) or its animal model, experimental autoimmune encephalopathy (EAE). The source of IL-10 was attributed to leukocytes that infiltrated from the vasculature. IL-10 synthesis would seem to be a likely and important anti-inflammatory response for such diseases. In the case of MS, several investigators found reduced levels of IL-10 in the cerebrospinal fluid (CSF) and peripheral blood cells from patients.[51-53] This suggests a mechanism of action of disease whereby decreased production of IL-10 leads to autoreactive T cells.[51]

Confounding results by Monteyne et al.[54] showed IL-10 mRNA levels in CSF cells are elevated in MS patients, which suggests IL-10's involvement in MS may be complex.[54-56] One would predict that a decrease in IL-10 would contribute to inflammation in the CNS based on its classification as an anti-inflammatory cytokine. In fact, Cannella et al.[57] found that intravenous injections of IL-10 did not affect or may have even worsened EAE. Other laboratories found IL-10 to be generated within the CNS during neuroinflammation.[58,59] These disparate examples of IL-10 in CNS pathologies suggest a diverse role possibly involving multiple factors, and are in need of further study.

One contributing confounding factor may be the cellular source of IL-10. The vast majority of the reports focus on the immune origin of IL-10, particularly in multiple sclerosis which involves a lymphoid invasion into the CNS.[51] Conversely, our studies and others have found neural and neuroendocrine origins for some IL-10s.[13,14] Mizuno et al.[60] showed that cultured mouse glial cells produce IL-10 and later Wong et al.[61] confirmed our findings of IL-10 in the neurohypophysis and the CNS. There is even some suggestion that IL-10 produced by glioblastoma cells may serve as a growth factor and an immune escape mechanism.[62] Therefore, non-immune sources of IL-10 may contribute to the immune system-related pathologies in the CNS, and later in this chapter some examples of nervous system effects will be discussed.

IL-10 PRODUCTION BY HPA TISSUES

The first published reports of IL-10 synthesis at non-immunological sites focused on the brain[41,60] and the pituitary.[13] IL-10 in the brain was associated with neuroinflammation and was assumed to be derived from invading T lymphocytes as discussed above[41] or produced by microglia, the macrophages of the brain.[60] In contrast, the IL-10 in the pituitary was found to be synthesized by the pituitary cells and was the first non-immune-related source of IL-10 to be identified.[13]

Our initial studies were aimed at determining the effects of IL-10 in tissue of neuroendocrine origin. Due to the inherent difficulties of utilizing isolated primary pituitary cells, we determined the effects of IL-10 *in vitro*, employing mouse pituitary tumor cells (AtT-20). These studies and our interest in novel expression of cytokines led to a reciprocal experiment to determine whether AtT-20 pituitary tumor cells also produced IL-10. IL-10 was quantified by an indirect ELISA in which IL-10 standards or samples believed to contain IL-10 were first bound to the plate.[13,63] Using this ELISA on supernatant fluids from untreated cells, we demonstrated a constitutive production of IL-10 from AtT-20 pituitary tumor cells. IL-10 was detected in both the supernatant fluids and the cellular lysates of these cells at levels of about 2 to 3 ng/ml. These levels are in the range utilized for IL-10 activity in other systems.[35,64,65]

To further determine whether IL-10 is involved in the induction of ACTH, AtT-20 cells were treated with or without CRF for 3 hours and 6 hours in the presence or absence of antibodies to IL-10, following which ACTH levels were measured by radioimmunoassay (RIA). In the absence of anti-IL-10, ACTH levels increased in a time- and dose-dependent fashion. However, ACTH levels were reduced in all samples treated with anti-IL-10, suggesting an intermediary role for IL-10 in CRF induction of ACTH. We also examined IL-10 mRNA synthesis in AtT-20 cells treated with CRF to determine whether the regulation occurred at the transcription level. It appeared that IL-10 mRNA is up-regulated in AtT-20 cells treated with 10 nM and 100 nM CRF for 2 hours (Hughes et al., unpublished data).

Immunohistochemical staining of normal murine pituitary tissue with antiserum to IL-10 showed that cells of the anterior pituitary that are histologically non-lymphoid in origin produced IL-10 (Figure 12.1) and cells in the same area produced ACTH. This shows that IL-10 production occurs in normal tissues and is not solely an artifact from transformation of pituitary cells. Authenticity of the pituitary-derived IL-10 was demonstrated by direct sequence analysis of cDNA fragments obtained from mouse splenocytes, AtT-20 pituitary tumor cells, and freshly isolated mouse pituitaries. Starting with identical amounts of RNA from each tissue, we utilized reverse transcriptase (RT)-coupled polymerase chain reaction (PCR) with custom-designed primers. The amplification products corresponding to the expected molecular weight were then subjected to direct sequencing by using the consensus primers as sequencing primers. The results of the RT-PCR amplification showed a major product at a molecular weight corresponding to 304 bp, which is the expected size product. When these fragments were excised from the gel and submitted to sequence analysis, 100% identity existed in sequences from all tissues tested. While this PCR is non-quantitative, identical amounts of RNA from each tissue were used in the amplification. Thus, the possibility that the 304-bp amplicon came solely from the small number of contaminating lymphocytes in the pituitary is unlikely, since similar amounts of amplification product were obtained from the lymphocyte-rich spleen preparations and the lymphocyte-negative AtT-20 cell line.[13]

We have shown that IL-10 can induce the production of ACTH in both mouse pituitary tumor cells (AtT-20) and mouse splenocytes; we have also shown that IL-10 is produced by AtT-20 cells and by freshly isolated mouse pituitaries. We next determined whether a similar phenomenon could be demonstrated in humans. Due to a lack of human pituitary cell lines, we tested pituitary and hypothalamus poly (A+) RNA (Clontech, Palo Alto, CA) derived from human postmortem samples for IL-10 mRNA.[14] Figure 12.2 shows that following RT-PCR with IL-10-specific primers, IL-10 transcripts could be detected in both the pituitary and the hypothalamus. The

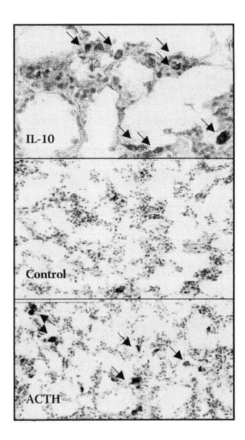

FIGURE 12.1 Immunohistochemical staining for IL-10 and ACTH in the anterior pituitary. Flash frozen sections of human anterior pituitary were stained for IL-10 and ACTH, as indicated, using standard horseradish peroxidase-based immunohistochemical procedures. Sections were initially hematoxylin–eosin stained. Control = isotype staining control. Arrows = IL-10 or ACTH positive staining.

specificity of this amplification was confirmed by Southern blot analysis of the PCR products with an oligonucleotide probe specific for IL-10.

Most of the IL-10 appeared to be produced by cells of the hypothalamus and pituitary rather than by lymphocytes in their vasculature. The levels of cDNA derived from equivalent amounts of RNA for IFN-γ, a lymphocyte-specific product, and IL-10 between the pituitary and the hypothalamus were compared with levels in peripheral blood leukocytes (PBLs).[14] G3PDH levels were monitored to ensure that equal amounts of amplification occurred in all tissues. A densitometric ratio of IFN-γ or IL-10 to G3PDH (a "housekeeping" gene present in all samples) was then determined. This ratio provided information as to the relative amounts of PCR product contributed by each tissue.

Figure 12.2 shows the RT-PCR and densitometric ratios for (A) IL-10/G3PDH and (B) IFN-γ/G3PDH in pituitary, hypothalamus, and PBLs. Relatively equivalent amounts of amplification occurred for G3PDH in all samples (lanes 4, 6, and 8). There was a

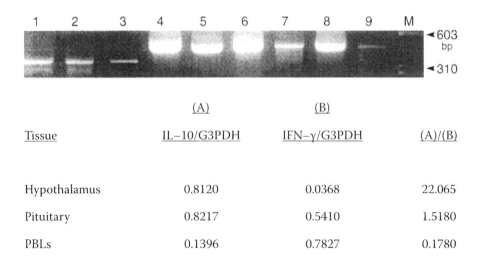

Tissue	(A) IL–10/G3PDH	(B) IFN–γ/G3PDH	(A)/(B)
Hypothalamus	0.8120	0.0368	22.065
Pituitary	0.8217	0.5410	1.5180
PBLs	0.1396	0.7827	0.1780

FIGURE 12.2 RT-PCR and densitometry of human pituitary and hypothalamus poly (A+) RNA utilizing IFN-γ, IL-10, and G3PDH specific primers. Integrated densitometry readings for each sample are in parentheses. Lane 1 = IL-10 pituitary (737,980). Lane 2 = IL-10 hypothalamus (675,300). Lane 3 = IL-10 PBLs (148,650). Lane 4 = G3PDH PBLs (1,064,800). Lane 5 = IFN- PBLs (833,420). Lane 6 = G3PDH pituitary (898,080). Lane 7 = IFN-γ pituitary (485,960). Lane 8 = G3PDH hypothalamus (831,650). Lane 9 = IFN-γ hypothalamus (30,567). M = molecular weight marker. (From Smith, E.M. et al. *J. Neuroimmunol.* 100, 140, 1999. With permission.)

minor amount of amplification for IFN-γ from the hypothalamus (lane 9), while a stronger signal occurred from the pituitary (lane 7). As expected, a large amount of amplification product was produced from PBLs (lane 5). RT-PCR for IL-10 indicated that greater amounts of amplification occurred for IL-10 in the pituitary and hypothalamus than in the PBLs (lanes 1 and 2 versus 3). When the densitometric ratios of (A) IL-10/G3PDH and (B) IFN-γ/G3PDH are compared between the tissues of (A/B), it can be seen that the ratio of the signals for IL-10 derived from the hypothalamus and the pituitary are about 124 and 8.5 times stronger, respectively, than that from the PBLs. Thus, while a component of the IL-10 RT-PCR product is probably derived from the lymphocytes in the vasculature, it appears that the majority is derived from the cells of the pituitary and hypothalamus.[14] Based on antigenicity, cDNA sequence, and bioactivity, it appears that the hypothalamus and pituitary synthesize bona fide IL-10.

IL-10 EFFECTS ON THE HYPOTHALAMUS

At the top of the HPA axis, IL-10 has been found to induce the production of CRF in hypothalamic median eminence (ME) tissue (Figure 12.3).[66] Treatment *in vitro* of rat ME fragments with IL-10 (1×10^{-8}M) for 10 minutes specifically stimulated CRF release. Pretreatment with inhibitors and direct measurement provided evidence that nitric oxide production was involved in the CRF release.[66] Therefore, not only is IL-10 synthesized in hypothalamic tissue, it appears able to act in an autocrine

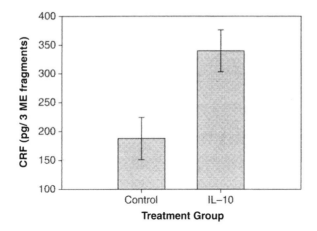

FIGURE 12.3 IL-10 induces the production of CRF from ME fragments exposed to an effective dose of IL-10 (10^{-8} M) for 10 minutes. Each separate experiment was performed in triplicate and the resulting mean ±SEM graphed. Supernatant fluids were assayed by RIA for CRF. (From Smith, E.M. et al. *J. Neuroimmunol.* 100, 140, 1999. With permission.)

fashion akin to its autoregulatory activities in the immune system[30] to induce CRF by the ME. Interestingly, Krueger et al.[67] recently showed IL-10 inhibited sleep in rabbits, as we found in rats,[68] and speculated that the mechanism of action may be through this induction of CRF in the ME.

IL-10 EFFECTS ON THE PITUITARY

The ability of IL-10 to induce ACTH production in AtT-20 pituitary cells was the first indication of what appear to be many effects throughout the HPA tissues. We treated AtT-20 cells with IL-10 at concentrations ranging from 10 to 100 ng/ml. These levels were chosen because they encompass effective concentrations described in the literature.[35,64,65] Following treatment for 6 hours, supernatant fluids were harvested and subjected to RIA for ACTH. A range of IL-10 concentrations induced the production of ACTH from AtT-20 pituitary tumor cells, with induction occurring in a dose-dependent fashion. The possibility of sequence or structural similarity between IL-10 and CRF was investigated. Computer-assisted amino acid sequence alignment and secondary structural comparisons (PC gene) revealed that this was not the case (data not shown) and presumably indicates that a different mechanism of induction of ACTH is occurring, such as through specific IL-10 receptors.

We also determined whether, as observed in AtT-20 cells, IL-10 induced splenocytes to produce ACTH. IL-10 (50 ng/ml) induced the production of ACTH from murine splenocytes, as detected by RIA, to rise from 30 pg/ml to 60 pg/ml after 48 hours. This also indicated that spleen cells, similar to AtT-20 cells, produce ACTH constitutively at low levels, which confirmed previous results.[69]

Indoleamine 2,3-dioxygenase (IDO) catalyzation of tryptophan is the first rate-limiting step of the kynurenine pathway in the majority of tissues. The kynurenine

pathway produces neurotoxic metabolites such as 3-hydroxykinurenine and quinolinic acid. IDO is inducible by the IFN-γ cytokine and has been proposed to mediate
the sickness behavior of patients with infectious or other inflammatory diseases.[70,71]
To better understand the neuroendocrine component of cytokine-induced sickness
behavior,[12] we determined the effects of the pro-inflammatory IFN-γ cytokine and
the anti-inflammatory IL-10 cytokine on IDO expression in cells derived from the
HPA axis: GT1-7, hypothalamic; AtT-20, pituitary; and Y-1, adrenal cells.[72] RT-PCR
was performed to check the IDO expression from IFN-γ- and IL-10-treated cells
such as GT1-7, AtT-20, and Y-1.

We found that IFN-γ induced IDO expression after 4 hours of treatment in GT1-7
and AtT-20 cells. IL-10 was also able to suppress IFN-γ-induced IDO expression in these
cells. In Y-1 adrenal cells, IFN-γ treatment had no effect on IDO expression. Our results
indicate that cytokines such as IFN-γ and IL-10 are able to regulate IDO expression in
cells of hypothalamic and pituitary origin. The ability of IL-10 to suppress IFN-γ-induced
IDO expression implies that IL-10 has a putative neuroprotective role in the HPA axis.
It could act at two levels, systemically by inhibiting sickness behavior-related Th1
cytokine synthesis and more centrally by inhibiting the kynurenine pathway.

IL-10 binds to a receptor complex that contains both R1 and R2 chains to activate
signaling. To further support the specificity of the IL-10 action in the induction of
ACTH by pituitary cells, it was necessary to determine that IL-10R was also present.
Using specific oligonucleotides for the mIL-10R1,[73] we examined AtT-20 cells for
expression of IL-10R1 mRNA by semi-quantitative RT-PCR.[15] Figure 12.4 is a
Southern blot indicating that the R1 receptor is expressed in AtT-20 cells. We also
noted a decrease in IL-10R1 cDNA expression following treatment with IL-10. The
IL-10 treatment did not seem to globally affect cell functions since relatively equiv-
alent amounts of amplification occurred for G3PDH in all samples.

Multiple publications have discussed transcription factor modulation in the signal transduction pathways following IL-10 treatment of lymphocytes.[4,38,43,45,46,48–50]
The principal signal transduction systems activated by IL-10 seem to be the
JAK/STAT pathway and activation of SOCS genes to suppress cytokine expression
as described above.[4,38,43,45–47,49] However, a number of studies have shown that IL-10
also inhibits NF-κB activation, which would be an effective alternate means to inhibit
cytokine expression.[48–50]

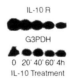

IL-10 R

G3PDH

0 20' 40' 60' 4h
IL-10 Treatment

FIGURE 12.4 Top: Southern blot analysis of murine IL-10R (R1, α) in AtT-20 pituitary
cells. An oligonucleotide probe was used to analyze IL-10R mRNA levels following IL-10
treatment. Bottom: Southern blot analysis of RT-PCR G3PDH internal control serving as a
semi-quantitative reference of equivalent amplification between samples. (From Smith, E.M.
et al. *J. Neuroimmunol.* 100, 140, 1999. With permission.)

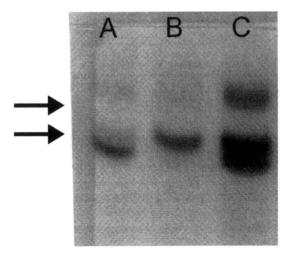

FIGURE 12.5 Effects of IL-10 on NF-κB activity in AtT-20 pituitary cells. Electrophoretic mobility shift assay (EMSA) was performed on nuclear lysates after 30 minutes of treatment. Lane A: mock control. Lane B: IL-10 (100 units/ml). Lane C: antibody to IL-10 (1:100). The cognate oligonucleotide was that of the kappa light chain obtained from Santa Cruz Biotech. (From Smith, E.M. et al. *J. Neuroimmunol.* 100, 140, 1999. With permission.)

To determine whether similar signaling pathways were modulated in neuroendocrine tissue, AtT-20 cells were treated with IL-10 or anti-IL10 antibody and examined for NF-κB-binding activity by electrophoretic mobility shift assays. Interestingly, IL-10 treatment did not alter NF-κB activity as determined by these assays (Figure 12.5). However, treatment of the AtT-20 cells with anti-IL-10 dramatically elevated NF-κB activity. This suggests that the endogenous IL-10 produced by the AtT-20 cells maximally inhibited NF-κB activity such that exogenous IL-10 had no increased effect. This further suggests that the IL-10 receptor on pituitary cells is coupled to similar intracellular signaling pathways as with lymphocytes.

IL-10 EFFECTS ON THE ADRENAL GLAND

The ability of IL-10 to induce hypothalamic CRF production and pituitary cells to produce ACTH suggested that IL-10 would induce an adrenal steroidogenic response *in vivo*. To determine IL-10's action *in vivo* on the HPA axis, we took advantage of commercially available IL-10-deficient (IL-10$^{-/-}$) mice as a novel, specific approach to investigate the relationship of IL-10 and systemic GCS levels. To test for IL-10-related control of HPA activity, normal and IL-10-deficient mice were compared in response to different stressors. One was a classical physiological stressor, a brief immersion in cold water (4°C). The second was an immune system stimulant, pI:C (poly I:C), a synthetic double-stranded RNA.

It is interesting to note that even when not particularly stressed, the IL-10-deficient mice had higher basal GCS levels (Figure 12.6 and Figure 12.7). The IL-10$^{-/-}$ mice following pI:C treatment produced three to five times the amount of corticosterone

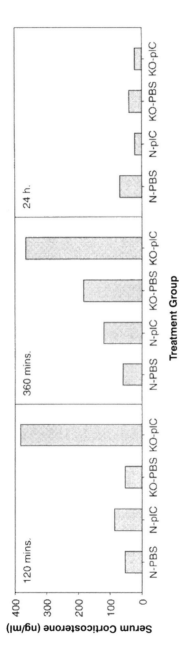

FIGURE 12.6 Preliminary studies showing endogenous IL-10 affects GCS levels following "immune stress" with pIC in IL-10$^{+/+}$ (normal = N) and IL-10$^{-/-}$ (KO). IL-10$^{+/+}$ and IL-10$^{-/-}$ mice were administered pIC intraperitoneally (0.1 mg per mouse) or vehicle (PBS). The animals were sacrificed 2, 6, and 24 hours later and serum GCS levels were determined by RIA. N = three or four mice per group, representative of three experiments. (From Smith, E.M. et al. *J. Neuroimmunol.* 100, 140, 1999. With permission.)

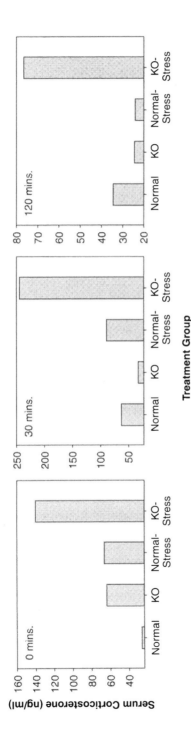

FIGURE 12.7 Preliminary studies indicating that endogenous IL-10 affects GCS levels following ice water immersion stress in IL-10$^{+/+}$ (normal) and IL-10$^{-/-}$ (knockout) mice. Mice in both groups were immersed in ice water for 45 to 60 seconds. They were sacrificed immediately, 30 minutes, or 120 minutes following immersion, and serum GCS levels were determined by RIA. N = three or four mice per group, representative of three experiments. (From Smith, E.M. et al. *J. Neuroimmunol.* 100, 140, 1999. With permission.)

when compared to similarly treated IL-10$^{+/+}$ controls (Figure 12.6). We would have predicted that the pI:C stressor might have exerted an effect because of its ability to induce cytokine production. It was surprising to find that in IL-10$^{-/-}$ mice, physiologic stress (ice water immersion for 45 to 60 seconds) also increased serum corticosterone levels nearly five-fold compared to IL-10$^{+/+}$ mice (Figure 12.7). Our data suggest that IL-10 may contribute to regulation of the endogenous corticosterone response, both tonically and following stressors.

How, if IL-10 stimulates the production of CRF and ACTH, does the inability to make IL-10 (IL-10$^{-/-}$) result in an elevated GCS? If it were by direct action of IL-10 on the adrenal tissue, it would mean that corticosterone production by the murine adrenal gland is inhibited. To test this mode of action, the effect of *in vitro*, IL-10 treatment on Y-1 pituitary tumor cells was determined. ACTH-treated Y-1 cells (that morphologically change from flat elongate to round when producing steroids) have almost three times the steroid response in the presence of anti-IL-10. Anti-IL-10 alone also significantly induced the rounding response (Table 12.1).

There are three major anatomical regions of the adrenal gland cortex: the zona glomerulosa, zona fasciculata, and zona reticularis. Each region is largely responsible for production of mineral corticoids (e.g., aldosterone), glucocorticocoids (e.g., corticosterone), and androgens (e.g., testosterone), respectively. The common precursor for each of these types of hormones is cholesterol and their synthesis is regulated by shared (e.g., 3-β-hydroxysteroid dehydrogenase; 3-β-HSD) and specific (e.g., 17-α-HSD) enzymes.

Considering our results observed with the IL-10 knockout mice, we determined the effects of IL-10 on adrenal cortex-associated enzymatic activity, and also determined the IL-10 receptor distributions in the various regions of the adrenal cortex. We found that IL-10 inhibits enzymes associated with corticosterone biosynthesis and that a preponderance of the IL-10 receptor is expressed in the region of the adrenal cortex that is largely responsible for corticosterone production, the zona

---

TABLE 12.1
Effect of IL-10 on Y-1 Adrenal Cell Response

Treatment	% of Control ± SEM
Control	100 ± 6
ACTH (1×10^{-8} M)	142 ± 7
IL-10 (30 ng/ml)	119 ± 9
Anti-IL-10 (30 ng/ml)	153 ± 8
ACTH + IL-10	153 ± 6
Anti-IL-10 + ACTH	208 ± 10

Note: Cells were treated with the indicated reagents in a microtiter plate (1×10^4 cells/well); 24 hours later, four microscopic fields of rounded cells were counted for each treatment as indicated in specific aim 3. One experiment representative of at least four is presented. Isotype control antibody had no effect.

---

fasciculata (Koldiz-Zivanovic et al., submitted for publication). Adrenal tissue also responds to IL-10 treatment and it appears to be through specific receptors as for the other HPA tissues.

IL-10 inhibits the expression of the steroidogenic enzyme 3-βHSD and the steroidogenic regulatory protein StAR in Y-1 cells. Corticosterone biosynthesis starts with the delivery of cholesterol to the side chain cleavage enzyme (P450ssc) on the inner mitochondrial membrane.[74,75] This rate limiting-step of corticosteroid synthesis is regulated by StAR.[75–77] Subsequent steps in corticosterone synthesis are catalyzed by 3-βHSD, 21-hydroxylase, and 11-βHSD. Microarray studies (data not shown) previously indicated that 3-βHSD was one of the transcripts in Y-1 cells that was down regulated following IL-10 treatment.

We used semi-quantitative RT-PCR to address whether IL-10 regulates the enzymes involved in corticosterone synthesis (P450ssc, 3-βHSD, 11-βHSD) (Koldiz-Zivanovic et al., submitted for publication). Y-1 cells do not express 21-hydroxylase (authors' RT-PCR data); therefore the effects of IL-10 on the expression of that particular enzyme were not addressed. Y-1 cells were treated with vehicle, IL-10, ACTH and/or IL-6. IL-10 inhibited the expression of 3-βHSD in Y-1 cells both by alone and with ACTH treatment. The expression of enzymes P450ssc and 11-HSD was not changed by IL-10 treatment. We used the same method to determine whether IL-10 influenced the expression of StAR regulatory protein and found that IL-10 treatment down-regulated StAR mRNA levels both alone and with ACTH.

To address the effects of IL-10 on the activities of proximal steroidogenic enzymes 450ssc and/or 3-βHSD, we used 22(R)-hydroxycholesterol (22R-HC, 25 μM), a membrane-permeable precursor for pregenolone synthesis. 22R-HC bypasses the transport within the mitochondrial membrane by the StAR protein, allowing the assessment of the influence of IL-10 on the activity of P450ssc and 3-HSD enzymes. Y-1 cells were treated with vehicle, IL-10, ACTH, and both IL-10 and ACTH in the presence and absence of 22R-HC, after which progesterone levels were measured by ELISA. IL-10 treatment did not change the activities of steroidogenic enzymes P450ssc and/or 3-βHSD. Thus, the expression and not the activity of the enzymes was affected. These studies show that IL-10 can inhibit enzymes in the metabolic pathway leading to GCS production. Therefore, even though IL-10 can potentially activate the HPA axis at the hypothalamic and pituitary levels, it can block one of the end products of the axis at the adrenal level and may explain the elevated GCS response in IL-10$^{-/-}$ mice.

OTHER NON-IMMUNE EFFECTS OF IL-10

SLEEP

IL-10 in the CNS, whether arising from infiltrating lymphocytes or neural cells, can clearly affect nervous system functioning. Intracerebroventricular (ICV) administration of 100 ng of gp120 [the major envelope glycoprotein of the human immunodeficiency virus (HIV)] into the central nervous systems of cannulated rats was found to induce the expression of both IL-1β and IL-10 mRNAs.[78] IL-10 mRNA was induced as early as 1 hour post-injection and remained elevated until at least 4 hours

TABLE 12.2
Effects of IL-10 on NREM Sleep in Rats

Experiment	Treatment	% Recording Time	% Difference
A	Vehicle	44.1 ± 1.5	
	IL-10 (50 ng)	36.4 ± 1.6	–17.5
B	Vehicle	51.8 ± 2.8	
	IL-10 (100 ng)	42.9 ± 3.0	–17.2

Note: Values represent percent of recording time for NREM sleep for a 4-hour period beginning 23 hours post-injection. IL-10 or vehicle at the indicated concentrations was injected ICV and sleep was monitored by EEG recordings.

Modified from Opp, M.D. et al. *Am. J. Physiol.*

following injection. IL-1β mRNA was not detectable until 2 hours post-injection. The expression of the two cytokines at different times suggests there may be some interplay regulating their expression.

Sleep patterns in the rats receiving gp120 were monitored and significant changes were seen when compared to control rats.[79] Percentages of time spent in both non-rapid eye movement sleep (NREMS) and rapid eye movement sleep (REMS) were initially enhanced and subsequently decreased after a 100-ng dose of gp120 that induced cytokine production. We were not able to measure the brain cytokine levels in these studies, but these data led us to speculate that the IL-1β induced by gp120 initially enhances sleep. Subsequently, the IL-10 reduces the NREMS and alters the degree of synchrony in electrocorticograms.

The direct effect of IL-10 on sleep was verified by ICV injection of IL-10 into rats instrumented with recording electrodes (EEG) and monitoring their sleep behavior. Table 12.2 summarizes the effects of IL-10 on NREMS. Both doses (50 or 100 ng) decreased NREMS by approximately 17%. Thus, it is likely that with the gp120 injections described above, it was the IL-10 that reduced the NREMS of the animals.

Other studies show IL-10's potential interaction with the nervous system. Van der Poll et al.[65] showed that epinephrine potentiates IL-10 production during human endotoxemia. Martinez et al.[80] provided evidence that vasoactive intestinal peptide will inhibit IL-10 production in murine T lymphocytes. Finally, IL-10 was shown to attenuate astroglial cell reactivity; probably through the inhibition of endogenous cytokine production.[64]

NOCICEPTION

Pro-inflammatory cytokines such as IL-1β, IL-6, and TNF-α are able to directly contribute to central and peripheral neuropathic pain.[81,82] Exogenous IL-10 has been shown to impede development of dynorphin-induced allodynia, presumably by inhibiting IL-1β.[83,84] To determine whether endogenous IL-10 had a role in pain perception, we compared the paw licking response as a measure of pain perception between IL-10-deficient and normal mice.[85] IL-10[+/+] and IL-10[–/–] mice were observed for latency times to paw licking using a hot plate test. Each animal was placed on a 55°C hotplate and the length of time until the mouse licked or shook its front paws was measured. Normal IL-10[+/+] mice had a latency time to paw licking of 11.1 ± 0.6 seconds. When IL-10-deficient mice were used, the latency times observed increased to 15.2 ± 0.7 seconds — a 40% increase (p <0.005). These results associated the absence of IL-10 with decreased nociception.

A genetic knockout of IL-10 is a long-term chronic deficiency and may be compensated for by the redundancy in the cytokine network. In an alternative approach, we injected wild-type mice with an antiserum to mouse IL-10 to acutely inactivate IL-10 prior to the nociceptive test. Figure 12.8 shows that the latency responses in the IL-10[+/+] mice receiving vehicle maintained an average 13-second latency period throughout the test. The antiserum-injected animals showed increases in latency time to a maximum of approximately 25 seconds at 2 hours post-antibody treatment. The responses returned to normal levels by 4 hours post-treatment. These results suggest that blockage of endogenous IL-10 is associated with decreased nociception. Furthermore, antibody blockage of endogenous IL-10 appears to decrease nociception to an even greater degree than knocking out the gene for IL-10; a possible explanation is that cytokine redundancy did not have time to develop in the acute (anti-IL-10-injected) knockouts.

The site and condition associated with the pain may be important factors determining IL-10's effect on pain. In contrast to our findings with IL-10-deficient mice, Watkins' laboratory found that injecting or expressing IL-10 at a site of spinal cord inflammation decreased pain sensitivity in IL-10[+/+] animals.[81] The IL-10 seemed to act in as an anti-inflammatory substance to counter IL-1, IL-6, and other pro-inflammatory

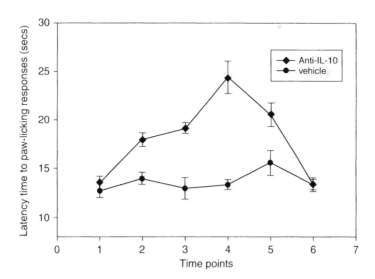

FIGURE 12.8 Antibody to IL-10 increases latency time to paw licking in IL-10[+/+] mice. N = five mice per group. Each mouse was tested at time points (0, 0.5, 1, 2, 3, and 4 hours) relative to anti-IL-10 administration. The latency times (seconds) were then measured (mean ± SEM). (From Tu, H. et al. *J. Neuroimmunol.* 139, 145, 2003. With permission.)

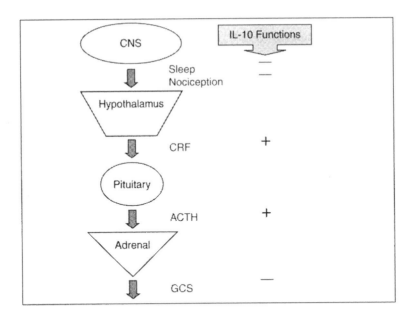

FIGURE 12.9 Major areas of impact of IL-10 on the HPA axis.

factors.[86] As with many activities of IL-10, the effect on pain is complex and may depend upon the IL-10 source, site, and target cells.

CONCLUSIONS AND IMPLICATIONS

IL-10 has been shown to be an important regulator in the immune system, especially in regard to Th1-mediated processes. In this review, we have summarized our data and those of others that indicate that, in addition to immunity, IL-10 directly impacts and appears to be part of normal HPA and CNS homeostasis. Figure 12.9 summarizes the major interactions of IL-10 associated with the HPA axis and some CNS effects.

The production and/or differential action of IL-10 in hypothalamic, pituitary, and adrenal tissue indicates that it can be associated with stress responses. The use of IL-10 knockout mice proved especially useful in this regard. Our unexpected finding of the IL-10 R1 distribution in the zona fasciculata region of the adrenal provided structural and functional evidence for an implicit role in regulating corticosterone biosynthesis. We also summarized findings that indicate that IL-10 is a player in the CNS. It appears to be involved in sleep processes and in nociception. Again, IL-10 knockout mice have proved useful tools in these studies.

Important questions remain as to the relative contributions of solid and/or immune-derived IL-10 in CNS and neuroendocrine responses. A potential approach to address this will be in the production of IL-10 chimera mice derived from using IL-10[+/+] and IL-10[-/-] mice. Our preliminary data indicate that IL-10 derived from solid tissue plays a significant role, but these studies must be interpreted with caution and need to be repeated. In conclusion, the cross-regulation of Th1 and Th2 cytokines in the neuroendocrine system appears to strongly mirror regulation in the immune system and provides an intriguing direction for research in this area.

ACKNOWLEDGMENTS

The authors wish to thank Drs. Patrick Cadet, Peter Rady, and Nina Koldiz-Zivanovic and Ms. Terry Juelich for their contributions to the studies reviewed in this chapter. This work was supported in part by grants from the National Institute of Neurological Disorders and Stroke (NS39974 and NS41495) and the John Sealy Memorial Endowment Fund of the University of Texas Medical Branch.

REFERENCES

1. Fiorentino, D.F.; Bond, M.A.; and Mosmann, T.R. Two types of mouse helper T-cells IV. The clones secrete a factor that inhibits cytokine production by Th1 cells. *Journal of Experimental Medicine* 170, 2081, 1989.
2. Howard, M.; O'Garra, A.; Ishida, H.; and de Vries, J. Biological properties of IL-10. *Journal of Clinical Immunology* 12, 239, 1992.
3. MacNeil, I.A.; Suda, T.; Moore, K.W.; Mosmann, T.R.; and Zlotnik, A. IL-10: a novel growth cofactor for mature and immature T-cells. *Journal of Immunology* 145, 4167, 1990.
4. Pestka, S.; Krause, C.D.; Sarkar, D.; Walter, M.R.; Shi, Y.; and Fisher, P.B. Interleukin-10 and related cytokines and receptors. *Annual Review of Immunology* 22, 929, 2004.
5. de Vries, J.E. Immunosuppressive and anti-inflammatory properties of IL-10. *Annals of Medicine* 27, 537, 1995.
6. Ho, A.S. and Moore, K.W. Interleukin-10 and its receptor. *Therapeutic Immunology* 1, 173, 1994.
7. Holland, G. and Zlotnik, A. Interleukin-10 and cancer. *Cancer Investigation* 11, 751, 1993.
8. Mosmann, T.R. Properties and functions of interleukin-10. *Advances in Immunology* 56, 1, 1994.
9. Munck, A. and Naray-Fejes-Toth, A. Glucocorticoids and stress: permissive and suppressive actions. *Annals of the New York Academy of Sciences* 746, 115, 1994.
10. Smith, E.M. Hormonal activities of cytokines. *Chemical Immunology* 52, 154, 1992.
11. Smith, E.M. Corticotropin and immunoregulation, in *Neuropeptides and Immunoregulation*. B. Scharrer; E.M. Smith; and G.B. Stefano, Eds. Springer-Verlag: Berlin, 1994; Ch. 3.
12. Kelley, K.W.; Bluthe, R.M.; Dantzer, R.; Zhou, J.H.; Shen, W.H.; Johnson, R.W.; and Broussard, S.R. Cytokine-induced sickness behavior. *Brain, Behavior, & Immunity* 17, Suppl. 1, S112, 2003.
13. Hughes, T.K.; Cadet, P.; Rady, P.L.; Tyring, S.K.; Chin, R.; and Smith, E.M. Evidence for the production and action of interleukin-10 in pituitary cells. *Cellular & Molecular Neurobiology* 14, 59, 1994.
14. Rady, P.L.; Smith, E.M.; Cadet, P.; Opp, M.R.; Tyring, S.K.; and Hughes, T.K., Jr. Presence of interleukin-10 transcripts in human pituitary and hypothalamus. *Cellular & Molecular Neurobiology* 15, 289, 1995.

15. Smith, E.M.; Cadet, P.; Stefano, G.B.; Opp, M.R.; and Hughes, T.K., Jr. IL-10 as a mediator in the HPA axis and brain. *Journal of Neuroimmunology* 100, 140, 1999.

16. Black, P.H. and Garbutt, L.D. Stress, inflammation and cardiovascular disease. *Journal of Psychosomatic Research* 52, 1, 2002.

17. Pawelec, G. Working together for robust immune responses in the elderly. *Nature Immunology* 1, 91, 2000.

18. Shearer, G.M. TH1/TH2 changes in aging. *Mechanisms of Ageing and Development* 94, 1, 1997.

19. Kim, J.M.; Brannan, C.I.; Copeland, N.G.; Jenkins, N.A.; Khan, T.A.; and Moore, K.W. Structure of the mouse IL-10 gene and chromosomal localization of the mouse and human genes. *Journal of Immunology* 148, 3618, 1992.

20. Yssel, H.; Grazia-Roncarolo, M.; Abrams, J.S.; Lahesmaa, R.; Spits, H.; and de Vries, J. IL-10 is produced by subsets of human CD4+ T-cell clones and peripheral blood T-cells. *Journal of Immunology* 149, 2378, 1992.

21. Vieira, P.; Dang, M.N.; Johnson, K.E.X.; Fiorentino, D.F.; deVries, J.E.; Roncarolo, M.G.; Mosmann, T.R.; and Moore, K.W. Isolation and expression of human cytokine synthesis inhibitory factor cDNA clones: homology to Epstein–Barr virus open reading frame BCRFI. *Proceedings of the National Academy of Sciences of the United States of America* 88, 1172, 1991.

22. Hsu, D.H.; Fiorentino, D.F.; Dang, M.N.X.; Vieira, P.; Spits, H.; Mosmann, T.R.; and Moore, K.W. Expression of interleukin-10 activity by Epstein–Barr virus protein BCRF1. *Science* 250, 830, 1990.

23. Moore, K.W.; Vieira, P.; Fiorentino, D.F.; Trounstine, M.L.; Khan, T.A.; and Mosmann, T.R. Homology of cytokine synthesis inhibitory factor (IL-10) to the Epstein–Barr virus gene BCRFI. *Science* 248, 1230, 1990 [published erratum: *Science* 250, 494, 1990].

24. Fleming, S.B.; McCaughan, C.A.; Andrews, A.E.; Nash, A.D.; and Mercer, A.A. A homolog of interleukin-10 is encoded by the poxvirus orf virus. *Journal of Virology* 71, 4857, 1997.

25. Kotenko, S.V.; Saccani, S.; Izotova, L.S.; Mirochnitchenko, O.V.; and Pestka, S. Human cytomegalovirus harbors its own unique IL-10 homolog (cmvIL-10). *Proceedings of the National Academy of Sciences* 97, 1695, 2000.

26. Bogdan, C.; Vodovotz, Y.; and Nathan, C. Macrophage deactivation by IL-10. *Journal of Experimental Medicine* 174, 1549, 1991.

27. Chen, W.F. and Zlotnik, A. A novel cytotoxic T-cell differentiation factor. *Journal of Immunology* 147, 528, 1990.

28. Thompson-Snipes, L.; Dhar, V.; Bond, M.W.; Mosmann, T.R.; Moore, K.W.; and Rennick, D. Interleukin-10: a novel stimulatory factor for mast cells and their progenitors. *Journal of Experimental Medicine* 173, 507, 1991.

29. Fiorentino, D.F.; Zlotnik, A.; Mosmann, T.R.; Howard, M.; and O'Garra, A. IL-10 inhibits cytokine production by activated macrophages. *Journal of Immunology* 147, 3815, 1991.

30. Waal-Malefyt, R.; Abrams, J.; Bennett, B.; Figdor, C.G.; and de Vries, J.E. Interleukin 10 (IL-10) inhibits cytokine synthesis by human monocytes: an autoregulatory role of IL-10 produced by monocytes. *Journal of Experimental Medicine* 174, 1209, 1991.

31. Go, N.F.; Castle, B.E.; Barrett, R.; Kastlestein, R.; Dang, W.; Mosmann, T. R.; Moore, K.W.; and Howard, M. Interleukin-10 (IL-10), a novel B-stimulatory factor: unresponsiveness of X-chromosome linked immunodeficient B-cells. *Journal of Experimental Medicine* 172, 1625, 1990.

32. Bancherau, J.; de Paoli, P.; Valle, A.; Garcia, E.; and Rousett, F. Long-term human B-cell lines dependent on interleukin-4 and antibody to CD40. *Science* 251, 70, 1991.

33. Defrance, T.; Vanbervliet, B.; Briere, F.; Durand, I.; Rousett, F.; and Bancherau, J. Interleukin-10 and TGF beta cooperate to induce anti-CD40 activated naive human B-cells to secrete immunoglobulin A. *Journal of Experimental Medicine* 175, 671, 1992.

34. Suda, T.; O'Garra, A.; MacNeil, I.; Fischer, M.; Bond, M.; and Zlotnik, A. Identification of a novel thymocyte growth promoting factor derived from B-cell lymphomas. *Cellular Immunology* 129, 228, 1990.

35. Sher, A.; Fiorentino, D.; Caspar, P.; Pearce, E.; and Mosmann, T.R. Production of IL-10 by CD4 T lymphocytes correlates with down-regulation of Th1 cytokine synthesis in helminth infection. *Journal of Immunology* 147, 2713, 1992.

36. Clerici, M. and Shearer, G.M. A TH1–TH2 switch is a critical step in the etiology of HIV infection. *Immunology Today* 14, 107, 1993.

37. Kuhn, R.; Lohler, J.; Rennick, D.; Rajewsky, K.; and Muller, W. Interleukin-10-deficient mice develop chronic enterocolitis. *Cell* 75, 263, 1993.

38. Donnelly, R.P.; Dickensheets, H.; and Finbloom, D.S. The interleukin-10 signal transduction pathway and regulation of gene expression in mononuclear phagocytes. *Journal of Interferon & Cytokine Research* 19, 563, 1999.

39. Kotenko, S.V.; Krause, C.D.; Izotova, L.S.; Pollack, B.P.; Wu, W.; and Pestka, S. Identification and functional characterization of a second chain of the interleukin-10 receptor complex. *EMBO Journal* 16, 5894, 1997.

40. Spencer, S.D.; Di Marco, F.; Hooley, J.; Pitts-Meek, S.; Bauer, M.; Ryan, A.M.; Sordat, B.; Gibbs, V.C.; and Aguet, M. The orphan receptor CRF2-4 is an essential subunit of the interleukin 10 receptor. *Journal of Experimental Medicine* 187, 571, 1998.

41. Gallo, P.; Sivieri, S.; Rinaldi, L.; Yan, X.B.; Loiil, F.; De Rossi, A.; and Tavolato, B. Intrathecal synthesis of interleukin-10 (IL-10) in viral and inflammatory diseases of the central nervous system. *Journal of Neurological Science* 126, 49, 1994.

42. Tan, J.C.; Indelicato, S.R.; Narula, S.K.; Zavodny, P.J.; and Chou, C.C. Characterization of interleukin-10 receptors on human and mouse cells. *Journal of Biological Chemistry* 268, 21053, 1993.

43. Finbloom, D.S. and Winestock. K.D. IL-10 induces the tyrosine phosphorylation of tyk2 and Jak1 and the differential assembly of STAT1 alpha and STAT3 complexes in human T-cells and monocytes. *Journal of Immunology* 155, 1079, 1995.

44. Kotenko, S.V.; Izotova, L.S.; Pollack, B.P.; Muthukumaran, G.; Paukku, K.; Silvennoinen, O.; Ihle, J.N.; and Pestka, S. Other kinases can substitute for Jak2 in signal transduction by interferon-gamma. *Journal of Biological Chemistry* 271, 17174, 1996.

45. Usacheva, A.; Kotenko, S.; Witte, M.M.; and Colamonici, O.R. Two distinct domains within the N-terminal region of Janus kinase 1 interact with cytokine receptors. *Journal of Immunology* 169, 1302, 2002.

46. Lehmann, J.; Seegert, D.; Strehlow, I.; Schindler, C.; Lohmann-Matthes, M.L.; and Decker, T. IL-10-induced factors belonging to the p91 family of proteins bind to IFN-gamma-responsive promoter elements. *Journal of Immunology* 153, 165, 1994.

47. Takeda, K.; Clausen, B.E.; Kaisho, T.; Tsujimura, T.; Terada, N.; Forster, I.; and Akira, S. Enhanced Th1 activity and development of chronic enterocolitis in mice devoid of Stat3 in macrophages and neutrophils. *Immunity* 10, 39, 1999.

48. Ehrlich, L.C.; Hu, S.; Peterson, P.K.; and Chao, C.C. IL-10 down-regulates human microglial IL-8 by inhibition of NF-κB activation. *Neuroreport* 9, 1723, 1998.

49. Wang, P.; Wu, P.; Siegel, M.I.; Egan, R.W.; and Billah, M.M. Interleukin (IL)-10 inhibits nuclear factor kappa B (NFκB) activation in human monocytes: IL-10 and IL-4 suppress cytokine synthesis by different mechanisms. *Journal of Biological Chemistry* 270, 9558, 1995.

50. Heyen, J.R.; Ye. S.; Finck, B.N.; and Johnson, R.W. Interleukin (IL)-10 inhibits IL-6 production in microglia by preventing activation of NF-kappa-B. *Brain Research & Molecular Brain Research* 77, 138, 2000.

51. Musette, P.; Benveniste, O.; Lim, A.; Bequet, D.; Kourilsky, P.; Dormont, D.; and Gachelin, G. The pattern of production of cytokine mRNAs is markedly altered at the onset of multiple sclerosis. *Research in Immunology* 147, 435, 1996.

52. Rudick, R.A.; Ransohoff, R.M.; Peppler, R.; VanderBrug, M.S.; Lehmann, P.; and Alam, J. Interferon beta induces interleukin-10 expression: relevance to multiple sclerosis. *Annals of Neurology* 40, 618, 1996.

53. Salmaggi, A.; Dufour, A.; Eoli, M.; Corsini, E.; La Mantia, L.; Massa, G.; Nespolo, A.; and Milanese, C. Low serum interleukin-10 levels in multiple sclerosis: further evidence for decreased systemic immunosuppression? *Journal of Neurology* 243, 13, 1996.

54. Monteyne, P.; Van Laere, V.; Marichal, R.; and Sindic, C.J. Cytokine mRNA expression in CSF and peripheral blood mononuclear cells in multiple sclerosis: detection by RT-PCR without *in vitro* stimulation. *Journal of Neuroimmunology* 80, 137, 1997.

55. Crucian, B.; Dunne, P.; Friedman, H.; Ragsdale, R.; Pross, S.; and Widen, R. Detection of altered T helper 1 and T helper 2 cytokine production by peripheral blood mononuclear cells in patients with multiple sclerosis utilizing intracellular cytokine detection by flow cytometry and surface marker analysis. *Clinical and Diagnostic Laboratory Immunology* 3, 411, 1996.

56. Gelati, M.; Lamperti, E.; Dufour, A.; Corsini, E.; Venegoni, E.; Milanese, C.; Nespolo, A.; and Salmaggi, A. IL-10 production in multiple sclerosis patients, SLE patients and healthy controls: preliminary findings. *Italian Journal of Neurological Sciences* 18, 191, 1997.

57. Cannella, B.; Gao, Y.L.; Brosnan, C.; and Raine, C.S. IL-10 fails to abrogate experimental autoimmune encephalomyelitis. *Journal of Neuroscience Research* 45, 735, 1996.

58. Chabot, S.; Williams, G.; Hamilton, M.; Sutherland, G.; and Yong, V.W. Mechanisms of IL-10 production in human microglia-T cell interaction. *Journal of Immunology* 162, 6819, 1999.

59. Jander, S.; Pohl, J.; D'Urso, D.; Gillen, C.; and Stoll, G. Time course and cellular localization of interleukin-10 mRNA and protein expression in autoimmune inflammation of the rat central nervous system. *American Journal of Pathology* 152, 975, 1998.

60. Mizuno, T.; Sawada, M.; Marunouchi, T.; and Suzumura, A. Production of interleukin-10 by mouse glial cells in culture. *Biochemical and Biophysical Research Communications* 205, 1907, 1994.

61. Wong, M.L.; Bongiorno, P.B.; Rettori, V.; McCann, S.M.; and Licinio, J. Interleukin (IL) 1-beta, IL-1 receptor antagonist, IL-10, and IL-13 gene expression in the central nervous system and anterior pituitary during systemic inflammation: pathophysiological implications. *Proceedings of the National Academy of Sciences of the United States of America* 94, 227, 1997.

62. Wagner, S.; Czub, S.; Greif, M.; Vince, G.H.; Suss, N.; Kerkau, S.; Rieckmann, P.; Roggendorf, W.; Roosen, K.; and Tonn, J.C. Microglial/macrophage expression of interleukin-10 in human glioblastomas. *International Journal of Cancer* 82, 12, 1999.

63. Voeller. A.; Bidwell, D.; and Bartlett, A. Microplate enzyme immunoassays for the immunodiagnosis of virus infections, in *Manual of Clinical Immunology*, N.R. Rose and H. Friedman, Eds., 1976; Ch. 69.

64. Balasingam, V. and Yong, V.W. Attenuation of astroglial reactivity by interleukin-10. *Journal of Neuroscience* 16, 2945, 1996.

65. van der Poll, T.; Coyle, S.M.; Barbosa, K.; Braxton, C.C.; and Lowry, S.F. Epinephrine inhibits tumor necrosis factor-alpha and potentiates interleukin-10 production during human endotoxemia. *Journal of Clinical Investigation* 97, 713, 1996.

66. Stefano, G.B.; Prevot, V.; Beauvillain, J.C.; and Hughes, T.K. Interleukin-10 stimulation of corticotrophin releasing factor median eminence in rats: evidence for dependence upon nitric oxide production. *Neuroscience Letters* 256, 167, 1998.

67. Kushikata, T.; Fang, J.; and Krueger, J.M. Interleukin-10 inhibits spontaneous sleep in rabbits. *Journal of Interferon & Cytokine Research* 19, 1025, 1999.

68. Opp, M.R.; Smith, E.M.; and Hughes, T.K., Jr. Interleukin-10 (cytokine synthesis inhibitory factor) acts in the central nervous system of rats to reduce sleep. *Journal of Neuroimmunology* 60, 165, 1995.

69. Smith, E.M.; Morrill, A.C.; Meyer, W.J., III; and Blalock, J.E. Corticotropin releasing factor induction of leukocyte-derived immunoreactive ACTH and endorphins. *Nature* 322, 881, 1986.

70. Stone, T.W. The neuroprotective effect of purines. *Journal of Alzheimer's Disease* 3, 4, 2001.

71. Stone, T.W. Endogenous neurotoxins from tryptophan. *Toxicon* 39, 61, 2001.

72. Tu, H.; Juelich, T.; Rady, P.L.; Tyring, S.K.; Smith, E.M.; and Hughes, T.K. Regulation of tryptophan metabolism by pro- and anti-inflammatory cytokines in cells derived from the hypothalamic–pituitary–adrenal (HPA) axis: implications for protective and toxic consequences in neuroendocrine regulation. *Cellular & Molecular Neurobiology*, in press, 2005.

73. Knolle, P.A.; Uhrig, A.; Protzer, U.; Trippler, M.; Duchmann, R.; Meyer zum Buschenfelde, K.H.; and Gerken, G. Interleukin-10 expression is autoregulated at the transcriptional level in human and murine Kupffer cells. *Hepatology* 27, 93, 1998.

74. Rainey, W.E.; Saner, K.; and Schimmer, B.P. Adrenocortical cell lines. *Molecular and Cellular Endocrinology* 228, 23, 2004.

75. Stocco, D.M. and Clark, B.J. Regulation of the acute production of steroids in steroidogenic cells. *Endocrine Reviews* 17, 221, 1996.

76. Clark, B.J.; Wells, J.; King, S.R.; and Stocco, D.M. The purification, cloning, and expression of a novel luteinizing hormone-induced mitochondrial protein in MA-10 mouse Leydig tumor cells: characterization of the steroidogenic acute regulatory protein (StAR). *Journal of Biological Chemistry* 269, 28314, 1994.

77. Sugawara, T.; Lin, D.; Holt, J.A.; Martin, K.O.; Javitt, N.B.; Miller, W.L.; Strauss, J.F. Structure of the human steroidogenic acute regulatory protein (StAR) gene: StAR stimulates mitochondrial cholesterol 27-hydroxylase activity. *Biochemistry* 34, 12506, 1995.

78. Opp, M.R.; Rady, P.L.; Hughes, T.K.; Cadet, P.; Tyring, S.K.; and Smith, E.M. Human immunodeficiency virus envelope glycoprotein 120 alters sleep and induces cytokine mRNA expression in rats. *American Journal of Physiology* 270, R963, 1996.

79. Opp, M.R.; Hughes, T.K.; Rady, P.L.; and Smith, E.M. Mechanisms of HIV-induced alterations in sleep: role of cytokines in the CNS. *Sleep Research Society Bulletin* 2, 31, 1996.

80. Martinez, C.; Delgado, M.; Gomariz, R.P.; and Ganea, D. Vasoactive intestinal peptide and pituitary adenylate cyclase-activating polypeptide-38 inhibit IL-10 production in murine T lymphocytes. *Journal of Immunology* 156, 4128, 1996.

81. Johnston, I.N.; Milligan, E.D.; Wieseler-Frank, J.; Frank, M.G.; Zapata, V.; Campisi, J.; Langer, S.; Martin, D.; Green, P.; Fleshner, M.; Leinwand, L.; Maier, S.F.; and Watkins, L.R. A role for proinflammatory cytokines and fractalkine in analgesia, tolerance, and subsequent pain facilitation induced by chronic intrathecal morphine. *Journal of Neuroscience* 24, 7353, 2004.

82. Watkins, L.R.; Wiertelak, E.P.; Goehler, L.E.; Smith, K.P.; Martin, A.; and Maier, S.F. Characterization of cytokine-induced hyperalgesia. *Brain Research* 654, 15, 1994.

83. Cunha, J.M.; Cunha, F.Q.; Poole, S.; and Ferreira, S.H. Cytokine-mediated inflammatory hyperalgesia limited by interleukin-1 receptor antagonist. *British Journal of Pharmacology* 130, 1418, 2000.

84. Laughlin, T.M.; Bethea, J.R.; Yezierski, R.P.; and Wilcox, G.L. Cytokine involvement in dynorphin-induced allodynia. *Pain* 84, 159, 2000.

85. Tu, H.; Juelich, T.; Smith, E.M.; Tyring, S.K.; Rady, P.L.; and Hughes, J. Evidence for endogenous interleukin-10 during nociception. *Journal of Neuroimmunology* 139, 145, 2003.

86. Chacur, M.; Milligan, E.D.; Sloan, E.M.; Wieseler-Frank, J.; Barrientos, R.M.; Martin, D.; Poole, S.; Lomonte, B.; Gutierrez, J.M.; Maier, S.F.; Cury, Y.; and Watkins, L.R. Snake venom phospholipase A2s (Asp49 and Lys49) induce mechanical allodynia upon peri-sciatic administration: involvement of spinal cord glia, proinflammatory cytokines and nitric oxide. *Pain* 108, 180, 2004.

13 Cytokines, Stress, and Depression

Adrian J. Dunn

CONTENTS

ABSTRACT

Depression has long been associated with stress. Stress has long been linked to the genesis of depression, and depression is viewed by many as a chronic state of stress. Cytokines became part of the system when it was discovered that interleukin-1 had the ability to activate the hypothalamo-pituitary-adrenocortical (HPA) axis, considered a major component of the stress response. Subsequently, it was discovered that IL-1 had the ability to induce other stress-like effects, including activation of the sympathoadrenal and brain noradrenergic systems, and, most important, the induction of behaviors characteristic of stress. The combination of these findings with some clinical data led to the hypothesis that cytokines caused major depression. The purpose of this chapter is to review the key scientific findings implicating cytokines in the stress associated with illness, and to critically evaluate the evidence supporting the hypothesis that cytokines may cause depressive illness.

STRESS

Stress was initially associated with catecholamines in the classic studies of Walter Cannon, who observed that cats stressed by barking dogs had markedly increased circulating concentrations of adrenaline.[1] It was subsequently learned that plasma concentrations of both adrenaline (epinephrine, Epi) and noradrenaline (norepinephrine, NE) were

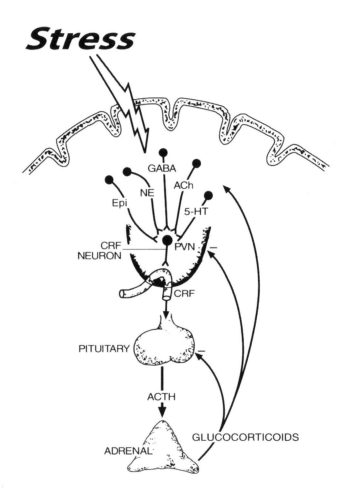

FIGURE 13.1 Relationships of the brain, the hypothalamic–pituitary–adrenocortical (HPA) axis, and immune cells. Interleukin-1 (IL-1) and possibly other cytokines produced by lymphocytes during the immune response activates noradrenergic (NE) projections from the brainstem to the hypothalamic paraventricular nucleus (PVN). This input activates the HPA axis, stimulating the release of corticotrophin-releasing factor (CRF) from the median eminence of the hypothalamus. CRF stimulates the secretion of adrenocorticotrophic hormone (ACTH) from the anterior lobe of the pituitary, which in turn activates the adrenal cortex to synthesize and secrete glucocorticoid hormones. The glucocorticoids may provide a negative feedback on cytokine production by lymphocytes. (Modified from Dunn, A.J., Neurochemistry of stress, in *Encyclopedia of Neuroscience*, G. Adelman, Ed., Birkhauser, Boston, 1989, pp. 1146–1148).

elevated (NE had not been identified in 1911), and that these catecholamines were secreted by the adrenal medulla (both Epi and NE) and the sympathetic nervous system (NE only).

Canon introduced the concept of the fight-or-flight response, and suggested that the catecholamines mobilized energy stores and redistributed the blood supply within the body to prepare an organism for fighting or fleeing. Some 20 years later, Hans Selye identified a second role for the adrenal gland in stress. He observed that when rats were subjected to various stressful treatments, certain morphological changes occurred in the adrenal cortex. He subsequently showed that these changes were associated with the synthesis and secretion of the glucocorticoid hormone, corticosterone.[2] The glucocorticoid hormones induced a number of adaptive changes including mobilization of energy stores and the production of glucose, and were responsible for many other physiological effects, most notably the involution (shrinking) of the thymus gland that had been recognized as an early manifestation of stress since the 19th century.

Subsequent studies revealed that the secretion of adrenal glucocorticoids is the final step in a cascade initiated by activation of corticotropin-releasing factor (CRF)-containing neurons with cell bodies in the paraventricular nucleus (PVN) of the hypothalamus (see Figure 13.1).

The CRF is secreted into the portal vessels associated with the median eminence region of the hypothalamus, and is carried in the vessels to the anterior pituitary gland, where it stimulates the secretion of adrenocorticotrophic hormone (corticotropin, ACTH) into the blood. ACTH then directly stimulates the adrenal cortex to synthesize and secrete glucocorticoids into the general circulation. This three-tiered system is known as the hypothalamo–pituitary–adrenocortical (HPA) axis (Figure 13.1). Thus physiologically, stress is characterized by a co-activation of the sympathoadrenal (catecholamine) system and the HPA axis.

The catecholamine activation in the periphery is echoed in the brain, primarily by the widespread activation of brain noradrenergic neurons,[3] although brain dopaminergic and serotonergic neurons may also be activated, depending on the nature and the intensity of the stress.[4] There may also be an activation of CRF-containing neurons in the brain outside the hypothalamus.

Not surprisingly, there are extensive interactions between these two major stress systems, many of which are still poorly understood. Most notably, brain, noradrenergic neurons innervating the PVN are major regulators of CRF secretion.[5] For example, during the development of the adrenal gland, glucocorticoids secreted from the cortex increase the proportion of epinephrine-containing cells in the adrenal medulla.[6]

STRESS AND DEPRESSION

Depressive illness in humans often occurs after a significant life stress. However, clinical studies suggest that an identifiable life stress is only present in approximately half the patients diagnosed with major depression.[7] The earliest hypothesis for the biological basis of depression was proposed around 40 years ago based on the observations that stimulant drugs, such as the amphetamines that increase catecholamine secretion, elevated mood, whereas amine-depleting drugs like reserpine depressed mood. This "catecholamine hypothesis of affective disorders" proposed that depression was associated with a hypoactivity of catecholaminergic (primarily noradrenergic) neurons, and conversely, that mania was associated with catecholaminergic hyperactivity. However, the sedation induced by reserpine did not truly resemble depression.

Animal studies indicated that stress was associated with activation of brain catecholaminergic systems, especially NE.[4,8] Consistent with this, clinical studies demonstrated increased concentrations of catabolites of NE in the cerebrospinal fluid (CSF) of depressed patients,[9] suggesting a hyperactivity of brain noradrenergic neurons. Most subsequent studies have found evidence consistent with increased noradrenergic activity in the brains of major depressives, for example, increased CSF concentrations of NE.[10] Thus depression appears to be associated with an activation of brain noradrenergic systems; whether this is a cause or a consequence of the depression is unresolved.

Depressive illness is also associated with activation of the HPA axis. A landmark study found that a majority of depressed patients exhibit elevated plasma concentrations of cortisol.[11] This observation has stood the test of time, although it occurs in only around two-thirds of patients diagnosed with major depression. Elevated cortisol is not useful for the diagnosis of depression, largely because plasma cortisol is rapidly elevated by any form of stress. Therefore, Carroll proposed a test using the potent glucocorticoid, dexamethasone, to inhibit pituitary ACTH secretion by activating the established endogenous negative feedback mechanism. When low doses of dexamethasone (1 mg) were given before patients went to sleep at night, plasma cortisol concentrations on waking the next morning were very low, and the normal morning rises in plasma cortisol did not occur. Some 60 to 70% of patients with major depression failed to suppress cortisol secretion in this dexamethasone suppression test (DST).[12] Although the overlap between patients who hypersecreted cortisol and those who failed to suppress cortisol secretion in the DST was considerable, the correlation is imperfect. In a subsequent refinement of this test, patients' responses to administration of CRF after dosing with dexamethasone was assessed in a combined CRF–dexamethasone test.[13] Depressed patients showed enhanced cortisol responses to CRF. This test appeared to have a greater ability to discriminate depressed patients than plasma cortisol alone or the DST.

CYTOKINES

The linking of stress with cytokines, or more specifically with interleukin-1 (IL-1), arose from the seminal discovery of Besedovsky et al. that intraperitoneal (ip) administration of small doses (1 μg) of recombinant human IL-1β to rats induced a substantial activation of the HPA axis.[14] This observation was rapidly confirmed, and somewhat surprisingly, it was subsequently shown that this activation did not occur by a direct action on the adrenal cortex or even the pituitary, but involved brain CRF.[15,16]

Thus, if HPA axis activation is regarded as defining stress, then IL-1 appears to act as a stressor. It is interesting that this effect of IL-1 uses the normal physiological pathway in the brain for the activation of the HPA axis, suggesting that it is important for the brain to be involved in initiating the HPA response, and possibly, that components of the HPA axis other than the glucocorticoids play important roles in stress.

Besedovsky et al.[14] noted that IL-1 production was universally induced very early in the induction of immune responses, and they speculated that IL-1 may act as a signal for pathological stress. Also, because it is well known that glucocorticoids are immunosuppressive, this activity of IL-1 would provide negative feedback to inhibit immune responses, for example, to limit or prevent autoimmunity.

It soon became apparent that activation of the HPA axis was not the only stress-like activity of IL-1. Administration of IL-1 to rats and mice also induced a modest increase in plasma catecholamines, apparently from both the adrenal medulla and the sympathetic nervous system.[17] Peripheral IL-1 administration also activated systems in the brain associated with stress, most notably a substantial activation of brain noradrenergic neurons.[18-20] This effect was most marked in the ventral projection system originating in the brain stem and innervating the hypothalamus, including the PVN. There were also changes in brain serotonergic systems, and increases in whole brain tryptophan.[18,19] Thus IL-1 is capable of activating the two major stress systems, the HPA axis and the catecholaminergic system.

The stress-like activities of IL-1 also extend to behavior. Endotoxin (lipopolysaccharide, LPS) has long been known to cause anorexia, and because IL-1 has similar effects, it was speculated that IL-1 might be responsible for this effect of endotoxin.[21] IL-1 has profound effects on locomotor activity.[22] It also decreases exploratory activity[23] and can cause anhedonia (inability to experience pleasure).[24] Sexual activity in female rats is also reduced.[25] Thus IL-1 has the ability to activate the two major physiological systems involved in stress and behavioral responses. Thus IL-1 could be construed as stress in a bottle!

The endocrine and neurochemical responses to IL-1 have been extended to certain other cytokines, although none is as potent or induces as widespread effects as IL-1. Interleukin-6 (IL-6) and tumor necrosis factor-α (TNF-α) can activate the HPA axis, but are far less potent than IL-1[26,27] (except perhaps for a relatively potent effect of IL-6 in humans[28]). IL-6 also activates brain serotonin metabolism[29,30] and TNF-α also has modest effects on NE and serotonin (for review see Dunn[26]).

These properties of IL-1 resemble those of many disease states. For example, infection with influenza virus activates the HPA axis and catecholaminergic systems[31] and also induces behaviors characteristic of sickness.[32] These characteristics can be mimicked by IL-1 administration, so that IL-1 is an excellent candidate as a mediator of sickness-induced stress. Indeed it has been touted as the major mediator of "immune stress." However, the responses to influenza virus infection can be only partially antagonized by IL-1 antagonists.[32,33] IL-1β knockout mice still exhibit some responses to LPS.[34] Thus, IL-1 cannot be the only factor involved, and other cytokines and unknown factors must contribute.[33]

CYTOKINE HYPOTHESIS OF DEPRESSION

The impetus for a relationship between cytokines and depression came from two sources. A primary stimulus derived from Hart's proposal that the behavior of sick animals was "not a maladaptive and undesirable effect of illness but rather a highly organized strategy that is at times critical to the survival of the individual."[35] In this classic review, Hart recognized that IL-1 induced several aspects of sickness behavior:

hyperthermia, hypomotility, hypophagia, decreased interest in exploring the environment, decreased libido, and increased sleep time. This led him to support Besedovsky's proposal that IL-1 was a signal, warning of an environmental stress, and suggested that it had the ability to induce the appropriate sickness behaviors. Smith[36] noted the similarity between some of the behavioral responses to IL-1 administration and depression in his macrophage theory of depression.

The other main impetus for a cytokine hypothesis of depression was the 50-year history of reports associating abnormalities of immune function with clinical depression[37,38] and the observations that various cytokine therapies (especially interferon-α [IFN]-α and IL-2) induced depression in some patients. Thus the cytokine hypothesis of depression was born. The hypothesis is *de facto* an IL-1 hypothesis of depression, because to date no other cytokine has been seriously implicated in depression. The only other candidate is IL-6, but the depression-like effects of IL-6 are limited (see below).

The evidence for an IL-1 hypothesis of depression is based on the following assertions:

- Treatment of patients with cytokines induces symptoms of depression.
- Activation of the immune system is observed in many depressed patients.
- Depression occurs more frequently in those with medical disorders associated with immune dysfunction.
- Activation of the immune system and administration of LPS or IL-1 to animals induces sickness behavior that resembles depression.
- Chronic treatment with antidepressants inhibits sickness behavior induced by LPS; IL-1, IL-6, TNF-α and IFN-α stimulate the HPA axis, which is commonly activated in depressed patients.
- IL-1 (and possibly TNF-α) activate cerebral noradrenergic systems, also commonly observed in depressed patients.
- IL-1 and IL-6 activate brain serotonergic systems implicated in major depressive illness and its treatment.

A brief discussion of the evidence for each of these tenets follows (for a more detailed analysis, see Dunn et al.[39]).

CYTOKINE THERAPY AND DEPRESSION

Neurobehavioral side effects occur frequently in patients treated with IFN-α and IL-2. Such patients often display influenza-like symptoms and nonspecific neuropsychiatric symptoms, some of which are characteristics of depression.[37,40,41] However, the incidence of depression associated with cytokine therapy is highly variable, ranging from 0% to 45% in the various studies (see de Beaurepaire et al.[38]).

The reasons for the variability relate to such factors as the disease under treatment and the cytokines and doses used, but the assessment measures, the patients' psychiatric histories, and the choice of comparison (control) subjects are also important factors.[38] Moreover, depression is not the most common symptom; fatigue is far more frequent.[42] Needless to say, depression may also occur independent of cytokine treatment.

Thus, the ability of cytokines to induce depression is not a particularly robust phenomenon[38] and has not been clearly linked to IL-1, the cytokine most commonly implicated in depression-like activity.

IMMUNE FUNCTION IN DEPRESSED PATIENTS

There appears to be a relatively high incidence of immune abnormalities in depressed patients, but no strong association between depression and specific immune abnormalities has been identified. In the earliest publications, depression was associated with deficient immune function, but more recent studies have argued for increased immune activity in depressed patients.[43,44] The data have been extremely variable and contradictions in the literature are common.[37,38,45] There are a number of obvious confounds. For example, a patient may be depressed because he knows he has a life-threatening disease (cancer, for example), and sometimes the immune abnormalities may be a direct consequence of the disease. It is also important that depression may occur in response to an undetected medical condition that also results in immune activation.

A few reports have cited elevated plasma concentrations of IL-1,[46,47] IL-6,[48,49] and interferon-γ [50] in patients with major depression. However, other studies failed to replicate these findings;[51,52] see review by Zorrilla et al.[53] Increased plasma concentrations of cytokines do not appear to be reliable biological markers of depression.

Other studies have assessed the ability of *in vitro* stimulation of isolated lymphocytes to synthesize and secrete IL-1 and IL-6 as a functional measure of immune activity, and increases of these measures have been reported in depressed patients.[44,54] However, the results have not proven to be particularly reliable,[55] and the biological significance of such *ex vivo* measures is not at all clear. A recent study in a small number of patients found elevated IL-1β in the CSF of depressed patients that correlated with the severity of the depression.[56] This is a promising finding, but it will need to be confirmed in a study with a substantially larger number of patients.

In an important meta-analysis of a large number of studies, Zorrilla et al.[53] concluded that patients with major depression exhibited the following immune abnormalities:

- An overall leukocytosis manifested as a relative neutrophilia and lymphopenia
- Increased CD4/CD8 ratios
- Increased circulating haptoglobin, prostaglandin E_2 (PGE_2), and IL-6 concentrations
- Reduced natural killer (NK) cell cytotoxicity
- Reduced lymphocyte proliferative responses to mitogens

Plasma concentrations of IL-1 were not consistently altered. This is important because IL-1 is the only cytokine that clearly induces depression-like symptoms. Zorrilla et al.[53] also commented that "the degree of heterogeneity of the studies' results raises questions about their robustness."

In a recent review, Pollmacher et al.[57] noted that several cytokines proposed to be implicated in depression (especially, IL-1β) are undetectable in human plasma under normal physiological conditions and even during experimental endotoxemia. They also noted that the physiological fluctuations of the detectable cytokines (IL-6 and TNF-α) are very poorly characterized in normal and pathological states, and the alterations of circulating cytokines observed in the depressed (as well as in immune-related medical conditions) are extremely modest compared with the concentrations of circulating cytokines that occur following cytokine treatments. It is also relevant that the magnitudes of the immune activations reported in depressed patients are very small compared to those observed when sickness behavior is induced by IL-1 or LPS or during infections with pathogens. These observations challenge the validity of a simple cytokine hypothesis of depression.

In sum, the evidence for activation of immune responses in patients with major depressive disorder is not very consistent,[37,45,53] although there are trends to leukocytosis; increased CD4/CD8 ratios; elevated plasma concentrations of haptoglobulin, IL-6, and PGE$_2$; and decreased NK cell activity and lymphocyte proliferative responses.[53] It seems that immune activation is not a general occurrence in patients with major depression.

IL-1-INDUCED SICKNESS BEHAVIOR

There are some compelling similarities between IL-1-induced sickness behavior and depression, but the match is far from perfect. First, although sickness behavior has been universally accepted to be a coping strategy and thus adaptive as proposed by Hart, it is far from clear that major depression in humans is a coping behavior (see, for example, Dubrovsky[58]).

The two critical symptoms for a DSM-IV diagnosis of major depressive illness are depressed mood and anhedonia. While both occur in sick humans, they cannot be assessed directly in animals. Certainly, IL-1-treated animals work less hard for food rewards or sweet solutions such as saccharin[59] and sweetened milk,[60] but whether this reflects hypophagia or anhedonia is difficult to assess. Some attempts have made to study anhedonia more directly using intracranial self-stimulation (ICSS). This technique involves implanting electrodes in the brains of laboratory animals; when a rat presses a bar, current is applied to the electrode, directly stimulating neurons in the brain. When the electrodes are placed in certain brain locations, most notably the medial forebrain bundle, animals will press the bar repeatedly, suggesting that such stimulation is pleasing. ICSS studies have not indicated any effects of systemic treatments with IL-1β or IL-6,[61,62] but IL-2 elevated ICSS thresholds when administered chronically, but not acutely .

The optional symptoms for a DSM-IV diagnosis of major depression (four are required) are significant loss of weight or appetite; insomnia; psychomotor agitation or retardation; fatigue or loss of energy; feelings of worthlessness; diminished ability to think or concentrate, or indecisiveness; and recurrent thoughts of death or suicidal ideation. It is clearly impractical to assess the ability of IL-1 to induce the last three symptoms in animals.

Anorexia and weight loss are universal responses to IL-1 and LPS,[21,60,63] but not to IL-6.[64] In depressed patients, hyperphagia and weight gain are more common than weight loss, but are regarded as atypical. In this respect, sickness behavior could be considered to parallel depression.

Administration of several cytokines (e.g., IL-1, TNF-α) to animals resulted in modest increases in slow-wave sleep.[65] Altered sleep patterns are common in depressed patients, but depressed patients are typically insomniacs.

It is not clear whether psychomotor retardation or agitation can be modeled in animals, but it could be regarded as related to decreases in overall activity observed after IL-1 and LPS administration.[60,66] On the other hand, the decreased activity could also be considered to reflect the fatigue listed in DSM-IV, but the assessment of fatigue is also difficult in animal studies.

Sickness behavior following administration of LPS, (and other immune activators, such as muramyl dipeptide [MDP] and poly I:C) and various pathogens closely resembled that induced by IL-1. However, IL-1 does not appear to be the only factor because IL-1 antagonists (such as antibodies and the IL-1-receptor antagonist protein, IL-1ra) failed to prevent the prevent the responses to these agents, although some attenuation may have occurred.[60,67]

Cognitive behavior following IL-1 has been less well researched. Sick animals may certainly show cognitive deficits, for example, in learning and memory tasks.[63,68] However, some of the characteristics of sickness behavior could explain the apparent cognitive deficits. IFN-α and IL-2 administration to cancer patients can affect cognitive functions, with effects reminiscent of the dysfunctions observed in neurodegenerative diseases.[40] On the other hand, clearly measurable responses to IL-1, such as the fever, are infrequently observed in depressed patients.[39] LPS and IL-1 induced a hypersensitivity to pain,[69] but depressed patients are not hypersensitive to pain and are more likely to suffer hypoalgesia.[38,39]

Several other observations are not compatible with a simple model of cytokine-induced depression. For example, IL-1 antagonists such as the IL-1-receptor antagonist (IL-1ra) can effectively prevent the hypophagic effects of exogenously administered IL-1, but the effects of LPS are only partially prevented, and those of influenza virus are only slightly attenuated.[60] Although the latter effects could be interpreted to indicate the involvement of cytokines other than IL-1, simultaneous blockade of IL-1, IL-6, and TNF-α also failed to prevent the effects of infection with influenza virus.[33] LPS also induced hypophagia in IL-1-knockout mice[34] and in IL-6-knockout mice.[64,70] Thus, although IL-1 is sufficient to induce sickness behaviors, it is not necessary and other factors must contribute to the behavioral responses.

The mechanisms involved in the expression of sickness behavior appear to be complex and must involve multiple mechanisms. It is certainly possible that these mechanisms involve cytokines other than IL-1, but no cytokine that induces sickness behavior as effectively as IL-1 has yet been identified.

One important aspect of sickness behavior is that it is adaptive and not stereotyped. Thus the expression of specific sickness behaviors varies according to the needs of the organism (see Larson and Dunn[71]). For example, although hypophagia is a typical symptom of sickness behavior, it may not be expressed if the food supply is limited or the animals are food-deprived.[68,72,73] It may also be diminished if there is only one source of food.[74] Priorities for food and warmth may also be altered.[75] Another example is sexual activity, which is inhibited by IL-1 and LPS in females, but not in males.[76] This presumably reflects the obvious danger for a sick gravid female and her offspring, but sickness presents no such threat for a male. In contrast, the symptoms in patients with major depression do not appear to be so readily adaptive.

CHRONIC ANTIDEPRESSANT TREATMENT AND SICKNESS BEHAVIOR

Yirmiya[59] proposed the use of ingestion of a saccharin solution by rats as a measure of hedonia. He showed that treatment of rats with LPS (which stimulates the production and secretion of IL-1, IL-6, TNF-α and IFN-γ) decreased the frequency with which rats pressed a bar to obtain the saccharin solution. This response was considered to reflect anhedonia, a cardinal symptom of depression. This hypothesis was tested by treating the rats chronically (for 3 to 5 weeks) with the tricyclic antidepressant, imipramine, which inhibits the reuptake of both NE and 5-HT. This treatment prevented the induction by LPS of the "anhedonia" in the rats. Similar results were obtained by Shen et al.[77] using the NE-selective reuptake inhibitor, desmethylimipramine, and by Yirmiya et al.[78] using the serotonin-selective re-uptake inhibitor (SSRI), fluoxetine, although in the latter case, the prevention was less complete.

However, Shen et al. observed no such effect of the SSRI, paroxetine, or venlafaxine (a 5-HT and NE reuptake inhibitor).[77] Thus, the effect of antidepressants appears to be less evident with the SSRIs than with tricyclic antidepressants.[24,77] Nevertheless, the atypical antidepressant, tianeptine was reported to be effective chronically but not acutely.[79] We failed to observe any effect of chronic imipramine or venlafaxine on the inhibitory effect on LPS on the drinking of sweetened milk in mice.[80] Yirmiya et al.[24] also indicated a failure to observe an effect of antidepressants on LPS-induced saccharin drinking in mice. Based on these studies, it appears that the effect of chronic antidepressant treatment is observed more clearly with LPS than IL-1, and the effects of the antidepressants are apparent in rats but not mice. Other evidence suggests that antidepressants may affect the induction of IL-1 production by LPS,[24,79,81] and reflect a peripheral rather than a central mechanism. Thus, Yirmiya's exciting observation has failed to provide strong support for an IL-1 hypothesis of depression.

In sum, although many similarities have been noted between sickness behavior and the behavior of patients suffering from major depressive disorder, there are many aspects in which sickness behavior does not resemble depression in humans. Furthermore, it has been shown that in experimental endotoxemia the fever and corticosterone responses occur at a time when there are no detectable increases in circulating endotoxin or cytokines.[82] These discrepancies suggest that cytokines may not be necessary for the activation of the endocrine and sickness responses, nor for major depressive disorders.

CYTOKINES AND THE HPA AXIS

The HPA-activating effect of IL-1 is shared by IL-6 and TNF-α, but IL-6 and TNF-α are markedly less potent than IL-1 and may have limited physiological significance, except perhaps in the absence of IL-1.[27,83] Treatment with antibodies to IL-6 and studies in IL-6-knockout mice indicate that IL-6 contributes only modestly to the elevation of plasma ACTH and corticosterone by LPS in mice.[70,84]

Administration of IFN-α, IFN-β, and IFN-γ has been reported to cause marked activation of the HPA axis in many (but not all) studies in humans.[85-87] However, administration of relatively high doses of IFN-α (human or mouse) to mice did not alter plasma corticosterone.[83,88] In rats, both peripheral (ip) and intracerebroventricular (icv) administration of hIFN-α decreased plasma ACTH and corticosterone,[89] although another study showed modest increases in ACTH and corticosterone following iv rat IFN-α.[90]

Maes et al.[48] argued that IL-1 may be responsible for the excess HPA axis activation in depressed patients. However, support for IL-1 as the mediator of the HPA axis activation in depression is diminished because IL-1 has not been shown clearly to be elevated in a substantial proportion of depressed patients (see above). Similar concerns apply for the interferons.

CYTOKINES AND BRAIN NORADRENERGIC SYSTEMS

Animal studies have shown clearly that central noradrenergic systems are markedly activated by IL-1 indicated by elevations of the NE catabolite, 3–methoxy,4-hydroxyphenylethyleneglycol (MHPG).[18,19,26] Microdialysis studies in rats confirmed the apparent increase in NE release.[91,92] IL-6 administration does not induce noradrenergic activation,[29] but TNF-α has an effect at high doses in mice.[93] The reported effects of the IFNs on brain NE have been extraordinarily inconsistent[83,94] and do not provide good evidence that IFNs activate brain NE.

IL-1, IL-6, and TNF-α do not induce consistent effects on dopamine (DA) metabolism, although small increases are occasionally observed with IL-1.[26] However, IL-2 (1 μg ip) induced a marked reduction in microdialysate concentrations of DA from the nucleus accumbens of the rat.[61] These effects of IL-1 on brain NE fit well with the reported increases in noradrenergic activity in the brains of depressed patients. However, the failure to observe consistent elevations of IL-1 in depressed patients weakens the case for a cytokine etiology.

CYTOKINES AND BRAIN SEROTONERGIC SYSTEMS

The IL-1, IL-6, and TNF-α cytokines have all been shown to activate brain serotonergic systems, increasing brain tryptophan concentrations and the metabolism of 5-HT as indicated by increases in the brain concentrations of its catabolite, 5-hydroxyindoleacetic acid (5-HIAA).[26] Apparent 5-HT release by peripherally administered IL-6 has also been indicated by microdialysis and *in vivo* chronoamperometry.[30]

There are few data on the effects of IFNs on brain 5-HT. Single icv injections of 200 or 2000 U hIFN-α were reported to decrease the 5-HT content of the frontal cortex, and both 5-HT and 5-HIAA were decreased in the midbrains and the striatum of rats.[95]

However, we observed no effects of ip human or mouse IFN-α on 5-HT or 5-HIAA in mice at doses (400 to 16000 U per mouse) that induced behavioral changes.[26] Nevertheless, in another study, a single icv injection of IFN-α (1000 U) increased 5-HIAA:5-HT ratios in the prefrontal cortex, but not in the striatum or the hippocampus of rats.[96]

Decreased plasma concentrations of tryptophan have been observed in depressed patients,[97] but low plasma tryptophan is not a reliable biologic marker for major depression.[98] Wichers and Maes[99] proposed that a decrease in plasma tryptophan may limit the availability of tryptophan to the brain, thus limiting serotonin synthesis and precipitating depression. Tryptophan depletion may also induce depression in susceptible individuals.[98] Lowering plasma tryptophan can precipitate a relapse in depressed patients treated with SSRIs,[100,101] but not in those treated with desmethylimipramine (whose primary mechanism of action is considered to be inhibition of NE re-uptake)[101] nor in those treated with cognitive therapy.[102] There is also evidence that individuals who exhibit mood changes in response to rapid tryptophan depletion may be at risk for depression.[103]

A significant problem for the hypothesis that cytokines induce depression by affecting brain serotonin is that these effects are apparently in the wrong direction. IL-1 and IL-6 increase brain tryptophan and activate serotonergic systems. However, the SSRIs appear to exert their antidepressant effects by increasing extracellular 5-HT. This discrepancy could perhaps be explained if the chronic effects of the cytokines differed from the acute ones. For example, the chronic elevation of cytokines might down-regulate 5-HT secretion. The effects of chronic administration of the cytokines on serotonin metabolism have not been studied extensively, but Hayley et al.[104] indicated that repeated TNF-α administration increased its effects on 5-HT metabolism. This effect is in the same direction as SSRI treatment, and thus TNF-α should be antidepressant. IL-1β has also been reported to activate the serotonin transporter,[105] which may decrease extracellular 5-HT and induce a depression-like activity.

Another mechanism by which infections may induce depression relates to the peripheral metabolism of tryptophan. Infections, especially viral ones, induce IFN-γ, which is a potent inducer of indoleamine 2,3-dioxygenase (IDO) in macrophages and certain other cells. IL-2 and IFN-α also induce IDO, but they are less potent than IFN-γ. IDO metabolizes tryptophan (to kynurenine), so that infections are typically associated with decreases in plasma tryptophan and increases in kynurenine and neopterin.

The catabolism of tryptophan decreasing its circulating concentrations (often observed during infections), is thought to be a mechanism to limit the availability of tryptophan for the synthesis of new proteins by invading pathogens. However, the decrease in plasma tryptophan may also limit its availability to the brain for the synthesis of serotonin. It is interesting therefore that IL-1 and LPS both elevate brain concentrations of tryptophan[18,19,26] so that we can speculate that this is a defensive mechanism to protect the brain's supply of tryptophan for protein and serotonin synthesis during infections. The mechanism of this increase in brain tryptophan uptake involves the sympathetic nervous system[106] and activation of β₂- and β₃-adrenoreceptors.[107]

There are several hypothetical mechanisms by which cytokines could act on brain serotonergic systems and thus contribute to the pathophysiology of depression. However, relationships between these potential mechanisms and depression remain to be demonstrated in depressed patients.

EFFECTS OF CYTOKINES IN ANIMAL TESTS FOR DEPRESSION

It is pertinent to assess the ability of the cytokines implicated in depressive illness in animal tests used to evaluate antidepressant and depression-inducing effects. The two tests most commonly used are the Porsolt forced swim test for both rats and mice[108,109] and the tail suspension test that can be used only in mice.[110]

Somewhat surprisingly, the literature on the effects of IL-1 in these tests is sparse and conflicting. del Cerro and Borrell[111] reported that IL-1 administered icv reduced floating in rats in the Porsolt test by more than two-fold. Such a response would normally be interpreted to indicate antidepressant activity. In contrast, Huang and Minor[112] reported (abstract form only) that icv injection of IL-1 significantly increased floating in rats in this test, and that this response was prevented by icv administration of the IL-1 receptor antagonist, IL-1ra. Jain et al.[113] found that systemically administered LPS increased floating in the forced swim test in mice, but they used a very high dose of LPS (50 µg), and did not report any assessment of locomotor activity. The increased floating was prevented by desmethylimipramine and fluoxetine, as well as cyclooxygenase inhibitors. Deak et al.[114] recently reported that the behavior of rats during the forced swim test was not affected by LPS (10 or 100 µg/kg ip), whereas social investigation of a juvenile was profoundly decreased.

We studied the behavior of mice in the Porsolt forced swim and the tail suspension tests, and observed that ip administration of IL-1β (30 to 300 ng) or LPS (1 to 5 µg) induced depression-like activity. However, the same doses of IL-1β and LPS induced profound decreases in locomotor activity.[66] This effect generally appeared at doses lower than those necessary to induce statistically similar results in both tests. Thus, it is difficult to dissociate these behavioral effects of IL-1 in the forced swim and tail suspension tests from a general reduction in activity.

CONCLUSIONS

The foregoing review indicates some associations between the appearance of cytokines and major depressive disorder. However, no clear causal relationship has been established. Administration of certain cytokines to humans (notably IFN-α and IL-2) induces symptoms of depression in some patients, but such responses occur in only a minority of patients, and many other neuropsychiatric symptoms may also be induced. Immune activation appears more frequently in depressed patients than in the general population, but is not observed in even a majority of depressed patients. Moreover, immune activation observed may reflect other medical conditions that themselves induce depression. Alternatively, depression may ensue when a patient learns he or she has a serious disease. Nevertheless, it is possible that excessive production of cytokines may induce symptoms of depression in some patients and exacerbate them in others.

There is evidence that depressed patients exhibit elevated plasma concentrations of some cytokines. Although IL-1 is the major cytokine associated with depression-like symptoms, the evidence for elevations of this cytokine in depressed patients is sparse. The major cytokine affected is IL-6. Elevations of IL-6 are not observed consistently, and are often relatively small. Plasma concentrations of IL-6 are frequently elevated during infections and other pathological conditions including stress. Thus there may not be any specific relationship between plasma IL-6 and depression. It is pertinent that when IL-6 is administered to rats and mice, it induces very little behavioral response and sickness behavior is not observed.

Sickness behavior induced by immune stimulation or IL-1 indeed has many similarities with the behavior of depressed patients. However, there are also important differences. For example, IL-1 increases body temperature, sensitivity to pain, and slow-wave sleep, none of which are typical of depression. Therefore it may be premature to consider experimentally induced sickness behavior as a good model for depressive illness, and the results obtained using this model should be interpreted conservatively. Moreover, experiments in which animals were treated chronically with antidepressant drugs failed to provide strong support for the concept that such treatments work by antagonizing the actions of cytokines.

A cytokine hypothesis of depression does not conflict with earlier hypotheses of depression such as those involving hyperactivity of the HPA axis or of noradrenergic systems because IL-1 activates the HPA axis via CRF and also activates brain noradrenergic systems. CRF appears to be involved in HPA axis responses to IL-1 because antibodies to CRF prevent IL-1-induced HPA activation in rats and mice, and HPA responses to IL-1 are minuscule in CRF knockout mice.

A cytokine hypothesis could also be consistent with a serotonin hypothesis of depression, because IL-1, IL-6, and TNF-α have all been shown to affect brain serotonergic transmission. However, IL-1, IL-6, and TNF-α administered acutely appear to increase 5-HT release, which would achieve an effect similar to that induced by the many commonly used antidepressants that inhibit 5-HT re-uptake, so that these cytokines ought to have antidepressant effects. Nevertheless, the chronic presence of elevated cytokines may down-regulate 5-HT release, which might contribute to depressive illness.

Drugs that inhibit serotonin re-uptake are currently the most useful for the treatment of depression, but there is no strong direct evidence that abnormalities in 5-HT *cause* depression. More research on the effects of antidepressants on functions of the immune system may be useful. The associations of abnormalities in tryptophan and serotonin with pathogen infection, immune activation, and depression, are potentially very significant. This is clearly an area in need of further investigation.

Our critique does not exclude a role for cytokines in depression. It is possible that increased cytokine production may induce depression in some patients, and certain cytokines may contribute to a variety of neuropsychiatric symptoms in patients with many diseases. Nevertheless, we can conclude that the actions of cytokines are unlikely to account for all depressive illness. It is also possible that by activating brain CRF systems and hence the HPA axis, as well as noradrenergic and serotonergic mechanisms, cytokines may complement or even synergize with other factors that induce depression.

ACKNOWLEDGMENT

The author's research reported in this article was supported by the U.S. National Institutes of Health (NS 35370).

REFERENCES

1. Cannon, W.B. and de la Paz, D., Emotional stimulation of adrenal secretion, *Am. J. Physiol.*, 28, 64–70, 1911.
2. Selye, H., Thymus and adrenals in the response of the organism to injuries and intoxications, *Brit. J. Exp. Pathol.*, 17, 234–248, 1936.
3. Stone, E.A., Stress and catecholamines, in *Catecholamines and Behavior*, Friedhoff, A.J., Ed., Plenum Press, New York, 1975, pp. 31–72.
4. Dunn, A.J. and Kramarcy, N.R., Neurochemical responses in stress: relationships between the hypothalamic–pituitary–adrenal and catecholamine systems, in *Handbook of Psychopharmacology*, Iversen, L.L., Iversen, S.D., and Snyder, S.H., Eds., Plenum Press, New York, 1984, pp. 455–515.
5. Plotsky, P.M., Cunningham, E.T., and Widmaier, E.P., Catecholaminergic modulation of corticotropin-releasing factor and adrenocorticotropin secretion, *Endocrine Rev.*, 10, 437–458, 1989.
6. Pohorecky, L.A. and Wurtman, R.J., Adrenocortical control of epinephrine synthesis, *Pharmacol. Rev.*, 23, 1–35, 1971.
7. van Praag, H.M., Can stress cause depression? *Prog. Neuropsychopharmacol. Biol. Psychiatr.*, 28, 891–907, 2004.
8. Stone, E.A., Stress and catecholamines, in *Catecholamines and Behavior*, Friedhoff, A.J., Ed., Plenum Press, New York, 1975, pp. 31–72.
9. Koslow, S.H., Maas, J.W., Bowden, C.L., Davis, J.M., Hanin, I., and Javaid, J., CSF and urinary biogenic amines and metabolites in depression and mania, *Arch. Gen. Psychiatr.*, 40, 999–1010, 1983.
10. Wong, M.L., Kling, M.A., Munson, P.J., Listwak, S., Licinio, J., Prolo, P., Karp, B., McCutcheon, I.E., Geracioti, T.D., DeBellis, M.D., Rice, K.C., Goldstein, D.S., Veldhuis, J.D., Chrousos, G.P., Oldfield, E.H., McCann, S.M., and Gold, P.W., Pronounced and sustained central hypernoradrenergic function in major depression with melancholic features: relation to hypercortisolism and corticotropin-releasing hormone, *Proc. Natl Acad. Sci. USA*, 97, 325–330, 2000.
11. Sachar, E.J., Hellman, L., Fukushima, D.K., and Gallagher, T.F., Cortisol production in depressive illness, *Arch. Gen. Psychiat.*, 23, 289–298, 1970.
12. Carroll, B.J., Martin, F.I.R., and Davies, B., Resistance to suppression by dexamethasone of plasma 11-OHCS levels in severe depressive illness, *Brit. Med. J.*, 3, 285–287, 1968.
13. Holsboer, F., Bardeleben, U.V., Gerken, A., Stalla, G.K., and Muller, O.A., Blunted corticotropin and normal cortisol response to human corticotropin-releasing factor in depression, *New Engl. J. Med.*, 311, 1127, 1984.
14. Besedovsky, H.O., del Rey, A., Sorkin, E., and Dinarello, C.A., Immunoregulatory feedback between interleukin-1 and glucocorticoid hormones, *Science*, 233, 652–654, 1986.
15. Sapolsky, R., Rivier, C., Yamamoto, G., Plotsky, P., and Vale, W., Interleukin-1 stimulates the secretion of hypothalamic corticotropin-releasing factor, *Science*, 238, 522–524, 1987.
16. Berkenbosch, F., van Oers, J., del Rey, A., Tilders, F., and Besedovsky, H., Corticotropin-releasing factor-producing neurons in the rat activated by interleukin-1, *Science*, 238, 524–526, 1987.

17. Berkenbosch, F., De Goeij, D.E.C., del Rey, A., and Besedovsky, H.O., Neuroendocrine, sympathetic and metabolic responses induced by interleukin-1, *Neuroendocrinology*, 50, 570–576, 1989.

18. Dunn, A.J., Systemic interleukin-1 administration stimulates hypothalamic norepinephrine metabolism parallelling the increased plasma corticosterone, *Life Sci.*, 43, 429–435, 1988.

19. Kabiersch, A., del Rey, A., Honegger, C.G., and Besedovsky, H.O., Interleukin-1 induces changes in norepinephrine metabolism in the rat brain, *Brain Behav. Immun.*, 2, 267–274, 1988.

20. Zalcman, S., Green-Johnson, J.M., Murray, L., Nance, D.M., Dyck, D., Anisman, H., and Greenberg, A.H., Cytokine-specific central monoamine alterations induced by interleukin-1, -2 and -6, *Brain Res.*, 643, 40–49, 1994.

21. McCarthy, D.O., Kluger, M.J., and Vander, A.J., Suppression of food intake during infections: is interleukin-1 involved? *Am. J. Clin. Nutr.*, 42, 1179–1182, 1985.

22. Dunn, A.J., Antoon, M., and Chapman, Y., Reduction of exploratory behavior by intraperitoneal injection of interleukin-1 involves brain corticotropin-releasing factor, *Brain Res. Bull.*, 26, 539–542, 1991.

23. Spadaro, F. and Dunn, A.J., Intracerebroventricular administration of interleukin-1 to mice alters investigation of stimuli in a novel environment, *Brain Behav. Immun.*, 4, 308–322, 1990.

24. Yirmiya, R., Weidenfeld, J., Pollak, Y., Morag, M., Morag, A., Avitsur, R., Barak, O., Reichenberg, A., Cohen, E., Shavit, Y., and Ovadia, H., Cytokines, "Depression due to a general medical condition" and antidepressant drugs, *Adv. Exp. Med. Biol.*, 461, 283–316, 1999.

25. Yirmiya, R., Avitsur, R., Donchin, O., and Cohen, E., Interleukin-1 inhibits sexual behavior in female but not in male rats, *Brain Behav. Immun.*, 9, 220–233, 1995.

26. Dunn, A.J., Effects of cytokines and infections on brain neurochemistry, in *Psychoneuroimmunology*, 3rd ed., Ader, R., Felten, D.L., and Cohen, N., Eds., Academic Press, New York, 2001, pp. 649–666.

27. Silverman, M.N., Pearce, B.D., and Miller, A.H., Cytokines and HPA axis regulation, in *Cytokines and Mental Health*, Kronfol, Z., Ed., Kluwer Academic Publishers, Boston, 2003, pp. 85–122.

28. Bornstein, S.R. and Chrousos, G.P., Clinical review 104: adrenocorticotropin (ACTH)- and non-ACTH-mediated regulation of the adrenal cortex: neural and immune inputs, *J. Clin. Endocrinol. Metab.*, 84, 1729–1736, 1999.

29. Wang, J.P. and Dunn, A.J., Mouse interleukin-6 stimulates the HPA axis and increases brain tryptophan and serotonin metabolism, *Neurochem. Int.*, 33, 143–154, 1998.

30. Zhang, J.-J., Terreni, L., De Simoni, M.-G., and Dunn, A.J., Peripheral interleukin-6 administration increases extracellular concentrations of serotonin and the evoked release of serotonin in the rat striatum, *Neurochem. Intl.*, 38, 303–308, 2001.

31. Dunn, A.J., Powell, M.L., Meitin, C., and Small, P.A., Virus infection as a stressor: influenza virus elevates plasma concentrations of corticosterone, and brain concentrations of MHPG and tryptophan, *Physiol. Behav.*, 45, 591–594, 1989.

32. Swiergiel, A.H., Smagin, G.N., and Dunn, A.J., Influenza virus infection of mice induces anorexia: comparison with endotoxin and interleukin-1 and the effects of indomethacin, *Pharmacol. Biochem. Behav.*, 57, 389–396, 1997.

33. Swiergiel, A.H. and Dunn, A.J., The roles of IL-1, IL-6 and TNFα in the feeding responses to endotoxin and influenza virus infection in mice, *Brain Behav. Immun.*, 13, 252–265, 1999.

34. Fantuzzi, G., Zheng, H., Faggioni, R., Benigni, F., Ghezzi, P., Sipe, J.D., Shaw, A.R., and Dinarello, C.A., Effect of endotoxin in IL-1β-deficient mice, *J. Immunol.*, 157, 291–296, 1996.

35. Hart, B.L., Biological basis of the behavior of sick animals, *Neurosci. Biobehav. Rev.*, 12, 123–137, 1988.

36. Smith, R.S., The macrophage theory of depression, *Med. Hypotheses*, 35, 298–306, 1991.

37. Kronfol, Z., Immune dysregulation in major depression: critical review of existing evidence, *Int. J. Neuropsychopharmacol.*, 5, 333–343, 2002.

38. de Beaurepaire, R., Swiergiel, A.H., and Dunn, A.J., Neuroimmune mediators: are cytokines mediators of depression, in *Biology of Depression*, Licinio, J. and Wong, M.-L., Eds., Wiley, Weinheim, 2005, pp. 557–581.

39. Dunn, A.J., Swiergiel, A.H., and de Beaurepaire, R., Cytokines as mediators of depression: what we can learn from animal studies? *Neurosci. Biobehav. Rev.*, 29, 891–909, 2005.

40. Meyers, C.A., Mood and cognitive disorders in cancer patients receiving cytokine therapy, *Adv. Exp. Med. Biol.*, 461, 75–81, 1999.

41. Capuron, L., Gumnick, J.F., Musselman, D.L., Lawson, D.H., Reemsnyder, A., Nemeroff, C.B., and Miller, A.H., Neurobehavioral effects of interferon-α in cancer patients: phenomenology and paroxetine responsiveness of symptom dimensions, *Neuropsychopharmacology*, 26, 643–652, 2002.

42. Cleeland, C.S., Bennett, G.J., Dantzer, R., Dougherty, P.M., Dunn, A.J., Meyers, C.A., Miller, A.H., Payne, R., Reuben, J.M., Wang, X.S., and Lee, B.-N., Are the symptoms of cancer and cancer treatment due to a shared biologic mechanism? A cytokine-immunologic model of cancer symptoms, *Cancer*, 97, 2919–2925, 2003.

43. Maes, M., Evidence for an immune response in major depression: a review and hypothesis, *Prog. Neuropsychopharmacol. Biol. Psychiatr.*, 19, 11–38, 1995.

44. Maes, M., Major depression and activation of the inflammatory response system, in *Cytokines, Stress, and Depression*, Dantzer, R., Wollman, E.E., and Yirmiya, R., Eds., Kluwer/Plenum New York, 1999, pp. 25–46.

45. Natelson, B.H., Denny, T., Zhou, X.D., LaManca, J.J., Ottenweller, J.E., Tiersky, L., DeLuca, J., and Gause, W.C., Is depression associated with immune activation? *J. Affect. Dis.*, 53, 179–184, 1999.

46. Griffiths, J., Ravindran, A.V., Merali, Z., and Anisman, H., Neuroendocrine measures and lymphocyte subsets in depressive illness: influence of a clinical interview concerning life experiences, *Psychoneuroendocrinology*, 22, 225–236, 1997.

47. Owen, B.M., Eccleston, D., Ferrier, I.N., and Young, A.H., Raised levels of plasma interleukin-1β in major and postviral depression, *Acta. Psychiatr. Scand.*, 103, 226–228, 2001.

48. Maes, M., Bosmans, E., Meltzer, H.Y., Scharpé, S., and Suy, E., Interleukin-1β: a putative mediator of HPA axis hyperactivity in major depression? *Am. J. Psychiatr.*, 150, 1189–1193, 1993.

49. Musselman, D.L., Miller, A.H., Porter, M.R., Manatunga, A., Gao, F., Penna, S., et al., Higher than normal plasma interleukin-6 concentrations in cancer patients with depression: preliminary findings, *Am. J. Psychiatr.*, 158, 1252–1257, 2001.

50. Maes, M., Scharpe, S., Meltzer, H.Y., Okayli, G., Bosmans, E., D'Hondt, P., Vanden Bossche, B.V., and Cosyns, P., Increased neopterin and interferon-gamma secretion and lower availability of L-tryptophan in major depression, further evidence for an immune response, *Psychiatr. Res.*, 54, 143–160, 1994.

51. Brambilla, F., Bellodi, L., Brunetta, M., and Perna, G., Plasma concentrations of interleukin-1β, interleukin-6 and tumor necrosis factor-a in anorexia and bulimia nervosa, *Psychoneuroendocrinology*, 23, 439–447, 1998.

52. Haack, M., Hinze-Selch, D., Fenzel, T., Kraus, T., Kuhn, M., Schuld, A., and Pollmacher, T., Plasma levels of cytokines and soluble cytokine receptors in psychiatric patients upon hospital admission: effects of confounding factors and diagnosis, *J. Psychiatr. Res.*, 33, 407–418, 1999.

53. Zorrilla, E.P., Luborsky, L., McKay, J.R., Rosenthal, R., Houldin, A., Tax, A., McCorkle, R., Seligman, D.A., and Schmidt, K., The relationship of depression and stressors to immunological assays: a meta-analytic review, *Brain Behav. Immun.*, 15, 199–226, 2001.

54. Anisman, H., Ravindran, A.V., Griffiths, J., and Merali, Z., Endocrine and cytokine correlates of major depression and dysthymia with typical or atypical features, *Molec. Psychiatr.*, 4, 182–188, 1999.

55. Landmann, R., Schaub, B., Link, S., and Wacker, H.R., Unaltered monocyte function in patients with major depression before and after three months of antidepressive therapy, *Biol. Psychiatr.*, 15, 675–681, 1997.

56. Levine, J., Barak, Y., Chengappa, K.N., Rapoport, A., Rebey, M., and Barak, V., Cerebrospinal cytokine levels in patients with acute depression, *Neuropsychobiology*, 40, 171–176, 1999.

57. Pollmächer, T., Haack, M., Schuld, A., Reichenberg, A., and Yirmiya, R., Low levels of circulating inflammatory cytokines: do they affect human brain functions? *Brain Behav. Immun.*, 16, 525–532, 2002.

58. Dubrovsky, B., Evolutionary psychiatry. Adaptationist and nonadaptationist conceptualizations, *Prog. Neuropsychopharmacol. Biol. Psychiatry*, 26, 1–19, 2002.

59. Yirmiya, R., Endotoxin produces a depressive-like episode in rats, *Brain Res.*, 711, 163–174, 1996.

60. Swiergiel, A.H., Smagin, G.N., Johnson, L.J., and Dunn, A.J., The role of cytokines in the behavioral responses to endotoxin and influenza virus infection in mice: effects of acute and chronic administration of the interleukin-1-receptor antagonist (IL-1ra), *Brain Res.*, 776, 96–104, 1997.

61. Anisman, H., Kokkinidis, L., and Merali, Z., Interleukin-2 decreases accumbal dopamine efflux and responding for rewarding lateral hypothalamic stimulation, *Brain Res.*, 731, 1–11, 1996.

62. Anisman, H., Kokkinidis, L., Borowski, T., and Merali, Z., Differential effects of interleukin (IL)-1β, IL-2 and IL-6 on responding for rewarding lateral hypothalamic stimulation, *Brain Res.*, 779, 177–187, 1998.

63. Dantzer, R., Bluthé, R.-M., Castanon, N., Chauvet, N., Capuron, L., Goodall, G., Kelley, K.W., Konsman, J.-P., Layé, S., Parnet, P., and Pousset, F., Cytokine effects on behavior, in *Psychoneuroimmunology*, 3rd ed., Ader, R., Felten, D., and Cohen, N., Eds., Academic Press, San Diego, 2001, pp. 703–727.

64. Swiergiel, A.H. and Dunn, A.J., Feeding, exploratory, anxiety- and depression-related behaviors are not altered in interleukin-6-deficient mice, *Behav. Brain Res.*, in press.

65. Krueger, J.M., Majde, J.A., and Obál, F., Sleep in host defense, *Brain Behav. Immun.*, 17, S41–S47, 2003.

66. Dunn, A.J. and Swiergiel, A.H., Effects of interleukin-1 and endotoxin in the forced swim and tail suspension tests in mice, *Pharmacol. Biochem. Behav.*, 81, 688–693, 2005.

67. Swiergiel, A.H., Burunda, T., Patterson, B., and Dunn, A.J., Endotoxin- and interleukin-1-induced hypophagia are not affected by noradrenergic, dopaminergic, histaminergic and muscarinic antagonists, *Pharmacol. Biochem. Behav.*, 63, 629–637, 1999.

68. Larson, S.J. and Dunn, A.J., Behavioral effects of cytokines, *Brain Behav. Immun.*, 15, 371–387, 2001.

69. Watkins, L.R., Wiertelak, E.P., Goehler, L.E., Smith, K.P., Martin, D., and Maier, S.F., Characterization of cytokine-induced hyperalgesia, *Brain Res.*, 654, 15–26, 1994.

70. Swiergiel, A.H. and Dunn, A.J., Feeding and anxiety-related behaviors are intact in IL-6 deficient mice, *Brain Behav. Immun.*, 17, 214, 2003.

71. Larson, S.J. and Dunn, A.J., Behavioral mechanisms for defense against pathogens, in *Natural Immunity*, Vol. 5, Bertók, L. and Chow, D.A., Eds., Elsevier, New York, 2005, pp. 351–368.

72. McCarthy, D.O., Kluger, M.J., and Vander, A.J., Effect of centrally administered interleukin-1 and endotoxin on food intake of fasted rats, *Physiol. Behav.*, 36, 745–749, 1986.

73. Kent, S., Rodriguez, F., Kelley, K.W., and Dantzer, R., Reduction in food and water intake induced by microinjection of interleukin-1β in the ventromedial hypothalamus of the rat, *Physiol. Behav.*, 56, 1031–1036, 1994.

74. Aubert, A., Kelley, K.W., and Dantzer, R., Differential effects of lipopolysaccharide on food hoarding behavior and food consumption in rats, *Brain Behav. Immun.*, 11, 229–238, 1997.

75. Aubert, A., Goodall, G., Dantzer, R., and Gheusi, G., Differential effects of lipopolysaccharide on pup retrieving and nest building in lactating mice, *Brain Behav. Immun.*, 11, 107–118, 1997.

76. Avitsur, R., Donchin, O., Barak, O., Cohen, E., and Yirmiya, R., Behavioral effects of interleukin-1β: modulation by gender, estrus cycle, and progesterone, *Brain Behav. Immun.*, 9, 234–241, 1995.

77. Shen, Y., Connor, T.J., Nolan, Y., Kelly, J.P., and Leonard, B.E., Differential effect of chronic antidepressant treatments on lipopolysaccharide-induced depressive-like behavioural symptoms in the rat, *Life Sci.*, 65, 1773–1786, 1999.

78. Yirmiya, R., Pollak, Y., Barak, O., Avitsur, R., Ovadia, H., Bette, M., Weihe, E., and Weidenfeld, J., Effects of antidepressant drugs on the behavioral and physiological responses to lipopolysaccharide (LPS) in rodents, *Neuropsychopharmacology*, 24, 531–544, 2001.

79. Castanon, N., Konsman, J.-P., Medina, C., Chauvet, N., and Dantzer, R., Chronic treatment with the antidepressant tianeptine attenuates lipopolysaccharide-induced Fos expression in the rat paraventricular nucleus and HPA axis activation, *Psychoneuroendocrinology*, 28, 19–34, 2003.

80. Dunn, A.J. and Swiergiel, A.H., The reductions in sweetened milk intake induced by interleukin-1 and endotoxin are not prevented by chronic antidepressant treatment, *Neuroimmunomodulation*, 9, 163–169, 2001.

81. Connor, T.J., Harkin, A., Kelly, J.P., and Leonard, B.E., Olfactory bulbectomy provokes a suppression of interleukin-1β and tumour necrosis factor-α production in response to an *in vivo* challenge with lipopolysaccharide: effect of chronic desipramine treatment, *Neuroimmunomodulation*, 7, 27–35, 2000.

82. Campisi, J., Hansen, M.K., O'Conner, K.A., Biedenkapp, J.C., Watkins, L.R., Maier, S.F., and Fleshner, M., Circulating cytokines and endotoxin are not necessary for the activation of the sickness or corticosterone response produced by peripheral E. coli challenge, *J. Appl. Physiol.*, 95, 1873–1882, 2003.

83. Dunn, A., Cytokine activation of the hypothalamo–pituitary–adrenal axis, in *Handbook of Stress and the Brain Part 2: Stress: Integrative and Clinical Aspects*, Steckler, T., Kalin, N., and Reul, J.M., Eds., Elsevier, Amsterdam, 2005, pp. 157–174.

84. Wang, J.P. and Dunn, A.J., The role of interleukin-6 in the activation of the hypothalamo–pituitary–adrenocortical axis induced by endotoxin and interleukin-1β, *Brain Res.*, 815, 337–348, 1999.

85. Shimizu, H., Ohtani, K.-I., Sato, N., Nagamine, T., and Mori, M., Increase in serum interleukin-6, plasma ACTH and serum cortisol levels after systemic interferon-α administration, *Endocr. J.*, 42, 551–556, 1995.

86. Capuron, L., Raison, C.L., Musselman, D.L., Lawson, D.H., Nemeroff, C.B., and Miller, A.H., Association of exaggerated HPA axis response to the initial injection of interferon-alpha with development of depression during interferon-alpha therapy, *Am. J. Psychiatr.*, 160, 1342–1345, 2003.

87. Holsboer, F., Stalla, G.K., von Bardeleben, U., Hammann, K., Müller, H., and Müller, O.A., Acute adrenocortical stimulation by recombinant gamma interferon in human controls, *Life Sci.*, 42, 1–5, 1988.

88. Dunn, A.J., The role of interleukin-1 and tumor necrosis factor α in the neurochemical and neuroendocrine responses to endotoxin, *Brain Res. Bull.*, 29, 807–812, 1992.

89. Saphier, D., Welch, J.E., and Chuluyan, H.E., α-Interferon inhibits adrenocortical secretion via μ_1-opioid receptors in the rat, *Eur. J. Pharmacol.*, 236, 183–191, 1993.

90. Menzies, R.A., Phelps, C.P., Wiranowska, M., Oliver, J., Chen, L.T., Horvath, E., and Hall, N.R.S., The effect of interferon-alpha on the pituitary-adrenal axis, *J. Interferon Cytokine Res.*, 16, 619–629, 1996.

91. Shintani, F., Kanba, S., Nakaki, T., Nibuya, M., Kinoshita, N., Suzuki, E., Yagi, G., Kato, R., and Asai, M., Interleukin-1β augments release of norepinephrine, dopamine, and serotonin in the rat anterior hypothalamus, *J. Neurosci.*, 13, 3574–3581, 1993.

92. Smagin, G.N., Swiergiel, A.H., and Dunn, A.J., Peripheral administration of inter-leukin-1 increases extracellular concentrations of norepinephrine in rat hypothalamus: comparison with plasma corticosterone, *Psychoneuroendocrinology*, 21, 83–93, 1996.

93. Ando, T. and Dunn, A.J., Mouse tumor necrosis factor-α increases brain tryptophan concentrations and norepinephrine metabolism while activating the HPA axis in mice, *Neuroimmunomodulation*, 6, 319–329, 1999.

94. Schaefer, M., Schwaiger, M., Pich, M., Lieb, K., and Heinz, A., Neurotransmitter changes by interferon-alpha and therapeutic implications, *Pharmacopsychiatry*, 36, Suppl. 3, S203–S206, 2003.

95. Kamata, M., Higuchi, H., Yoshimoto, M., Yoshida, K., and Shimizu, T., Effect of single intracerebroventricular injection of α-interferon on monoamine concentrations in the rat brain, *Europ. Neuropsychopharmacol.*, 10, 129–132, 2000.

96. De La Garza, R. and Asnis, G.M., The non-steroidal anti-inflammatory drug diclofenac sodium attenuates IFN-α induced alterations to monoamine turnover in prefrontal cortex and hippocampus, *Brain Res.*, 977, 70–79, 2003.

97. Coppen, A. and Wood, K., Tryptophan and depressive illness, *Psychol. Med.*, 8, 49–57, 1978.

98. Bell, C., Abrams, J., and Nutt, D., Tryptophan depletion and its implications for psychiatry, *Br. J. Psychiat.*, 178, 399–405, 2001.

99. Wichers, M.C. and Maes, M., The role of indoleamine 2,3-dioxygenase (IDO) in the pathophysiology of interferon-alpha-induced depression, *J. Psychiatr. Neurosci.*, 29, 11–17, 2004.

100. Delgado, P.L., Price, L.H., Miller, H.L., Salomon, R.M., Aghajanian, G.K., Heninger, G.R., and Charney, D.S., Serotonin and the neurobiology of depression: effects of tryptophan depletion in drug-free depressed patients, *Arch. Gen. Psychiatr.*, 51, 865–874, 1994.

101. Delgado, P.L., Miller, H.L., Salomon, R.M., Licinio, J., Krystal, J.H., Moreno, F.A., Heninger, G.R., and Charney, D.S., Tryptophan-depletion challenge in depressed patients treated with desipramine or fluoxetine: implications for the role of serotonin in the mechanism of antidepressant action, *Biol. Psychiatr.,* 46, 212–220, 1999.

102. O'Reardon, J.P., Chopra, M.P., Bergan, A., Gallop, R., DeRubeis, R.J., and Crits-Christoph, P., Response to tryptophan depletion in major depression treated with either cognitive therapy or selective serotonin reuptake inhibitor antidepressants, *Biol. Psychiatr.,* 55, 957–959, 2004.

103. Moreno, F.A., Heninger, G.R., McGahuey, C.A., and Delgado, P.L., Tryptophan depletion and risk of depression relapse: a prospective study of tryptophan depletion as a potential predictor of depressive episodes, *Biol. Psychiatr.,* 48, 327–329, 2000.

104. Hayley, S., Wall, P., and Anisman, H., Sensitization to the neuroendocrine, central monoamine and behavioural effects of murine tumor necrosis factor-α: peripheral and central mechanisms, *Eur. J. Neurosci.,* 15, 1061–1076, 2002.

105. Morikawa, O., Sakai, N., Obara, H., and Saito, N., Effects of interferon-a, interferon-g and cAMP on the transcriptional regulation of the serotonin transporter, *Eur. J. Pharmacol.,* 349, 317–324, 1998.

106. Dunn, A.J. and Welch, J., Stress- and endotoxin-induced increases in brain tryptophan and serotonin metabolism depend on sympathetic nervous system activation, *J. Neurochem.,* 57, 1615–1622, 1991.

107. Lenard, N.R., Gettys, T.W., and Dunn, A.J., Activation of β_2- and β_3-adrenergic receptors increases brain tryptophan, *J. Pharmacol. Exp. Ther.,* 305, 653–659, 2003.

108. Porsolt, R.D., Bertin, A., and Jalfre, M., Behavioural despair in mice: a primary screening test for antidepressants, *Arch. Int. Pharmacodyn.,* 229, 327–336, 1977.

109. Porsolt, R.D., Le Pichon, M., and Jalfre, M., Depression: a new animal model sensitive to antidepressant treatments, *Nature,* 266, 730–732, 1977.

110. Steru, L., Chermat, R., Thierry, B., and Simon, P., The tail suspension test: a new method for screening antidepressants in mice, *Psychopharmacology (Berlin),* 85, 367–370, 1985.

111. del Cerro, S. and Borrell, J., Interleukin-1 affects the behavioral despair response in rats by an indirect mechanism which requires endogenous CRF, *Brain Res.,* 528, 162–164, 1990.

112. Huang, Q. and Minor, T.R., Adenosine mediates interleukin-1-beta induced behavioral depression in rats, *Brain Behav. Immunol.,* 14, 101, 2000.

113. Jain, N.K., Kulkarni, S.K., and Singh, A., Lipopolysaccharide-mediated immobility in mice: reversal by cyclooxygenase enzyme inhibitors, *Meth. Find. Exp. Clin. Pharmacol.,* 23, 441–444, 2001.

114. Deak, T., Bellamy, C., D'Agostino, L.G., Rosanoff, M., McElderry, N.K., and Bordner, K.A., Behavioral responses during the forced swim test are not affected by anti-inflammatory agents or acute illness induced by lipopolysaccharide, *Behav. Brain Res.,* 160, 125–134, 2005.

14 Immunoconversion in Acute Phase Response

Istvan Berczi, Andres Quintanar-Stephano, and Kalman Kovacs

CONTENTS

ABSTRACT

Mild infection or sub-lethal dose of endotoxin elicit a brief elevation of growth hormone (GH) and prolactin (PRL) in the serum. These hormones are pro-inflammatory and immunostimulatory. In severe trauma, sepsis and shock, GH, and PRL are suppressed, whereas glucocorticoids and catecholamines are elevated. Under these conditions an acute phase response is induced by immune-derived cytokines, primarily IL-1, IL-6, and TNFα, which elicit a neuroendocrine response and initiate major metabolic alterations. Fever and catabolism prevails, whereas the synthesis of acute phase proteins in the liver, cell proliferation in the bone marrow, and protein synthesis by leukocytes are elevated. This is an emergency reaction to save the organism after the adaptive immune system has failed to contain and eliminate the infectious agent. During sepsis and endotoxin shock the systemic activation of the complement system and of leukocyte-derived releasing enzymes, tissue-derived break-down products, and highly toxic cytokines seriously threaten survival. Glucocorticoids and cathecolamines regulate pro-inflammatory cytokine production and potentiate the secretion of liver-derived acute phase proteins into the serum. Some of these proteins, such as C reactive protein, LPS binding protein, and mannose binding protein are designed to combine with micro-organisms and trigger their destruction by the activation of the complement system and of phagocytes. The increased production of some complement components also helps host resistance. The rise in serum fibrinogen promotes blood clotting. A number of enzyme inhibitors are produced as acute phase proteins, which are likely to serve to curb the nonspecific damage inflicted by enzymes released from activated phagocytes and from damaged cells. Serum leptin is also increased, which regulates energy metabolism and is a major stimulator of the immune system.

If the acute phase reaction fails to protect the host, shock will develop and death may follow. During the acute phase response, the T-cell regulated adaptive immune response is switched off and natural immune mechanisms are amplified several hundred to a thousand times within 24 to 48 hours. This phenomenon has been designated as *immunoconversion*. Immunoconversion is initiated by immune-derived cytokines, glucocorticoids, and cathecolamines, and involves profound neuroendocrine and metabolic changes, all in the interest of host defense. Once the cause of acute illness has been eliminated by the immune system, healing and recovery (immunoreversion) follow. Here we present data indicating that *vasopressin* may regulate the recovery from acute illness. Thus, natural immunity is essential for the first and the last line of host defence. It is also clear that the neuroendocrine system is the ultimate regulator of both the adaptive and the natural immune system.

INTRODUCTION

Cannon was the first to recognize that higher organisms exert a neuroendocrine reaction when in pain or faced with danger. The reaction is known as the fight-or-flight response.[226] Hans Selye discovered that a variety of noxious agents cause a profound involution of the thymus, spleen, and lymph nodes, and enlargement of the adrenal gland. Selye showed that these changes were mediated by the activation of the pituitary–adrenal axis and that glucocorticoids were responsible for the lymphoid involution observed.[1] Physical, chemical, and biological agents, and even emotional factors can evoke this neuroendocrine response. Selye designated the factors as *stressors* and their effect as *stress*. He called the body's reaction to stress a *general adaptation syndrome*. A stressed animal or individual shows an initial *alarm reaction* followed by a period of resistance or *adaptation*.

Adapted animals show resistance toward stressors and to various other insults in general. Eventually, with lasting stress, a breakdown due to *exhaustion* may occur and can lead to death.[2,3] Selye also discovered the inhibitory effects of glucocorticoids on inflammation[4] and made observations indicating that immune reactions are also subject to stress-induced alterations.[5] He demonstrated the influence of sex steroid hormones on lymphoid organs.[6]

RESPONSE TO INJURY

It is now apparent that Selye's general adaptation syndrome is analogous to the intensive and highly coordinated emergency defense reactions of humans and higher animals that frequently manifest in *febrile illness* — now designated the *acute phase response* (APR).[7–12] In a broad sense, the agents capable of causing injury and subsequent APR may be classified into physical, chemical, and biological categories. Without exception, injured cells release chemokines and cytokines that in turn attract and activate leukocytes that secrete cytokines. The cytokines then elicit neuroendocrine and metabolic responses characteristic of APR.

Among the physical agents studied in this respect are ultraviolet irradiation of the skin, x-irradiation, cold and burn injuries, and major surgical operations. In severe cases, injuries led to APR.[11,13–15] Chemical agents causing toxic injuries exert similar effects.[16] Biological injuries are caused by infectious agents, toxins, or immune effector mechanisms. Substances that are otherwise harmless to the body may cause severe injuries if an abnormal immune response (hypersensitivity) is directed against them. Tissue injuries may be mediated by IgE antibodies (immediate hypersensitivity, allergy, asthma, anaphylaxis), by sensitized T lymphocytes (delayed hypersensitivity, contact dermatitis, cytotoxicity), by immune complexes, and by phagocytic cells activated by antibodies or cytokines. Humoral or cell-mediated immune reactions may also be directed against self-antigens that could lead to autoimmune disease.[11,17,18–23]

ACUTE PHASE RESPONSE

Wannemacher et al.[24] isolated a protein from leukocytes and named it leukocytic endogenous mediator (LEM). It stimulates the uptake of amino acids by the liver in adrenalectomized (ADX), hypophysectomized (hypox), thyroidectomized, and diabetic rats. Similar stimulation could not be duplicated by pharmacological doses of a large variety of hormones. LEM augmented RNA synthesis and enhanced the hepatic production of a number of acute phase plasma globulins. Because the best known experimental model of APR is the syndrome elicited by bacterial endotoxin, we discuss first the characteristics of this reaction.

RESPONSE TO BACTERIAL ENDOTOXIN

Lipopolysaccharide (LPS), also known as *endotoxin,* is a constant component of the outer cell membranes of Gram-negative bacteria. Biochemically it can be divided into polysaccharide and lipid regions. The core glycolipid, *lipid A,* and the core polysaccharide are *obligatory components* of the bacterial cell wall; mutants lacking this component are not viable.

In contrast, polysaccharide chain sugars show great variation. They differ from one bacterial strain to another and provide epitopes for adaptive immune reactions and for the serological classification of Gram-negative bacteria.[25] The capsular polysaccharides present in bacteria, forming "smooth" colonies and providing the so-called K antigens and O-specific polysaccharides of LPS, contain *heterologous epitopes.* These are recognized specifically by the adaptive immune system according to the individual bacterial strains. On the other hand, lipid A is highly conserved evolutionarily and shows extensive cross-reactivity among all Gram-negative bacterial strains, whether pathogenic or saprophytic. This antigenic determinant may be classified as a *homologous epitope* or *homotope* for short. Lipid A is recognized by both the natural and the adaptive immune systems. It is possible to produce anti-lipid A antibodies, including monoclonal antibodies, with deliberate immunization.[7,25]

It has long been established that lipid A is a toxic moiety of endotoxin that is capable of a massive activation of the immune system and, in turn, immune-derived cytokines may induce shock and death.[12] Lipopolysaccharide binding protein (LBP) is present in the serum, which is produced by the liver. LBP has been identified in the sera of multiple species including rabbits, rats, mice, pigs, cattle, non-human primates, and humans. It combines with lipid A after Gram-negative infection or LPS injection.[26] LBP is a 60-kDa glycoprotein present in normal serum at concentrations of 0.5 to 10 μg/ml, and its level may surpass 200 μg/ml during APR.[27] Its specificity is directed toward the hydrophobic lipid A portion of LPS with an affinity of 10^{-9} M for both smooth and rough forms of LPS.[28]

LBP acts as an opsonin for LPS-bearing particles by enhancing its interaction with the CD14 cell surface molecules present on the surfaces of monocytes, macrophages, and neutrophilic granulocytes. LBP serves as a lipid transfer protein that facilitates the rate of transfer of LPS to CD14. This enables a cell to respond to extremely low levels of LPS that otherwise are unable to elicit a biological response.[29] Another serum protein that mediates LPS recognition by CD14 is septerin.[30]

CD14 is a 55-kDa glycoprotein present on the surfaces of monocytes, macrophages, and neutrophils. It lacks a transmembrane sequence.[31] CD14 plays an important role in mediating the induction of cytokines by LPS such as tumor necrosis factor-α (TNFα), IL-6, and IL-8, in monocytes and macrophages. 1-25-Dehydroxyvitamin D_3 (VD$_3$) induced CD14 expression in a premonocytic cell line. IL-4 decreased CD14 expression, and IL-4 or interferon-γ (IFN-γ) inhibited soluble CD14 release by monocytes. TNFα and LPS enhanced CD14 expression by monocyte cell lines. In human neutrophils, TNFα, granulocyte-macrophage colony stimulating factor (GM-CSF), G-CSF, and formyl peptide all increased CD14 expression. In addition to mediating the LPS response, CD14 appears to participate in diverse cellular responses that involve cell-to-cell contact.[32]

The serum concentration of CD14 in normal human plasma is 6 μg/ml; it increases in hospitalized patients, especially in those suffering from autoimmune disease. LPS and TNF increase the release of CD14, whereas IL-4 decreases its release *in vitro* from normal peripheral blood monocytes. Soluble CD14 inhibits the biological activities of LPS and is assumed to present LPS to endothelial cells.[32] Toll-like receptor 4 is required for signal transduction by complexes of LPS and membrane-bound CD14, which leads to nuclear factor (NF)κB activation.[33] Serum CD14 is an acute phase protein and its production is stimulated by IL-6 in the liver.[34]

The sensitivity to LPS toxicity differs considerably among various species of mammals. Lower vertebrates such as frogs and fish show extreme resistance.[35] Nevertheless, some observations suggest that at least some species of fish (*Tilapia oreochnomis mossanbicus* and Teleosti) react to LPS and show integumental and cortisol responses.[36] In contrast, the horseshoe crab (*Limulus polyphemus*) responds to LPS with fatal intravascular coagulation. This is due to the activation by endotoxin of a clottable protein of Limulus blood produced by circulating amebacytes.[37-39]

It seems apparent that lipid A has no inherent toxicity, but is rather a highly conserved *homologous epitope* that was singled out during evolution by vertebrate and some invertebrate animals for defense against Gram-negative bacterial infections.[7,35,40] Lipid A — the specific *homotope* involved — is recognized by serum proteins and cell surface receptors that are capable of activating the coagulation and complement systems and various members of the leukocyte series. This enables an animal to mount a rapid and effective immune defense reaction against all Gram-negative pathogens.[7-12]

In mice, approximately 7% of genes are mobilized during hepatic APR response to LPS. The extensive metabolic adjustments include suppression of pathways for cholesterol, fatty acid, and phospholipid synthesis. Increased expression of genes for innate defense was accompanied by coordinate induction of the major histocompatibility complex (MHC) class I antigen presentation machinery, illustrating an intersection of innate and adaptive immunity.[41]

Cytokine Response to Endotoxin

After systemic administration of LPS to mice, TNFα was significantly increased in the blood at 1 to 2 hours, followed by a decline; the TNF level returned to normal at around 4 hours. Exaggerated TNF responses occurred in adrenalectomized (ADX) animals. TNF levels in the plasma rose approximately 60 times higher and sensitivity to the lethal effects of TNF increased approximately 500 times over levels observed in normal control animals after LPS injection. This excessive response and increased mortality can be prevented if the animals are pretreated with dexamethasone. The inhibition of cortisone synthesis in the adrenals by metyrapone also led to increased susceptibility (~15 times) to LPS.[40-42] Similar kinetics of TNF release appeared in humans after LPS infusion.[44]

Interleukin-1 also rose in the blood of mice after endotoxin administration, reaching the maximum at about 4 hours; elevated levels remained up to 24 hours.[43,44] Circulating IL-6 increased significantly after LPS administration. In humans, IL-6 peaked at 120 minutes after LPS administration and was not inhibited by glucocorticoids or repeated LPS administration.[11,45,46]

Leukemia inhibitory factor (LIF) rose moderately in mice after sub-lethal injections of LPS and rose progressively during lethal septic shock induced by *Escherichia coli*.

LIF administered to mice induced catabolism and had a protective effect if given prior to the administration of the bacteria.[47]

Additional cytokines and mediators including interleukin-8,[48] interleukin-10,[49] interferon-γ,[50] TNF synthesis inhibitor,[51] interleukin receptor antagonist,[52] platelet activating factor, colony stimulating factor, prostaglandins, and thromboxanes[11,12,53] also play a role in endotoxin shock.

Neuroendocrine Response to Endotoxin

Wexler et al.[54] observed for the first time the stimulation of adrenocorticotropic hormone (ACTH) in rats by endotoxin as detected by the depletion of ascorbic acid and cholesterol in the adrenal glands. LPS was ineffective in causing these changes in the adrenal glands of hypophysectomized rats.

Endotoxin, infectious disease, and various forms of injury all elicit neuroendocrine responses via the stimulation of cytokines.[11,12] Profound changes occur in serum hormone levels. It is clear that dynamic and diurnal changes of hormones should be taken into consideration. Much remains to be elucidated about the significance of these hormonal alterations. Nevertheless, it is certain that the hypothalamus-pituitary-adrenal (HPA) axis exerts a powerful suppressive effect on the adaptive immune system and controls the levels of inflammatory cytokines. Through the activation of this axis, specific immune reactions are profoundly suppressed, whereas the induction of acute phase proteins in the liver and natural antibody production are augmented by glucocorticoids and catecholamines, which are also elevated.

Therefore, the conversion of the immune system from the adaptive mode of reactivity to the amplification of natural immunity is largely due to the activation of the HPA axis and of the sympathetic nervous system, e.g., sympathetic outflow.[12,54-57] Prolactin and growth hormone stimulate the adaptive immune system and usually rise within the first hour after endotoxin injection, followed by a decline; the level may become low normal to subnormal in serious cases of endotoxin shock. Luteinizing hormone (LH), follicle stimulating hormone (FSH), estrogens, androgens, progesterone, and thyroid hormones all decline during infection and endotoxin shock as a rule. Insulin, glucagon, α-melanocyte stimulating hormone (MSH), endorphin, leptin, corticotropin releasing hormone (CRH), and arginine vasopressin are increased during endotoxemia.[11,12,40,58-62] See Table 14.1 and Figure 14.1.

PRL receptor (PRLR) mRNA and protein levels were down-regulated in hepatic tissues after intraperitoneal (ip) LPS injection. A suppressive effect on mRNA expression was also observed in prostate, seminal vesicle, kidney, heart, and lung tissues. PRLR mRNA levels were increased in the thymus, and did not change in the spleen. The proportion of transcripts for the different receptor isoforms (long, S1, S2, and S3) in liver and thymus was not altered by LPS injection.[63]

Peripherally administered LPS induced anorexia, which is prevalent in females. Estradiol is capable of inducing this response. Estradiol affects meal frequency.[64] Hepatic dehydroepiandrosterone (DHEA) sulfotransferase (Sult2A1) activity and serum levels of DHEA sulfate were significantly decreased in LPS-treated animals. TNF and IL-1 caused a significant decrease in the mRNA level of Sult2A1 in Hep3B human hepatoma cells.[65]

TABLE 14.1
Major Neuroendocrine Changes Induced by Endotoxins

HPT and GLH	Responses	HPA Axis	Response	Gonadotropin Response
TRH ↑↓	↓	CRF	↑	LH
TSH ↓	0↓	VP/AVP	↑	FSH
T4 ↑↓	↓	ACTH	↑	E2
T3 ↑↓	↓	GC	↑	TS
PRL ↓?	↑↓	MSH	↑	DHEA
GH ↑↓	↑↓	END	↑	PS
IGF-I	↓	CAT	↑	
	IN	↑		
GLU	↑			
LEP	↑			

0 = no effect.
See list of abbreviations at end of chapter.

Source: Modified from Berczi, I. et al., Ann. NY Acad. Sci. 917, 248, 2001. (With permission.)

Endotoxin Shock

Geller et al.[66] observed that the administration of cortisone, a glucocorticoid (GC), to mice before or simultaneously with a lethal dose of LPS protected the majority of the animals from death. No protection ensued when cortisone was administered after LPS injection. The protective effect of GC against endotoxin shock has been observed repeatedly in various species.[67,68]

No correlation was found between TNF serum levels and the lethal effects induced by different types of LPS in rats.[69] The co-treatment of rats with low doses of TNF and LPS resulted in the rapid demise of the animals, leading to 100% mortality within 4 hours.[70] Pre-treatment of rats with a single low intravenous (iv) doses of TNF prevented subsequent death from a lethal dose of TNF or of LPS applied 24 hours later.[71] The lethal effect of endotoxin could be inhibited in various animal models by naloxone, an opioid antagonist, and also by indomethacin, monoclonal antibodies to TNFα, and pharmacological inhibition of platelet activating factor (PAF).[11] Anti-inflammatory cytokines such as the IL-1 receptor antagonist,[71] the TNF synthesis inhibitor,[72] IL-10,[73] and leukemia inhibitory factor[74] all participate in the down-regulation of the noxious effects of endotoxin. Interferon-γ antagonizes the development of endotoxin tolerance.[75]

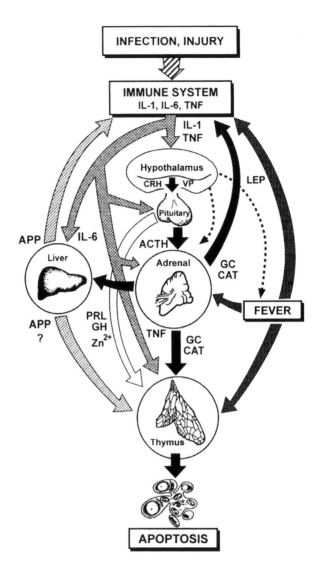

FIGURE 14.1 Immunoconversion during acute phase response (APR). APR is a systemic inflammatory reaction. Fever is a hallmark of the APR of febrile illness. Immune-derived cytokines, primarily IL-1, IL-6 and TNF-α, are released by the immune system and act either on nerve terminals or the brain. The cytokine signals eventually are registered in the hypothalamus and a powerful neuroendocrine and metabolic response to the infection or injury is initiated. Corticotrpoin releasing hormone (CRH) and vasopressin (VP) are secreted from the hypothalamus during APR. Both peptides stimulate the HPA axis. In addition, VP has the capacity to stimulate prolactin (PRL) secretion. Initially CRH prevails and activation of the HPA axis is dominant. This is coupled with sympathetic outflow from the adrenal gland. The increased levels of glucocorticoids (GC) and catecholamines (CAT) along with TNF-α are of prime importance for inducing thymus involution (e.g., by inducing apoptosis of CD8+4+ thymocytes)

In vitro observations revealed that the direct exposure of macrophages to LPS also led to decreased activation and cytokine production upon re-exposure to LPS.[76,77] Previte et al.[78] discovered that the exposure of endotoxin to ionizing radiation resulted in significant loss of toxicity. Subsequently Bertok and colleagues[79] demonstrated over a number of years that radiodetoxified endotoxin is capable of boosting host resistance against infectious agents, radiation, septic shock, tourniquet shock, intestinal ischemic shock, hemorrhagic shock, x-irradiation, and even against immunosuppression by anti-lymphocytic serum.[80,81] Radiodetoxified endotoxin has been tested clinically for the treatment of infectious disease in humans.[81] Monophosphoryl lipid A preparations of low toxicity were also studied in animals and humans related to boosting host resistance to infections and traumatic events.[82,83]

PATHOMECHANISMS OF APR

Clinically, APR is characterized by fever, loss of appetite, inactivity, and sleepiness. Changes in sleep are hallmarks of the acute phase response to infectious challenge. The regulation of these responses involves a cytokine cascade including IL-1, TNF, and several other substances such as growth hormone releasing hormone, PRL, nitric oxide, and NFκB within the brain. These substances are also involved in the regulation of normal spontaneous sleep.[84]

Cytokines and Hormones

Acute febrile illness (e.g., APR) is mediated by cytokines, GCs, and catecholamines. Cytokines appear in the circulation and function as acute phase hormones affecting the central nervous system (CNS), the neuroendocrine system, and virtually the functions of every other tissue and organ. IL-1, IL-6, and TNFα have been identified

FIGURE 14.1 **(Continued)** and inhibiting the T cell-dependent adaptive immune system. Other factors likely to contribute to this suppression are the down-regulation of growth hormone and prolactin synthesis and zinc deficiency. During APR, the synthesis of acute phase proteins (APP) is amplified in the liver by IL-6, GC, and CAT. Serum C-reactive protein (CRP) will increase as much as 1000 times the basal level within 24 to 48 hours. CRP is capable of recognizing pathogenic organisms and activating complement and leukocytes for phagocytosis and cytotoxicity. Other serum proteins with similar biology are lipopolysaccharide-binding protein (LBP) and mannan binging protein (MBP). Additional acute phase proteins (APP) are fibrinogen and a number of anti-inflammatory and enzyme inhibitory proteins that also increase in serum during APR. Natural antibodies that are poly-specific (similarly to CRP LBP, and MBP) are also stimulated during APR and serve to identify pathogenic agents, followed by immune activation. The essence of febrile illness is to switch the immune system from the adaptive (T cell-dependent) mode of reactivity to the activation of innate/natural immune mechanisms. The process is called *immunoconversion*. During the chronic phase of inflammmatory disease, CRH will subside and VP will take over regulation of the HPA axis. Because VP also stimulates PRL secretion, it is hypothesized that VP alters the neuroendocrine milieu to favor restoration of adaptive immunocompetence. This process is called *immunoreversion* and it leads to recovery from acute illness.

as major mediators of the endocrine and metabolic changes characteristic of APR. However, several other cytokines have been found to be inducers of acute phase proteins (APPs).[7,9,12,85] ACTH and GC, leptin (LEP), epinephrine (EP), norepineprine (NEP), glucagon (GLN), vasopressin (VP), and aldosterone (ALD) are elevated during the APR, whereas growth hormone (GH), prolactin (PRL), estrogens, androgens, insulin (IN), and thyroid hormones may be either elevated or suppressed, depending on the severity of the condition.[7-12,85,86]

A subset of marrow-derived brain macrophages, known as *perivascular cells*, synthesize prostanoids after systemic cytokine or endotoxin challenges. These brain macrophages are critically involved in the IL-1-induced HPA axis activation. This suggests a two-way interaction between perivascular and endothelial cells in monitoring circulating cytokine signals.[87]

In most burn patients, bone density dropped significantly 6 and 12 months post-injury, indicating bone resorption. Cortisol was elevated, both in blood and in urine (free cortisol). Very low testosterone, dihydrotestosterone (DHT), and free testosterone levels were found in the blood of males, but not of females. 17β-Estradiol was elevated in many burned males, but was generally normal in burned females. DHEA-S levels were generally low. Triiodothyronine (T3) and free thyroxine (FT4) were very low. Increased and even very high PTH values were occasionally present. hGH and IGF-1 were generally normal. Total and ionized calcium levels were low after burn; 25-0H vitamin D was usually low or low normal. Osteocalcin levels were initially low to low normal, and later increased to normal levels. In most instances, elevated levels of TNFα, IL-2, IL-6, and IL-8 levels were found. The use of anabolics, of vitamin D, calcium, and calcitonin was suggested for treatment.[88]

During APR (e.g., sepsis), the serum level of leptin rises rapidly. Cytokines, especially TNFα, cause this elevation. LEP inhibits glucocorticoid and IL-6 production. The levels of LEP in serum correlate positively with the survival of patients with septicemia. LEP stimulates the production of IL-1 receptor antagonist, which protects against LPS toxicity in mice. LEP stimulated the production of IL-1β in murine glial cells. Exogenous LEP up-regulated both phagocytosis and the production of pro-inflammatory cytokines in animals. Leptin is also involved in wound healing and angiogenesis.[89-98] Chronic leptin deficiency in *ob/ob* mice interfered with adequate control of zymosan-induced arthritis.[98]

Acute Phase Proteins

An alteration of protein synthesis by the liver is most characteristic for APR. The synthesis of acute phase proteins (APPs) is initiated, whereas the synthesis of some normal serum constituents such as albumin and transferrin is decreased. The concentration of APP increased dramatically in serum. For example, in humans, C-reactive protein (CRP) and serum amyloid A (SAA) may increase over 1000-fold within 24 to 48 hours. Fibrinogen, 1-antitrypsin, and certain complement and properdin components (factor B and C3) show a more moderate increase.[7,12] In humans, IL-6 exerted a hyperglycemic effect, whereas IL-2 induced a decrease in blood glucose concentration.[100]

CRP binds to C-type pneumococcal cell walls in the presence of Ca^{2+}. CRP has been identified in multiple species, including mammals, chickens, fish, and crabs. In the serum, CRP consists of five identical subunits that form a ring-shaped molecule named pentraxin. This term now also stands for a protein family. Human serum amyloid P also belongs to this family. The mature subunits consist of 206 amino acids with 23 kDa molecular weight.[101]

CRP recognizes specifically several homotopes, such as phosphocholine, with polysaccharides containing galactose, with some biologic polycations, such as protamine, poly-L-lysin and with myelin basic protein. CRP is in its pentameric form, if Ca^{2+} is present and binds phosphocholine and galactans, whereas in the absence of Ca^{2+}, it becomes monomeric and binds various polycations.

These homotope determinants are frequently present on the surfaces of bacteria, fungi, parasites, and damaged cells and tissues. After combination with the specific ligand, CRP activates complement by the classical pathway, induces chemotaxis, and enhances phagocytosis by neutrophilic leukocytes and monocytes and elicits tumoricidal activity in macrophages, all of which are complement-dependent. In addition, CRP stimulates the synthesis of IL-1 and TNFα, and potentiates the cytotoxic activities of T lymphocytes, natural killer (NK) cells, and platelets. CRP localizes *in vivo* at sites of inflammation. It binds platelet activating factor (PAF) and blocks its activity. The clinical determination of CRP is diagnostic for the presence of infectious and inflammatory disease.[101–104]

CRP influences polymorphonuclear (PMN) cell adhesion and migration and expression of CD11b/CD18 and fibronectin receptors. It can modulate the action of IL-8 on PMN attachment to endothelium and fibronectin, and on PMN traffic through the extracellular matrix during transendothelial migration.[105]

Upon denaturation or after attachment onto polystyrol plates, free CRP subunits attain a third conformation referred to as neoCRP. NeoCRP is a membrane protein on NK cells and macrophages and functions as galactose-specific receptor. It also accumulates at injured sites of tissue. Monocytes and macrophages express a specific CRP receptor. Proteolytic fragments of CRP activate macrophages and neutrophils.[101] Human CRP protected mice from an otherwise lethal *Streptococcus pneumoniae* infection.[104]

LBP shows a 100-fold increase (from 0.5 to 50 µg/ml) in serum during an APR. LBP is capable of opsonizing LPS-bearing particles, and thus may be required for the activation of complement by endotoxin through the alternate pathway. LBP–LPS complexes are also potent stimulators of cytokines from monocytes and macrophages after combining with CD14 on the surfaces of these cells.[26]

High-dose LBP (hd-LBP) suppressed the binding of both R-type and S-type LPS to CD14 and inhibited LPS-induced nuclear translocation of NFκB in humans. This inhibitory effect of serum could be mimicked by purified high-density lipoprotein (HDL) in serum-free medium, indicating an LBP-mediated transfer of preferentially S-type LPS to plasma lipoproteins such as HDL.[106]

Haptoglobin is an acute phase protein that binds hemoglobin, thus preventing iron loss and renal damage. It is an antioxidant, has antibacterial activity, and plays a role in modulating many aspects of the APR.[107] Haptoglobin selectively antagonized LPS effects *in vitro* by suppressing monocyte production of TNFα, IL-10, and

IL-12, but failed to inhibit the production of IL-6, IL-8, and IL-1 receptor antagonist. Haptoglobin knockout mice were more sensitive to LPS effects than their wild-type counterparts.[108]

The acute phase proteins α1-acid glycoprotein and α1-antitrypsin exert anti-apoptotic and anti-inflammatory effects and contribute to the delayed type of protection associated with ischemic preconditioning in the kidney and in other insults.[109]

Mannose-binding lectin (MBL) is a serum protein characterized by both collagenous regions and lectin domains; it plays an important role in innate immune defense. It binds to the repeating sugar arrays on many microbial surfaces through multiple lectin domains. Following binding, MBL is able to activate the complement system via an associated serum protease, MASP-2. There is an increased incidence of infections in individuals with mutations of MBL and an association with the systemic lupus erythematosus (SLE) and rheumatoid arthritis autoimmune disorders.[110] MBL activates the complement cascade and inflammation following binding to carbohydrate structures. The serum concentration of MBL is subject to large individual differences. Growth hormone influences MBL levels.[111]

Mouse MBL-A and MBL-C were studied in various strains and in APR. The MBL-A and MBL-C levels in 10 laboratory mice strains were found to vary from 4 µg/ml to 12 µg/ml and from 16 µg/ml to 118 µg/ml, respectively. After the induction of APR by ip injection of casein or LPS, MBL-A was found to increase approximately two-fold, with a maximum after 32 hours; MBL-C did not increase significantly. Serum amyloid A peaked at 15 hours with an approximate 100-fold increase.[112]

Other APP are proteinase inhibitors, such as α2-macroglobulin, α1-acid glycoprotein, antithrombin III, α1-acute phase globulin, and α1-proteinase inhibitor that are abundant in rats. Kupffer cells stimulate α2-macroglobulin synthesis by hepatocytes *in vitro* in the presence of 10^{-9} M DEX. Fibrinogen is also an APP with an important role in blood clotting and healing. α-Macrofetoprotein (α-MFP) is a strong inhibitor of inflammatory mediators such as histamine, bradykinin, serotonin, and PGE2 and also inhibits polymorphonuclear chemotaxis.[113]

Regulation of APP Production

Catecholamines and GC induce α-MFP in normal rats. The α-MFP levels induced by catecholamines (CATs) were very high, comparable to those observed in the post-injury phase, whereas the effect of GC was moderate. In ADX rats, the effect of CAT on α-MFP synthesis was greatly diminished, whereas the moderate effect of GC remained. The combination of GC and CAT induced extremely high α-MFP levels in ADX animals. Other APPs such as haptoglobin and α1-major acute phase protein were affected differently by these hormones.[114]

Glucocorticoids (GCs) exert a stimulatory effect on a variety of inflammatory response components. This is usually observed at near-basal GC concentrations. For example, such stimulation was observed for the hepatic APR, for cytokine secretion, expression of cytokine/chemokine receptors, and for the pro-inflammatory mediator, macrophage migration inhibition factor.[115]

IL-1 and TNF induced a full range of APPs *in vivo*, but only a limited number of APPs were induced by these cytokines in cultured liver cells compared with crude cytokine preparations from macrophages. This led to the discovery of IL-6 as a major inducer of APP synthesis. Additional cytokines, namely IFN-γ, leukemia inhibitory factor, TGF-β, and oncostatin M, were found to be active as direct inducers of APP from the liver. IL-6 activates the genes of APP through the DNA binding protein called NF-IL-6. NF-IL-6 is a pleiotropic mediator of many inducible genes involved in the acute, immune, and inflammatory responses, similarly to NFκB. Both NF-IL-6 and NFκB binding sites are present in the inducible genes such as IL-6, IL-8 and several acute phase genes.[116] In rats, adrenalin evokes a high level of IL-6 that can be antagonized by propranolol. When IL-6 release is blocked, the fast reacting APP, α2-macroglobulin, and cysteine protease inhibitor are strongly depressed. Isoprenalin, a β2-adrenergic receptor agonist, also causes very high levels of IL-6, indicating that β2 receptors are involved.[117]

During chronic liver injury induced by biweekly application of CCl_4, deletion of the gp130 receptor in nonparenchymal liver cells (and not hepatocytes) resulted in fibrosis progression. This indicates the involvement of IL-6 in the pathogenesis of liver diseases and suggests a protective role of IL-6/gp130-dependent pathways in nonparenchymal liver cells during fibrosis progression in chronic liver disease.[118]

The relationship between spontaneously occurring activation of the acute phase response and leptin levels were examined in 29 chronic hemodialysis patients. When CRP was elevated, leptin levels were significantly reduced, as were the negative acute phase proteins albumin and transferrin. Serum amyloid A, ceruloplasmin, α-(1)-acid glycoprotein, and IL-6 were all significantly increased at the maximum CRP level, compatible with general activation of the acute phase response. The change in leptin correlated negatively with the change in CRP, as did changes in albumin.[119] Pro-inflammatory cytokines, especially TNFα, induce inflammatory hyperleptinemia. This is an integral part of APR and necessary for comprehensive immunocompetence. It indicates the existence of an integrated communication network to coordinate the energy status of an animal with the ability to fight pathogens.[120]

The thymus is severely affected by stress and APR. This rapidly leads to the loss of thymocytes manifesting in profound involution. The thymus is a central primary lymphoid organ responsible for the generation of mature, functional, thymus-derived (T) lymphocytes. In turn T lymphocytes govern adaptive immune reactions through their regulatory function. The thymus also exerts endocrine functions, the significance of which is not yet fully appreciated. A large body of evidence attests to a complex neuroendocrine control of thymus physiology and consistent observations indicate that the thymus becomes involuted during the stress response. During stress, and more forcefully during APR, the HPA axis is activated. This results in the suppression of the T cell-dependent adaptive immune response supported further by the suppression of the hormones essential for the maintenance of the thymus and of T lymphocytes, e.g., PRL, GH, and IGF-I. Catecholamines and glucocorticoids released in large quantities during APR induce apoptosis in the thymus with striking efficiency. The elevated level of TNFα and zinc deficiency that develop during APR also contribute to thymic involution and to the suppression of the adaptive immune system (Figure 14.1).[9]

Cytokine-induced hyperlipoproteinemia, clinically designated the lipemia of sepsis, represents an innate, non-adaptive host immune response to infection. Triglyceride (TG)-rich lipoproteins (VLDL and chylomicrons [CMs]) bind and neutralize LPS.

CM-bound LPS attenuates the hepatocellular response to pro-inflammatory cytokines. Primary rodent hepatocytes pretreated with CM-LPS complexes for 2 hours
demonstrated a near 70% reduction in cytokine-induced nitric oxide (NO). The
lipemia of sepsis likely represents a mechanism by which the host combats sporadic,
non-life-threatening episodes of endotoxemia. Also, it may indicate a negative regulatory mechanism for the hepatic response to sepsis, serving to effectively down-
regulate the acute phase response.[121]

The multiple organ failure induced by critical illness was suggested to be a primarily
functional, rather than structural, abnormality with a potentially protective mechanism.
The decline in organ function is triggered by decreases in mitochondrial activity and
in oxidative phosphorylation, leading to reduced cellular metabolism. This may be the
consequence of acute phase changes in hormones and inflammatory mediators.[122]

RECOVERY FROM ACUTE PHASE RESPONSE

Most people develop febrile illnesses on numerous occasions during a lifetime. These
febrile episodes normally subside and are followed by healing and return to health
and to normal adaptive immunocompetence. We now understand how the APR
develops and what it does, but we know little about the recovery phase. We would
expect that in accord with the tight neuroendocrine regulation of APR, the recovery
phase also would be regulated by neuroendocrine mechanisms. Some recent observations on the role of vasopressin in immune function and in APR provide indications
of the mechanism of recovery known as *immunoreversion*.

Vasopressin is primarily a neurohypophysial hormone, produced in magnocel-
lular neurones of the hypothalamic paraventricular and supraoptic nuclei, but parvocellular CRH neurones also co-express VP. VP acts as a second releasing factor
for ACTH along with CRH. Aminergic, cholinergic, GABAergic, glutamatergic, and
peptidergic inputs have all been implicated in the regulation of CRH/VP neurones.
VP is also expressed within the immune system.[123,124]

Vasopressin in Acute Phase Response

The activation of the HPA axis has a fundamental role in the stress response. Stressors
increase the secretion of epinephrine and norepinephrine from the sympathetic
nervous system and adrenal medulla and the release of CRH and VP from parvice-
llular neurons into the portal circulation. These processes are followed seconds later
by the secretion of ACTH, leading to secretion of GC by the adrenal gland. CRH
coordinates the endocrine, autonomic, behavioral, and immune responses to stress
and also acts as a neurotransmitter or neuromodulator in the amygdala, dorsal raphe
nucleus, hippocampus, and locus ceruleus.

Vasopressin, serotonin (5-hydroxytryptamine or 5-HT), and catecholamines
are additional classical mediators. Other neuropeptides/neuromodulators involved are
substance P, vasoactive intestinal polypeptide, neuropeptide Y, and cholecystokinin.
Cytokines such as interleukin-1 stimulate CRH and vasopressin gene expression, and
are implicated in immune–neuroendocrine regulation. Expression profiles of the CRH
and VP genes are not uniform after stress exposure, and the VP gene appears to be

more sensitive to glucocorticoid suppression.[124,125] Cytokine-induced CRF and VP synthesis and/or release are modulated by catecholamines, prostaglandins (PGs), and NO.[126]

In Lewis rats, IL-1 priming markedly suppressed the neurological symptoms of experimental allergic encephalomyelitis (EAE), without affecting the onset or duration of the disease. Measurement of VP and CRH in the external zone of the median eminence revealed that, as compared to Wistar rats, Lewis rats exhibited low vasopressin and identical CRH. IL-1 priming increased (0.001) vasopressin without affecting CRH stores; this is consistent with a shift to vasopressin-dominated control of ACTH secretion as described in Wistar rats under conditions of HPA hyper(re)activity. IL-1 priming of Lewis rats attenuated the ACTH responses to an IL-1 challenge 11 days later, which may relate to an increase in resting corticosterone levels. There was no effect on immune reactivity. The conclusion is that IL-1-induced elevation of resting corticosterone levels may influence the development of EAE.[127]

Total contents of immunoreactive (ir)-CRH in the spleen and thymus were not altered following the induction of arthritis, although a significant decrease was observed in splenic extracts from arthritis rats compared to controls. Low levels of VP were also detected in immune tissues, with contents significantly increased in spleens from arthritis animals, compared to controls. Thymic contents of VP were not altered by arthritis.[128]

Elevated plasma VP levels were noted in seven patients with status asthmaticus during the acute illness. These values returned to normal with resolution of the disease.[129]

Thirteen patients with multiple sclerosis (MS) were studied at baseline and with provocative tests of HPA axis function (ovine CRH, VP, and ACTH stimulation). Compared to matched controls, patients with MS had significantly higher plasma cortisol levels at baseline. Despite this, patients with MS showed normal, rather than blunted, plasma ACTH responses to ovine CRH. They had blunted ACTH responses to VP stimulation and normal cortisol responses to high and low dose ACTH stimulation.[130]

Plasma VP values were significantly higher during pneumonia than after recovery. A positive correlation between plasma VP and minimum urine osmolality was found during pneumonia. These defects varied in severity, depending on the extent of the pneumonia, and persisted until clearing of alveolar opacities, accounting for the protracted courses in some patients.[131]

Vasopressin in Chronic Inflammation and Stress

In Sprague–Dawley (SD), and Piebald–Viral–Glaxo (PVG) rats that had been immunized to induce adjuvant arthritis (AA), VP increased in portal blood continuously from day 7 through 11 and day 16 through 21, which was coincident with the progression of inflammation in the PVG rats. VP, but not CRF mRNA, was increased in the medial parvocellular divisions of the hypothalamic paraventricular nuclei (PVN) of arthritic SD rats. CRF binding was decreased and VP binding was increased to anterior pituitary membranes, indicating changes in receptor expression. Basal ACTH secretion *in vitro* was similar in both control and arthritic SD rats, but PVG rat pituitaries contained significantly more ACTH than the respective controls (436 ± 91 versus 167 ± 23 pg/tube). The ACTH responses of pituitaries of arthritic PVG rats to CRF or the combination of CRF and VP were significantly higher compared with the controls, although the ACTH responses of arthritic SD rat pituitaries were unchanged.[132]

During chronic inflammatory conditions, such as adjuvant-induced arthritis of rats, CRF does not act as the major ACTH-releasing factor. This is also true for EAE, eosinophilia myalgia syndrome, systemic lupus erythematosus, and leishmaniasis. During chronic inflammation, arginine vasopressin takes over as the major regulator of the HPA axis.[133]

A number of other studies support the importance of VP in the regulation of pituitary corticotrophs in chronic stress. Chronic intermittent exposure to immobilization, insulin-induced hypoglycemia, or psychological stress stimuli has been shown to increase the number of CRF cells containing VP and the ratio of VP to CRF within the zona externa of the median eminence.[134–137] In chronically restrained rats, exogenous VP but not CRF was found to increase plasma levels of both ACTH and corticosterone.[138]

Chronic inflammatory stress is associated with much larger stimulation of VP than other stress models. Activation of CRH does not appear to play a role under these conditions. However, only CRH (and not VP) can stimulate POMC transcription.[139] VP has been less potent than CRF in producing ACTH release from rat pituitaries. The effect of VP on CRF-mediated ACTH release is either synergistic or additive.[140,141]

Vasopressin and Cytokines

IL-1β (100 U/ml) significantly potentiated acetylcholine-induced VP release. This effect was completely blocked in the presence of neutralizing antibodies to IL-1β, atropine, or mecamylamine.[142] In IL-1β-treated rats, changes in body temperature and ventral septal area VP release were negatively correlated.[143] In male rats, the ACTH responses to IL-1β were significantly reduced by both anti-CRH and anti-VP antisera, compared to the levels after normal rabbit serum.[144] Similarly, in rats, IL-6-induced ACTH responses were significantly suppressed by both anti-CRH and anti-VP antibodies. The TNFα-induced ACTH responses were not significantly affected by anti-VP antibody, although anti-CRH antibody could suppress the response.[145] IL-6 potentiated acetylcholine-induced VP release in rats.[146]

A single injection of recombinant mouse IL-2 (rmIL-2) caused a significant increase in VP and oxytocin (OT) mRNA levels in the hypothalamus of nude mice. This effect was specific to nude mice.[147] IL-2 released VP from the hypothalamus and amygdala of rats *in vitro*. The IL-2-and acetylcholine-induced VP release was antagonized by Ng-methyl-L-arginine, indicating a role for NO in this VP release.[146] IL-2 caused a dose-dependent stimulation of VP, but not CRH, secretion from both the intact rat hypothalamus *in vitro* and hypothalamic cell cultures.[148] Centrally administered leukemia inhibitory factor significantly increased plasma VP concentrations from 5 to 60 minutes after injection.[149]

Mechanisms of Action of VP in APR

VP significantly attenuated the febrile responses of rabbits to bacterial pyrogen. As the body temperature rose in response to the pyrogen, the level of VP in the perfusate collected from the septal area decreased.[150] Endotoxin may stimulate endogenous pathways that lead to the generation of NO, which in turn inhibits CRH. In addition, it generates CO, which modulates the release of VP. These gases are thus potential counter-regulatory controls to the activation of the HPA.[151]

Inhibitors of phenylethanolamine-N-methyltransferase (PNMT) which are active either peripherally (SKF 29661) or both peripherally and centrally (SKF 64139), thus lowering epinephrine (EPI) synthesis] were studied. In adult male rats, SKF 64139 pretreatment significantly ($p < 0.05$) enhanced basal medial basal hypothalamus (MBH) and basal median eminence VP contents. LPS administration significantly ($p < 0.05$) decreased MBH AVP in CTRL and SKF-29661-pretreated rats and diminished ($p < 0.05$ versus basal values) ME AVP in all groups.[152]

In rats, 3 to 4 hours following iv LPS injection (100 µg/kg), CRH gene transcription was up-regulated in the PVN. Transcripts of CRH receptors type A were present in the hypothalamus 6 hours after endotoxin treatment. However, no alterations in cytoplasmic VP mRNA levels were noted in rats injected with LPS. Because the dose of LPS we used stimulates ACTH secretion within 30 minutes, our results suggest that systemic LPS acts first within the median eminence, where it stimulates peptidic nerve terminals.[153]

In alert, normally behaving ewes, endotoxin potently stimulated CRH and VP secretion into portal blood of the pituitary gland, and cortisol and progesterone into peripheral blood. Both CRH and VP generally rose and fell simultaneously, although the peak of the VP response was approximately 10-fold greater than that of CRH. This stimulation coincided with significant suppression of GnRH and LH pulsatile secretion in these same ewes and with the generation of fever.[154]

In Holstein steers, LPS increased body temperature, plasma ACTH and cortisol ($p < 0.05$). Abundance of anterior pituitary VP receptor V3 mRNA was decreased at 2, 4, and 12 hours following LPS administration ($p < 0.05$) and returned to basal by 24 hours. A similar temporal regulation of pituitary CRFR1 mRNA ($p < 0.05$), but not pituitary pro-opiomelanocortin (POMC) mRNA, was observed following LPS administration. Similar down-regulation of CRFR1 mRNA was not observed in other brain regions (cerebellum, hypothalamus) following LPS administration.[155]

Regulation of Pituitary Hormones by Vasopressin

The ACTH response to exogenous administration of VP was impaired in V1bR–/– mice, while CRH-stimulated ACTH release in V1bR–/– mice was not significantly different from that in the V1bR+/+ mice. VP-induced ACTH release from primary cultured pituitary cells in V1bR–/– mice was also blunted. The increase in ACTH after a forced swim stress was significantly suppressed in V1bR–/– mice.[156]

In conscious male rats, icv infusion of histamine (HA)-induced PRL secretion was inhibited by pretreatment with a specific antiserum to VP. A VP antagonist also inhibited the PRL response to HA and inhibited the PRL response to restraint stress. In contrast, pretreatment with a specific oxytocin (OT) antagonist had no effect on the HA- or stress-induced PRL release.[157] Vasopressin antiserum (VP-Ab) was administered iv to lactating rats 15 minutes before permitting their previously isolated pups to suckle and to continuously suckled rats. The suckling-induced rise in plasma PRL levels was significantly less in VP-Ab-treated mothers when compared to rats receiving similar amounts of normal rabbit serum (NRS).[158]

Anterior pituitary cells derived from juvenile female turkeys were incubated with posterior pituitary extracts or test substances for 3 hours. Posterior pituitary extracts contained potent substances that stimulated PRL release in a concentration-dependent manner. Antisera to VP and vasoactive intestinal peptide (VIP) (1:500) completely abolished the PRL-releasing activities of their respective peptides but partially reduced (p <0.05) the PRF activity of the posterior pituitary.[159]

CRH or VP released ACTH and immunoreactive β-endorphin (β-ENDir) in response to histamine and restraint stress. Pretreatment with CRH antiserum abolished the ACTH response to stress and inhibited the β-ENDir response by 60%. Immunoneutralization with VP antiserum had only half the inhibitory effect of that seen with CRH antiserum. CRH (100 pmol iv) increased the plasma levels of ACTH and β-ENDir. This effect was abolished by pretreatment with CRH antiserum, whereas pretreatment with VP antiserum prevented the CRH-induced ACTH release and inhibited the β-ENDir response by 50%. VP (24 to 800 pmol iv) stimulated ACTH and β-ENDir in a dose-dependent manner. CRH or VP antisera prevented the effect of VP (800 pmol) on ACTH secretion, whereas the β-ENDir response to VP was only inhibited by about 60% by the antisera.[157]

Endogenous oxytocin plays a role in the control of basal GH release, probably by stimulating somatostatin secretion and/or inhibiting GH-releasing hormone secretion. Endogenous VP and oxytocin play a physiologically significant stimulatory role in the control of basal ACTH release.[160]

The novel high-affinity non-peptide CRH 1 receptor antagonist R121919 significantly inhibits stress-induced corticotropin release and displays anxiolytic effects in rats selectively bred for high anxiety-related behavior. R121919 attenuates the stress-induced release of corticosterone, prolactin, and oxytocin. Moreover, the decrease in plasma testosterone following exposure to stress is abolished by R121919. Our data indicate that antagonism of CRH 1 receptors may prevent stress-associated endocrine alterations.[161] In rats with paraventricular nucleus lesions, LPS was able to activate the hypophysial–adrenal system in the absence of hypophysiotrophic neuropeptides of paraventricular origin.[162]

Vasopressin and Immune Response

Morphofunctional immune disorders were revealed in vasopressin-deficient Brattleboro rats with diabetes insipidus during ontogeny. Permanent decreases in the number of blood lymphocytes, increases in neutrophil count, reduced activities of macrophages, early involution of the thymus and spleen, and suppression of antibody production were observed.[163] Brattleboro (DI) rats are homozygous for diabetes insipidus. They lack vasopressin and were derived from Long–Evans (LE) rats. NK cell activity in DI rats was significantly higher than in LE rats. Vasopressin replacement normalized water intake in DI rats, but had no significant effect on NK cell activity. DI rats exhibited lower plasma corticosterone levels that were not elevated by vasopressin replacement. The results suggest that the lack of vasopressin in DI rats elevates baseline NK cell activity, probably via mechanisms that are secondary to the vasopressin deficiency (e.g., lower corticosterone levels).[164]

In mice with the disruption of the VP receptor 1a (v1a) gene, a shift from IgM(high)/IgD(high) to the more mature IgM(low)/IgD(high) B cells, splenic B cells proliferation was significantly greater in response to anti-IgM stimulation, and enhanced IgG1 and IgG2b production in response to immune challenge with T-dependent antigen was demonstrated. B-1 cells were increased in v1a(−/−) mice. T cell differentiation and activation were normal in v1a(−/−) mice.[165]

The AVP-binding nonapeptide has the sequence Thr-Met-Lys-Val-Leu-Thr-Gly-Ser-Pro (binding peptide). AVP and its 6-amino acid N-terminus cyclic ring pressinoic acid (PA) are both capable of replacing the IL-2 requirement for IFN- production by mouse splenic lymphocytes. We showed that the AVP-binding peptide specifically and reversibly blocks AVP help in IFN- production, but fails to block the helper signal of PA. Thus the intact AVP molecule and not just the N-terminal cyclic ring is important for interaction with the binding peptide.[166,167] VP enhances the autologous mixed lymphocyte response. Enhanced proliferation appears to be a specific response influenced by arginine residues in position 8 of this nonapeptide.[168]

In rats, the icv administration of VP suppressed the proliferative responses of splenic T cells and NK cytotoxicity in an adrenal-independent manner. These effects were completely reversed by icv preadministration of the V1 receptor antagonist.[169] V1 vasopressin receptor agonist (V1 agonist) induces a complex intracellular Ca^{2+} signaling cascade in cortical astrocytes. V1 agonist dramatically decreased the mRNA level of five cytokines. IL-1β and TNFα expression was confirmed with reverse transcriptase PCR. IL-1β and TNFα secretion was also decreased in response to V1 agonist.[170]

Our Observations

We investigated the effect of NIL on immune function in rats. NIL rats have low plasma levels of VP and oxytocin.[171,172] In NIL animals, the adrenal glands were enlarged, whereas the thymuses and spleens decreased in size in some experiments but not in others (Organista-Espartz et al.[173] and Quintanar-Stephano unpublished observations). If thyroidectomies were performed in NIL animals, the increases in adrenal weight and decreases in thymus and spleen weights were exaggerated (Table 14.2). In addition, NIL inhibited immune function including the decreased antibody IgG and IgM responses to sheep red blood cells[174] and to *Salmonella typhimurium* (Campos et al., unpublished data), and delayed type cell-mediated immunity to dinitrochlorobenzene and the Arthus reaction.[175] Decreased incidence and severity of EAE[176] and decreased incidence of adjuvant-induced arthritis were also observed in NIL animals.

We also studied the effects of desmopressin, a synthetic analog of VP, on immune responses and on the HPA axis activity during EAE. The results showed that (1) DP treatment restores immune function in NIL animals; (2) the decreased incidence and severity of the EAE by the NIL is accompanied by an unresponsive HPA axis; and (3) DP treatment restores the susceptibility of the NIL animals to EAE and stimulates the HPA axis. Thus a high clinical score of EAE is accompanied by high ACTH and corticosterone plasma levels.[174]

Comments

This survey indicates that VP participates in immunoregulation, both by regulating pituitary hormones and by direct effect on immunocytes. It seems certain that VP is required for the maintenance of adaptive immunocompetence. Growth and lactogenic

TABLE 14.2
Immunoregulation by Vasopressin

	Intact Control	Sham	Sham + DP	HYPOX	HYPOX + DP	NIL	NIL + DP	NIL + TX
Adrenal weight		≠	↑	↓↓↓	↓	←→	↑←	↑←
Thymus weight		≠	≠	→	↑ compared to HYPOX	↑→→	≠→	↓↓↓
Spleen weight		≠	↑↓	↓↓↓	↑ compared to HYPOX	↑→→	≠→	
Serum anti-SRBC agglutinin	↑←	↑←		→		→		
Serum anti-SRBC hemolysin	↑←	↑←		→		→		
Serum anti-SRBC IgG, IgM	↑←	↑←		→		→		
Arthus reaction (SRBC)	↑←	↑←		→		→		
Serum IgG and IgM and intestinal IgA anti-*S. typhi*								
Contact sensitivity to DNCB	↑←	↑←	→	→		→↓	←↑	
EAE: clinical score	↑←	↑←	←	←	↑↑↑	↓↓		
EAE: ACTH and corticosterone plasma levels		↑←	→	↓↓↓↓	↓↓↓	≠	↑	
Arthritis	↑←	≠		≠	≠	≠	≠	
Adeno-hypophyseal cell counts						GH↓ LH↓		TSH↑↑↑ GH↓↓↓ PRL↓↓↓

Abbreviations listed at end of chapter. See text for detailed explanation.

↑ = Increase compared to intact control or sham operated control.

↓ = Decrease in relation to controls.

≠ = No change with respect to controls.

↑↓ = Variable response.

GH, PRL, TSH, and LH producing cell types were detected by immunocytochemistry.

In long-surviving NIL rats (8 months), adrenal weight increased 30% whereas thymus weight decreased 50% when compared to intact control. Oral infection was used in experiments with *Salmonella typhimurium*.

hormones are responsible for the maintenance of thymus function and of the T cell-regulated adaptive immune system in a competent state. It is clear that VP has the capacity to stimulate both the HPA axis and PRL in a balanced fashion. This is in contrast with CRH which stimulates the HPA axis only.

In APR, CRH is dominant because of its resistance to GC inhibition, whereas VP is in the background. However, as established, during chronic inflammatory disease, VP will take over the regulation of the HPA axis. Moreover, VP has the capacity to stimulate PRL synthesis which is suppressed during APR. PRL is an important immunostimulant, and restores adaptive immunocompetence that sets the stage for recovery and healing. Additional studies are required to support this hypothesis.

CLINICAL RELEVANCE

In patients with APR, the GH-IGF-I axis is suppressed, growth hormone (GH) action is attenuated, and the adaptive immune response is grossly impaired.[177] These facts prompted clinical trials of GH treatment aimed at preventing the severe catabolic state and improving immunocompetence. Results to date are not encouraging. A controlled clinical trial on patients with acute critical illness showed that the proportion of patients who did not survive after GH treatment was significantly elevated.[178] Deaths attributed to "septic shock or uncontrolled infection" occurred nearly four times more often in GH-treated patients compared to placebos receiving controls. Although no data were given regarding immune parameters, the authors suggested that alterations in immune functions contributed to the fatalities.

Although there is no clear-cut consensus concerning the interpretation of this important clinical trial, one must keep in mind that patients with acute critical illness (APR) were involved. APR is a massive neuroimmune and metabolic response that mobilizes all the resources of the body in the interest of host defense and survival. The findings of Takala and colleagues[178] suggest strongly that the suppression of the GH-IGF-I axis in APR is required for intense catabolism to take place. A rapid release of nutrients and energy is necessary under these conditions in order to support maximally the defense system that includes the HPA axis, sympathetic nervous system, bone marrow, CD5+ B lymphocytes, leukocytes, and the liver.[7,9,10-12,85,86]

The adaptive immune system is controlled by thymus-derived (T) lymphocytes and it needs several days to a week to develop an effective response. During APR, no time is available for an adaptive immune reaction, and therefore this system is shut down, primarily by the cytokine and endocrine alterations that take place. Thymus and T cell function is heavily dependent on the GH/PRL/IGF-I axis and it is suppressed profoundly by elevated levels of glucocorticoids and catecholamines.[7,9,10-12,85,86] Recent observations showed that GH inhibits the production of acute phase proteins in rats with burn injuries and in human hepatocytes.[9,179,180] One may argue that the most efficient way to fuel the intensive systemic effort for survival in APR is the rapid breakdown of body tissues.

GH is a powerful anabolic hormone that supports the T lymphocyte-dependent immune system and acts as an antagonist of the HPA axis that promotes APR.[7,9,10-12,85,86,181,182] The results of this controlled trial support the hypothesis that the inhibition of the HPA axis and of catabolism by GH treatment in APR hampers the body's defense mechanisms, increasing susceptibility to infectious disease. This is supported by the studies of GH treatment of burn injuries discussed below.

However, GH as a potent anabolic hormone, can be administered with minimal risk of untoward side effects to children with burn injuries. GH reduces the catabolic effects of trauma through stimulation of protein synthesis. Accelerated wound healing and reduction in tissue wasting are clear benefits that reduce the overall morbidity associated with burn injuries in children.[183] Twenty-eight thermally injured children received either 0.2 mg/kg/day of recombinant human growth hormone (rHGH) or saline within 3 days of admission for at least 25 days. IGF-I and IGFBP-3 increased with rHGH treatment, whereas IGFBP-1 decreased in serum compared with placebo (p <0.05). Burned children treated with rHGH required significantly less albumin substitution and demonstrated decreases in serum CRP amyloid-A and increases in retinol-binding protein compared with placebo (p <0.05). rHGH decreased serum TNFα and IL-1β, whereas no changes were found for serum IL-1α, IL-6, and IL-10 compared with placebo (p <0.05). Free fatty acids were elevated in burned children who received rHGH (p <0.05).[184] Severely burned children receiving IGF-I/BP-3 showed decreases in IL-1β and TNFα, followed by decreases in type I APPs. This was associated with concomitant increases in constitutive hepatic proteins.[185]

GH attenuated IL-1β- or IL-6-induced APP gene expression associated with increased expression of SOCS-3. This study suggests that SOCS-3 plays an important role in the suppression of cytokine signaling by GH in down-regulating APR after injury.[186] Some hepatic acute phase and constitutive proteins remain abnormal even 2 years after injury. GH treatment during convalescence had no effect on hepatic APP changes.[187]

Insulin therapy exerts a powerful anti-inflammatory effect during critical illness; this at least partially explains improvements in morbidity and mortality. Possible adverse effects of low baseline mannose binding lectin are overcome by insulin therapy.[188] Insulin administration decreased pro-inflammatory cytokines and proteins while increasing constitutive hepatic proteins (p <0.05). Burned children receiving insulin required significantly less albumin substitution to maintain normal levels compared with control (p <0.05). Insulin decreased free fatty acids and serum triglycerides when compared with controls (p <0.05). Serum IGF-I and IGFBP-3 significantly increased with insulin administration (p <0.05).[189]

Growth factors such as recombinant human growth hormone, insulin-like growth factor-I, hepatocyte growth factor, and insulin exert anabolic effects and restore the inflammatory hepatic metabolism toward homeostasis during inflammation.[190] Fever has been associated with improved survival and shortened disease duration in non-life-threatening infections. However, the influence of fever and the effects of antipyresis in patients with sepsis has not been prospectively studied.[191] Elderly subjects showed more prolonged fever in response to LPS compared to young individuals. TNF, soluble TNF receptors (sTNFR-I), IL-6, IL-8, IL-10, and IL-1ra in plasma increased markedly in both groups. The elderly group showed larger initial increases in TNF and sTNFR-I levels and prolonged increased levels of sTNFR-I. Monocyte concentrations decreased in both groups, with the elderly group showing a more rapid decrease and a slower subsequent increase. The elderly group had more rapid increases in CRP than did the young group.[192]

Cachexia is the clinical consequence of a chronic systemic inflammatory response. The changes seen are multidimensional and highly coordinated. Most obvious is a redistribution of the body's protein content, with preferential depletion of skeletal muscle and an increase in the synthesis of APP involved in APR. The physiologic, metabolic, and behavioral changes of cachexia are tightly regulated by cytokines that signal the synthesis of APP as well as changes in intermediary metabolism that provide substrate and energy. The increase in the rate of protein degradation limits the ability of hypercaloric feeding to reverse the depletion of lean mass.[193]

The anorexia of infection is part of the host's APR that is beneficial in the beginning and deleterious if long lasting. Bacterial cell wall compounds (e.g., LPS, peptidoglycans), microbial nucleic acids, and viral glycoproteins trigger the APR and anorexia by stimulating the production of proinflammatory cytokines (e.g., interleukins, TNFα, interferons) that serve as endogenous mediators.

Cytokines increase leptin and may contribute to but are not essential for the anorectic effects of microbial products and cytokines. Cytokines can reach the CNS through the circumventricular organs and through active or passive transport mechanisms or they can act through receptors on endothelial cells of the brain vasculature and stimulate the release of subsequent mediators such as eicosanoids. De novo CNS cytokine synthesis also occurs in response to peripheral infections. The central mediators of anorexia during infection appear to be neurochemicals involved in the normal control of feeding, such as serotonin, dopamine, histamine, CRF, neuropeptide Y, and αMSH. Reciprocal, synergistic, and antagonistic interactions between various pleiotropic cytokines and between cytokines and neurochemicals form a complex network that mediates anorexia during infection.[194]

Other clinical conditions in which APR play a role are acute coronary syndromes,[195] obesity, sleep disturbance, depression, chronic fatigue, and low levels of physical activity.[196] In many people aging is associated with increased inflammatory activity, increased circulating levels of TNFα, IL-6, cytokine antagonists, and APPs.[197] The metabolic syndrome is characterized by cardiovascular and diabetes risk factors generally linked to insulin resistance, and obesity. Biological evidence suggests that chronic activation of the innate immune system may underlie the metabolic syndrome.[198] In 574 nondiabetic elderly men and women, insulin strongly and significantly (p <0.001) correlated with the markers of inflammation, C-reactive protein, α-1-antichymotrypsin, and IL-6, when adjusted for age and gender. Insulin also correlated with soluble ICAM-1. This indicates that low grade inflammation and the cellular adhesion molecule soluble ICAM-1 are integral parts of insulin resistance in nondiabetic elderly.[199] An IL-6 promoter polymorphism was found to be associated with insulin resistance in Pima Indians and in Caucasians.[200]

Adipocyte-derived mediators, adipokines, are involved in inflammation (e.g., TNFα, IL-1β, IL-6, IL-8, IL-10, TGFβ, NGF) and in APR (e.g., plasminogen activator inhibitor-1, haptoglobin, serum amyloid A). The production of these mediators by adipose tissue is increased in obesity.[201] Free cortisol index is a better measurement than serum total cortisol in determining HPA status in patients undergoing surgery.[202]

BIOLOGICAL SIGNIFICANCE OF ACUTE PHASE RESPONSE

Although host defense comes into mind when one considers the acute phase response (APR), it is clear that the cytokines and APPs are produced under physiological conditions and therefore are expected to fulfill important functions in healthy animals and humans. Some examples that illustrate this point are given below.

Proinflammatory cytokines such as IL-1β and IL-6 have been implicated as mediators in labor.[203] In newborn babies, there was an increase in IL-6 during the first day, followed by increases in CRP, serum amyloid A, and procalcitonin on the second postnatal day. The level of prealbumin fell after birth, reaching its lowest value at 3 days of age. Interleukin-1β remained unchanged.[204]

Strenuous exercise increased plasma levels of TNFα, IL-1, IL-6, IL-1 receptor antagonist, TNF receptors, IL-10, IL-8, and macrophage inflammatory protein-1. IL-6 increased up to 100-fold after a marathon race and the increase was tightly related to the duration and intensity of the exercise. IL-6 is produced in the skeletal muscles in response to exercise and it has growth factor abilities.[205] Exercise induces immune changes and also alters neuroendocrinological factors including catecholamines, growth hormone, cortisol, β-endorphin, and sex steroids. Exercise-associated muscle damage initiates the inflammatory cytokine cascade.[206] LPS enters the circulation in athletes after ultra-endurance exercise and may, together with muscle damage, be responsible for the increased cytokine response and hence GI complaints.[207]

Traditionally it is held that endotoxin is harmful and causes disease. However, LPS alone is devoid of toxicity in some lower animal species. The enormous differences in toxicity for various species are due to the ability of LPS to activate the immune system. Therefore, the immune system and not LPS kills the host. Many other microbial pathogens are able to activate the immune system nonspecifically (often called "polyclonal lymphocyte activation").[208] Some of these immunogens are known as superantigens.[209-211] The immunobiology of superantigens is complex and is beyond the scope of this chapter. However, many superantigens are pyrogenic substances[212] and therefore capable of activating APR.

It should be clear that acute immune activation is beneficial to a host in a natural setting. It represents a rapid and efficient way of mounting a massive immune defense against the pathogens right at the site of invasion. The target is promptly identified by the immune system locally at the infection site, where complement, blood clotting, or various subsets of white blood cells are activated.[7,9,10-12,85,86]

When the immune system fails to control an infection or insult locally, APR will develop. A severe febrile illness represents the mobilization of all resources of the host in the interest of defeating or eliminating the pathogen and achieving survival and recovery. This ancient defense mechanism is very demanding on the body, but by and large is very successful. In an overwhelming majority of cases, febrile illness will lead to recovery and healing. On this basis, one may suggest that APR is truly beneficial and only in rare and extreme cases will it result in severe disease, shock, and death.

LPS exerts an effect on the central nervous system, on other endocrine organs, and on many other tissues and organs.[213–216] The various organs and tissues contain "resident macrophages" or related structures such as the glia cells in the CNS, Kupffer cells in the liver, and Langerhans cells in the skin that have the capacity to react to LPS with cytokine production.[217,218] Therefore, systemically applied LPS has the capacity to activate the immune and the neuroendocrine systems and also the liver via locally induced cytokines. Indirect activation by blood-borne cytokines is supplemented by direct activation by LPS of the key organs necessary to execute an APR. This is complemented also by neural communication. For instance, the vagus nerve plays a role in the activation of the ACTH–adrenal axis and the initiation of a behavioral response after the ip injection of LPS.[219,220] Indeed increasing evidence indicates that in addition to cytokines nerves are also capable of rapidly transmitting pyrogenic signals from the periphery toward the CNS.[221]

Endotoxin is always present in the gastrointestinal tract, even in germ-free animals. However, endotoxin does not absorb from the guts of rats even when mucosal damage is inflicted.[222] The reason is that bile acids destroy the integrity of lipid A, which leads to the loss of biological activity. If bile is diverted from the gastrointestinal tract, oral intoxication with LPS can readily be achieved.[223] The liver is an important clearance organ of LPS via bile secretion.[224] Bertok suggested that bile functions as a physico-chemical defense barrier against endotoxin toxicity in vertebrate animals.[225]

LPS has enormous potential to boost host resistance and the APR is capable of efficiently protecting a host. On this basis, it is possible to suggest that evolution has produced a pathophysiological mechanism that utilizes intestinal LPS for the rapid conversion of the immune system from adaptive reactivity to acute phase host defense by the amplification of natural immunity. This *immunoconversion* may be achieved simply by the control of bile secretion. Indeed, there is ample evidence in the literature to illustrate that intestinal endotoxin readily absorbs after x-irradiation, trauma, or even after stressful situations.[7,85]

We note in this chapter for the first time that recovery from APR, regeneration, and healing are also under hypothalamic control. VP appears to have the capacity to restore PRL secretion after APR, leading to anabolic activities and the restoration of normal cell growth and function in all tissues and organs, including the *restoration of adaptive immunocompetence*. This process is called *immunoreversion*.

One may conclude on the basis of evidence reviewed here that the APR makes use of evolutionarily preserved elements of ancient defense mechanisms of lower animals in combination with the highly evolved cytokine and neuroendocrine systems of higher animals. These elements were integrated physiologically to create a rapid, highly coordinated, and very efficient acute immune response, during which profound catabolism takes place in order to maximally support host defense. There can be little doubt that a detailed understanding of febrile illness will lead to new insights into human diseases and better patient care.

List of Abbreviations

    AA = adjuvant arthritis
ACTH = adrenocorticotropic hormone
 ADX = adrenalectomy
 ALD = aldosterone
 APP = acute phase protein
 APR = acute phase response
 CAT = catecholamine
CD14 = cluster designation 14
  CM = chylomicron
 CNS = central nervous system
 CRF = corticotropin releasing factor
 CRH = corticotropin releasing hormone
 CRP = C-reactive protein
DHEA = dehydroepiandrosterone
 DHT = dehydrotestosterone
DNCB = dinitrochlorobenzene
  DP = desmopressin
  E2 = estradiol
 EAE = experimental autoimmune encephalomyelitis
 END = endorphin
  EP = epinephrine
 FSH = follicle stimulating hormone
 FT4 = free thyroxin
  GC = glucocorticoid
  GH = growth hormone
 GLN = glucagon
 HDL = high density lipoprotein
 HPA = hypothalamus–pituitary–adrenal axis
Hypox = hypophysectomy
5-HT = 5-hydroxytryptamin/serotonin
 IFN = interferon
  IL = interleukin
  IN = insulin
 LBP = lipopolysaccharide binding protein
 LEM = leukocyte-derived endogenous mediator
 LEP = leptin
  LH = luteinizing hormone
 LIF = leukemia inhibitory factor
 LPS = lipopolysaccharide/endotoxin
 MBH = medial basal hypothalamus
 MBL = mannose binding lectin
 MFP = α-macrofetoprotein
 MHC = major histocompatibility complex
  MS = multiple sclerosis

MSH = α-melanocyte stimulating hormone
NEP = norepinephrine
NFκB = nuclear factor κB
NIL = neurointermediate pituitary lobectomy
NO = nitric oxide
OT = oxytocin
PAF = platelet activating factor
PG = prostaglandin
PMN = polymorphonuclear leukocyte
PRL = prolactin
PRLR = prolactin receptor
PS = progesterone
PVN = paraventricular nucleus
SAA = serum amyloid A
SRBC = sheep red blood cell
T = thymus-derived (lymphocyte)
T3 = tri-iodo-thyronine
T4 = thyroxin
TNF = tumor necrosis factor
TS = testosterone
TX = thyroidectomy
VD_3 = vitamin D_3
VLDL = very low density lipoprotein
VP/AVP = vasopressin/arginine vasopressin

REFERENCES

1. Selye, H. A syndrome produced by diverse nocuous agents. *Nature* 138, 32, 1936.
2. Selye, H. Thymus and the adrenals in response of the organism to injuries and intoxications. *Br. J. Exp. Pathol.* 17, 234, 1936.
3. Selye, H. The general adaptation syndrome and the diseases of adaptation. *J. Clin. Endocrinol.* 6, 117, 1946.
4. Selye, H. Effect of ACTH and cortisone upon an "anaphylactoid reaction." *Can. Med. Assoc. J.* 61, 553, 1949.
5. Karady, S., Selye, H., and Brownie, J.S.L. The influence of the alarm reaction on the development of anaphylactic shock. *J. Immunol.* 35, 335, 1938.
6. Selye, H. Morphological changes in fowl following chronic overdosage with various steroids. *J. Morphol.* 73, 401, 1943.
7. Berczi, I. Neurohormonal host defence in endotoxin shock. *Ann. NY Acad. Sci.* 840, 787, 1998.
8. Berczi, I. The stress concept and neuroimmunoregulation in modern biology. *Ann. NY Acad. Sci.* 851, 3, 1998.
9. Haeryfar, S.M.M. and Berczi, I. The thymus and the acute phase response. *Cell. Mol. Biol.* 47, 145, 2001.
10. Berczi, I., Bertok, L., and Chow, D. Natural immunity and neuroimmune host defence. *Ann. NY Acad. Sci.* 917, 248, 2001.

11. Berczi, I. and Nagy, E. Neurohormonal control of cytokines during injury, in *Brain Control of Responses to Trauma*, Rothwell, N.J. and Berkenbosch, F., Eds., Cambridge University Press, Cambridge, 1994, p. 32.

12. Berczi, I. and Szentivanyi, A. The acute phase response, in *Neuroimmmune Biology, Vol. 3, The Immune-Neuroendocrine Circuitry: History and Progress*. Berczi, I. and Szentivanyi, A., Eds., Elsevier, Amsterdam, 2003, p. 463.

13. O'Flaherty, L. and Bouchier-Hayes, D.J. Immunonutrition and surgical practice. *Proc. Nutr. Soc.* 58, 831, 1999.

14. Moses, A.G., Dowidar, N., Holloway, B., Waddell, I., Fearon, K.C., and Ross, J.A. Leptin and its relation to weight loss, ob gene expression and the acute-phase response in surgical patients. *Br. J. Surg.* 88, 588, 2001.

15. Maruna, P., Gurlich, R., Fried, M., Frasko, R., Chachkhiani, I., and Haluzik, M. Leptin as an acute phase reactant after non-adjustable laparoscopic gastric banding. *Obes. Surg.* 11, 609, 2001.

16. Hoshiya, T., Watanabe, D., Akagi, K., Mizoguchi, Y., Kamiya, K., Mizuguchi, H., Kumahara, M., Toya, H., Nagashima, Y., and Okaniwa, A. Acute phase response in toxicity studies. I. Survey of beagle dogs subjected to single-dose toxicity studies. *J. Toxicol. Sci.* 26, 95, 2001.

17. Janeway C.A., Travers, P., Walport, M., and Shlomchik, M.J. Failures of host defence mechanisms, in *Immunobiology*, 6th ed., Garland Scientific, New York, 2005, p. 461.

18. Berczi, I. and Szentivanyi, A. Autoimmune disease, in *Neuroimmmune Biology, Vol. 3, The Immune-Neuroendocrine Circuitry: History and Progress*. Berczi, I. and Szentivanyi, A., Eds., Elsevier, Amsterdam, 2003, p. 495.

19. Eastman, A. and Barry, M.A. The origins of DNA breaks: a consequence of DNA damage, DNA repair, or apoptosis. *Cancer Invest.* 10, 229, 1992.

20. Banck, G. and Forsgren, A. Many bacterial species are mitogenic for human blood lymphocytes. *Scand. J. Immunol.* 8, 347, 1978.

21. Sibbald, W.J., Short, A., Chohen, M.P., and Wilson, R.F. Variations in adrenocortical responsiveness during severe bacterial infections: unrecognized adrenocortical insufficiency in severe bacterial infections. *Ann. Surg.* 186, 29, 1977.

22. Rothwell, P.M., Udwadia, Z.F., and Lawler, P.G. Cortisol response to corticotropin and survival in septic shock. *Lancet* 337, 582, 1991.

23. Leshin, L.S. and Malven, P.V. Bacteremia-induced changes in pituitary hormone release and effect of naloxone. *Am. J. Physiol.* 247, E585, 1984.

24. Wannemacher, R.W., Jr., Pekarek, R.S., Thompson, W.L., Curnow, R.T., Beall, F.A., Zenser, T.V., deRubertis, R.F., and Beisel, W.R. A protein from polymorphonuclear leukocytes (LEM) which affects the rate of hepatic amino acid transport and synthesis of acute-phase globulins. *Endocrinology* 96, 651, 1975.

25. Westphal, O., Jann, K., and Himmelspach, K. Chemistry and immunochemistry of bacterial lipopolysaccharides as cell wall antigens and endotoxins. *Prog. Allergy* 33, 9, 1983.

26. Raetz, C.R.H., Ulevitch, R.J., Wright, S.D., Sibley, C.H., Ding, A., and Nathan, C.F. Gram-negative endotoxin: an extraordinary lipid with profound effects on eukaryotic signal transduction. *FASEB J.* 5, 2652, 1991.

27. Tobias, P.S., Mathison, J., Mintz, D., Lee, J.D., Kravchenko, V., Kato, K., Pugin, J., and Ulevitch, R.J. Participation of lipopolysaccharide-binding protein in lipopolysaccharide-dependent macrophage activation. *Am. J. Respir. Cell. Mol. Biol.* 7, 239, 1992.

28. Schumann, R.R. Function of lipopolysaccharide (LPS)-binding protein (LBP) and CD14, the receptor for LPS/LBP complexes: a short review. *Res. Immunol.* 143, 11, 1992.

29. Mathison, J.C., Tobias, P.S., Wolfson, E., and Ulevitch, R.J. Plasma lipopolysaccharide (LPS)-binding protein: a key component in macrophage recognition of Gram-negative LPS. *J. Immunol.* 149, 200, 1992.

30. Wright, S.D., Ramos, R.A., Patel, M., and Miller, D.S. Septin: a factor in plasma that opsonizes lipopolysaccharide-bearing particles for recognition by CD14 on phagocytes. *J. Exp. Med.* 176, 719, 1992.

31. Haziot, A,, Chen, S., Ferrero, E., Low, M.G., Silber, R., and Goyert, S.M. The monocyte differentiation antigen, CD14, is anchored to the cell membrane by a phosphatidylinositol linkage. *J Immunol.* 141, 547, 1988.

32. Kielian, T.L., and Blecha, F. CD14 and other recognition molecules for lipopolysaccharide: a review. *Immunopharmacology* 29, 187, 1995.

33. Rivest, S., Nadeau, S., Lacroix, S., and Laflamme, N. Proinflammatory signal transduction pathways in the CNS during systemic immune response, in *New Foundation of Biology, Neuroimmune Biology,* Vol. 1, Berczi, I. and Gorczynski R.M., Eds., Elsevier, Amsterdam, 1991, p. 163.

34. Bas, S., Gauthier, B.R., Spenato, U., Stingelin, S., and Gabay, C. CD14 is an acute-phase protein. *J. Immunol.* 172, 4470, 2004.

35. Berczi, I., Bertok, L., and Bereznay, T. Comparative studies on the toxicity of *Escherichia coli* lipopolysaccharide endotoxin in various animal species. *Can. J. Microbiol.* 12, 1070, 1966.

36. Balm, P.H., van Lieshout, E., Lokate, J., and Wendelaar-Bonga, S.E. Bacterial lipopolysaccharide (LPS) and interleukin 1 (IL-1) exert multiple physiological effects in the tilapia *Oreochromis mossambicus* (Teleostei). *J. Comp. Physiol. [B].* 165, 85, 1995.

37. Bang, F.B. A bacterial disease of *Limulus polyphemus. Bull. Johns Hopkins Hosp.* 98, 325, 1956.

38. Levin, J. and Bang, F.B. A description of cellular coagulation in the Limulus. *Bull. Johns Hopkins Hosp.* 115, 337, 1964.

39. Levin, J. and Bang, F.B. The role of endotoxin in the extracellular coagulation of limulus blood. *Bull. Johns Hopkins Hosp.* 115, 265, 1964.

40. Ramachandra, R.N., Sehon, A.H., and Berczi, I. Neuro-hormonal host defense in endotoxin shock. *Brain Behav. Immun.* 6, 157, 1992.

41. Yoo, J.Y. and Desiderio, S. Innate and acquired immunity intersect in a global view of the acute-phase response. *Proc. Natl. Acad. Sci. USA* 100, 1157, 2003.

42. Parant, M., Le Contel, C., Parant, F., and Chedid, L. Influence of endogenous glucocorticoid on endotoxin-induced production of circulating TNF-alpha. *Lymphokine Cytokine Res.* 10, 265, 1991.

43. Zuckerman, S.H., Shellhaas, J., and Butler L.D. Differential regulation of lipopolysaccharide-induced interleukin 1 and tumor necrosis factor synthesis: effects of endogenous and exogenous glucocorticoids and the role of the pituitary-adrenal axis. *Eur. J. Immunol.* 19, 301, 1989.

44. Richardson, R.P., Rhyne, C.D., Fong, Y., Hesse, D.G., Tracey, K.J., Marano, M.A., Lowry, S.F., Antonacci, A.C., and Calvano, S.E. Peripheral blood leukocyte kinetics following *in vivo* lipopolysaccharide (LPS) administration to normal human subjects: influence of elicited hormones and cytokines. *Ann. Surg.* 210, 239, 1989.

45. Flohe, S., Heinrich, P.C., Schneider, J., Wendel, A., and Flohe, L. Time course of IL-6 and TNF alpha release during endotoxin-induced endotoxin tolerance in rats. *Biochem. Pharmacol.* 41, 1607, 1991.

46. Barber, A.E., Coyle, S.M., Marano, M.A., Fischer, E., Calvano, S.E., Fong, Y., Moldawer, L.L., and Lowry, S.F. Glucocorticoid therapy alters hormonal and cytokine responses to endotoxin in man. *J Immunol.* 150, 1999, 1993.

47. Waring, P.M., Waring, L.J., Billington, T., and Metcalf, D. Leukemia inhibitory factor protects against experimental lethal *Escherichia coli* septic shock in mice. *Proc. Natl. Acad. Sci. USA* 92, 1337, 1995.

48. Granowitz, E.V., Porat, R., Mier, J.W., Orencole, S.F., Kaplanski, G., Lynch, E.A., Ye, K., Vannier, E., Wolff, S.M., and Dinarello, C.A. Intravenous endotoxin suppresses the cytokine response of peripheral blood mononuclear cells of healthy humans. *J. Immunol.* 151, 1637, 1993.

49. Berg, D.J., Kuhn, R., Rajewsky, K., Muller, W., Menon, S., Davidson, N., Grunig, G., and Rennick, D. Interleukin-10 is a central regulator of the response to LPS in murine models of endotoxic shock and the Shwartzman reaction but not endotoxin tolerance. *J. Clin. Invest.* 96, 2339, 1995.

50. Matic, M., and Simon, S.R. Effects of gamma interferon on release of tumor necrosis factor alpha from lipopolysaccharide-tolerant human monocyte-derived macrophages. *Infect. Immun.* 60, 3756, 1992.

51. Schade, F.U., Franke, C., Schlegel, J., and Rietschel, E.T. Formation of a TNF synthesis inhibitor in endotoxin tolerance. *Prog. Clin. Biol. Res.* 392, 513, 1995.

52. Henricson, B.E., Neta, R., Vogel, S.N. An interleukin-1 receptor antagonist blocks lipopolysaccharide-induced colony-stimulating factor production and early endotoxin tolerance. *Infect. Immun.* 59, 1188, 1991.

53. Berczi, I. and Szentivanyi, A. The pituitary gland, psychoneuroimmunology and infectious disease, in *Psychoneuroimmunology, Stress and Infectious Disease*. Friedman, H., Klein, T., and Friedman, A.L., Eds., CRC Press, Boca Raton, FL, 1996, p. 79.

54. Wexler, B.C., Dolgin, A.E., and Tryczynski, E.W. Effects of bacterial polysaccharide (piromen) on the pituitary-adrenal axis: adrenal ascorbic acid, cholesterol and histological alterations. *Endocrinology* 61, 300, 1957.

55. Wilder, R.L. Neuroendocrineñimmune system interactions and autoimmunity. *Annu Rev. Immunol.* 13, 307, 1995.

56. Torpy, D.J. and Chrousos, G.P. The three-way interaction between the hypothalamic–pituitary–adrenal and gonadal axes and the immune system. *Bailliere Clin. Rheumatol.* 10, 181, 1996.

57. Berczi, I., Chalmers, I.M., Nagy, E. and Warrington, R.J. The immune effects of neuropeptides. *Bailliere Clin. Rheumatol.* 10, 227, 1996.

58. Nagy, E. and Berczi, I. Prolactin and contact sensitivity. *Allergy* 36, 429, 1981.

59. Berczi, I., Nagy, E., Kovacs, K., and Horvath, E. Regulation of humoral immunity in rats by pituitary hormones. *Acta Endocrinol.* 98, 506, 1981.

60. Berczi, I. and Nagy, E. A possible role of prolactin in adjuvant arthritis. *Arthritis Rheum.* 25, 591, 1982.

61. Nagy, E., Berczi, I., and Friesen, H.G. Regulation of immunity in rats by lactogenic and growth hormones. *Acta Endocrinol.* 102, 351, 1983.

62. Nagy, E., Berczi, I., Wren, G.E., Asa, S.L., and Kovacs, K. Immunomodulation by bromocriptine. *Immunopharmacology* 6, 231, 1983.

63. Corbacho, A.M., Valacchi, G., Kubala, L., Olano-Martin, E., Schock, B.C., Kenny, T.P., and Cross, C.E. Tissue-specific gene expression of prolactin receptor in the acute-phase response induced by lipopolysaccharides. *Am. J. Physiol. Endocrinol. Metab.* 287, E750, 2004.

64. Geary, N., Asarian, L., Sheahan, J., and Langhans, W. Estradiol-mediated increases in the anorexia induced by intraperitoneal injection of bacterial lipopolysaccharide in female rats. *Physiol. Behav.* 82, 251, 2004.

65. Kim, M.S., Shigenaga, J., Moser, A., Grunfeld, C., and Feingold, K.R. Suppression of DHEA sulfotransferase (Sult2A1) during the acute-phase response. *Am J Physiol Endocrinol Metab.* 287, E731, 2004.

66. Geller, P., Merrill, E.R., and Jawetz, E. Effects of cortisone and antibiotics on lethal action of endotoxins in mice. *Proc. Soc. Exp. Biol. Med.* 86, 716, 1954.

67. Jansen, N.J.G., Vanoeveren, W., Hoiting, B.H., and Wildevuur, C.R.H. Methylprednisolone prophylaxis protects against endotoxin-induced death in rabbits. *Inflammation* 15, 91, 1991.

68. Izumi, T. and Bakhle, Y.S. Modification by steroids of pulmonary oedema and prostaglandin E2 pharmacokinetics induced by endotoxin in rats. *Brit. J. Pharmacol.* 93, 955, 1988.

69. Sanchez-Cantu, L., Rode, H.N., Yun, T.J., and Christou, N.V. Tumor necrosis factor alone does not explain the lethal effect of lipopolysaccharide. *Arch. Surg.* 126, 231, 1991.

70. Ciancio, M.J., Hunt, J., Jones, S.B., and Filkins, J.P. Comparative and interactive *in vivo* effects of tumor necrosis factor and endotoxin. *Circ. Shock* 33, 108, 1991.

71. Henricson, B.E., Neta, R., and Vogel, S.N. An interleukin-1 receptor antagonist blocks lipopolysaccharide-induced colony-stimulating factor production and early endotoxin tolerance. *Infect. Immun.* 59, 1188, 1991.

72. Schade, F.U., Franke, C., Schlegel, J., and Rietschel, E.T. Formation of a TNF synthesis inhibitor in endotoxin tolerance. *Prog. Clin. Biol. Res.* 392, 513, 1995.

73. Berg, D.J., Kuhn, R., Rajewsky, K., Muller, W., Menon, S., Davidson, N., Grunig, G., and Rennick, D. Interleukin-10 is a central regulator of the response to LPS in murine models of endotoxic shock and the Shwartzman reaction but not endotoxin tolerance. *J. Clin. Invest.* 96, 2339, 1995.

74. Waring, P.M., Waring, L.J., Billington, T., and Metcalf, D. Leukemia inhibitory factor protects against experimental lethal *Escherichia coli* septic shock in mice. *Proc. Natl. Acad. Sci. USA* 92, 1337,1995.

75. Matic, M. and Simon, S.R. Effects of gamma interferon on release of tumor necrosis factor alpha from lipopolysaccharide-tolerant human monocyte-derived macrophages. *Infect. Immun.* 60, 3756, 1992.

76. Seatter, S.C., Bennet, T., Li, M.H., Bubrick, M.P., and West, M.A. Macrophage endotoxin tolerance: tumor necrosis factor and interleukin-1 regulation by lipopolysaccharide pretreatment. *Arch. Surg.* 129, 1263, 1994.

77. Li, M.H., Seatter, S.C., Manthei, R., Bubrick, M., and West, M.A. Macrophage endotoxin tolerance: effect of TNF or endotoxin pretreatment. *J. Surg. Res.* 57, 85, 1994.

78. Previte, J.J., Chang, Y., and El-Bisi, H.M. Detoxification of *Salmonella typhimurium* lipopolysaccharide by ionizing radiation. *J. Bacteriol.* 93, 1607, 1967.

79. Fust, G., Bertok, L., and Juhasz-Nagy, S. Interactions of radio-detoxified *Escherichia coli* endotoxin preparations with the complement system. *Infect. Immun.* 16, 26, 1977.

80. Bertok, L. Stimulation of nonspecific resistance by radiation-detoxified endotoxin, in *Beneficial Effects of Endotoxin.* Nowotny, A., Ed., Plenum Press, New York, 1983, p. 213.

81. Banhegyi, D., Varnai, F., Horvath, A., and Bertok, L. Treatment of severe immune deficiency with radio-detoxified endotoxin. *J. Med.* 23, 154, 1992.

82. Gustafson, G.L., Rhodes, M.J., and Hegel, T. Monophosphoryl lipid A as a prophylactic for sepsis and septic shock. *Prog. Clin. Biol. Res.* 392, 567, 1995.

83. Astiz, M.E., Rackow, E.C., Still, J.G., Howell, S.T., Cato, A., Von Eschen, K.B., Ulrich, J.T., Rudbach, J.A., McMahon, G., Vargas, R., et al. Pretreatment of normal humans with monophosphoryl lipid A induces tolerance to endotoxin: a prospective, double-blind, randomized, controlled trial. *Crit. Care Med.* 23, 9, 1995.

84. Krueger, J.M., Majde, J.A., and Obal, F. Sleep in host defense. *Brain Behav. Immun.* 17, Suppl. 1, S41, 2003.

85. Berczi, I. Neuroendocrine defence in endotoxin shock (review). *Acta Microbiol. Hung.* 40, 265, 1993.

86. Berczi, I. Neuroendocrine regulation of natural immunity, in *Natural Immunity, Neuroimmune Bilogy*, Vol. 5, Bertok, L. and Chow, D.A., Eds., Elsevier, Amsterdam, 2005, in press.

87. Schiltz, J.C. and Sawchenko, P.E. Signaling the brain in systemic inflammation: the role of perivascular cells. *Front. Biosci.* 8, s1321, 2003.

88. Dolecek, R., Tymonova, J., Adamkova, M., Kadlcik, M., Pohlidal, A., and Zavodna, R. Endocrine changes after burns: the bone involvement. *Acta Chir. Plast.* 45, 95, 2003.

89. Bornstein, S.R., Licinio, J., Tauchnitz, R., Engelmann, L., Negrao, A.B., Gold, P., and Chrousos, G.P. Plasma leptin levels are increased in survivors of acute sepsis: associated loss of diurnal rhythm in cortisol and leptin secretion. *J. Clin. Endocrinol. Metab.* 83, 280, 1998.

90. Giovambattista, A., Chisari, A.N., Corro, L., Gaillard, R.C., and Spinedi, E. Metabolic, neuroendocrine and immune functions in basal conditions and during the acute-phase response to endotoxic shock in undernourished rats. *Neuroimmunomodulation* 7, 92, 2000.

91. Okamoto, S., Irie, Y., Ishikawa, I., Kimura, K., Masayuki, S. Central leptin suppresses splenic lymphocyte functions through activation of the corticotropin-releasing hormone-sympathetic nervous system. *Brain. Res.* 855, 192, 2000.

92. Chautard, T., Spinedi, E., Voirol, M., Pralong, F.P., and Gaillard, R.C. Role of glucocorticoids in the response of the hypothalamo-corticotrope, immune and adipose systems to repeated endotoxin administration. *Neuroendocrinology* 69, 360, 1999.

93. Torpy, D.J., Bornstein, S.R., and Chrousos G.P. Leptin and interleukin-6 in sepsis. *Horm. Metab. Res.* 30, 726, 1998.

94. Faggioni, R., Fantuzzi, G., Gabay, C., Moser, A., Dinarello, C.A., Feingold, K.R., and Grunfeld, C. Leptin deficiency enhances sensitivity to endotoxin-induced lethality. *Am. J. Physiol.* 276, R136, 1999.

95. Takahashi, N., Waelput, W., and Guisez, Y. Leptin is an endogenous protective protein against the toxicity exerted by tumor necrosis factor. *J. Exp. Med.* 189, 207, 1999.

96. Finck, B.N., Kelley, K.W., Dantzer, R., and Johnson, R.W. *In vivo* and *in vitro* evidence for the involvement of tumor necrosis factor-alpha in the induction of leptin by lipopolysaccharide. *Endocrinology* 139, 2278, 1998.

97. Loffreda, S., Yang, S.Q., Lin, H.Z., Karp, C.L., Brengman, M.L., Wang, D.J., Klein, A.S., Bulkley, G.B., Bao, C., Noble, P.W., Lane, M.D., and Diehl, A.M. Leptin regulates proinflammatory immune responses. *FASEB J.* 12, 57, 1998.

98. Fantuzzi, G. and Faggioni, R. Leptin in the regulation of immunity, inflammation, and hematopoiesis. *J. Leukoc. Biol.* 68, 437, 2000.

99. Bernotiene, E., Palmer, G., Talabot-Ayer, D., Szalay-Quinodoz, I., Aubert, M.L., and Gabay, C. Delayed resolution of acute inflammation during zymosan-induced arthritis in leptin-deficient mice. *Arthritis Res. Ther.* 6, R256, 2004.

100. Harnish, M.J., Lange, T., Dimitrov, S., Born, J., and Fehm, H.L. Differential regulation of human blood glucose level by interleukin-2 and -6. *Exp. Clin. Endocrinol. Diabetes* 113, 43, 2005.

101. Kolb-Bachofen, V. A review on the biological properties of C-reactive protein. *Immunobiology* 183, 133, 1991.

102. Ballou, S.P. and Kushner, I. C-reactive protein and the acute phase response. *Adv. Intern. Med.* 37, 313, 1992.

103. Young, B., Gleeson, M., and Cripps, A.W. C-reactive protein: a critical review. *Pathology* 23, 118, 1991.

104. Mold, C., Nakayama, S., Holzer, T.J., Gewurz, H., and Du Clos, T.W. C-reactive protein is protective against *Streptococcus pneumoniae* infection in mice. *J. Exp. Med.* 154, 1703, 1981.

105. Galkina, E.V., Nazarov, P.G., Polevschikov, A.V., Berestovaya, L.K., Galkin, V.E., and Bychkova, N.V. Interactions of C-reactive protein and serum amyloid P component with interleukin-8 and their role in regulation of neutrophil functions. *Russ. J. Immunol.* 5, 363, 2000.

106. Hamann, L., Alexander, C., Stamme, C., Zahringer, U., and Schumann, R.R. Acute-phase concentrations of lipopolysaccharide (LPS)-binding protein inhibit innate immune cell activation by different LPS chemotypes via different mechanisms. *Infect. Immun.* 73, 193, 2005.

107. Wassell, J. Haptoglobin: function and polymorphism. *Clin. Lab.* 46, 547, 2000.

108. Arredouani, M.S., Kasran, A., Vanoirbeek, J.A., Berger, F.G., Baumann, H., and Ceuppens, J.L. Haptoglobin dampens endotoxin-induced inflammatory effects both *in vitro* and *in vivo*. *Immunology* 114, 263, 2005.

109. Daemen, M.A., Heemskerk, V.H., van't Veer, C., Denecker, G., Wolfs, T.G., Vandenabeele, P., and Buurman, W.A. Functional protection by acute phase proteins alpha(1)-acid glycoprotein and alpha(1)-antitrypsin against ischemia/reperfusion injury by preventing apoptosis and inflammation. *Circulation* 102, 1420, 2000.

110. Liu, H., Jensen, L., Hansen, S., Petersen, S.V., Takahashi, K., Ezekowitz, A.B., Hansen, F.D., Jensenius, J.C., and Thiel, S. Characterization and quantification of mouse mannan-binding lectins (MBL-A and MBL-C) and study of acute phase responses. *Scand. J. Immunol.* 53, 489, 2001.

111. Hansen, T.K., Thiel, S., Wouters, P.J., Christiansen, J.S., and Van den Berghe, G. Intensive insulin therapy exerts antiinflammatory effects in critically ill patients and counteracts the adverse effect of low mannose-binding lectin levels. *J. Clin. Endocrinol. Metab.* 88, 1082, 2003.

112. Turner, M.W. and Hamvas, R.M. Mannose-binding lectin: structure, function, genetics and disease associations. *Rev. Immunogenet.* 2, 305, 2000.

113. Bauer, J., Birmelin, M., Northoff, G.H., Northemann, W., Tran-Thi, T.A., Ueberberg, H., Decker, K., and Heinrich, P. Induction of rat alpha2-macroglobulin *in vivo* and in hepatocyte primary cultures: synergistic action of glucocorticoids and a Kupffer cell-derived factor. *FEBS Lett.* 177, 89, 1984.

114. van Gool, J., Boers, W., Sala, M., and Ladiges, N.C. Glucocorticoids and catecholamines as mediators of acute-phase proteins, especially rat alpha-macrofoetoprotein. *Biochem. J.* 220, 125, 1984.

115. Yeager, M.P., Guyre, P.M., and Munck, A.U. Glucocorticoid regulation of the inflammatory response to injury. *Acta Anaesthesiol. Scand.* 48, 799, 2004.

116. Akira, S. and Kishimoto, T. IL-6 and NF-IL6 in acute-phase response and viral infection. *Immunol. Rev.* 127, 26, 1992.

117. Van Gool, J., Van Vugt, H., Helle, M., and Aarden, L.A. The relation among stress, adrenalin, interleukin-6, and acute phase proteins in the rat. *Clin. Immunol. Immunopathol.* 57, 200, 1990.

118. Streetz, K.L., Tacke, F., Leifeld, L., Wustefeld, T., Graw, A., Klein, C., Kamino, K., Spengler, U., Kreipe, H., Kubicka, S., Muller, W., Manns, M.P., and Trautwein, C. Interleukin 6/gp130-dependent pathways are protective during chronic liver diseases. *Hepatology* 38, 218, 2003.

119. Don, B.R., Rosales, L.M., Levine, N.W., Mitch, W., and Kaysen, G.A. Leptin is a negative acute phase protein in chronic hemodialysis patients. *Kidney Int.* 59, 1114, 2001.

120. Finck, B.N. and Johnson, R.W. Tumor necrosis factor-alpha regulates secretion of the adipocyte-derived cytokine, leptin. *Microsc. Res. Tech.* 50, 209, 2000.

121. Harris, H.W., and Kasravi, F.B. Lipoprotein-bound LPS induces cytokine tolerance in hepatocytes. *J. Endotoxin Res.* 9, 45, 2003.

122. Singer, M., De Santis, V., Vitale, D., and Jeffcoate, W. Multiorgan failure is an adaptive, endocrine-mediated, metabolic response to overwhelming systemic inflammation. *Lancet* 364, 545, 2004.

123. Ekman, R., Gobom, J., Persson, R., Mecocci, P., and Nilsson, C.L. Arginine vasopressin in the cytoplasm and nuclear fraction of lymphocytes from healthy donors and patients with depression or schizophrenia. *Peptides* 22, 67, 2001.

124. Itoi, K., Jiang, Y.Q., Iwasaki, Y., and Watson, S.J. Regulatory mechanisms of corticotropin-releasing hormone and vasopressin gene expression in the hypothalamus. *J. Neuroendocrinol.* 16, 348, 2004.

125. Carrasco, G.A. and Van de Kar, L.D. Neuroendocrine pharmacology of stress. *Eur. J. Pharmacol.* 463, 235, 2003.

126. Turnbull, A.V., Lee, S., and Rivier C. Mechanisms of hypothalamic–pituitary–adrenal axis stimulation by immune signals in the adult rat. *Ann. NY Acad. Sci.* 840, 434, 1998.

127. Huitinga, I., Schmidt, E.D., van der Cammen, M.J., Binnekade, R., and Tilders, F.J. Priming with interleukin-1-beta suppresses experimental allergic encephalomyelitis in the Lewis rat. *J. Neuroendocrinol.* 12, 1186, 2000.

128. Chowdrey, H.S., Larsen, P.J., Harbuz, M.S., Jessop, D.S., Aguilera, G., Eckland, D.J., and Lightman, S.L. Evidence for arginine vasopressin as the primary activator of the HPA axis during adjuvant-induced arthritis. *Br. J. Pharmacol.* 116, 2417, 1995.

129. Baker, J.W., Yerger, S., and Segar, W.E. Elevated plasma antidiuretic hormone levels in status asthmaticus. *Mayo Clin. Proc.* 51, 31, 1976.

130. Michelson, D., Stone, L., Galliven, E., Magiakou, M.A., Chrousos, G.P., Sternberg, E.M., and Gold, P.W. Multiple sclerosis is associated with alterations in hypothalamic–pituitary–adrenal axis function. *J. Clin. Endocrinol. Metab.* 79, 848, 1994.

131. Dreyfuss, D., Leviel, F., Paillard, M., Rahmani, J., and Coste, F. Acute infectious pneumonia is accompanied by a latent vasopressin-dependent impairment of renal water excretion. *Am. Rev. Respir. Dis.* 138, 583, 1988.

132. Chowdrey, H.S., Larsen, P.J., Harbuz, M.S., Jessop, D.S., Aguilera, G., Eckland D.J.A. and Lightman, S.L.. Evidence for arginine vasopressin as the primary activator for the HPA axis during adjuvant-induced arthritis. *Br. J. Pharmacol.* 116, 2417, 1995.

133. Harbuz, M.S., Chover-Gonzalez, A.J. and Jessop, D.S. Hypothalamo–pituitary–adrenal axis and chronic immune activation. *Ann. NY Acad. Sci.* 992, 99, 2003.

134. DeGoeij, D., Kvetnansky, R., Whitnall, M.H., Jesova, D., Bekenbosch, F., and Tilders, F.J.H. Repeated stress activation of corticotropin releasing factor neurons enhances vasopressin stores and colocalization with corticotropin-releasing factor in the median eminence of rats. *Neuroendocrinology* 53, 150, 1991.

135. DeGoeij, D., Binnekade, R., aand Tilders, F. Chronic intermittent stress enhances vasopressin but not corticotropin releasing factor secretion during hypoglycemia. *Am. J. Physiol.* 263, E394, 1992.

136. DeGoeij, D., Dijkstra, H., and Tilders, F. Chronic psychological stress enhances vasopressin but not corticotropin releasing factor, in the external zone of the median eminence of male rats: relationship to subordinate status. *Endocrinology* 131, 847, 1992

137. DeGoeij, D., Jezova, D., and Tilders F.J.H. Repeated stress enhances vasopressin synthesis in corticotropin releasing factor neurons in the paraventricular nucleus. *Brain Res.* 577, 165, 1992.

138. Hashimoto, K., Suemaru, S., Takao, T., Sugarwara, M., Makino, S., and Ota, S. Corticotropin-releasing hormones and pituitary-adrenocortical response in chronically stressed rats. *Regul. Pept.* 23, 117, 1988.

139. Levin, N., Blum, M., and Roberts, J.L. Modulation of basal and corticotropin-releasing factor-stimulated proopiomelanocortin gene expression by vasopressin in rat anterior pituitary. *Endocinology* 125, 2957, 1989.

140. Antoni, E.A. Hypothalamic control of adrenocorticotropin secretion: advances since the discovery of 41-residue corticotropin releasing factor. *Endocrinol. Rev.* 7, 351, 1986.

141. Gilles, G., Linton, E.A., and Lowry, P.F. Corticotropin releasing activity of the new CRF is potentiated several times by vasopressin. *Nature* 299, 355, 1982.

142. Raber, J., Pich, E.M., Koob, G.F., and Bloom F.E. IL-1-beta potentiates the acetylcholine-induced release of vasopressin from the hypothalamus *in vitro*, but not from the amygdala. *Neuroendocrinology* 59, 208, 1994.

143. Wilkinson, M.F., Horn, T.F., Kasting, N.W., and Pittman Q.J. Central interleukin-1 beta stimulation of vasopressin release into the rat brain: activation of an antipyretic pathway. *J. Physiol.* 481 (Pt 3), 641, 1994.

144. Sasaki, S., Watanobe, H., and Takebe, K. The role of arginine vasopressin in interleukin-1 beta-induced adrenocorticotropin secretion in the rat. *Neuroimmunomodulation* 2, 134, 1995.

145. Kageyama, K., Watanobe, H., and Takebe, K. *In vivo* evidence that arginine vasopressin is involved in the adrenocorticotropin response induced by interleukin-6 but not by tumor necrosis factor-alpha in the rat. *Neuroimmunomodulation* 2, 137, 1995.

146. Raber, J., and Bloom, F.E. IL-2 induces vasopressin release from the hypothalamus and the amygdala: role of nitric oxide-mediated signaling. *J. Neurosci.* 14, 6187, 1994.

147. Pardy, K., Murphy, D., Carter, D., and Hui, K.M. The influence of interleukin-2 on vasopressin and oxytocin gene expression in the rodent hypothalamus. *J. Neuroimmunol.* 42, 131, 1993.

148. Hillhouse, E.W. Interleukin-2 stimulates the secretion of arginine vasopressin but not corticotropin-releasing hormone from rat hypothalamic cells *in vitro*. *Brain Res.* 650, 323, 1994.

149. Ishizaki, S., Murase, T., Sugimura, Y., Banno, R., Arima, H., Miura, Y., and Oiso, Y. Leukemia inhibitory factor stimulates vasopressin release in rats. *Neurosci. Lett.* 359, 77, 2004.

150. Malkinson, T.J., Bridges, T.E., Lederis, K., and Veale, W.L. Perfusion of the septum of the rabbit with vasopressin antiserum enhances endotoxin fever. *Peptides* 8, 385, 1987.

151. Kostoglou-Athanassiou, I., Costa, A., Navarra, P., Nappi, G., Forsling, M.L., and Grossman, A.B. Endotoxin stimulates an endogenous pathway regulating corticotropin-releasing hormone and vasopressin release involving the generation of nitric oxide and carbon monoxide. *J. Neuroimmunol.* 86, 104, 1998.

152. Giovambattista, A., Chisari, A.N., Gaillard, R.C., and Spinedi, E. Modulatory role of the epinergic system in the neuroendocrine-immune system function. *Neuroimmunomodulation* 8, 98, 2000.

153. Lee, S., Barbanel, G., and Rivier, C. Systemic endotoxin increases steady-state gene expression of hypothalamic nitric oxide synthase: comparison with corticotropin-releasing factor and vasopressin gene transcripts. *Brain Res.* 705, 136, 1995.

154. Battaglia, D.F., Brown, M.E., Krasa, H.B., Thrun, L.A., Viguie, C., and Karsch, F.J. Systemic challenge with endotoxin stimulates corticotropin-releasing hormone and arginine vasopressin secretion into hypophyseal portal blood: coincidence with gonadotropin-releasing hormone suppression. *Endocrinology* 139, 4175, 1998.

155. Qahwash, I.M., Cassar, C.A., Radcliff, R.P., and Smith, G.W. Bacterial lipopolysaccharide-induced coordinate down-regulation of arginine vasopressin receptor V3 and corticotropin-releasing factor receptor 1 messenger ribonucleic acids in the anterior pituitary of endotoxemic steers. *Endocrine* 18, 13, 2002.

156. Tanoue, A., Ito, S., Honda, K., Oshikawa, S., Kitagawa, Y., Koshimizu, T.A., Mori, T., and Tsujimoto, G. The vasopressin V1b receptor critically regulates hypothalamic-pituitary-adrenal axis activity under both stress and resting conditions. *J. Clin. Invest.* 113, 302, 2004.

157. Kjaer, A., Knigge, U., Bach, F.W., and Warberg, J. Histamine- and stress-induced secretion of ACTH and beta-endorphin: involvement of corticotropin-releasing hormone and vasopressin. *Neuroendocrinology* 56, 419, 1992.

158. Nagy, G.M., Gorcs, T.J., and Halasz, B. Attenuation of the suckling-induced prolactin release and the high afternoon oscillations of plasma prolactin secretion of lactating rats by antiserum to vasopressin. *Neuroendocrinology* 54, 566, 1991.

159. el Halawani, M.E., Silsby, J.L., Koike, T.I., and Robinzon, B. Evidence of a role for the turkey posterior pituitary in prolactin release. *Gen. Comp. Endocrinol.* 87, 436, 1992.

160. Franci, C.R., Anselmo-Franci, J.A., Kozlowski, G.P., and McCann S.M. Actions of endogenous vasopressin and oxytocin on anterior pituitary hormone secretion. *Neuroendocrinology* 57, 693, 1993.

161. Keck, M.E., Welt, T., Muller, M.B., Landgraf, R., and Holsboer, F. The high-affinity non-peptide CRH1 receptor antagonist R121919 attenuates stress-induced alterations in plasma oxytocin, prolactin, and testosterone secretion in rats. *Pharmacopsychiatry* 36, 27, 2003.

162. Elenkov, I.J., Kovacs, K., Kiss, J., Bertok, L., and Vizi, E.S. Lipopolysaccharide is able to bypass corticotrophin-releasing factor in affecting plasma ACTH and corticosterone levels: evidence from rats with lesions of the paraventricular nucleus. *J Endocrinol.* 133, 231, 1992.

163. Khegai, I.I., Gulyaeva, M.A., Popova, N.A., Zakharova, L.A., and Ivanova, L.N. Immune system in vasopressin-deficient rats during ontogeny. *Bull. Exp. Biol. Med.* 136, 448, 2003.

164. Yirmiya, R., Shavit, Y., Ben-Eliyahu, S., Martin, F.C., Weiner, H., and Liebeskind, J.C. Natural killer cell activity in vasopressin-deficient rats (Brattleboro strain). *Brain Res.* 479, 16, 1989.

165. Hu, S.B., Zhao, Z.S., Yhap, C., Grinberg, A., Huang, S.P., Westphal, H., and Gold, P. Vasopressin receptor 1a-mediated negative regulation of B cell receptor signaling. *J. Neuroimmunol.* 135, 72, 2003.

166. Johnson, H.M. and Torres, B.A. A novel arginine vasopressin-binding peptide that blocks arginine vasopressin modulation of immune function. *J. Immunol.* 141, 2420, 1988.

167. Torres, B.A. and Johnson, H.M. Arginine vasopressin-binding peptides derived from the bovine and rat genomes differ in their abilities to block arginine vasopressin modulation of murine immune function. *J. Neuroimmunol.* 27, 191, 1990.

168. Bell, J., Adler, M.W., Greenstein, J.I., and Liu-Chen, L.Y. Identification and characterization of [125 I] arginine vasopressin binding sites on human peripheral blood mononuclear cells. *Life Sci.* 52, 95, 1993.

169. Shibasaki, T., Hotta, M., Sugihara, H., and Wakabayashi, I. Brain vasopressin is involved in stress-induced suppression of immune function in the rat. *Brain Res.* 808, 84, 1998.

170. Zhao, L. and Brinton, R.D. Suppression of proinflammatory cytokines interleukin-1beta and tumor necrosis factor-alpha in astrocytes by a V1 vasopressin receptor agonist: a cAMP response element-binding protein-dependent mechanism. *J. Neurosci.* 24, 2226, 2004.

171. Moll, J., and De Wied, D. Observations on the hypothalamo-posthypophyseal system of the posterior lobectomized rat. *Gen. Comp. Endocrinol.* 2, 215, 1962.

172. Miller, R.E., Yueh-Chien, H., Wiley, M.K., and Hewitt, R. Anterior hypophysial function in the posterior-hypophysectomised rat: normal regulation of the adrenal system. *Neuroendocrinology* 14, 233, 1974.

173. Organista-Esparza, A., Tinajero-Ruelas, M., Medina-Fernández, M., Sánchez-Herrera, I.O., and Quintanar-Stephano, A. Efectos de la lobectomía neurointermedia hipofisiaria y la hipofisectomía sobre la respuesta inmune humoral en la rata Wistarp (Effects of neurointermediate pituitary lobectomy and hypophysectomy on humoral immune response in the Wistar rat). In *XLVI National Congress of Physiological Sciences,* Mexican Society of Physiological Sciences, Aguascalientes, 2003, p. 96.

174. Quintanar-Stephano, A., Kovacs, K., and Berczi, I. Effects of neurointermedate pituitary lobectomy on humoral and cell-mediated immune responses in the rat. *Neuroimmunomodulation* 11, 233, 2004.

175. Quintanar-Stephano, A., Organista-Esparza, A., Tinajero-Ruelas, M., Chavira-Ramírez, R., Gonzalez-Delgado, E., Garcia, D., Ramirez, E., Rodriguez, E., Berczi, I., and Kovacs, K. Protection against adjuvant-induced arthritis (AIA) by the excision of the neuro-intermediate pituitary lobe (NIL) in Lewis rats. FASEB 2005. Meeting, San Diego, CA, Abstract 7407.

176. Quintanar-Stephano, A., Chavira-Ramírez, R., Kovacs, K., and Berczi, I. Neurointermediate pituitary lobectomy decreases the incidence and severity of experimental autoimmune encephalomyelitis in Lewis rats. *J. Endocrinol.* 184, 51, 2005.

177. Bergad, P.L., Schwarzenberg, S.J., Humbert, J.T., Morrison, M., Amarasinghe, S., Towle, H.C., and Berry, S.A. Inhibition of growth hormone action in models of inflammation. *Am. J. Physiol. Cell. Physiol.* 279, C1906, 2000.

178. Takala, J., Ruokonen, E., Webster, N.R., et al. Increased mortality associated with growth hormone treatment in critically ill adults. *New Engl. J. Med.* 341, 785, 1999.

179. Jaschke, M.G., Herndon, D.N., Wolf, S.E., et al. Recombinant human growth hormone alters acute phase reactant proteins, cytokine expression, and liver morphology in burned rats. *J. Surg. Res.* 83, 122, 1999.

180. Derfalvi, B., Igaz, P., Fulop, K.A., Szalai, C., and Falus, A. Interleukin-6-induced production of type II acute phase proteins and expression of junB gene are down-regulated by human recombinant growth hormone in vitro. *Cell Biol. Int.* 24, 109, 2000.

181. Berczi, I., Nagy, E., Asa, S.L., and Kovacs, K. Pituitary hormones and contact sensitivity in rats. *Allergy* 38, 325, 1983.

182. Berczi, I., Nagy, E., Asa, S.L., and Kovacs K. The influence of pituitary hormones on adjuvant arthritis. *Arthritis Rheum.* 27, 682, 1984.

183. Ramirez, R.J., Wolf, S.E., and Herndon, D.N. Is there a role for growth hormone in the clinical management of burn injuries? *Growth. Horm. IGF Res.* 8, Suppl. B, 99, 1998.

184. Jaschke, M.G., Barrow, R.E., and Herndon, D.N. Recombinant human growth hormone treatment in pediatric burn patients and its role during the hepatic acute phase response. *Crit. Care Med.* 28, 1578, 2000.

185. Jaschke, M.G., Herndon, D.N., and Barrow, R.E. Insulin-like growth factor I in combination with insulin-like growth factor binding protein 3 affects the hepatic acute phase response and hepatic morphology in thermally injured rats. *Ann. Surg.* 231, 408, 2000.

186. Wu, X., Herndon, D.N., and Wolf, S.E. Growth hormone down-regulation of Interleukin-1beta and Interleukin-6 induced acute phase protein gene expression is associated with increased gene expression of suppressor of cytokine signal-3. *Shock* 19, 314, 2003.

187. Thomas, S., Wolf, S.E., Chinkes, D.L., and Herndon, D.N. Recovery from the hepatic acute phase response in the severely burned and the effects of long-term growth hormone treatment. *Burns* 30, 675, 2004.

188. Hansen, T.K. Growth hormone and mannan-binding lectin: emerging evidence for hormonal regulation of humoral innate immunity. *Minerva Endocrinol.* 28, 75, 2003.

189. Jeschke, M.G., Klein, D., and Herndon, D.N. Insulin treatment improves the systemic inflammatory reaction to severe trauma. *Ann. Surg.* 239, 553, 2004.

190. Jeschke, M.G. and Herndon, D.N. Effect of growth factors as therapeutic drugs on hepatic metabolism during the systemic inflammatory response syndrome. *Curr. Drug Metab.* 5, 399, 2004.

191. Hasday, J.D., Fairchild, K.D., and Shanholtz, C. The role of fever in the infected host. *Microbes Infect.* 2, 1891, 2000.

192. Krabbe, K.S., Bruunsgaard, H., Hansen, C.M., Moller, K., Fonsmark, L., Qvist, J., Madsen, P.L., Kronborg, G., Andersen, H.O., Skinhoj, P., and Pedersen, B.K. Ageing is associated with a prolonged fever response in human endotoxemia. *Clin. Diagn. Lab. Immunol.* 8, 333, 2001.

193. Kotler, D.P. Cachexia. *Ann. Intern. Med.* 133, 622, 2000.

194. Langhans, W. Anorexia of infection: current prospects. *Nutrition* 16, 996, 2000.

195. Yudkin, J.S., Kumari, M., Humphries, S.E., and Mohamed-Ali, V. Inflammation, obesity, stress and coronary heart disease: is interleukin-6 the link? *Atherosclerosis* 148, 209, 2000.

196. Kushner, I. C-reactive protein elevation can be caused by conditions other than inflammation and may reflect biologic aging. *Cleve. Clin. J. Med.* 68, 535, 2001.

197. Bruunsgaard, H., Pedersen, M., and Pedersen, B.K. Aging and proinflammatory cytokines. *Curr. Opin. Hematol.* 8, 131, 2001.

198. Duncan, B.B. and Schmidt, M.I. Chronic activation of the innate immune system may underlie the metabolic syndrome. *Sao Paulo Med. J.* 119, 122, 2001.

199. Hak, A.E., Pols, H.A., Stehouwer, C.D., Meijer, J., Kiliaan, A.J., Hofman, A., Breteler, M.M., and Witteman, J.C. Markers of inflammation and cellular adhesion molecules in relation to insulin resistance in nondiabetic elderly: the Rotterdam study. *J. Clin. Endocrinol. Metab.* 86, 4398, 2001.

200. Vozarova, B., Fernandez-Real, J.M., Knowler, W.C., Gallart, L., Hanson, R.L., Gruber, J.D., Ricart, W., Vendrell, J., Richart, C., Tataranni, P.A., and Wolford J.K. The interleukin-6 (-174) G/C promoter polymorphism is associated with type-2 diabetes mellitus in Native Americans and Caucasians. *Hum. Genet.* 112, 409, 2003.

201. Trayhurn, P. and Wood, I.S. Adipokines: inflammation and the pleiotropic role of white adipose tissue. *Br. J. Nutr.* 92, 347, 2004.

202. le Roux, C.W., Chapman, G.A., Kong, W.M., Dhillo, W.S., Jones, J., and Alaghband-Zadeh, J. Free cortisol index is better than serum total cortisol in determining hypothalamic-pituitary-adrenal status in patients undergoing surgery. *J. Clin. Endocrinol. Metab.* 88, 2045, 2003.

203. Schmid, B., Wong, S., and Mitchell, B.F. Transcriptional regulation of oxytocin receptor by interleukin-1beta and interleukin-6. *Endocrinology* 142, 1380, 2001.

204. Marchini, G., Berggren, V., Djilali-Merzoug, R., and Hansson, L.O. The birth process initiates an acute phase reaction in the fetus-newborn infant. *Acta Paediatr.* 89, 1082, 2000.

205. Pedersen, B.K. Special feature for the Olympics: effects of exercise on the immune system: exercise and cytokines. *Immunol. Cell Biol.* 78, 532, 2000.

206. Pedersen, B.K. and Hoffman-Goetz, L. Exercise and the immune system: regulation, integration, and adaptation. *Physiol. Rev.* 80, 1055, 2000.

207. Jeukendrup, A.E., Vet-Joop, K., Sturk, A., Stegen, J.H., Senden, J., Saris, W.H., and Wagenmakers, A.J. Relationship between gastrointestinal complaints and endotoxaemia, cytokine release and the acute-phase reaction during and after a long-distance triathlon in highly trained men. *Clin. Sci.*, 98, 47, 2000.

208. Banck, G. and Forsgren, A. Many bacterial species are mitogenic for human blood B lymphocytes. *Scand. J. Immunol.* 8, 347, 1978.

209. Fleischer, B., Gerlach, D., Fuhrmann, A., and Schmidt, K.H. Superantigens and pseudosuperantigens of Gram-positive cocci. *Med. Microbiol. Immunol.* 184, 1, 1995.

210. Levinson, A.I., Kozlowski, L., Zheng, Y., and Wheatley, L. B-cell superantigens: definition and potential impact on the immune response. *J. Clin. Immunol.* 15 (6 Suppl.), 26S, 1995.

211. Zumla, A. Superantigens, T cells and microbes. *Clin. Infect. Dis.* 15, 313, 1992.

212. Kotb, M. Bacterial pyrogenic exotoxins as superantigens. *Clin. Microbiol. Rev.* 8, 411, 1995.

213. Spangelo, B.L., deHoll, P.D., Kalabay, L., Bond, B.R., and Arnaud, P. Neurointermediate pituitary lobe cells synthesize and release interleukin-6 *in vitro*: effects of lipopolysaccharide and interleukin-1 beta. *Endocrinology* 135, 556, 1994.

214. Chao, H.S., Poisner, A.M., Poisner, R., and Handwerger, S. Lipopolysaccharides inhibit prolactin and renin release from human decidual cells. *Biol. Reprod.* 50, 210, 1994.

215. Di Santo, E., Sironi, M., Pozzi, P., Gnocchi, P., Isetta, A.M., Delvaux, A., Goldman, M., Marchant, A., and Ghezzi, P. Interleukin-10 inhibits lipopolysaccharide-induced tumor necrosis factor and interleukin-1 beta production in the brain without affecting the activation of the hypothalamus–pituitary–adrenal axis. *Neuroimmunomodulation* 2, 149, 1995.

216. Faggioni, R., Fantuzzi, G., Villa, P., Buurman, W., van Tits, L.J., and Ghezzi, P. Independent down-regulation of central and peripheral tumor necrosis factor production as a result of lipopolysaccharide tolerance in mice. *Infect. Immun.* 63, 1473, 1995.

217. Das, K.P., McMillian, M.K., Bing, G., and Hong, J.S. Modulatory effects of [Met5]-enkephalin on interleukin-1 beta secretion from microglia in mixed brain cell cultures. *J. Neuroimmunol.* 62, 9, 1995.

218. Scotte, M., Hiron, M., Masson, S., Lyoumi, S., Banine, F., Teniere, P., Lebreton, J.P., and Daveau, M. Differential expression of cytokine genes in monocytes, peritoneal macrophages and liver following endotoxin- or turpentine-induced inflammation in rat. *Cytokine* 8, 115, 1996.

219. Gaykema, R.P., Dijkstra, I., and Tilders, F.J. Subdiaphragmatic vagotomy suppresses endotoxin-induced activation of hypothalamic corticotropin-releasing hormone neurons and ACTH secretion. *Endocrinology* 136, 4717, 1995.

220. Laye, S., Bluthe, R.M., Kent, S., Combe, C., Medina, C., Parnet, P., Kelley, K., and Dantzer, R. Subdiaphragmatic vagotomy blocks induction of IL-1 beta mRNA in mice brain in response to peripheral LPS. *Am. J. Physiol.* 268 (5 Pt 2), R1327, 1995.

221. Blatteis, C.M., Fever and host defence, in *The Brain and Host Defence, Neuroimmune Biology,* Vol. 9, Buckingham, J., Arnason B., and Berczi, I., Eds., Elsevier, Amsterdam, 2005, in press.

222. Berczi, I., Bertok, L., Baintner, K., Jr., and Veress, B. Failure of oral *Escherichia coli* endotoxin to induce either specific tolerance or toxic syndromes in rats. *J. Path. Bact.* 96, 481, 1968.

223. Kocsar, L.T., Bertok, L., and Varteresz, V. Effect of bile acids on the intestinal absorption of endotoxin in rats. *J. Bacteriol.* 100, 220, 1969.

224. Mimura, Y., Sakisaka, S., Harada, M., Sata, M., and Tanikawa, K. Role of hepatocytes in direct clearance of lipopolysaccharide in rats. *Gastroenterology* 109, 1969, 1995.

225. Bertok, L. Physico-chemical defence of vertebrate organisms: the role of bile acids in defence against endotoxins. *Persp. Biol. Med.* 21, 70, 1977.

226. Cannon W.B. The emergency function of the adrenal medulla in pain and in the major emotions. *Am. J. Physiol.* 33, 356, 1914.

15 Interferon in Health and Disease

Nachum Dafny, Pamela B. Yang, and Stanley A. Brod

CONTENTS

INTRODUCTION

Interferons were discovered by Drs. Isaacs and Lindenmann [1957] who had been studying the effects of different agents on viral growth. They infected egg membranes with live viruses and found that the viruses failed to grow. They concluded that something had interfered with the growth processes of the viruses. They isolated this protein and called it interferon (IFN) because it interfered with viruses' growth. IFNs are also produced by cells when a subject is invaded by viruses. The IFN is released into the blood stream and intercellular fluid to induce the production of an enzyme that counters the viral infection by preventing the viruses from replicating in the body [Bocci, 1992]. Beside the activation of immunity, IFN produces a broad spectrum of non-immunological host defenses in the countered response to infection, including fever, anorexia, and sleep. It was found that a variety of stimuli act on different cells and organ systems to give rise to various endogenous types of IFNs.

Three different families of IFNs are produced. They initially were classified as leukocyte, fibroblast, and immune IFNs according to their supposed production by particular cell and organ sites. These three classes are now classified differently on the basis of the antigenicities of their proteins and their biological properties: alpha (α), beta (β), and gamma (γ) [Bocci, 1985, 1988a,b, 1992; Makino et al., 2000; Paulesu et al., 1985; Yasuda, 1993]. Alpha-interferon (α-IFN) is produced by epithelial cells. Beta-interferon (β-IFN) is produced by fibroblast cells, whereas gamma-interferon (γ-IFN) is produced by cells of the immune system.

α-IFN is a protein with immunomodulatory, antiproliferative, and antiviral properties. It plays a critical role in maintaining the balance of the immune system by stimulating natural killer (NK) cells and is used in the treatment of hairy cell leukemia, AIDS-related Kaposi's sarcoma, and sarcoma. Exogenous α-IFN was induced initially by infection of white blood cells in cultures. The human α-IFN gene family contains at least 20 distinct members. Some of these genes are non-allelic variants; others are allelic variants [Kirchner, 1984].

β-IFN shares about 60% homology with α-IFN and exists in the form of a single molecule. In vivo, β-IFN is produced by fibroblasts that are stimulated by viruses or by synthetic inducers. β-IFN is an immunoregulatory cytokine that reduces relapse frequency in multiple sclerosis (MS) and ameliorates experimental autoimmune neuritis. Recent observations suggest that β-IFN treatment is beneficial in chronic inflammatory demyelinating polyradiculoneuropathy [Creange et al., 1998; Hadden et al., 1999; Pritchard et al., 2003; Schaller et al., 2001; Vallat et al., 2003; Zou et al., 1999].

γ-IFN is a macrophage-activating protein that modulates a variety of biological pathways potentially relevant to muscle wasting and immune dysfunction and plays a fundamental role in mediating the hypercatabolic states of multiple cell types following burn trauma. γ-IFN has no homology to α-IFN or β-IFN. The human γ-IFN appears to exist in the form of a single molecule and is produced by T lymphocytes. The γ-IFN gene possesses several introns, whereas the genes of the other IFN subtypes are devoid of introns [Gray and Goeddel, 1982]. γ-IFN is a prototype of two classes of substances: lymphokines and interferons [Kirchner, 1984].

The doses of IFN used in patient treatment at clinics are in International Units (IU). An IU of IFN is defined as the amount that inhibits viral replication by 50% [Bendtzen, 2003; Kirchner, 1984].

Since IFN used in immunologic therapy is synthesized and released naturally in the body, it was thought to be nontoxic [Goldstein et al., 1988]. However, several adverse effects such as sensory and motor abnormality, fever, anorexia, confusion, and depression have been reported as results of exogenous IFN treatment. All these symptoms are central nervous system (CNS)-mediated phenomena [Ackerman et al., 1984; Cantell et al., 1980; Hori et al., 1991; Iivanainen et al., 1985; Mattson et al., 1983; Smedley et al., 1983]. Therefore, this review will focus on the role of IFN in CNS activity.

INTERFERON RECEPTORS AND INTERFERON BINDING IN THE CNS

Interferon receptors have been identified in the CNS, immune system, and endocrine system [Aguet, 1980; Pestka et al., 1987]. IFN participates in the regulation of various cellular processes and exerts effects on the neuroendocrine system, CNS, and immune system [Aguet and Mogensen, 1983; Aguet, 1980; Besedovsky and del Rey, 2002; Blalock and Smith, 1981b; Dafny et al., 1985a, 2004; Langer et al., 1996; Pestka et al., 1987].

Interferon receptors are found in macrophages, monocytes, T-lymphocytes, glia, and neurons. Interferons modulate gene expression via simple, direct signaling pathway containing receptors for JAK tyrosine kinases and STAT transcription factors. Tyrosine kinase activation is a common mechanism for triggering eukaryotic signaling pathways [Pestka, 2000; Yan et al., 1998]. Interferons bind to specific receptors on cell surfaces, resulting in a complex cellular response associated with changes in the expression of a large number of genes [Samuel, 1991]. This binding elicits a variety of cellular responses. The IFN receptors have extracellular ligand-binding domains and intracellular kinase domains that are activated following ligand-induced dimerization [Pestka, 2000].

More recently, IFNs have been classified into at least five classes: alpha (α), beta (β), gamma (γ), tau (τ), and omega (ω) [Pestka, 2000]. In general, the IFN family is divided into two groups: types I and II. α-IFN and β-IFN belong to the type I IFN family of cytokines [Baron et al., 1991; Campbell et al., 1999; Pestka et al., 1987]. Type I IFNs share a common receptor and exhibit similar biological activities [Pestka, 2000]. The type I α-IFN and β-IFN (α/β-IFN) are comprised of the products of multiple α-IFN genes (up to 12) and a single β-IFN gene [Biron, 2001]. Type II IFN, also known as γ-IFN, activates the JAK/STAT pathway via its α and β subunit receptors [Kaur et al., 2003; Stark et al., 1998] that activate JAK1 and JAK2 kinases, followed by tyrosine phosphorylation of STAT1 [Boehm et al., 1997; Shuai et al., 1993; Stark et al., 1998].

The brain is relatively isolated from the immune system due to the presence of the blood–brain barrier (BBB) that limits the penetration of circulating cytokines and antibodies [Darling et al., 1981]. However, a small amount of exogenous IFNs does penetrate the brain [Cathala and Baron, 1970; Habif et al., 1975; Mattson et al., 1983; Vass and Lassman, 1990]. Systemically, α-IFN administration enters the brain through areas where the BBB is more permeable [Bocci, 1985, 1992; Janicki, 1992; Scott et al., 1981; Smith et al., 1985, 1986; Wiranowska et al., 1989; Zimmerman and Krivoy, 1973]. α-IFN binds to brain tissue, and this binding varies among brain regions. The existence of specific binding sites within the CNS may, however, represent the link between α-IFN and its effects on neuronal activity. α-IFN also binds to opiate sites on biological membranes and in experiments using radiolabeled opioid receptor ligand. Moreover, α-IFN inhibits dihydromorphine binding in mouse brain homogenates [Blalock, 1989] and α-IFN treatment also exhibits inhibitory effects on the binding of [^{3}H] naloxone and enkephalin of rat brain membrane *in vitro* [Menzies et al., 1992], suggesting interactions between IFNs and the opioid system.

INTERFERON AND OPIOID

Drug dependence has been considered primarily a CNS phenomenon [Jaffe, 1990; Dafny, 1999]. One means whereby the degree of opioid dependence is assessed is by administering an opioid antagonist such as naloxone in animals treated chronically with opiate to precipitate stereotypical withdrawal behavior [Dafny, 1983b,c; Wei, 1971]. It was found that selective destruction of specific brain sites in morphine-dependent animals attenuated the severity of systemically naloxone-precipitated withdrawal [Kerr and Pozuelo, 1971; Laschka et al., 1976; Teitelbaum et al., 1974]. Moreover, intracerebral microinjection of naloxone only to specific brain areas of opiate-dependent animals precipitated withdrawal identical to that following systemic naloxone administration [Louria, 1969], indicating that several specific brain areas are involved in the withdrawal behavior [Dafny and Reyes-Vazquez, 1987].

The involvement of the immune system in various aspects associated with the chronic use of opioids was suggested a long time ago by Andral in 1844 [Cohen et al., 1965] and more recently by others [Dafny et al., 1985b, 1988b]. The cells of the immune system possess opiate receptors [Hazum et al., 1984] that, when activated, induce a variety of functional modifications such as the establishment of profound immune suppression following chronic opiate treatment [Jaffe, 1990; Pellis et al., 1986]. The ability of the immune system and the CNS to communicate and interact with each other was demonstrated [Blalock, 1989; Dafny, 1998; Dafny et al., 1985a, 1988b, 2004; Dafny and Reyes-Vazquez, 1987]. Hypothalamic lesions or ablations modulate immune components and reactions [Jankovic and Isakovic, 1973; Spector and Korneva, 1981] and hypothalamic neurons alter their neuronal firing rates following an immune challenge [Besedovsky et al., 1986; Spector and Korneva, 1981].

The participation of the immune system in modulating central opioid actions has been recognized by the finding that various immunomodulator agents such as IFN [Dafny, 1983b,c; Dafny, 1998; Dafny and Reyes-Vazquez, 1984; Dafny et al., 1985b, 1988b, 1989, 2004], cyclophosphamide, cortisol [Montgomery and Dafny, 1987], cyclosporine [Dafny et al., 1985b], and immune suppressive doses of gamma irradiation [Dafny and Pellis, 1986; Meisheri and Isom, 1978] attenuate the severity of naloxone-precipitated withdrawal in opiate-dependent rats. These observations provide additional evidence that the immune system and immunomodifiers such as IFNs participate in opiate activity.

In addition, the neuronal activities of the cortex, hypothalamus, and hippocampus neurons were modulated following systemic or local IFN application or manipulation of the immune system [Dafny, 1983a; Dafny et al., 1985a, 1988b; Jankovic and Isakovic, 1973; Prieto-Gomez et al., 1983; Reyes-Vazquez and Dafny, 1984; Reyes-Vazquez et al., 1982, 1984a,b, 1994; Spector and Korneva, 1981]. These studies suggest that the immune system compartments or immune cell products (immunomodulator agents) act on the CNS and are involved in regulating function including the opiate-mediated response [Dafny et al., 1989], and that there is a reciprocal pathway of communication between the immune system and the CNS.

Interferon was reported to modulate opiate-mediated phenomena by a direct action within the CNS, thus directly supporting the contention that immune-derived peptide can convey information from the immune system to the CNS [Calvet and Gresser, 1979; Dafny, 1983b,c; Dafny et al., 1983, 1985a, 1988b; Dafny and Reyes-Vazquez, 1984; Dougherty et al., 1986a,b; Reite et al., 1987; Reyes-Vazquez and Dafny, 1984]. Using neurophysiological recording procedures, Dafny et al. [1985a] and Reyes-Vazquez et al. [1984a] demonstrated that α-IFN administration resulted in an alteration of the neuronal activity of brain regions participating in the expression of opioid activities when IFN was given alone and in the presence of opioid [Dafny, 1998].

It is important to emphasize that IFN exerts its effects upon opioid receptor and upon a distinct receptor complex [Dafny, 1998; Dafny et al., 1988b, 2004; Reyes-Vazquez et al., 1984a]. α-IFN modulates opioid activity at the level of single neurons in discrete CNS sites and modifies behavioral paradigms, supporting the concept that α-IFN is a neuromodulator of immunologic origin [Dafny, 1998; Dafny et al., 1988b, 2004]. Thus, α-IFN is one of the cytokine products released by the immune system that possesses immunological, endocrinological, and neuromodulatory properties.

The administration of morphine resulted in decreased levels of endogenous circulating α-IFN and decreased the capability of cells to produce α-IFN [Vilcek et al., 1968]. The level of α-IFN inhibition was directly related to the morphine dosage [Hung et al., 1973]. α-IFN shares some pharmacologic properties similar to β-endorphin, such as the production of analgesia and catatonia as well as affinity for [3H]-morphine binding sites in mouse brain membranes [Blalock and Smith, 1980, 1981a]. We conclude that this reduction in endogenous IFN resulted in morphine-dependent addiction [Dafny, 1984, 1985] and hypothesize that α-IFN is the endogenous cytokine that serves to prevent the development of tolerance and dependence to the endogenous opioids.

In a series of experiments, α-IFN given intracerebroventrically (icv) and systemically (ip) dramatically attenuated the severity of opiate withdrawal behaviors [Dafny, 1983b,c; Dafny et al., 1983, 1985a, 1988b; Dougherty et al., 1987]. Using several electrophysiological procedures such as sensory evoked potential, EEG, single neuron recording, microiontophoretic and systemic application of IFNs, morphine, and naloxone [Dafny, 1983a, 1985; Dafny et al., 1985a, 1988b; Prieto-Gomez et al., 1983; Reyes-Vazquez et al., 1982, 1984a,b, 1994] suggests the presence of at least three different functional and/or receptor sites for α-IFN within the CNS: (1) a site where α-IFN caused excitation and this excitation is blocked or reversed by the opiate antagonist naloxone, which may represent the κ or δ opiate receptor type [Nakashima et al., 1987], (2) a site where α-IFN caused reduction (inhibition) in neuronal activities and this effect is also antagonized by naloxone which may represent the μ receptor type, and (3) a site where α-IFN caused excitation in neuronal activity but naloxone was unable to antagonize the α-IFN-induced excitation [Dafny et al., 1985a; Reyes-Vazquez et al., 1984a].

In an experiment using molecular procedures, it was demonstrated that icv injection of α-IFN suppressed the cytotoxic activities of the cells in the spleens of mice, and this effect was prevented by pretreatment with naloxone [Take et al., 1992a,b, 1993]. Moreover, in *in vivo* preparations from rat brain membrane, α-IFN treatment has been shown to inhibit the binding of [3H] naloxone [Menzies et al., 1992], demonstrating a competition between α-IFN and naloxone for membrane binding sites. This observation may explain the mechanism of how α-IFN attenuates withdrawal behaviors in morphine-dependent animals [Menzies et al., 1992; Dafny, 1998]. In conclusion, α-IFN and opioids are modulatory agents mediating brain endocrine and immune interaction through complex mechanisms involving multiple receptors and sites and acting at different levels of integration [Dougherty et al., 1986a,b; Dougherty and Dafny, 1991; Roda et al., 1996].

INTERFERON AND SLEEP

Sleep is a behavioral state that alternates with waking. An ascending brainstem projection regulates the sleep–waking cycle. The output of the ascending reticular activating system (ARAS) divides into the thalamocortical, thalamohypothalamus, and thalamoforebrain systems. Therefore, a day sleep modulation agent has effects on the ARAS. It is known that cytokines such as IFN are somnogenic and are involved in the sleep–wake regulation via altering the neuroendocrine system, neurotransmitters, and nitric oxide [Kruger and Majde, 1995].

The primary determinant in identifying stages of sleep is the electroencephalogram (EEG). The EEG is a gross potential recorded from the surface of the scalp of a human and can be recorded from cortical and subcortical structures [Dafny, 1983a]. The frequencies of the EEG potentials recorded varied from 1 to 40 Hz with amplitudes ranging from 20 to 100 µV, i.e., the behavioral signs of sleep vary regularly during sleep time among the following stages: (1) the wake stage is indicated by low amplitude desynchronized fast (30 Hz) EEG activity; (2) the drowsy stage indicated by a 7- to 13-Hz alpha wave is known as stage 1 sleep; (3) the high amplitude–low frequency 4- to 7-Hz theta wave is classified as the step 2 sleep spindle; (4) an EEG recording exhibiting 12 to 14 Hz that includes the sleep spindle and K complexes indicates the stage known as step 3 sleep; (5) the next stage (stage 4) is defined by deep sleep of 1- to 4-Hz high amplitude waves; and (6) the last stage (REM sleep) is characterized by activity similar to the awake state, such as low amplitude desynchronized fast activity. The electromyogram (EMG) activity of the head, neck and general skeletal muscles is dramatically reduced except for the middle ear muscle and the eyes that exhibit rapid eye movement (REM).

α-IFN given to a healthy human [Spath-Schwalbe et al., 1999] impaired the quality of night sleep, suppressed the slow wave sleep, and increased the time spent in shallow sleep. The time spent in REM sleep was also decreased, suggesting that α-IFN may be a factor responsible for alterations of sleep [Spath-Schwalbe et al., 1999]. EEG and EEG-like activity recording from several cortical and subcortical sites in albino Sprague–Dawley rats before and after systemic α-IFN injection resulted in alteration of the EEG recording first in the hypothalamus, followed by somatosensory cortex, limbic structures, and motor cortex, respectively [Dafny, 1983a]. This effect of α-IFN in modifying the ARAS that results in output signals is the underlying cause of its diverse effects on the 24-hour rhythms in physiology and behavior like sleep [Koyanagi and Ohdo, 2002].

The somnogenic actions of α- and β-IFN were initially reported [Birmanns et al., 1990; Dafny 1983a; De Sarro et al., 1990; Kidron et al., 1989; Krueger et al., 1987; Kuriyama et al., 1990; Mattson et al., 1983; Reite et al., 1987; Saphier et al., 1987, 1988; Shoham et al., 1987; Smedley, 1983]. It was only recently recognized that γ-IFN also elicits a dose-dependent increase in non-rapid eye movement sleep (N-REM) accompanied with slow wave EEG activity [Kubota et al., 2001].

Changes in sleep patterns are common symptoms of an infectious disease. The initial sleep alterations induced by infection are increases in N-REM sleep and in the delta wave activity of the EEG [Fang et al., 1995; Kimura-Takenchi et al., 1992; Toth and Kruger, 1988; Kubota et al., 2001]. Similar observations were obtained following IFN injection [Kruger et al., 1987]. For example, α- and β-IFN enhanced EEG synchronization in rats, rabbits, and humans [Birmanns et al., 1990; Dafny, 1983a; DeSarrato et al., 1990; Krueger et al., 1987], while γ-IFN promoted N-REM sleep in humans [Kubota et al., 2001]. Men with difficulty maintaining normal sleep had significantly lower γ-IFN to IL ratios by a factor of 4 [Sakami et al., 2002–2003). Alcoholic subjects showed profound sleep disturbances, with γ-IFN to IL ratios of 10. They also exhibited reduced levels of NK cell activity coupled with losses of delta sleep and increased REM sleep [Redwine et al., 2003]. All these observations suggest that the IFN modulates sleep patterns by altering the ascending reticular activating system.

INTERFERON AND TEMPERATURE

Fever is regulated by the central nervous system (CNS), mainly in two sites within the hypothalamus: the hypothalamic preoptic (PO) area and the anterior hypothalamic (AH) area. The PO/AH area contains three types of neurons sensitive to cold only, to heat only, and to different degrees of temperature. These neurons are involved in determining the temperature set point. Therefore, the PO/AH area is suggested as the site of regulating temperature [Ackerman et al., 1984; Dinarello et al., 1984]. Fever is initiated by the activation of these thermosensitive neurons. Hypothermia is a thermoregulatory response to systemic inflammation that is often regarded as maladaptive to the host [Leon, 2004]. The mechanisms regulating hypothermia are not fully understood, but cytokines such as the IFNs have been shown to modulate the neuronal activities of temperature sensitive neurons in the PO/AH area.

Local application of interleukin-1 (IL-1) and α-IFN to thermosensitive neurons in the PO/AH area altered PO/AH neuronal activity [Blatteis et al., 1991; Kidron et al., 1989; Kuriyama et al., 1990; Nakashima et al., 1981, 1987, 1988; Saphier et al., 1988] that resulted in induction of fever. Therefore, α-IFN is considered an endogenous pyrogen [Dinarello, 1988, 1989; Hori et al., 1991]. The PO/AH area is the most probable site of the pyrogenic action of IFN [Ackermann et al., 1984; Dinerello et al., 1984].

Fever is a host's defensive response to various exogenously pathogenic organisms and their products such as lipopolysaccharides; it is mediated centrally by endogenous pyrogens that include the IFN family [Blatteis et al., 1991]. The production of pyrogenic endogenous cytokines results from a host's defensive response to various exogenously pathogenic organisms [Blatteis et al., 1991]. The terms *granulocytic* and *endogenous pyrogen* were used to describe substances with biological properties of fever induction. It became evident that pyrogenicity is a fundamental biologic property of several cytokines including the IFN family [Leon, 2004]. The iv or intracerebroventricular (icv) injection of α-IFN in rodents, cats, and rabbits elicited fever without the production and involvement of the endogenously pyrogenic IL-1; this leads to the suggestion that α-IFN is an endogenous pyrogen [Dinarello, 1988; Dinarello et al., 1984].

It was reported that the IFN-induced fever resulted from its effects on PO/AH thermosensitive neurons. These activities are blocked by naloxone, an opiate antagonist, and failed to respond to antipyrogenic agents such as sodium salicylate, which is known to block the neuronal responses to endotoxin and leukocytic pyrogen [Blatteis et al., 1991; Hori et al., 1991; Kuriyama et al., 1990; Nakashima et al., 1987, 1988]. This suggests that α-IFN induces fever, at least in part by direct effects on PO/AH thermosensitive neurons, which involve also the opiate receptor mechanism [Nakayama et al., 1981; Nakashima et al., 1988] and led to the postulation that IFN in the brain produces fever by a two-step mechanism. The first step is the immediate action on opioid receptors on PO/AH thermosensitive neurons follow by the release of prostaglandin that elicits fever [Blatteis et al., 1991; Hori et al., 1988, 1991].

INTERFERON AND FOOD REGULATION

Eating is a regulatory behavior that contributes to caloric homeostasis. Food intake provides nutrients to support the continuous energy demands and maintains stable body weight. Stereotaxic lesions of distinct brain regions in rats such as the ventromedial hypothalamus (VMH) or lateral hypothalamus (LH) resulted in obese or aphagic animals [Dafny et al., 1988a; Dafny and Jacobson, 1975; Schanzer et al., 1978; Tempel et al., 1993]. For example, bilateral VMH lesion or deafferentiation resulted in marked hyperphagia (and obesity); faster gastric emptying resulted in more frequent eating [Dafny et al., 1988a]. Bilateral LH lesions elicited aphagia (absence of eating) and reduced parasympathetic tone, which resulted in reducing the rate of gastric emptying and prolonging the time interval between eating, similar to anorexia.

Local application of α-IFN using a microiontophoretic procedure with a multibarrel electrode on VMH and LH neurons [Dafny et al., 1985a; Prieto-Gomez et al., 1981, 1983] elicited different responses, i.e., decreased activity of LH neurons and increased VMH neuronal activity. Similar observations were obtained using coronal brain slice sections [Dafny et al., 1996; Reyes-Vazquez et al., 1994, 1997] containing both the VMH and LH areas and recording single neuronal activity simultaneously in both sites with glass microelectrodes before and after glucose and α-IFN administration. It was observed that glucose perfusion elicited mainly a decrease in firing rate in the VMH, but elicited mainly an increase in firing rate in the LH. When α-IFN was perfused alone, the opposite effects were observed, mainly a decrease neuronal activity in LH and an increase in neuronal discharges in the VMH. When both agents were given simultaneously, the presence of α-IFN prevented the glucose effects, i.e., the glucose-elicited decrease in the firing rate in LH was prevented [Hori et al., 1988, 1991; Kow and Pfaff, 1985; Mattson et al., 1983; Plata-Salaman et al., 1989; Prieto-Gomez et al., 1983; Reyes-Vazquez et al., 1994]. Similar observations were reported by others using different preparations [Dafny et al., 1985a; Hori et al., 1991; Kerr et al., 1974; Prieto-Gomez et al., 1981, 1983; Reyes-Vazquez et al., 1994]. The reciprocal interaction of VMH and LH in the mechanism of food intake was reported previously using different approaches [Dafny et al., 1988b; Schanzer et al., 1978]. These observations suggest that endogenous IFN in the brain [Bocci, 1988a,b, 1992; Marcovitz et al., 1984] is involved in feeding regulation as a neurotransmitter or a neuroregulator.

Other cytokines such as tumor necrosis factor (TNF) and IL-1 exert effects similar to IFN in inhibiting glucose-sensitive neurons in the so-called *hunger center* (or LH), resulting in feeding suppression [Kow and Pfaff, 1985; Plata-Salaman, 1989, 1991].

Most of the glucose-sensitive neurons altering their activity to IL-1 or TNF were also sensitive to α-IFN [Hori et al., 1988, 1991; Plata-Salaman 1989]. It has been reported [Reyes-Vazquez et al., 1994; Rohatiner et al., 1983; Saphier et al., 1988] that patients treated daily with α-IFN show prominent side effects such as anorexia by losing more than 10% of their body weight [Adams et al., 1984; Crnic and Segall, 1992; Meyers and Valentine, 1995; Rohatiner et al., 1983; Smedley et al., 1983]. The anorexic state produced by α-IFN is reversible. After discontinuation of α-IFN therapy, patients usually return to their normal weights within 7 to 10 days [Rohatiner et al., 1983]. Similar decreases in food intake were observed in animals following IFN treatment [Crnic and Segall, 1992; Plata-Salaman, 1989; Reyes-Vazquez et al., 1994; Saphier et al., 1988; Segall and Crnic, 1990]. The weight losses presumably were the results of increased VMH activity and decreased LH activity.

Although cytokines such as IFN suppress food intake independently of fever, it is possible that the increase in temperature caused by IFN treatment results in the inhibition of feeding, and the fever modulates the activities of glucose-responsive neurons in the VMH and LH [Hori et al., 1988; Nakayama et al., 1981]. Since IFN also produces sleep and sleep prevents eating, less eating results in weight loss. This is another possible explanation of how IFN affects feeding behavior [Birmanns et al., 1990; Dafny et al., 1988a; De Sarro et al., 1990; Krueger et al., 1987; Plata-Salaman 1991; Saphier et al., 1988].

Plasma IFN levels in healthy subjects increased after eating during the day with peak levels at 18:00 hours and the lowest levels in early morning [Bocci et al., 1985; Paulesu et al., 1985]. These daily variations of endogenous IFN levels in healthy humans are linked to external cues such as physical activity, feeding, and sleep [Paulesu et al., 1985]. Such observations can explain how IFN elicits feeding suppression and anorexia [Hori et al., 1991; Krueger et al., 1987; Mattson et al., 1983].

INTERFERON AND ENDOCRINE SYSTEM

The detection of adrenocorticotrophic hormone (ACTH) and endorphin-like substances from lymphocytes infected with the Newcastle disease virus (NDV) was one of the first studies demonstrating that the immune system produces peptides and that these peptides interact with the neuroendocrine system [Blalock, 1989; Dinarello, 1988, 1989; Reder, 1992]. Leukocyte IFN provides an afferent link between the immune and endocrine systems [Blalock and Smith, 1980; McCain et al., 1982]. Moreover, it was shown that α-IFN shares a common binding site to specific receptors such as ACTH [Aguet, 1980; Aguet and Mogensen, 1983;

Blalock and Smith, 1981a,b; Blalock and Stanton, 1980]. Cytokine production including α-IFN is not restricted to the immune cells. Cytokines are also produced and released by the CNS and the endocrine system [Blalock, 1989; Dinarello, 1988, 1989; Reder, 1992]. These cytokines exert direct effects on the CNS, the immune system, and the endocrine system [Dinarello, 1988; Kidron et al., 1989; Reder, 1992].

Sequential similarities of α-IFN, ACTH, and melanotrophic stimulation hormone (MSH) have been reported [Cantell et al., 1980; Krueger et al., 1982; Root-Bernstein, 1984; Vernikos-Danellis et al., 1977]. The similarities of these structures may explain the presence of common functional characteristics found in MSH, ACTH, α-IFN and immunological activity. Moreover, α-IFN stimulates ACTH secretion [Blalock and Smith, 1980; D'Urso et al., 1991; Root-Bernstein, 1984; Smith and Blalock, 1981]. Systematic (ip), central (icv), and local (microiontophoretic) treatment of α-IFN within the paraventricular hypothalamic nucleus (PVN) inhibited the hypo-thalamus–pituitary–adrenocortical (HPA) axis [Kidron et al., 1989; Saphier et al., 1993, 1994], such as the glucocorticoid hormones that modulate immune activity [Reder, 1992; Saphier et al., 1994]. It was demonstrated in electrophysiologically identified neurosecretory PVN neurons regulating adrenocortical secretion that α-IFN treatment decreased their neuronal activities. This decrease in PVN neuronal activity indicates that α-IFN participates in the regulation of adrenocortical release and secretion.

The CNS, immune system, and endocrine system contain IFN receptors. More-over, these three systems synthesize and release IFNs. The experiments reviewed in this chapter suggest that the CNS, immune system, and endocrine system communicate with each other. Some environmental cues such as stress or mental disorders lead to alteration of these three systems, resulting in the modification of immunocompetence and incidence of disease [Besedovsky and Del Rey, 1987; Bullock, 1985; Dunn, 1989; Felten et al., 1987; Solomon, 1987]. In turn, activation of the endocrine system or the immune system results in production and release of α-IFN; this stimulates the CNS and modulates its neuronal activity. The change in neuronal activity following IFN results in altering the neuroendocrine system and thereby providing feedback to regulate the immune system [Besedovsky et al., 1975, 1977; Dafny et al., 1985a; Dunn, 1989; Saphier et al., 1987, 1988, 1994]. In conclusion, all these studies support the notion that the IFNs are neuroregulators and suggest that they are the messengers that provide communications among the CNS, the immune system, and the endocrine system.

CLINICAL UTILITIES OF INTERFERONS

α/β-IFN and ω/τ-IFN (type I IFNs) and γ-IFN (type II IFN) have different primary structures. Therefore, the two types of IFN induce or suppress the synthesis of numerous disparate proteins. α/β-IFN stimulate natural killer (NK) cells, whereas γ-IFN stimulates mainly macrophages. α/β-IFN is stable at pH 2.0 while γ-IFN is acid labile. γ-IFN, unlike α/β-IFN, is not constitutively produced [Tovey et al., 1987].

α-IFN administered subcutaneously (sc) demonstrated a surprisingly wide range of efficacy in hematologic malignancies including tumors of presumed B-cell,

T-cell, and myeloid lineages. In some diseases, e.g., hairy cell leukemia and chronic myelogenous leukemia, α-IFN was broadly effective [Spiegel, 1987; Stuart-Harris et al., 1992]. However, at present, interferon has a relatively limited role in the treatment of hairy cell leukemia, and it is reserved for selected patients who failed nucleoside analogue therapy [Ahmed and Rai, 2003].

Kaposi's Sarcoma (KS)

High dose (27 to 36 million IU) recombinant α-IFN2a (rα-IFN2a) qd achieved major responses in 12 of 26 evaluable KS patients; 5 showed histologically confirmed complete responses [de Wit et al., 1988] with dose and blood levels important factors in responses [Sawyer et al., 1990]. The addition of zidovudine in AIDS-associated KS added to the efficacy of interferon [de Wit et al., 1991; Shepherd et al., 1998]. HIV-seropositive subjects with biopsy-confirmed cutaneous KS randomized to receive either low (1 million IU) or intermediate (10 million IU) doses of α-IFN2b once daily with twice daily doses of didanosine achieved similar response rates without optimal antiretroviral therapy [Krown et al., 2002].

Lymphoma

α-IFN2b plus chlorambucil was superior to chlorambucil alone in treating advanced follicular lymphoma [Price et al., 1991] and low-grade lymphoma [Aviles et al., 1995; Cole et al., 1998]. IFN maintenance therapy in diffuse large cell lymphoma improved duration of complete remission and survival [Aviles et al., 1992] and prolonged remission after fludarabine monophosphate therapy in low-grade non-Hodgkin's lymphoma [Zinzani et al., 1997]. However, α-IFN as maintenance therapy was not useful in aggressive malignant lymphoma when more intensive chemotherapy (CHOP-BLEO regimens) was employed during induction [Aviles et al., 2001].

Polycythemia Vera (PCV)

α-IFN was superior to phlebotomy in controlling the pathologic expansion of erythroid elements and all the clinical aspects of PCV [Sacchi et al., 1994] and corrected peripheral thrombocytosis in essential thrombocythemia [Middelhoff and Boll, 1992]. Summarized treatment results of 279 patients participating in 16 prospective nonrandomized studies and three case reports showed that phlebotomies were reduced in 82% of the patients and complete remissions were achieved in 50%. In addition, reduction of splenomegaly was seen in 77% and control of pruritus was achieved in 81% of the patients, demonstrating that IFN is an effective alternative to the present forms of treatment of PV [Lengfelder, 2000].

Chronic Myelogenous Leukemia (CML)

α-IFN exerted significant activity in CML, with best results at dosages of 5 million IU/m2/day. Early stage Philadelphia[+] CML hematologic response rates were 70 to 80% and cytogenetic response rates were 50% (approximately 20% of which were complete) [Guilhot et al., 1997; Wetzler et al., 1995]. α-IFN2a given daily continuously and intermittent low-dose cytosine arabinoside (Ara-C) proved superior to the results using IFN alone in CML [Arthur and Ma, 1993]. IFN also effectively treated CML relapse in the chronic phase after bone marrow transplantation [Higano et al., 1993]. Cytoreductive/myeloablative treatment followed by unmanipulated peripheral blood stem cell transplantation and low-dose α-IFN can result in long-term survival in newly diagnosed CML patients [Meloni et al., 2001]. A randomized trial compared the combination of IFN and hydroxyurea versus hydroxyurea (HU) monotherapy (CML Study II) showed complete hematologic response rates higher in IFN/HU-treated patients versus HU monotherapy (59 versus 32%) [Hehlmann et al., 2003].

Hairy Cell Leukemia

α-IFN, by its direct action on hairy cells [Pralle et al., 1988; Sigaux et al., 1987] was shown to be extraordinarily effective at doses as low as 150,000 to 500,000 IU/m2/day [Zinzani et al., 1991], a level sufficient to maximize biomarker neopterin levels [Aulitzky et al., 1985].

Virus Infections

IFN acts too slowly to arrest acute viral infections, but α-IFN has proved useful in certain chronic viral infections. Some patients form neutralizing antibodies that block the effects of the IFN; these appear to be relatively more common after rα-IFN-2 than after IFN derived from human cells [Finter et al., 1991].

Hepatitis C

In randomized controlled trials using sc IFN, 3 million IU α-IFN-2b tiw normalized aminoleucine transferase (ALT) levels and eliminated hepatitis C virus (HCV) RNA in 53% of treated patients and no untreated patients [Lampertico, 1994]. Comparing rα-IFN2a to no treatment, 20 treated cases (66.7%) had normalized serum aminotransferase levels within the first 4 months of treatment, compared with one case in the untreated group. However, reactivation or breakthrough frequently occurred afterward (20% in both cases) [Diodati et al., 1994]. Reinforced regimens (6 million IU qd × 12 days, 6 million IU tiw × 22 weeks, and 3 million IU tiw × 24 weeks) as opposed to the standard regimen (3 million IU tiw × 24 weeks) produced sustained responses (ALT normalizations) in a limited number (18%) of previously untreated patients and reduced the risk of cirrhosis (1%) after 18 months [Degos et al., 1998].

In patients with compensated HCV-related cirrhosis, 3 million IU α-IFN2b tiw showed biochemical responses in 6 of 47 treated patients and 0 of 39 controls. However, a 48-week course of IFN therapy usually failed to achieve sustained responses and did not significantly improve 3-year outcomes [Valla et al., 1999].

Serum HCV RNA is better than ALT for predicting long term cure after α-IFN therapy in chronic hepatitis C (CHC) [Chemello et al., 1999]. Pegylated α-IFN2b provided higher virologic responses in patients infected with genotype 1 [Lindsay et al., 2001]. In patients with CHC, weekly pegylated α-IFN2a plus ribavirin was tolerated as well as α-IFN2b plus ribavirin and produced significant improvements in rates of sustained virologic response as compared with α-IFN2b plus ribavirin or pegylated α-IFN2a alone [Fried et al., 2002].

Certain features of hepatitis C infections predict success or failure of IFN therapy. Clinical and serum biochemical response to α-IFN in CHC is associated with a loss of detectable HCV genome from serum [Shindo et al., 1991]. Short-term and sustained responses were independently predicted by lobular structure on pre-treatment liver biopsy and by short disease duration [Pagliaro, 1994]. IFN does not seem to affect overall or event-free survival of patients with hepatitis C virus-related cirrhosis while it seems to prevent the development of hepatocellular carcinoma [Gramenzi et al., 2001].

Hepatitis C virus genotype and viral loads are important predictors for sustained virologic response (SVR) to α-IFN therapy for CHC. Patients with tailored dose regimens had significantly higher rates of SVR than those receiving fixed dose α-IFN (46.7 versus 29.3%). Low pretreatment viral loads and tailored dose IFN regimens were significantly associated with higher SVR [Yu et al., 2004].

HEPATITIS B

In randomized controlled trials, 10 million IU/m2 α-IFN2a administered tiw for 6 months was significantly better than no treatment in producing sustained losses of HBeAg in hepatitis B virus (HBV) chronic carriers [Brook et al., 1989; Finter et al., 1991; Perrillo, 1993]. Ten of 31 (32%) patients treated for 4 months and only 1 of 14 (7%) control patients became negative for serum HBV DNA/DNAp that can induce remission in about one third of chronic HBV patients [Perrillo, 1993]. Treatment with 5 million IU rα-IFN2b for 12-weeks decreased viral replication and tripled sponta-neous seroconversion rates observed in chronic HBV active viral replication patients [Coppens et al., 1989]. However, α-IFN therapy induced HBeAg seroconversion in only about one third of patients, thus leaving the majority with persistent disease [Finter et al., 1991; Perrillo, 1993]. Data from three previously published multicenter, randomized, controlled trials were insufficient to establish a presumed beneficial effect of α-IFN2a on disease progression and survival [Krogsgaard, 1998].

MULTIPLE SCLEROSIS

High dose intramuscular (im) rα-IFN2a (9 million IU qod) reduced the multiple sclerosis (MS) relapse rate by 83% and active MRI scans over 6 months [Durelli et al., 1995]. However, attack rates rapidly returned to pretreatment values when therapy was stopped [Durelli et al., 1996]. The apparent difference between the results of this small but well conducted Italian study and prior studies with α-IFN in MS relates to IFN doses used in earlier trials: 1 million IU α-IFN sc qd [Knobler et al., 1984]; 3 million IU α-IFN sc twice weekly for 2 months, then weekly [AUSTIMS Research Group, 1989]; and 2 million IU rα-IFN2 sc tiw [Camenga et al., 1986]. The difference also relates to differences in trial design [Knobler et al., 1984] and the selection of more severely affected patients with secondary progressive multiple sclerosis (SPMS) [Kastrukoff et al., 1990; Kinnunen et al., 1993].

Ingested α-IFN may have activity in MS. In a phase I trial, there were significant decreases in peripheral blood mononuclear cells (PMNCs), IL-2, and γ–IFN production after ingestion of α-IFN. Ingested α-IFN showed no toxicity in normal volunteers or patients with relapsing remitting (RR) MS at doses ranging from 300 to 100,000 units. In subjects with RRMS, significant decreases in concanavalin A (Con A)-mediated proliferation and serum soluble intercellular adhesion molecule-1 (sICAM-1), a surrogate measure for disease activity in MS, were found after ingestion of 10,000 and 30,000 IU α-IFN. The RRMS subjects also showed decreased IL-2 secretion after ingesting 10,000 IU α-IFN, and decreased γ–IFN, β-TGF, and IL-10 production after ingesting 30,000 IU α-IFN. Our studies suggest that ingested human α-IFN is a biological response modifier in humans [Brod et al., 1997].

In a phase II randomized, placebo-controlled, double-blind trial, we investigated whether ingested α-IFN2a was safe and whether treatment reduced the number of gadolinium-enhanced lesions on serial MRIs of patients with active RRMS. Entry criteria included clinically definite RRMS and one or more gadolinium-enhanced lesions on a screening MRI. Of 80 patients screened, 33 were eligible and 30 of them enrolled for treatment. Patients were randomized (10 per group) to placebo, 10,000 or 30,000 IU α-IFN2a ingested on alternate days for 9 months. They were evaluated clinically and cerebral MRIs were performed monthly. Sample size projections were based on the assumption of a parenteral *IFN-like effect*, a 90% reduction of enhancing lesions evident within 1 month of the initiation of treatment in the active treatment groups sustained over the 9-month study as the primary outcome variable. There was no significant effect on enhancing lesions overall. However, by direct monthly comparison of the placebo and 10,000-IU groups after 5 months of treatment, there were 73% (p <0.05) fewer enhancements in the 10,000-IU group compared to the placebo group. There was a decrease of α-TNF protein secretion at months 4 and 5. γ-IFN cytokine secretion in the 10,000-IU group at month 5 showed a significant decrease that corresponded with the effect of ingested α-IFN on decreasing gadolinium enhancements. Relapses and adverse events were not different among the treatment groups. Ingested α-IFN2a did not induce systemic anti-α-IFN antibodies. Because we detected changes in immune responses and post hoc analysis suggested that a smaller dose could have an effect, ingested α-IFN deserves additional study in dose-response experiments in MS using biological response markers [Brod et al., 2001].

BETA-INTERFERON (β-IFN)

The use of β-IFN has been largely confined to MS. A phase III study in RRMS showed that 8 million IU of rβ-IFN1b (Betaseron) sc qod decreased attacks by 30% and decreased brain inflammation as assessed by serial quantitative MRI [IFNB, 1995]. Another phase III clinical trial using 6 million IU rβ-IFN1a im weekly (30 μg Avonex) showed a 38% reduction in the proportion showing progression, an 18% reduction in relapse rate, and a 33% reduction in average number of active (gadolinium-enhancing) lesions on MRI [Jacobs et al., 1994]. Patients receiving sc β-IFN1a (Rebif), 22 or 44 μg tiw in a phase III study had reduced relapse rates for 4 years with reduced new T2 lesion number and lesion burden [PRISMS-4, 2001].

However, 6% to 40% of β-IFN-treated patients generated neutralizing antibodies who appeared to lose both clinical benefits and MRI-defined responses [IFNB, 1995; PRISMS-4, 2001].

GAMMA-INTERFERON (γ-IFN)

Immune interferon (γ-IFN) acts in the defense of an organism against foreign pathogens via cellular immunity mediated by macrophages. It is a product of T-helper 1 (Th1) cells that can modulate the function of Th2 lymphocytes. In general, Th1 cytokines stimulate the body's cellular immunity in viral infections. γ-IFN is potentially antiviral, antibacterial, anti-proliferative, anti-tumor, and anti-allergic.

However, the clinical use of sc γ-IFN has been relatively limited. γ-IFN can decrease healing time by 50% to 60% in human papillomaviruses (condylomata acuminata) [Rockley and Tyring, 1995]. It can clear the damage caused by refractory nontuberculous mycobacterium infection [Holland et al., 1994] and can have a beneficial effect in chronic granulomatous disease [Curnutte, 1993]. Inducible nitric oxide (NO) synthase can be amplified by γ-IFN in murine macrophages. NO production increased to 132% of that for controls, and on day 3 it reached 360% of that for controls with bactericidal capacity of PMNs increased on day 3. Increase in NO release could be instrumental in augmenting host defense [Ahlin et al., 1999]. γ-IFN is contraindicated in MS [Panitch et al., 1987]. In general, MS lymphocytes secrete excess amounts of γ-IFN [Beck et al., 1988; Bever et al., 1991; Hirsch et al., 1985].

The IFNs, primarily type I IFNs, have surprisingly wide applications in biology because of their pleiotropic activities. New parenteral delivery systems that allow sustained serum levels and novel delivery systems that avoid systemic side effects may well increase the applicability of these interesting biologic compounds.

REFERENCES

Ackerman S.K., Hochstein, H.D., Zoon K., Browne, W., Rivera E., Elisberg B. Interferon fever: absence of human leukocytic pyrogen response to recombinant α-interferon. *J Leukoc Biol* 1984; 36: 17–25.

Adams F., Quesada J.R., Gutterman J.U. Neuropsychiatric manifestations of human leukocyte interferon therapy in patients with cancer. *JAMA* 1984; 252: 938–941.

Aguet M. High affinity binding of ^{125}I-labelled mouse interferon to a specific cell surface receptor. *Nature* 1980; 284: 459–461.

Aguet M., Mogensen K.E. Interferon receptors, in *Interferon*, Vol. 5, Gresser, Ed., Academic Press, London, 1983, pp. 1–22.

Ahlin A., Larfars G., Elinder G., Palmblad J., Gyllenhammar H. Gamma interferon treatment of patients with chronic granulomatous disease is associated with augmented production of nitric oxide by polymorphonuclear neutrophils. *Clin Diagn Lab Immunol* 1999; 6: 420–424.

Ahmed S., Rai K.R. Interferon in the treatment of hairy-cell leukemia. *Best Pract Res Clin Haematol* 2003; 16: 69–81.

Arthur C.K., Ma D.D. Combined interferon alfa-2a and cytosine arabinoside as first-line treatment for chronic myeloid leukemia. *Acta Haematol* 1993; 89, Suppl 1: 15–21.

Aulitzky W., Gastl G., Troppmair J., Tilg H., Abbrederis K., Nerl C., Flener R., Rokos H., Huber C. Results of a phase II study on the treatment of hairy cell leukemias with various doses of alpha-2-recombinant interferon. *Acta Med Austr* 1985; 12: 115–121.

AUSTIMS Research Group. Interferon-alpha and transfer factor in the treatment of multiple sclerosis: a double-blind, placebo-controlled trial. *J Neurol Neurosurg Psychiatr* 1989; 52: 566.

Aviles A., Diaz-Maqueo J.C., Garcia E.L., Talavera A., Guzman R. Maintenance therapy with interferon alfa 2b in patients with diffuse large cell lymphoma. *Invest New Drugs* 1992; 10: 351–355.

Aviles A., Talavera A., Guzman R., Cuadra I. Treatment of refractory low grade lymphoma with chlorambucil alternating with interferon and radiotherapy. *Cancer Biother* 1995; 10: 273–277.

Aviles A., Cleto S., Huerta-Guzman J., Neri N. Interferon alfa 2b as maintenance therapy in poor risk diffuse large B-cell lymphoma in complete remission after intensive CHOP-BLEO regimens. *Eur J Haematol* 2001; 66: 94–99.

Baron S., Tyring S.K., Fleischmann W.R., Coppenhaver D.H., Niesel D.W., Klimpel G.R., Stanton G.J., Hughes T.K. The interferons: mechanisms of action and clinical applications. *JAMA* 1991; 266: 1375–1383.

Beck J., Rondot P., Catinot L., Falcoff E., Kirchner H., Wietzerbin J. Increased production of interferon-gamma and tumor neurons factor precedes clinical manifestations in multiple sclerosis: do cytokines trigger off exacerbations?. *Acta Neurol Scand* 1988; 78: 318–323.

Bendtzen K. Anti-IFN BAb and Nab antibodies: a minireview. *Neurology* 2003; 61, Suppl 5: S6–S10.

Besedovsky H., Sorkin E., Keller M., Muller J. Changes in blood hormone levels during the immune response. *Proc Soc Exp Biol Med* 1975; 150: 466–470.

Besedovsky H., Sorkin E., Felix D., Haas H. Hypothalamic changes during the immune response. *Eur J Immunol* 1977; 7: 323–325.

Besedovsky H., del Rey A., Sorkin E., Dinarello C.A. Immuno-regulatory feedback between interleukin-1 and glucocorticoid hormones. *Science* 1986; 233: 652–654.

Besedovsky H., del Rey A. Neuroendocrine and metabolic response induced by interleukin-1. *J Neurosci Res* 1987; 18: 172–178.

Besedovsky H.O., del Rey A. Introduction: immune-neuroendocrine network. *Front Horm Res* 2002; 29: 1–14.

Bever C.T., Panitch H.S., Levy H.B., McFarlin D.E., Johnson K.P. Gamma-interferon induction in patients with chronic progressive MS. *Neurology* 1991; 41: 1124–1127.

Birmanns B., Saphier D., Abramsky O. Alpha-interferon modifies cortical EEG activity: dose-dependence and antagonism by naloxone. *J Neurol Sci* 1990; 100: 22–26.

Biron C.A. Interferons and as immune regulators: a new look. *Immunity* 2001; 14: 661–664.

Blalock J.E., Stanton J.D. Common pathways of interferon and hormonal action. *Nature* 1980; 283: 406–408.

Blalock J.E., Smith E.M. Human leukocyte interferon: structural and biological relatedness to adrenocotropic hormone and endorphins. *Proc Nat Acad Sci USA* 1980; 77: 5972–5974.

Blalock J.E., Smith E.M. Human leukocyte interferon (HuIFN-α): potent endorphin-like opioid activity. *Biochem Biophys Res Commun* 1981a; 101: 472–478.

Blalock J.E., Smith E.M. Structure and function of interferon (IFN) and neuroendocrine hormones, in *The Biology of the Interferon System*, De Maeyer E., Galasso G., Schellekens H., Eds., Elsevier, Amsterdam, 1981b, pp. 93–99.

Blalock J.E. A molecular basis for bidirectional communication between the immune and neuroendocrine systems. *Physiol Rev* 1989; 69: 1–32.

Blatteis C.M., Xin L., Quan N. Neuromodulation of fever: apparent involvement of opioids. *Brain Res Bull* 1991; 26: 219–223.

Bocci V., Paulesu L., Muscettola M., Viti A. The physiologic interferon response. VI. Interferon activity in human plasma after a meal and drinking. *Lymphokine Res* 1985; 4: 151–158.

Bocci V. The physiological interferon response. *Immunol Today* 1985; 6: 7–9.

Bocci V. Central nervous system toxicity of interferons and other cytokines. *J Biol Regul Homeost Agents* 1988a; 2: 107–118.

Bocci V. What are the roles of interferons in physiological conditions? *NIPS* 1988b; 3: 201–203.

Bocci V. Physicochemical and biologic properties of interferons and their potential uses in drug delivery systems. *Crit Rev Ther Drug Carrier Syst* 1992; 9: 91–133.

Boehm U., Klamp T., Groot M., Howard J.C. Cellular responses to interferon-gamma. *Annu Rev Immunol* 1997; 15: 749–795.

Brod S.A., Kerman R.H., Nelson L.D., Marshall G.D., Henninger E.M., Khan M., Jin R., Wolinsky J.S. Ingested IFN-alpha has biological effects in humans with relapsing-remitting multiple sclerosis. *Mult Scler* 1997; 3: 1–7.

Brod S.A., Lindsey J.W., Vriesendorp F.S., Ahn C., Henninger E., Narayana P.A., Wolinsky J.S. Ingested IFN-alpha: results of a pilot study in relapsing-remitting MS. *Neurology* 2001; 57: 845–852.

Brook M.G., McDonald J.A., Karayiannis P., Caruso L., Forster G., Harris J.R., Thomas H.C. Randomised controlled trial of interferon alfa 2A (rbe) (Roferon-A) for the treatment of chronic hepatitis B virus (HBV) infection: factors that influence response. *Gut* 1989; 30: 1116–1122.

Bullock K. Neuroanatomy of lymphoid tissue: a review, in *Neural Modulation of Immunity*, Guillemin R., Cohn M., Melnechuk T., Eds., Raven Press, New York, 1985, pp. 111–128.

Calvet M.C., Gresser I. Interferon enhances the excitability of cultured neurons. *Nature* 1979; 278: 558–560.

Camenga D.L., Johnson K.P., Alter M., Engelhardt C.D., Fishman P.S., Greenstein J.I., Haley A.S., Hirsch R.L., Kleiner J.E., Kofie V.Y. et al. Systemic recombinant alpha-2 interferon therapy in relapsing multiple sclerosis. *Arch Neurol* 1986; 43: 1239–1246.

Campbell I.L., Krucker T., Steffensen S., Akwa Y., Powell H.C., Lane T., Carr D.J., Gold L.H., Henriksen S.J., Siggins G.R. Structural and functional neuropathology in transgenic mice with CNS expression of IFN-alpha. *Brain Res* 1999; 835: 46–61.

Cantell K., Pulkkinen E., Elosuo R., Suominen J. Effect of interferon on severe psychiatric diseases. *Ann Clin Res* 1980; 12: 131–132.

Cathala F., Baron S. Interferon in rabbit brain, cerebrospinal fluid and serum following administration of polyinosinic-polycytidylic acid. *J Immunol* 1970; 104: 1355–1358.

Chemello L., Cavalletto L., Bernardinello E., Boccato S., Casarin P., Cavinato F., Urban F., Pontisso P., Cecchetto A., Gatta A., Alberti A. Comparison of thrice weekly versus daily human leucocyte interferon-alpha therapy for chronic hepatitis C. *J Viral Hepat* 1999; 6: 321–327.

Cohen M., Keats A.S., Krivoy W., Ungar G. Effect of actinomycin D on morphine tolerance. *Proc Soc Exp Biol Med* 1965; 119: 381–384.

Cole B.F., Solal-Celigny P., Gelber R.D., Lepage E., Gisselbrecht C., Reyes F., Sebban C., Sugano D., Tendler C., Goldhirsch A. Quality-of-life-adjusted survival analysis of interferon alfa-2b treatment for advanced follicular lymphoma: an aid to clinical decision making. *J Clin Oncol* 1998; 16: 2339–2344.

Coppens J.P., Cornu C., Lens E., Lamy M., Geubel A. Prospective trial of recombinant leucocyte interferon in chronic hepatitis B: a 10-month follow-up study. *Liver* 1989; 9: 307–313.

Creange A., Lerat H., Meyrignac C., Degos J.D., Gherardi R.K., Cesaro P. Treatment of Guillain–Barre syndrome with interferon-beta. *Lancet* 1998; 352: 368–369.

Crnic L.S., Segall M.A. Behavioral effects of mouse interferon-alpha and -gamma and human interferon-alpha in mice. *Brain Res* 1992; 590: 277–284.

Curnutte J.T. Conventional versus interferon-gamma therapy in chronic granulomatous disease. *J Infect Dis* 1993; 167, Suppl 1: S8–S12.

Dafny N., Jacob R.H., Jacobson E.D. Gastrointestinal hormones and neural interaction within the central nervous system. *Experientia* 1975; 31: 658–660.

Dafny N. Interferon modifies EEG and EEG-like activity recorded from sensory, motor, and limbic system structures in freely behaving rats. *Neurotoxicology* 1983a; 4: 235–240.

Dafny N. Modification of morphine withdrawal by interferon. *Life Sci* 1983b; 32: 303–305.

Dafny N. Interferon modifies morphine withdrawal phenomena in rodents. *Neuropharmacology* 1983c; 22: 647–651.

Dafny N., Zielinksi M., Reyes-Vazquez C. Alteration of morphine withdrawal to naloxone by interferon. *Neuropeptides* 1983; 3: 453–463.

Dafny N., Reyes-Vazquez C. Three different types of alpha-interferon alter naloxone-induced abstinence in morphine-addicted rats. *Immunopharmacology* 1985; 9: 13–17.

Dafny N. Interferon: a candidate as the endogenous substance preventing tolerance and dependence to brain opioids. *Prog Neuropsychopharmacol Biol Psychiatry* 1984; 8: 351–357.

Dafny N. Interferon as an endocoids candidate preventing and attenuating opiate addiction, in *Endocoids*, Lal H., Labella F., Lane J., Eds., Alan R. Liss, Inc., New York, 1985, pp. 269–276.

Dafny N., Prieto-Gomez B., Reyes-Vazquez C. Does the immune system communicate with the central nervous system? Interferon modifies central nervous system activity. *J Neuroimmunol* 1985a; 9: 1–12.

Dafny N., Wagle V.G., Drath D.B. Cyclosporine alters opiate withdrawal in rodents. *Life Sci* 1985b; 36: 1721–1726.

Dafny N., Pellis N.R., Evidence that opiate addiction is in part an immune response: destruction of immune system by irradiation altered opiate withdrawal. *Neuropharmacology* 1986; 25: 815–818.

Dafny N., Reyes-Vazquez C. Single injection of three different preparations of alpha-interferon modifies morphine abstinence signs for a prolonged period. *Int J Neurosci* 1987; 32: 953–961.

Dafny N., Gillman M.A., Lichtigfeld F.J. Cholecystokinin: induced suppression of feeding in fed, fasting and hypothalamic island rats. *Brain Res Bull* 1988a; 21: 225–231.

Dafny N., Lee J.R., Dougherty P.M. Immune response products alter CNS activity: interferon modulates central opioid functions. *J Neurosci Res* 1988b; 19: 130–139.

Dafny N., Dougherty P.M., Pellis N.R. The immune system and opiate withdrawal. *Int J Immunopharmacol* 1989; 11: 371–375.

Dafny N., Prieto-Gomez B., Reyes-Vazquez C. Effects of interferon on central nervous system, in *Interferon Therapy in Multiple Sclerosis*, Reder A.T., Ed., Marcel Dekker, 1996, pp. 115–137.

Dafny N. Is interferon- a neuromodulator? *Brain Res* 1998; 26: 1–15.

Dafny N. Interferon and the central nervous system, in *Cytokines: Stress and Immunity*, Plotnikoff N.P., Ed., CRC Press, Boca Raton, 1999, pp. 221–232.

Dafny N., Yang P.B., Brod S.A. Interferons, in *Encyclopedia of Endocrine Diseases*, Martini L., Ed., Academic Press, San Diego, 2004, pp. 53–59.

Darling J.J., Hoyle N.R., Thomas D.G.T. Self and non-self in the brain. *Immunol Today* 1981; 2: 176–181.

Degos F., Daurat V., Chevret S., Gayno S., Bastie A., Riachi G., Bartolomei-Portal I., Barange K., Moussalli J., Naveau S., Bailly F., Chaumet-Riffaud P., Chastang C. Reinforced regimen of interferon alfa-2a reduces the incidence of cirrhosis in patients with chronic hepatitis C: a multicentre randomised trial. *J Hepatol* 1998; 29: 224–232.

De Sarro G.B., Masuda Y., Ascioti C., Audino M.G., Nistico G. Behavioral and ECoG spectrum changes induced by intracerebral infusion of interferons and interleukin 2 in rats are antagonized by naloxone. *Neuropharmacology* 1990; 29: 167–179.

de Wit R., Schattenkerk J.K., Boucher C.A., Bakker P.J., Veenhof K.H., Danner S.A. Clinical and virological effects of high-dose recombinant interferon-alpha in disseminated AIDS-related Kaposi's sarcoma. *Lancet* 1988; 2: 1214–1217.

de Wit R., Danner S.A., Bakker P.J., Lange J.M., Eeftinck Schattenkerk J.K., Veenhof C.H. Combined zidovudine and interferon-alpha treatment in patients with AIDS-associated Kaposi's sarcoma. *J Intern Med* 1991; 229: 35–40.

Dinarello C.A. Interleukin-1. *Ann NY Acad Sci* 1988; 546: 122–132.

Dinarello C.A. Interleukin-1 and its biologically related cytokines. *Adv Immunol* 1989; 44: 153–205.

Dinarello C.A., Bernheim H.A., Duff G.W., Le H.V., Nagabhushan T.L., Hamilton N.C., Coceani F. Mechanisms of fever induced by recombinant human interferon. *J Clin Invest* 1984; 74: 906–913.

Diodati G., Bonetti P., Noventa F., Casarin C., Rugge M., Scaccabarozzi S., Tagger A., Pollice L., Tremolada F., Davite C. et al. Treatment of chronic hepatitis C with recombinant human interferon-alpha 2a: results of a randomized controlled clinical trial. *Hepatology* 1994; 19: 1–5.

Dougherty P.M., Aronowski J., Samorajaski T., Dafny N. Opiate antinociception is altered by immunomodification: the effects of interferon, cyclosporine and radiation-induced immune suppression upon acute and long-term morphine activity. *Brain Res* 1986a; 385: 401–404.

Dougherty P.M., Harper C., Dafny N. The effect of alpha-interferon, cyclosporine A and radiation-induced immune suppression on morphine-induced hypothermia and tolerance. *Life Sci* 1986b; 39: 2191–2197.

Dougherty P.M., Pearl J., Krajewski K.J., Pellis N.R., Dafny N. Differential modification of morphine and methadone dependence by interferon-alpha, *Neuropharmacology* 1987; 26: 1595–1600.

Dougherty P.M., Dafny N. Interaction of immune cytokines and CNS opioids: a possible interface for stress-induced immune suppression, in: *Stress and Immunity,* Wybran J., Faith R., McCain H.W., Plotnikoff N.P., Eds., Plenum Press, New York, 1991, pp. 373–385.

Dunn A.J. Psychoneuroimmunology for the psychoneuroendocrinologist: a review of animal studies of nervous system–immune system interactions. *Psychoendocrinology* 1989; 14: 251–274.

Durelli L., Bongioanni M.R., Caballo R., Ferrero B., Ferri R., Verdun E., Bradac G.B., Riva A., Geuna M., Bergamini L. et al. Interferon alpha treatment of relapsing-remitting multiple sclerosis: long-term study of the correlations between clinical and magnetic resonance imaging results and effects on the immune function. *Mult Scler* 1995; 1: S32–S37.

Durelli L., Bongioanni M.R., Ferraro B., Ferri R., Imperiale D., Bradac G.B., Bergui M., Geuna M., Bergamini L., Bergamasco B.. Interferon alpha-2a treatment of relapsing-remitting multiple sclerosis: disease activity resumes after stopping treatment. *Neurology* 1996; 47: 123–129.

D'Urso R., Falaschi P., Canfalone G., Carusi E., Proietti A., Barnaba V., Balsano F. Neuroendocrine effects of recombinant -interferon administration in humans. *Prog Neuroendocrin Immunol* 1991; 4: 20–29.

Fang J., Sanborn C.K., Renegar K.B., Majde J.A., Krueger J.M. Influenza viral infections enhance sleep in mice. *Proc Soc Exp Biol Med* 1995; 210: 242–252.

Felten D.L., Felten S.Y., Bellinger D.L., Carlson S.L., Ackerman K.D., Madden K.S., Olschowki J.A., Livnat S. Noradrenergic sympathetic neural interactions with the immune system: structure and function. *Immunol Rev* 1987; 100: 225–260.

Finter N.B., Chapman S., Dowd P., Johnston J.M., Manna V., Sarantis N., Sheron N., Scott G., Phua S., Tatum P.B. The use of interferon-alpha in virus infections. *Drugs* 1991; 42: 749–765.

Fried M.W., Shiffman M.L., Reddy K.R., Smith C., Marinos G., Goncales F.L., Haussinger D., Diago M., Carosi G., Dhumeaux D., Craxi A., Lin A., Hoffman J., Yu J. PEG interferon alfa-2a plus ribavirin for chronic hepatitis C virus infection. *New Engl J Med* 2002; 347: 975–982.

Goldstein D., Laszlo J. The role of interferon in cancer therapy: a current perspective. *Cancer J Clin* 1988; 38: 258–277.

Gramenzi A., Andreone P., Fiorino S., Camma C., Giunta M., Magalotti D., Cursaro C., Calabrese C., Arienti V., Rossi C., Di Febo G., Zoli M., Craxi A., Gasbarrini G., Bernardi M. Impact of interferon therapy on the natural history of hepatitis C virus related cirrhosis. *Gut* 2001; 48: 843–848.

Gray P.W., Goeddel D.V. Structure of the human immune interferon gene. *Nature* 1982; 298: 859–863.

Guilhot F., Chastang C., Michallet M., Guerci A., Harousseau J.L., Maloisel F., Bouabdallah R., Guyotat D., Cheron N., Nicolini F., Abgrall J. F., Tanzer J. Interferon alfa-2b combined with cytarabine versus interferon alone in chronic myelogenous leukemia. *New Engl J Med* 1997; 337: 223–229.

Habif D.V., Lipton R., Cantell K. Interferon crosses blood-cerebrospinal fluid barrier in monkeys. *Proc Soc Exp Biol Med* 1975; 149: 287–289.

Hadden R.D., Sharrack B., Bensa S., Soudain S.E., Hughes R.A. Randomized trial of interferon beta-1a in chronic inflammatory demyelinating polyradiculoneuropathy. *Neurology* 1999; 53: 57–61.

Hazum E., Chang K.J., Cuatrecasas P. Specific non-opiate receptors for -endorphin. *Science* 1979; 205: 1033–1035.

Hehlmann R., Berger U., Pfirrmann M., Hochhaus A., Metzgeroth G., Maywald O., Hasford J., Reiter A., Hossfeld D.K. et al. Randomized comparison of interferon alpha and hydroxyurea with hydroxyurea monotherapy in chronic myeloid leukemia (CML-study II): prolongation of survival by the combination of interferon alpha and hydroxyurea. *Leukemia* 2003; 17: 1529–1537.

Higano C. S., Raskind W. H., Singer J. W. Use of interferon alfa-2a to treat hematologic relapse of chronic myelogenous leukemia after bone marrow transplantation. *Acta Haematol* 1993; 89, Suppl 1: 8–14.

Hirsch R.L., Panitch H.S., Johnson K.P. Lymphocytes from multiple sclerosis patients produce elevated levels of gamma interferon *in vitro*. *J Clin Immunol* 1985; 5: 386–389.

Holland S.M., Eisenstein E.M., Kuhns D.B., Turner M.L., Fleisher T.A., Strober W., Gallin J.I. Treatment of refractory disseminated nontuberculous mycobacterial infection with interferon gamma: preliminary report. *New Engl J Med* 1994; 330: 1348–1355.

Hori T., Kuriyama K., Nakashima T. Thermal responsiveness of neurons in the ventromedial nucleus of hypothalamus. *J Physiol Soc Jpn* 1988; 50: 619.

Hori T., Nakashima T., Take S., Kaizuka Y., Mori T., Katafuchi T. Immune cytokines and regulation of body temperature, food intake and cellular immunity. *Brain Res Bull* 1991; 27: 309–313.

Hung C.Y., Lefkowitz S.S., Geber W.F. Interferon inhibition by narcotic analgesics. *Proc Soc Exp Biol Med* 1973; 142: 106–111.

IFNB Multiple Sclerosis Study Group, University of British Columbia MS/MRI Analysis Group. Interferon beta-1b in the treatment of multiple sclerosis: final outcome of the randomized controlled trial. *Neurology* 1995; 45: 1277.

Iivanainen M., Laaksonen R., Niemi M.L., Farkkila M., Bergstrom L., Mattson K., Niiranen A., Cantell K. Memory and psychomotor impairment following high dose interferon treatment in amyotrophic lateral sclerosis. *Acta Neurol Scand* 1985; 72: 475–480.

Isaacs A., Lindenmann J. Virus interference. I. The interferon. *Proc R Soc Lond B Biol Sci* 1957; 147: 258–267.

Jacobs L., Cookfair D., Rudick R., Herndon R., Richert J., Salazar A., Fischer J., Granger C., Simon J., Goodkin D., Granger C., Simon J., Alam J., Bartoszak D., Bourdette D., Braiman J. et al. Intramuscular interferon beta-1a for disease progression in relapsing multiple sclerosis. *Ann Neurol* 1996; 39: 285–294.

Jaffe J.H. Drug addiction and drug abuse, in *The Pharmacological Basis of Therapeutics*, 8th ed., Gilman A.G., Rall T.W., Nies A.S., Taylor P., Eds., Macmillan, New York, 1990, pp. 435–521.

Janicki P.K. Binding of human alpha-interferon in the brain tissue membranes of rat. *Res Commun Chem Pathol Pharmacol* 1992; 75: 117–120.

Jankovic B.D., Isakovic K. Neuroendocrine correlates of the immune response. I. Effects of brain lesions on antibody production, Athus reactivity and delayed hypersensitivity in the rat. *Int Arch Allergy Appl Immunol* 1973; 45: 360–372.

Kastrukoff L.F., Oger J.J., Hashimoto S.A., Sacks S.L., Li D.K., Palmer M.R., Koopmans R.A., Petkau A.J., Berkowitz J., Paty D.W. Systemic lymphoblastoid interferon therapy in chronic progressive multiple sclerosis I. Clinical and MRI evaluation. *Neurology* 1990; 40: 479–486.

Kaur N., Kim I.J., Higgins D., Halvorsen S.W. Induction of an interferon- Stat3 response in nerve cells by pre-treatment with gp130 cytokines. *N Neurochem* 2003; 87: 437–447.

Kerr F.W., Pozuelo J. Suppression of physical dependence and induction of the hypersensitivity to morphine by stereotaxic hypothalamus lesions in addicted rats: a new theory of addiction. *Mayo Clin Proc* 1971; 46: 653–665.

Kerr F.W., Triplett J.N., Beeler G.W. Reciprocal (push–pull) effects of morphine on single units in the ventromedian and lateral hypothalamus and influences on other nuclei: with a comment on methadone effects during withdrawal from morphine. *Brain Res* 1974; 74: 81–103.

Kidron D., Saphier D., Ovadia H., Wiedenfeld J., Abramsky O. Central administration of immunomodulatory factors alters neural activity and adrenocortical secretion. *Brain Behav Immun* 1989; 3: 15–27.

Kimura-Takeuchi M., Majde J.A., Toth L.A., Krueger J.M. Influenza virus-induced changes in rabbit sleep and acute phase responses. *Am J Physiol* 1992; 263: R1115–R1121.

Kinnunen E., Timonen T., Pirttila T., Kalliomaki P., Ketonen L., Matikainen E., Sepponen R., Juntunen J. Effects of recombinant alpha-2b-interferon therapy in patients with progressive MS. *Acta Neurol Scand* 1993; 87: 457–460.

Kirchner H. Interferon gamma. *Prog Clin Biochem* 1984; 1: 169–203.

Knobler R.L., Panitch H.S., Braheny S.L., Sipe J.C., Rice G.P., Huddlestone J.R., Francis G.S., Hooper C.J., Kamin-Lewis R.M., Johnson K.P., Oldstone M.B.A., Merigan T.C. Systemic alpha-interferon therapy in multiple sclerosis. *Neurology* 1984; 34: 1273–1279.

Kow L.M., Pfaff D.W. Actions of feeding-relevant agents on hypothalamic glucose-responsive neurons *in vitro*. *Brain Res Bull* 1985; 15: 509–513.

Koyanagi S., Ohdo S. Alteration of intrinsic biological rhythms during interferon treatment and its possible mechanism. *Mol Pharmacol* 2002; 62: 1393–1399.

Krogsgaard K. The long-term effect of treatment with interferon-alpha 2a in chronic hepatitis B. *J Viral Hepat* 1998; 5: 389.

Krown S.E., Li P., Von Roenn J.H., Paredes J., Huang J., Testa M.A. Efficacy of low-dose interferon with antiretroviral therapy in Kaposi's sarcoma: a randomized phase II AIDS clinical trials group study. *J Interferon Cytokine Res* 2002; 22: 295–303.

Krueger J.M., Pappenheimer J.R., Karnovsky M.L. The composition of sleep-promoting factor isolated from human urine. *J Biol Chem* 1982; 257: 1664–1669.

Krueger J.M., Dinarello C.A., Shoham S., Davenne D., Walter J., Kubillus S. Interferon alpha-2 enhances slow-wave sleep in rabbits. *Int J Immunopharmacol* 1987; 9: 23–30.

Krueger J.M., Majde J.A. Cytokines and sleep. *Int Arch Allergy Immunol* 1995; 106: 97–100.

Kubota T., Majde J.A., Brown R.A., Krueger J.M. Tumor necrosis factor receptor fragment attenuates interferon-induced non-REM sleep in rabbits. *J Neuroimmunol* 2001; 119: 192–198.

Kuriyama K., Hori T., Mori T., Nakashima T. Actions of interferon- on the activity of preoptic thermosensitive neurons in tissue slices. *Brain Res* 1988; 454: 361–367.

Lampertico P., Rumi M., Romeo R., Craxi A., Soffredini R., Biassoni D., Colombo M. A multicenter randomized controlled trial of recombinant interferon-alpha 2b in patients with acute transfusion-associated hepatitis C. *Hepatology* 1994; 19: 19–22.

Langer J., Garotta G., Pestka S. Interferon receptors. Biotherapy 1996; 8:163–174.

Laschka E., Herz A., Blasig J. Sites of action of morphine involved in the development of physical dependence in rats I. Comparison of precipitated morphine withdrawal after intraperitoneal and intraventricular injection of morphine antagonists. *Psychopharmacologia* 1976; 46: 133–139.

Lengfelder E., Berger U., Hehlmann R. Interferon alpha in the treatment of polycythemia vera. *Ann Hematol* 2000; 79: 103–109.

Leon L.R. Hypothermia in systemic inflammation: role of cytokines. *Front Biosci* 2004; 9: 1877–1888.

Lindsay K.L., Trepo C., Heintges T., Shiffman M.L., Gordon S.C., Hoefs J.C., Schiff E.R., Goodman Z.D., Laughlin M., Yao R., Albrecht J.K. A randomized, double-blind trial comparing pegylated interferon alfa-2b to interferon alfa-2b as initial treatment for chronic hepatitis C. *Hepatology* 2001; 34: 395–403.

Louria D.B. Medical complications of pleasure-giving drugs. *Arch Intern Med* 1969; 123: 82–87.

Makino M., Kitano Y., Komiyama C., Hirohashi M., Kohno M., Moriyama M., Takasuna K. Human interferon-α induces immobility in the mouse forced swimming test: involvement of the opioid system. 2000; 852: 482–484.

Marcovistz R., Tsiang H., Hovanessian A.G. Production and action of interferon in mice affected with rabies virus. *Ann Virol* 1984; 135E: 19–33.

Mattson K., Niiranen A., Iivanainen M., Farkkila M., Bergstrom L., Holsti L.R., Kauppinen HL, Cantell K. Neurotoxicity of interferon. *Cancer Treat Rep* 1983; 67: 958–961.

McCain H.W., Lamster I.B., Bozzone J.M., Grbic J.T. β-endorphin modulates human immune activity via non-opiate receptor mechanisms. *Life Sci* 1982; 31: 1619–1624.

Meisheri K.D., Isom G.E. Influence of immune stimulation and suppression on morphine physical dependence and tolerance. *Res Commun Chem Pathol Pharmacol* 1978; 19: 85–99.

Meloni G., Capria S., Vignetti M., Alimena G., de Fabritiis P., Montefusco E., Mandelli F. Ten-year follow-up of a single center prospective trial of unmanipulated peripheral blood stem cell autograft and interferon-alpha in early phase chronic myeloyd leukemia. *Haematologica* 2001; 86: 596–601.

Menzies R.A., Patel R., Hall N.R., O'Grady M.P., Rier S.E. Human recombinant interferon alpha inhibits naloxone binding to rat brain membranes. *Life Sci* 1992; 50: PL227–PL232.

Meyers C.A., Valentine A.D. Neurological and psychiatric adverse effects of immunological therapy. *CNS Drugs* 1995; 3: 56–68.

Middelhoff G., Boll I. A long-term clinical trial of interferon alpha-therapy in essential thrombocythemia. *Ann Hematol* 1992; 64: 207–209.

Montgomery S.P., Dafny N. Cyclophosphamide and cortisol reduce the severity of morphine withdrawal. *Int J Immunopharmacol* 1987; 9: 453–457.

Nakashima T., Hori T., Kuriyama K., Kiyohara T. Naloxone blocks the interferon-α induced changes in hypothalamic neuronal activity. *Neurosci Lett* 1987; 82: 332–336.

Nakashima T., Hori T., Kuriyama K., Matsuda T. Effects of interferon-α on the activity of preoptic thermosensitive neurons in tissue slices. *Brain Res* 1988; 454: 361–367.

Nakayama T., Yamamoto K., Ishikawa Y., Imai K. Effects of preoptic thermal stimulation on the ventromedial hypothalamic neurons in rats. *Neurosci Lett* 1981; 26: 177–181.

Pagliaro L., Craxi A., Cama C., Tine F., Di Marco V., Lo Iacono O., Almasio P. Interferon-alpha for chronic hepatitis C: an analysis of pretreatment clinical predictors of response. *Hepatology* 1994; 19: 820–828.

Panitch H.S., Hirsch R.L., Haley A.S., Johnson K.P. Exacerbations of multiple sclerosis in patients treated with gamma interferon. *Lancet* 1987; 1: 893–895.

Paulesu L., Muscettola M, Bocci V., Viti A. Daily variations of plasma interferon levels in the rat. *IRCS Med Sci* 1985; 13: 993–994.

Pellis N.R., Harper C., Dafny N. Suppression of the induction of delayed hypersensitivity in rats by repetitive morphine treatments. *Exp Neurol* 1986; 93: 92–97.

Perrillo R.P. Interferon for hepatitis B: US experience. *Gut* 1993; 34: S95–S96.

Pestka S., Langer J.A., Zoon K.C., Samuel C.E. Interferons and their actions. *Annu Rev Biochem* 1987; 56: 727–777.

Pestka S. The human interferon species and receptors. *Biopolymers* 2000; 55: 254–287.

Plata-Salaman C.R. Immunoregulators in the nervous system. *Neurosci Biobehav Rev* 1991; 15: 185–215.

Plata-Salaman C.R. Immunomodulators and feeding regulation: a humoral link between the immune and nervous systems. *Brain Behav Immun* 1989; 3: 193–213.

Pralle H., Bartel A., Boedewadt-Radzun S., Bross K., Bruhn H.D., Dorken B., Drees N., Essers U., Fuhr H., Gamm H. et al. Alpha interferon in the therapy of hairy cell leukemia: results of three prospective multicenter studies in West Germany. *Onkologie* 1988; 11: 44–47.

Price C.G., Rohatiner A.Z., Steward W., Deakin D., Bailey N., Norton A., Blackledge G., Crowther D., Lister T.A. Interferon alfa-2b in addition to chlorambucil in the treatment of follicular lymphoma: preliminary results of a randomized trial in progress. *Eur J Cancer* 1991; 27, Suppl 4: S34–S36.

Prieto-Gomez B., Reyes-Vazquez C., Dafny N. Microiontophoretic application of morphine and naloxone to neurons in hypothalamus of rat. *Neuropharmacology* 1984; 23: 1081–1089.

Prieto-Gomez B., Reyes-Vazquez C., Dafny N. Differential effects of interferon on ventromedial hypothalamus and dorsal hippocampus. *J Neurosci Res* 1983; 10: 273–278.

PRISMS-4. Long-term efficacy of interferon-beta-1a in relapsing MS. *Neurology* 2001; 56: 1628.

Pritchard J., Gray I.A., Idrissova Z.R., Lecky B.R., Sutton I.J., Swan A.V., Willison H.J., Winer J.B., Hughes R.A. A randomized controlled trial of recombinant interferon-beta 1a in Guillain–Barre syndrome. *Neurology* 2003; 61: 1282–1284.

Reder A.T. Regulation of production of adrenocorticotropin-like proteins in human mononuclear cells. *Immunology* 1992; 77: 436–442.

Redwine L., Dang J., Hall M., Irwin M. Disordered sleep, nocturnal cytokines, and immunity in alcoholics. *Psychosom Med* 2003; 65: 75–85.

Reite M., Laudenslager M., Jones J., Crnic L., Keamingk K. Interferon decreases REM latency. *Biol Psychiatr* 1987; 22: 104–107.

Reyes-Vazquez C., Prieto-Gomez B., Dafny N. Novel effects of interferon on the brain: microiontophoretic application and single cell recording in the rat. *Neurosci Lett* 1982; 34: 201–206.

Reyes-Vazquez C., Dafny N. Microiontophoretically applied morphine and naloxone on single cell activity in the parafasciculus nucleus of naïve and morphine-dependent rats. *J Pharmacol Exp Ther* 1984; 229: 583–588.

Reyes-Vazquez C., Prieto-Gomez B., Georgiades J.A., Dafny N. Alpha and gamma interferons effects on cortical and hippocampal neurons: microiontophoretic application and single cell recording. *Int J Neurosci* 1984a; 25: 113–121.

Reyes-Vazquez C., Weisbrodt N., Dafny N. Does interferon exert its action through opiate receptors? *Life Sci* 1984b; 35: 1015–1021.

Reyes-Vazquez C., Prieto-Gomez B., Dafny N. Alpha-interferon suppresses food intake and neuronal activity of the lateral hypothalamus. *Neuropharmacology* 1994; 33: 1545–1552.

Reyes-Vazquez C., Mendoza-Fernandez V., Herrera-Rhiz M., Dafny N. Interferon modulates glucose-sensitive neurons in the hypothalamus. *Exp Brain Res* 1997; 116; 519–524.

Rockley P.F., Tyring S.K. Interferons alpha, beta and gamma therapy of anogenital human papillomavirus infections. *Pharmacol Ther* 1995; 65: 265–287.

Roda L.G., Bongiorno L., Trani E., Urbani A., Marini M. Positive and negative immunomodulation by opioid peptides. *Int J Immunopharmacol* 1996; 18: 1–16.

Rohatiner A.Z., Prior P.F., Burton A.C., Smith A.T., Balkwill F.R., Lister T.A. Central nervous system toxicity of interferon. *Br J Cancer* 1983; 47: 419–422.

Root-Bernstein R.S. "Molecular sandwiches" as a basis for structural and functional similarities of interferons, MSH, ACTH, LHRH, myelin basic protein, and albumins. *FEBS Lett* 1984; 168: 208–212.

Sacchi S., Leoni P., Liberati M., Riccardi A., Tabilio A., Tartoni P., Messora C., Vecchi A., Bensi L., Rupoli S. et al. A prospective comparison between treatment with phlebotomy alone and with interferon-alpha in patients with polycythemia vera. *Ann Hematol* 1994; 68: 247–250.

Sakami S., Ishikawa T., Kawakami N., Haratani T., Fukui A., Kobayashi F., Fujita O., Araki S., Kawamura N. Coemergence of insomnia and a shift in the Th1/Th2 balance toward Th2 dominance. *Neuroimmunomodulation* 2002-2003; 10: 337–343.

Samuel C.E. Antiviral actions of interferon: interferon-regulated cellular proteins and their surprisingly selective antiviral activities. *Virology* 1991; 183: 1–11.

Saphier D., Kidron D., Ovadia H., Weidenfeld J., Abramsky O., Burstein Y., Pecht M., Trainin N. Preoptic area (POA) multiunit activity (MUA) and cortical EEG changes following intracerebroventricular (ICV) administration of-interferon (IFN), thymic humoral factor (THF), histamine (HIS), and interleukin-1 (IL-1). *Rev Clin Basic Pharmacol* 1987; 6: 265–278.

Saphier D., Kidron D., Ovadia H., Trainin N., Pecht M., Burstein Y., Abramsky O. Neurophysiological changes in the brain following central administration of immunomodulatory factors. *Isr J Med Sci* 1988; 24: 261–263.

Saphier D., Welch J.E., Chuluyan H.E. Alpha-interferon inhibits adrenocortical secretion via μ_1-opioid receptors in the rat. *Eur J Pharmacol* 1993; 236: 183–191.

Saphier D., Roerig S.C., Ito C., Vlasak W.R., Farrar G.E., Broyles J.E., Welch J.E. Inhibition of neural and neuroendocrine activity by α-interferon: neuroendocrine, electrophysiological, and biochemical studies in the rat. *Brain Behav Immun* 1994; 8: 37–56.

Sawyer L.A., Metcalf J.A., Zoon K.C., Boone E.J., Kovacs J.A., Lane H.C., Quinnan G.V. Effects of interferon-alpha in patients with AIDS-associated Kaposi's sarcoma are related to blood interferon levels and dose. *Cytokine* 1990; 2: 247–252.

Schaller B., Radziwill A.J., Steck A.J. Successful treatment of Guillain–Barre syndrome with combined administration of interferon-beta-1a and intravenous immunoglobulin. *Eur Neurol* 2001; 46: 167–168.

Schanzer M.C., Jacobson E.D., Dafny N. Endocrine control of appetite: gastrointestinal hormonal effects on CNS appetite structures. *Neuroendocrinology* 1978: 25: 329–342.

Scott G.M., Secher D.S., Flowers D., Bate J., Cantell K., Tyrrell D.A. Toxicity of interferon. *Br Med J* 1981; 282: 1345–1348.

Segall M.A., Crnic L.S. An animal model for the behavioral effects of interferon. *Behav Neurosci* 1990; 104: 612–618.

Shepherd F.A., Beaulieu R., Gelmon K., Thuot C.A., Sawka C., Read S., Singer J. Prospective randomized trial of two dose levels of interferon alfa with zidovudine for the treatment of Kaposi's sarcoma associated with human immunodeficiency virus infection: a Canadian HIV Clinical Trials Network study. *J Clin Oncol* 1998; 16: 1736–1742.

Shindo M., Di Bisceglie A.M., Cheung L., Shih J.W., Cristiano K., Feinstone S.M., Hoofnagle J.H. Decrease in serum hepatitis C viral RNA during alpha-interferon therapy for chronic hepatitis C. *Ann Intern Med* 1991; 115: 700–704.

Shoham S., Davenne D., Cady A.B., Dinarello C.A., Krueger J.M. Recombinant tumor necrosis factor and interleukin 1 enhance slow wave sleep. *Am J Physiol* 1987; 253: R142–R149.

Shuai K., Stark G.R., Kerr I.M., Darnell J.E. A single phosphotyrosine residue of Stat91 required for gene activation by interferon-gamma. *Science* 1993; 261: 1744–1746.

Sigaux F., Castaigne S., Lehn P., Dupuy E., Billard C., Gluckman J. C., Boiron M., Falcoff E., Flandrin G., Degos L. Alpha-interferon in hairy cell leukaemia: direct effects on hairy cells or indirect cytotoxicity? *Int J Cancer Suppl* 1987; 1: 2–8.

Smedley H., Katrak M., Sikora K., Wheeler T. Neurological effects of recombinant human interferon. *Br Med J* 1983; 286: 262–264.

Smith E.M., Blalock J.E. Human lymphocyte production of corticotrophin and endorphin-like substances: association with leukocyte interferon. *Proc Natl Acad Sci USA* 1981; 78: 7530–7534.

Smith R.A., Norris F., Palmer D., Bernhardt L., Wills R.J. Distribution of alpha interferon in serum and cerebrospinal fluid after systemic administration. *Clin Pharmacol Ther* 1985; 37: 85–88.

Smith R.A., Landel C., Cornelius C.E., Revel M. Mapping the action of interferon on primate brain. *J Interferon Res* 1986; 6, Suppl. 1: 140.

Solomon G.F. Psychoneuroimmunology: interactions between central nervous system and immune system. *J Neurosci Res* 1987; 18: 1–9.

Spath-Schwalbe E., Lange T., Perras B., Fehm H.L., Born J. Interferon-α acutely impairs sleep in healthy humans. *Cytokine* 2000; 12: 518–521.

Spector N.H., Korneva E.A. Neurophysiology/immunopharmacology and neuroimmuno-modulation, in *Psychoneuroimmunology*, Ader R., Ed., Academic Press, New York, 1981, pp. 449–473.

Spiegel R. J. Clinical overview of alpha interferon: studies and future directions. *Cancer* 1987; 59: 626–631.

Stark G.R., Kerr I.M., Williams B.R., Silverman R.H., Schreiber R.D. How cells respond to interferons. *Annu Rev Biochem* 1998; 67: 227–264.

Stuart-Harris R. C., Lauchlan R., Day R. The clinical application of the interferons: a review. *Med J Aust* 1992; 156: 869–872.

Take S., Katafuchi T., Ando D., Uchimura Y., Kanemitsu Y., Ichijo T., Shimizu N., Hori T., Kosaka T. Hypothalamic interferon-α reduces splenic NK cytotoxicity. *Soc Neurosci Abstr* 1992a; 18: 681.

Take S., Mori T., Kaizuka T., Katafuchi T., Hori T. Central interferon suppresses the cytotoxic activity of natural killer cells in the mouse spleen. *Ann NY Acad Sci* 1992b; 650: 46–50.

Take S., Mori T., Katafuchi T., Hori T. Central interferon inhibits natural killer cytotoxicity through sympathetic innervation. *Am J Physiol* 1993; 265: R453–R459.

Teitelbaum H., Catravas G.N., McFarland W.L. Reversal of morphine tolerance after medial thalamic lesions in the rat. *Science* 1974; 185: 449–451.

Tempel D.L., Kim T., Leibowitz S.F. The paraventricular nucleus is uniquely responsive to the feeding stimulatory effects of steroid hormones. *Brain Res* 1993; 614: 197–204.

Tovey M. G., Streuli M., Gresser I., Gugenheim J., Blanchard B., Guymarho J., Vignaux F., Gigou M. Interferon messenger RNA is produced constitutively in the organs of normal individuals. *Proc Natl Acad Sci USA* 1987; 84: 5038–5042.

Toth L.A., Krueger J.M. Alteration of sleep in rabbits by *Staphylococcus aureus* infection. *Infect Immun* 1988; 56: 1785–1791.

Valla D.C., Chevallier M., Marcellin P., Payen J.L., Trepo C., Fonck M., Bourliere M., Boucher E., Miguet J.P., Parlier D., Lemonnier C., Opolon P. Treatment of hepatitis C virus-related cirrhosis: a randomized, controlled trial of interferon alfa-2b versus no treatment. *Hepatology* 1999; 29: 1870–1875.

Vallat J.M., Hahn A.F., Leger J.M., Cros D.P., Magy L., Tabaraud F., Bouche P., Preux P.M. Interferon beta-1a as an investigational treatment for CIDP. *Neurology* 2003; 60: S23–S28.

Vass K., Lassmann H. Intrathecal application of interferon gamma: progressive appearance of MHC antigens within the rat nervous system. *Am J Pathol* 1990; 137: 789–800.

Vernikos-Danellis J., Kellar K.J., Kent D., Gonzales C., Gerger P.A., Barchas J.D. Serotonin involvement in pituitary-adrenal function. *Ann NY Acad Sci* 1977; 297: 518–526.

Vilcek J., Ng M.H., Friedman-Kien A.E., Krawciw T. Induction of interferon synthesis by synthetic double-stranded polynucleotides. *J Virol* 1968; 2: 648–650.

Wei E. Quantification of precipitated abstinence in morphine dependent rats. *Fed Proc* 1971; 31: 527.

Wetzler M., Kantarjian H., Kurzrock R., Talpaz M. Interferon-alpha therapy for chronic myelogenous leukemia. *Am J Med* 1995; 99: 402–411.

Wiranowska M., Wilson T.C., Thompson K., Prockop L.D. Cerebral interferon entry in mice after osmotic alteration of blood–brain barrier. *J Interferon Res* 1989; 9: 353–362.

Yan H., Piazza F., Krishnan K., Pine R., Krolewski J.J. Definition of the interferon receptor-binding domain on the TYK2 kinase. *J Biol Chem* 1998; 273: 4046–4051.

Yasuda K. Sustained release formulation of interferon. *Biomed Ther* 1993; 27: 1221–1223.

Yu M.L., Dai C.Y., Chen S.C., Lee L.P., Huang J.F., Lin Z.Y., Hsieh M.Y., Wang L.Y., Chuang W.L., Chang W.Y. A prospective study on treatment of chronic hepatitis C with tailored and extended interferon-alpha regimens according to pretreatment virological factors. *Antiviral Res* 2004; 63: 25–32.

Zimmermann E., Krivoy W. Antagonism between morphine and the polypeptides ACTH, $ACTH_{1-24}$, and beta-MSH in the nervous system. *Prog Brain Res* 1973; 39: 383–392.

Zinzani P.L., Lauria F., Raspadori D., Buzzi M., Benfenati D., Bocchia M., Rondelli D., Tura S. Comparison of low-dose versus standard-dose alpha-interferon regimen in the hairy cell leukemia treatment. *Acta Haematol* 1991; 85: 16–19.

Zinzani P.L., Bendandi M., Magagnoli M., Rondelli D., de Vivo A., Benni M., Zamagni E., Cavo M., Tura S. Results of a fludarabine induction and alpha-interferon maintenance protocol in pretreated patients with chronic lymphocytic leukemia and low-grade non-Hodgkin's lymphoma. *Eur J Haematol* 1997; 59: 82–88.

Zou L.P., Ma D.H., Wei L., van der Meide P.H., Mix E., Zhu J. IFN-beta suppresses experimental autoimmune neuritis in Lewis rats by inhibiting the migration of inflammatory cells into peripheral nervous tissue. *J Neurosci Res* 1999; 56: 123–130.

16 Neuropeptide Precursor Processing in Immunocytes: Involvement in Neuroimmune Communication

Robert Day and Michel Salzet

CONTENTS

INTRODUCTION

Communication among and reciprocal regulation of the nervous, endocrine, and immune systems are essential for the stability of an organism. Among others, cytokines, hormones, and neuropeptides have been identified as signaling molecules mediating communications among the three systems. Neuropeptides, originally described in the central nervous system (CNS), were also found to be expressed by immune cells and exhibit a number of immunomodulatory properties [Stefano and Salzet 1999; Salzet, Vieau et al. 2000; Blalock 2005; Elmquist et al. 1997].

283

In the past few years, various animal models have served to study neuroimmune mechanisms, confirming the view of communication between the neuroendocrine and immune systems via neuropeptide signaling [Stefano and Salzet 1999; Salzet, Vieau et al. 2000; Blalock 2005]. Another emerging function of neuropeptides within the immune system is their direct role in defense. Peptides with antibacterial properties have been shown to be derived from neuropeptide precursors such as proenkephalin and chromogranin B [Salzet and Stefano 1997; Salzet, Vieau et al. 2000; Salzet 2001; Salzet 2002; Metz-Boutigue, Kieffer et al. 2003]. The role of neuropeptide precursors in immunity, through the release of antibacterial peptides, is an entirely novel concept [Day and Salzet 2002]. Antibacterial peptides implicated in the innate immune response also derive from processing of "true" proantibacterial peptide precursors like prodefensin [Salzet 2002]. Therefore, enzymatic processing, including differential processing events, is a key mechanism to generate an antimicrobial defense in tissues.

The biosynthetic pathway that leads to the production of biologically active neuropeptides begins with the synthesis of large inactive precursor proteins that are cleaved at specific paired or single basic residues within the Golgi secretory pathway [Bergeron et al. 2000]. It is a family of subtilase-like pro-protein convertases (PCs) that is largely responsible for these processing events that activate precursor proteins into neuropeptides [Bergeron et al. 2000].

The PCs have been extensively studied in both the neural and endocrine systems. However, much less is known concerning their expression, regulation, and role within the immune system at the basal level or their function during microbial challenge [Padros et al. 1989; Vindrola et al. 1990; Vindrola et al. 1994; Saravia et al. 1998]. Understanding PC function is important since differential expression of PCs and the resulting cleavage patterns determine the nature and biological activity of the peptide products. Thus, depending on the pattern of PC expression, a single protein precursor can give rise to different peptides with diverse biological activities.

PRO-PROTEIN CONVERTASES (PCS)

There are presently seven known genes that give rise to convertases: furin, PC1/3, PC2, PC4, PACE4, PC5/6, and PC7 [Bergeron et al. 2000]. There is now a large body of evidence demonstrating that these enzymes are critical for the formation of neuropeptides. In particular, it has been established that PC2 and PC1/3 enter the regulated secretory pathway. Thus, these enzymes fulfill a primary prerequisite, since most neuropeptides are assembled and matured within the regulated pathway of secretion.

In PC2 null mice [Zhu et al. 2002], neuropeptide processing was also severely affected, while the processing of a number of other precursors such as growth factors and enzymes that transit the constitutive pathway was unaffected. In humans, a naturally occurring PC1/3 gene inactivation resulted in the impairment of the processing of neuropeptide precursors such as POMC and proinsulin, leading to various endocrine disorders [Day and Salzet 2002]. These data lead us to the notion that convertases such as PC2 and PC1/3 are tightly linked to the regulated secretory pathway and thus to the biosynthetic pathway of neuropeptides.

It has recently been shown that two peptides "specifically" expressed in endocrine and neural cells may influence PC2 and PC1/3 activity. The first one, 7B2, is a bifunctional molecule that acts via distinct domains both as a chaperone-like molecule and a specific inhibitor of PC2 [Martens et al. 1994]. The second one, proSAAS, has just been characterized and seems to behave as a specific PC1/3 endogenous inhibitor [Fricker et al. 2000; Qian et al. 2000]. The exact function of proSAAS on PC1/3 activity remains to be determined and it cannot be ruled out that, in the same manner as 7B2, it may also act as a chaperone-like molecule.

NEUROIMMUNE CONNECTION

Neuroimmune interactions can be essentially considered as bidirectional exchanges of information carried out by classes of molecules that were originally thought to be restricted to either neural, endocrine, or immune systems [Elmquist et al. 1997; Day and Salzet 2002; Blalock 2005]. These include neuropeptides such as corticotrophin releasing hormone (CRH), adrenocorticotrophic hormone (ACTH), monoamines (epinephrine, norepinephrine, and dopamine), glucocorticoids, free radicals, cytokines such as interleukin (IL)-1, IL-6, and tumor necrosis factor (TNF), opioid peptides, opiates, and endocannabinoids [Elmquist et al. 1997; Stefano and Salzet 1999; Salzet, Breton et al. 2000; Salzet 2001; Day and Salzet 2002; Blalock 2005].

Cytokines were originally described as small proteins that coordinate the activities of leukocytes and vascular elements during infection and inflammation. Neuropeptides, originally described in the CNS, were also found to be expressed by immune cells and exhibit a number of immunomodulatory properties [Dantzer 2004a,b]. A consequence of these observations has been a comparison of various immunocytes from evolutionarily diverse organisms with neuroendocrine cells [Stefano and Salzet 1999]. Immunocytes were shown to bear "receptors" for several neurohormones and hypothalamic releasing factors. In addition, they have the ability to produce neurohormones after processing by PCs in response to neuroendocrine and/or immune stimuli (Figure 16.1) [Stefano, Salzet et al. 1998; Stefano and Salzet 1999]. Such overlapping elements between classic neuroendocrine and immune systems strongly suggest a level of cross-talk mediated by a common currency of signaling molecules and a key role of processing enzymes such as PCs.

PCS IN IMMUNE CELLS

PC1/3 expression was demonstrated in THP-1 cells [LaMendola et al. 1997]. PC1/3, PC2, and 7B2 are present in macrophages, monocytes, granulocytes, and lymphocytes of the blood and within inflamed subcutaneous paw tissue [Mousa et al. 2004]. PC2 and PC1/3 have also been detected in immune effector organs like the spleen and their expression increases after bacteria infection [Salzet, Vieau et al. 2000]. Immunoelectron microscopy revealed that opioids are localized within secretory granules packed in membranous structures in macrophages, monocytes, granulocytes, and lymphocytes [Mousa et al. 2004].

Endorphin is released by noradrenaline from immune cells *in vitro*, indicating that immune cells express the entire machinery required for pro-opiomelanocortin (POMC)

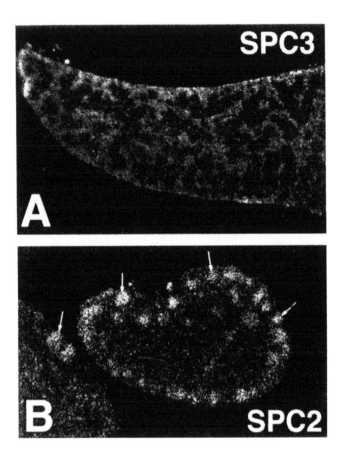

FIGURE 16.1 Photomicrographs of *in situ* hybridization study showing expression of (A) SPC3 mRNA in rat splenocytes within the red pulp and (B) SPC2 mRNA in rat lymph node follicles (see small arrows). With permission of *Trends in Neurosciences.*

processing into functionally active peptides such as endorphin and are able to release these peptides from secretory granules [Brack et al. 2004; Mousa et al. 2004]. Similarities in expression of enzymes involved in the conversion of neuroendocrine precursors such as opioids into functionally mature peptides underscore the potential of human immunocytes to express certain neuroendocrine cell characteristics.

NEUROPEPTIDES AS SOURCES OF ANTIMICROBIAL PEPTIDES

PROENKEPHALIN-DERIVED ANTIBACTERIAL PEPTIDES

Secretory granules from adrenal medullary chromaffin cells contain a complex mixture of low molecular mass constituents such as catecholamines, ascorbate, nucleotides, calcium, and several water-soluble peptides and proteins [Metz-Boutigue, Kieffer et al. 2003]. These components are released into the circulation in response to splanchnic nerve stimulation. It has long been known that relatively large amounts of proenkephalin and chromogranin-derived peptides are also found in the bovine adrenal medulla.

Metz-Boutique's group has shown that antibacterial activity is present within the intragranular chromaffin granule matrix and the extracellular medium following exocytosis [Strub, Garcia-Sablone et al. 1995; Goumon, Strub et al. 1996; Strub, Hubert et al. 1996; Goumon, Lugardon et al. 1998; Metz-Boutigue, Goumon et al. 1998; Goumon, Lugardon et al. 2000; Metz-Boutigue, Lugardon et al. 2000; Lugardon, Chasserot-Golaz et al. 2001; Metz-Boutigue, Goumon et al. 2003; Metz-Boutigue, Kieffer et al. 2003; Briolat et al. 2005]. These peptides inhibit the growth of Gram-positive bacteria (*Micrococcus luteus* and *Bacillus megaterium*) at micromolar concentrations.

In addition, antibacterial assays on soluble chromaffin granule material recovered from HPLC indicate the presence of several other endogenous peptides with potent antibacterial activities against Gram-positive and -negative bacteria in bovines [Strub, Garcia-Sablone et al. 1995; Goumon, Strub et al. 1996; Strub, Hubert et al. 1996; Goumon, Lugardon et al. 1998; Metz-Boutigue, Goumon et al. 1998; Goumon, Lugardon et al. 2000; Metz-Boutigue, Lugardon et al. 2000; Lugardon, Chasserot-Golaz et al. 2001; Metz-Boutigue, Goumon et al. 2003; Metz-Boutigue, Kieffer et al. 2003; Briolat et al. 2005]. These new antibacterial peptides derived from chromogranin B and proenkephalin precursors are stored with catecholamines and released during stress [Metz-Boutigue, Kieffer et al. 2003].

Bactericidal activities of the bovine chromogranin B- or proenkephalin-derived peptides are modulated by the degree of maturation of the precursor and by the presence of post-translational modifications (phosphorylation, O-glycosylation). Natural processing of these precursors at the N- and C- terminals generates most of these peptides [Metz-Boutigue, Kieffer et al. 2003]. This points out the key role of adrenals and the processing mechanism present in the chromaffin cells. Lack of adrenals dramatically reduces resistance against sepsis, supporting the concept of the involvement of Toll-like receptors (TLRs) in this endocrine tissue. In fact, TLRs are key elements in the innate immune response, functioning as pattern-recognition receptors for the detection of and response to endotoxins and other microbial ligands.

Inflammatory cytokines play an important role in the activation of the hypothalamic–pituitary–adrenal (HPA) axis during inflammation and sepsis. The newly recognized major role of TLR2 and TLR4 and the adrenal stress response during critical illnesses such as inflammation and sepsis demands comprehensive analysis of their interactions [Scocchi, Wang et al. 1997; Scocchi, Wang et al. 1998; Scocchi, Bontempo et al. 1999]. Western blot analysis demonstrated the expression of TLR2 and TLR4 in the human adrenocortical cell line NCI-H295 [Scocchi, Wang et al. 1997; Scocchi, Wang et al. 1998; Scocchi, Bontempo et al. 1999]. Immunohistochemical analysis of normal human adrenal glands revealed TLR2 and TLR4 expression in the adrenal cortex, but not in the adrenal medulla [Scocchi, Wang et al. 1997; Scocchi, Wang et al. 1998; Scocchi, Bontempo et al. 1999].

Considering the crucial role of the HPA axis and the innate immune response during acute sepsis or septic shock, elucidating the functional interaction of these systems should be of great clinical relevance. Moreover, C3H/HeJ mice lacking TLR-4 and consequently endotoxin hyporesponsive have recently been shown to be resistant to glucocorticoid protection against live *Escherichia coli*. Effective antibiotic intervention as an additional parameter and with concomitant administration of glucocorticoid allows for expected antibiotic protection and also for glucocorticoid protection against *E. coli* or *Staphylococcus aureus* of mice sensitized to tumor necrosis factor-α regardless of the status of the TLR-4 receptor. TLRs, including but not limited to TLR-2, may be involved in glucocorticoid protective efficacy against Gram-positive and Gram-negative sepsis [Scocchi, Wang et al. 1997; Scocchi, Wang et al. 1998; Scocchi, Bontempo et al. 1999]. Overlapping and possibly endotoxin-independent signaling may become important considerations.

Human leukocytes also contain proenkephalin and chromogranin-derived peptides [Tasiemski, Salzet et al. 2000; Tasiemski, Hammad et al. 2002] like peptide B and secretolytin. Levels of both peptides are significantly increased in response to lipopolysaccharides (LPS), surgical trauma, and bacterial exposure [Tasiemski, Salzet et al. 2000].

In invertebrates such as leeches and the *Mytilus edulis* mollusks [Salzet and Stefano 1997; Stefano and Salzet 1999], such proenkephalin-derived [Tasiemski, Verger-Bocquet et al. 2000] and chromogranin-derived [Tasiemski, Hammad et al. 2002; Salzet and Stefano 2003] peptides were detected in hemolymph. Furthermore, invertebrate and vertebrate peptideB/enkelytin was found to be very similar, exhibiting high sequence homology (95 to 98%) [Tasiemski, Salzet et al. 2000]. Peptide B/enkelytin is strongly antibacterial as indicated by *in vivo* and *in vitro* experiments [Tasiemski, Salzet et al. 2000; Salzet 2001; Salzet and Tasiemski 2001]. It should be noted that the C-terminus of peptide B contains the opioid heptapeptide Met-enkephalin-Arg-Phe [Tasiemski, Salzet et al. 2000; Salzet 2001; Salzet and Tasiemski 2001]. This is similar to what is found in amphibian dermal glands after stress [Amiche et al. 1998]. There are also a variety of antibacterial peptides and neuropeptides related to opioids (for example, dermorphin and dermenkephalin) [Amiche et al. 1998]. In *Caenorhabditis elegans*, such a family precursor has also recently been discovered in the genome [Couillault et al. 2004]. This precursor contains multiple copies of YGGFR or YGGFG peptides as well as antimicrobial peptides containing these sequences [Couillault et al. 2004]. According to genome analyses, Drosophila also contains such a precursor [Couillault et al. 2004]. These peptides seem to be released independently of TLR activation [Couillault et al. 2004], reflecting a new source of antimicrobial peptides and the ancient origins of such molecules.

MODEL OF UNIFIED NEUROIMMUNE RESPONSE

Met-enkephalin-Arg-Phe stimulates immunocytes, but does not have antibacterial properties. It binds to the δ₂ opioid receptor subtype [Stefano, Scharrer et al. 1996], as does amphibian dermenkephalin [Amiche et al. 1998]. Incubation of peptide B with neutral endopeptidase (NEP)-containing immunocytes resulted in activation of antimicrobial function, a phenomenon that can be blocked with the NEP inhibitor phosphoramidon [Shipp et al. 1991], indicating that it is processed to Met-enkephalin-Arg-Phe. An important point for our understanding of the significance of this molecule in diverse organisms is the fact that LPS, surgical trauma, and electric shocks directed to neural tissues cause increases in circulating levels of peptide B/enkelytin and Met-enkephalin. Stefano's group demonstrated that electrical shocks stress Mytilus, which activates immunocytes via the secretion of Met-enkephalin [Stefano and Salzet 1999].

We can now add peptide B to this stress response. In the aggregate, these data lead us to surmise that the co-processing and liberation of peptide B and Met-enkephalin represents a unified neuroimmune protective response to an immediate threat to an organism, regardless of the specific stimulus [Stefano, Salzet et al. 1998].

Since microbial infection often accompanies physical injury, peptide B is released to deal with real or potential microbial threat, whereas Met-enkephalin stimulates or activates immunocytes during the initial stages of the response. Therefore, this unified neuroimmune response provides a highly beneficial survival strategy when it is most needed — at the beginning of the host defense response [Stefano, Salzet et al. 1998]. A simultaneous presence of Met-enkephalin is equally important for this response.

Both human and invertebrate immunocytes contain δ opioid receptors that appear to mediate activation of these cells [Stefano, Scharrer et al. 1996; Stefano, Salzet et al. 1998; Salzet and Tasiemski 2001]. In this regard, Met-enkephalin can be envisioned to activate immunocytes and to provide a chemotactic signal for further immunocyte recruitment [Stefano, Scharrer et al. 1996; Stefano, Salzet et al. 1998; Salzet and Tasiemski 2001]. However, this process may take many minutes to accomplish, hence the presence of bactericidal peptide B to act during this period of latency. In this scenario, as peptide B breaks down with time, it first liberates the heptapeptide Met-enkephalin-Arg-Phe or the antibacterial peptide, enkelytin. Met-enkephalin-Arg-Phe can further interact with the δ_2 opioid receptor, ensuring a continuation of the immunocyte-activated state including chemotaxis. This enhancement is required, since human granulocytes and invertebrate immunocytes contain NEP, which appears to be the critical enzyme in this process [Salzet 2001].

SOURCES OF ANTIBACTERIAL PEPTIDES

In models in which inflammatory processes occur in the absence of bacterial infection, such as during intra-surgical cardiac bypass, time-course experiments have shown the presence of enkelytin, peptide B, opioids (met-enkephalin and met-enkephalin-Arg-Phe) [Tasiemski, Salzet et al. 2000], and other new antibacterial peptides derived from fibrinopeptide A, chromogranins, or aplipoprotein CIII in plasma before surgery [Salzet, unpublished data]. Their amounts are greatly increased just after surgical trauma (skin incision). Moreover, the peptides identified are also contained within chromaffin granules in cells of the adrenal medulla [Metz-Boutigue, Kieffer et al. 2003].

Chromaffin cells are innervated by preganglionic fibers conveyed by the splanchnic nerves, which pass through the celiac and renal sympathetic nerve plexuses and are under the control of stress-sensitive supraspinal centers in the brain [Metz-Boutigue, Kieffer et al. 2003]. Thus, the presence and the increase in peptide levels we observed may be due to the release of adrenal chromaffin granules induced by a systemic stress response to endothelial injury. Additionally, pituitary adenylate cyclase activating polypeptide (PACAP) containing neuronal cell bodies located in the sensory neurons of dorsal root ganglia can be activated by sensory receptors located in the skin. This suggests that an incision may also cause the release of these peptides from the adrenal medulla. This is in agreement with the significant increase of these peptides during surgery [Metz-Boutigue, Kieffer et al. 2003].

Interestingly, the other source of antibacterial peptides may be the skin itself, possibly from macrophages located in the dermis [Brogden, De Lucca et al. 1996; Brogden, Ackermann et al. 1997; Brogden, Ackermann et al. 1998; Brogden, Ackermann et al. 1999; Brogden, Ackermann et al. 2003; Brogden 2005] In fact, opioids, like several epithelial peptide antibiotics, are constitutively expressed. Others are inducible, either by the presence of microorganisms through yet poorly characterized elicitor receptors or by endogenous pro-inflammatory cytokines [Nissen and Kragballe 1997; Nissen, Lund et al. 1997]. However, considering the fact that monocytes contain pro-enkephalin, we cannot exclude the possibility that autocrine or paracrine pathways also exist to release pro-inflammatory peptides [Nissen and Kragballe 1997; Nissen, Lund et al. 1997].

We recently demonstrated that the chromogranin B gene is present in monocytes like proenkephalin (Figure 16.2). Its processing into secretolytin is stimulated by IL-6 which is released in circulation [Tasiemski, Hammad et al. 2002]. Secretolytin is released from monocytes upon IL-6 stimulation, evoking a systemic action while peptide B [Tasiemski, Hammad et al. 2002] like defensins [Befus et al. 1999] would act intracellularly (Figure 16.3). Neither secretolytin nor peptide B is excreted from neutrophils [Tasiemski, Hammad et al. 2002].

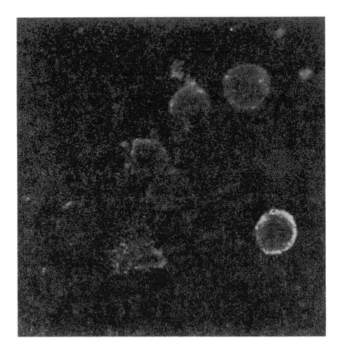

FIGURE 16.2 Photomicrograph of human monocytes in confocal microscopy study showing monocytes expressing chromogranin B-derived peptide and monocytes expressing both chromogranin B-derived (secretolytin) and proenkephalin-derived (enkelytin) peptides.

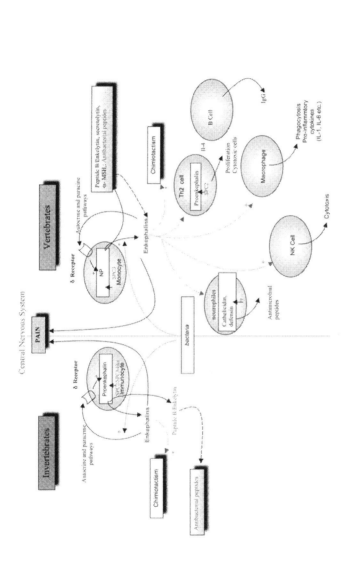

FIGURE 16.3 Precursor processing in vertebrates and invertebrates immunocytes after bacteria challenge. Immune level: An infection produced experimentally provokes enkephalin synthesis by SPCs attacking neuropeptide precursor to lead neuropeptide-derived peptides. Enkephalins induce immunocyte chemotaxis and the release of other signaling molecules (i.e., cytokines), whereas peptideB/enkelytin exerts an antibacterial action. Within minutes, enkelytin is processed to yield [Met]enkephalin-Arg-Phe that further augments the immunocyte response. Enkephalins also stimulate Th2 lymphocyte responses via CD3, coupled to Ca^{2+} intracellular release that conducts IL-4 release. Thus, enkephalins act as immune messengers, so-called cytokines. They also stimulate cathelicidin and defensin precursor processing in order to raise antimicrobial peptides in a systemic response. At the present time processing enzymes are unknown.

OTHER NEUROPEPTIDES AS SOURCES OF ANTIMICROBIAL ACTIVITIES

Another opioid-derived peptide, le α-melanostimulating hormone (MSH), is also known to exert antimicrobial activity [Cutuli et al. 2000; Grieco et al. 2003]. α-MSH and its carboxy-terminal tripeptide (11–13, KPV) have been determined to have antimicrobial influences against two major and representative pathogens, i.e., *Staphylococcus aureus* and *Candida albicans*. α-MSH peptides significantly inhibited *S. aureus* colony formation and reversed the enhancing effect of urokinase on colony formation.

Antimicrobial effects occurred over a broad range of concentrations including the physiological (picomolar) range. Small concentrations of α-MSH peptides likewise reduced viability and germ tube formation of the *C. albicans* yeast. Antimicrobial influences of α-MSH peptides could be mediated by their capacity to increase cellular cAMP. This messenger was significantly augmented in peptide-treated yeast and the potent adenylyl cyclase inhibitor dideoxyadenosine partly reversed the killing activity of α-MSH peptides. Reduced killing of pathogens is a detrimental consequence of therapy with anti-inflammatory drugs. α-MSH peptides that combine antipyretic, anti-inflammatory, and antimicrobial effects could be useful in treatment of disorders in which infection and inflammation coexist.

Chromogranin precursors contain chromogranin A and chromogranin B, two peptides that have antibacterial activities [Strub, Garcia-Sablone et al. 1995; Strub, Hubert et al. 1996; Metz-Boutigue, Goumon et al. 2003; Metz-Boutigue, Kieffer et al. 2003]. C-terminal processing at basic resides in chromogranin B forms the antibacterial peptide secretolytin and the N-terminal part of chromogranin A contains vasostatin and chromofungin [Strub, Garcia-Sablone et al. 1995; Strub, Hubert et al. 1996; Metz-Boutigue, Goumon et al. 2003; Metz-Boutigue, Kieffer et al. 2003]. Chromofungin is an antifungal peptide corresponding to chromogranin A (47–66) that can bind calmodulin in the presence of calcium and induce inhibition of calcineurin, a calmodulin-dependent enzyme [Lugardon et al. 2001].Vasostatin-1 and secretolytin initially present in plasma at low levels and are released just after skin incision [Metz-Boutigue, Kieffer et al. 2003].

PROTEOLYSIS AND ACTIVATION OF CATIONIC ANTIMICROBIAL PEPTIDES

Most antimicrobial peptides are cationic and are produced in propeptide forms. Another family of cationic molecules, the cathelicidins, has been demonstrated in vertebrate neutrophils [Zanetti et al. 1995]. These peptides constitute a family of antimicrobial peptides formed like neuropeptide precursors [Zanetti et al. 1995]. Initially they are synthesized as prepropeptides with highly conserved prepro regions of 128 to 143 residues including a putative 29- to 30-residue signal peptide and a cathelin-like propeptide of 99 to 114 residues containing 4 invariant cysteine residues and a variable C-terminal antimicrobial region ranging in length from 12 to 100 residues [Zanetti et al. 1995].

The cathelin domain is similar to cystatin domains present in the precursors of such inflammation-related peptides. Studies of bovine and porcine cathelicidins

[Scocchi, Wang et al. 1997; Scocchi, Wang et al. 1998; Scocchi, Bontempo et al. 1999] identified neutrophil elastase as the enzyme that processes cathelicidins in these two animal species. Inhibitors of neutrophil elastase have been used to show that the antimicrobial activity of porcine inflammatory fluids is dependent to a large extent on the secretion of proprotegrin, a porcine cathelicidin precursor, and its activation by neutrophil elastase.

Another well-known family of antimicrobial peptides synthesized in neutrophils are defensins [Ganz 2004]. In fact, during the development of neutrophil precursors in the bone marrow, polypeptides with primary antimicrobial function are synthesized, post-translationally processed, and stored in granules. Defensins are 29- to 50-amino acid antimicrobial peptides that are abundant effector molecules of phagocytes and epithelia involved in host defense [Ganz 2004]. α-Defensins are expressed in human and other mammalian neutrophils and Paneth cells of the small intestine. They are synthesized as 90- to 100-amino acid pre-prodefensins, with 19-amino acid signal sequences, ~45-amino acid anionic propieces, and 29- to 40-amino acid C-terminal mature cationic defensins [Valore and Ganz 1992; Valore, Martin et al. 1996]. The removal of the anionic propiece is an activation step that converts the inert prodefensin to antimicrobial mature defensin [Valore and Ganz 1992; Valore, Martin et al. 1996]. The enzymes that process prodefensins to defensins in neutrophil precursors have not yet been characterized.

The identification of enzymes that convert prodefensins to defensins would greatly advance the studies of the biological functions of these peptides. The processing of neutrophil defensins bears some resemblance to that of various peptide hormones. Many peptide hormones are processed by SPCs that recognize a dibasic motif N-terminal to the cleavage site and frequently act with a carboxypeptidase to liberate the mature active hormone. For neutrophil prodefensins, there is a lysine or arginine in the propiece 0 to 3 residues from the N-terminus of the mature defensin, suggesting that an enzyme recognizing this cationic site could be involved in the cleavage, perhaps followed by aminopeptidases.

CONCLUSION

Taken together, these data strongly suggest that the same processing enzymes are expressed in leukocytes as in the neuroendocrine system to accomplish this task. Furthermore, differential processing has also been observed in immune system, leading to the production of peptides with biological functions such as antimicrobial activities. While there is strong evidence to suggest that the PCs fulfill an important role in the immune system, their functions remain only poorly characterized.

ACKNOWLEDGMENTS

This work was supported in part by the MNERT, the CNRS, the FEDER, the Conseil Régional de la région Nord-Pas De Calais, the INSERM, the FRSQ and the IRSC.

REFERENCES

Amiche, M., A. Delfour, et al. (1998). Opioid peptides from frog skin. *Exs* 85: 57–71.

Befus, A.D., C. Mowat, et al. (1999). Neutrophil defensins induce histamine secretion from mast cells: mechanisms of action. *J Immunol* 163 (2): 947–953.

Bergeron, F., R. Leduc, et al. (2000). Subtilase-like pro-protein convertases: from molecular specificity to therapeutic applications. *J Mol Endocrinol* 24 (1): 1–22.

Blalock, J.E. (2005). The immune system as the sixth sense. *J Intern Med* 257 (2): 126–138.

Brack, A., H.L. Rittner, et al. (2004). Mobilization of opioid-containing polymorphonuclear cells by hematopoietic growth factors and influence on inflammatory pain. *Anesthesiology* 100 (1): 149–157.

Briolat, J., S.D. Wu, et al. (2005). New antimicrobial activity for the catecholamine release-inhibitory peptide from chromogranin A. *Cell Mol Life Sci* 62 (3): 377–385.

Brogden, K.A. (2005). Antimicrobial peptides: pore formers or metabolic inhibitors in bacteria? *Nat Rev Microbiol* 3: 238–250.

Brogden, K.A., M. Ackermann, et al. (1997). Small, anionic, and charge-neutralizing propeptide fragments of zymogens are antimicrobial. *Antimicrob Agents Chemother* 41 (7): 1615–1617.

Brogden, K.A., M. Ackermann, et al. (1998). Detection of anionic antimicrobial peptides in ovine bronchoalveolar lavage fluid and respiratory epithelium. *Infect Immun* 66 (12): 5948–5954.

Brogden, K.A., M. Ackermann, et al. (2003). Antimicrobial peptides in animals and their role in host defences. *Int J Antimicrob Agents* 22 (5): 465–478.

Brogden, K.A., M.R. Ackermann, et al. (1999). Differences in the concentrations of small, anionic, antimicrobial peptides in bronchoalveolar lavage fluid and in respiratory epithelia of patients with and without cystic fibrosis. *Infect Immun* 67 (8): 4256–4259.

Brogden, K.A., A.J. De Lucca, et al. (1996). Isolation of an ovine pulmonary surfactant-associated anionic peptide bactericidal for *Pasteurella haemolytica*. *Proc Natl Acad Sci USA* 93 (1): 412–416.

Couillault, C., N. Pujol, et al. (2004). TLR-independent control of innate immunity in *Caenorhabditis elegans* by the TIR domain adaptor protein TIR-1, an ortholog of human SARM. *Nat Immunol* 5 (5): 488–494.

Cutuli, M., S. Cristiani, et al. (2000). Antimicrobial effects of alpha-MSH peptides. *J Leukoc Biol* 67 (2): 233–239.

Dantzer, R. (2004). Cytokine-induced sickness behaviour: a neuroimmune response to activation of innate immunity. *Eur J Pharmacol* 500 (1–3): 399–411.

Dantzer, R. (2004). Innate immunity at the forefront of psychoneuroimmunology. *Brain Behav Immun* 18 (1): 1–6.

Day, R. and M. Salzet (2002). The neuroendocrine phenotype, cellular plasticity, and the search for genetic switches: redefining the diffuse neuroendocrine system. *Neuroendocrinol Lett* 23 (5–6): 447–451.

Elmquist, J.K., T.E. Scammell, et al. (1997). Mechanisms of CNS response to systemic immune challenge: the febrile response. *Trends Neurosci* 20 (12): 565–570.

Fricker, L.D., A.A. McKinzie, et al. (2000). Identification and characterization of proSAAS, a granin-like neuroendocrine peptide precursor that inhibits prohormone processing. *J Neurosci* 20 (2): 639–648.

Ganz, T. (2004). Defensins: antimicrobial peptides of vertebrates. *C R Biol* 327 (6): 539–549.

Goumon, Y., K. Lugardon, et al. (2000). Processing of proenkephalin-A in bovine chromaffin cells: identification of natural derived fragments by N-terminal sequencing and matrix-assisted laser desorption ionization-time of flight mass spectrometry. *J Biol Chem* 275 (49): 38355–38362.

Goumon, Y., K. Lugardon, et al. (1998). Characterization of antibacterial COOH-terminal proenkephalin-A-derived peptides (PEAP) in infectious fluids: importance of enkelytin, the antibacterial PEAP209-237 secreted by stimulated chromaffin cells. *J Biol Chem* 273 (45): 29847–29856.

Goumon, Y., J.M. Strub, et al. (1996). The C-terminal bisphosphorylated proenkephalin-A-(209–237)-peptide from adrenal medullary chromaffin granules possesses antibacterial activity. *Eur J Biochem* 235 (3): 516–525.

Grieco, P., C. Rossi, et al. (2003). Novel alpha-melanocyte stimulating hormone peptide analogues with high candidacidal activity. *J Med Chem* 46 (5): 850–855.

LaMendola, J., S.K. Martin, et al. (1997). Expression of PC3, carboxypeptidase E and enkephalin in human monocyte-derived macrophages as a tool for genetic studies. *FEBS Lett* 404 (1): 19–22.

Lugardon, K., S. Chasserot-Golaz, et al. (2001). Structural and biological characterization of chromofungin, the antifungal chromogranin A-(47–66)-derived peptide. *J Biol Chem* 276 (38): 35875–35882.

Martens, G.J., J.A. Braks, et al. (1994). The neuroendocrine polypeptide 7B2 is an endogenous inhibitor of prohormone convertase PC2. *Proc Natl Acad Sci USA* 91 (13): 5784–5787.

Metz-Boutigue, M.H., Y. Goumon, et al. (1998). Antibacterial peptides are present in chromaffin cell secretory granules. *Cell Mol Neurobiol* 18 (2): 249–266.

Metz-Boutigue, M.H., Y. Goumon, et al. (2003). Antimicrobial chromogranins and proenkephalin-A-derived peptides: antibacterial and antifungal activities of chromogranins and proenkephalin-A-derived peptides. *Ann NY Acad Sci* 992: 168–178.

Metz-Boutigue, M.H., A.E. Kieffer, et al. (2003). Innate immunity: involvement of new neuropeptides. *Trends Microbiol* 11 (12): 585–592.

Metz-Boutigue, M.H., K. Lugardon, et al. (2000). Antibacterial and antifungal peptides derived from chromogranins and proenkephalin-A: from structural to biological aspects. *Adv Exp Med Biol* 482: 299–315.

Mousa, S.A., M. Shakibaei, et al. (2004). Subcellular pathways of beta-endorphin synthesis, processing, and release from immunocytes in inflammatory pain. *Endocrinology* 145 (3): 1331–1341.

Nissen, J.B. and K. Kragballe (1997). Enkephalins modulate differentiation of normal human keratinocytes *in vitro*. *Exp Dermatol* 6 (5): 222–229.

Nissen, J.B., M. Lund, et al. (1997). Enkephalin-like immunoreactivity in human skin is found selectively in a fraction of CD68-positive dermal cells: increase in enkephalin-positive cells in lesional psoriasis. *Arch Dermatol Res* 289 (5): 265–271.

Padros, M.R., O. Vindrola, et al. (1989). Mitogenic activation of the human lymphocytes induces the release of proenkephalin derived peptides. *Life Sci* 45 (19): 1805–1811.

Qian, Y., L.A. Devi, et al. (2000). The C-terminal region of proSAAS is a potent inhibitor of prohormone convertase 1. *J Biol Chem* 275 (31): 23596–23601.

Salzet, M. (2001). Neuroimmunology of opioids from invertebrates to human. *Neurondocrinol Lett* 22 (6): 467–474.

Salzet, M. (2002). Antimicrobial peptides are signaling molecules. *Trends Immunol* 23 (6): 283–284.

Salzet, M., C. Breton, et al. (2000). Comparative biology of the endocannabinoid system: possible role in the immune response. *Eur J Biochem* 267 (16): 4917–4927.

Salzet, M. and G. Stefano (2003). Chromacin-like peptide in leeches. *Neuroendocrinol Lett* 24 (3–4): 227–232.

Salzet, M. and G. B. Stefano (1997). Invertebrate proenkephalin: delta opioid binding sites in leech ganglia and immunocytes. *Brain Res* 768 (1–2): 224–232.

Salzet, M. and A. Tasiemski (2001). Involvement of pro-enkephalin-derived peptides in immunity. *Dev Comp Immunol* 25 (3): 177–185.

Salzet, M., D. Vieau, et al. (2000). Crosstalk between nervous and immune systems through the animal kingdom: focus on opioids. *Trends Neurosci* 23 (11): 550–555.

Saravia, F., M.R. Padros, et al. (1998). Differential response to a stress stimulus of proen-kephalin peptide content in immune cells of naive and chronically stressed rats. *Neuropeptides* 32 (4): 351–359.

Scocchi, M., D. Bontempo, et al. (1999). Novel cathelicidins in horse leukocytes. *FEBS Lett* 457 (3): 459–464.

Scocchi, M., S. Wang, et al. (1998). Cloning and analysis of a transcript derived from two contiguous genes of the cathelicidin family. *Biochim Biophys Acta* 1398(3): 393–396.

Scocchi, M., S. Wang, et al. (1997). Structural organization of the bovine cathelicidin gene family and identification of a novel member. *FEBS Lett* 417(3): 311–315.

Shipp, M.A., G.B. Stefano, et al. (1991). CD10 (CALLA)/neutral endopeptidase 24.11 mod-ulates inflammatory peptide-induced changes in neutrophil morphology, migration, and adhesion proteins and is itself regulated by neutrophil activation. *Blood* 78 (7): 1834–1841.

Stefano, G.B., B. Salzet, et al. (1998). Enkelytin and opioid peptide association in invertebrates and vertebrates: immune activation and pain. *Immunol Today* 19 (6): 265–268.

Stefano, G.B. and M. Salzet (1999). Invertebrate opioid precursors: evolutionary conservation and the significance of enzymatic processing. *Int Rev Cytol* 187: 261–286.

Stefano, G. B., M. Salzet, et al. (1998). Delta2 opioid receptor subtype on human vascular endothelium uncouples morphine stimulated nitric oxide release. *Int J Cardiol* 64, Suppl 1: S43–S51.

Stefano, G.B., B. Scharrer, et al. (1996). Opioid and opiate immunoregulatory processes. *Crit Rev Immunol* 16 (2): 109–144.

Strub, J.M., P. Garcia-Sablone, et al. (1995). Processing of chromogranin B in bovine adrenal medulla. Identification of secretolytin, the endogenous C-terminal fragment of resi-dues 614-626 with antibacterial activity. *Eur J Biochem* 229 (2): 356–368.

Strub, J.M., P. Hubert, et al. (1996). Antibacterial activity of secretolytin, a chromogranin B-derived peptide (614-626), is correlated with peptide structure. *FEBS Lett* 379 (3): 273–278.

Tasiemski, A., H. Hammad, et al. (2002). Presence of chromogranin-derived antimicrobial peptides in plasma during coronary artery bypass surgery and evidence of an immune origin of these peptides. *Blood* 100 (2): 553–559.

Tasiemski, A., M. Salzet, et al. (2000). The presence of antibacterial and opioid peptides in human plasma during coronary artery bypass surgery. *J Neuroimmunol* 109 (2): 228–235.

Tasiemski, A., M. Verger-Bocquet, et al. (2000). Proenkephalin A-derived peptides in inver-tebrate innate immune processes. *Brain Res Mol Brain Res* 76 (2): 237–252.

Valore, E.V. and T. Ganz (1992). Post-translational processing of defensins in immature human myeloid cells. *Blood* 79 (6): 1538–1544.

Valore, E.V., E. Martin, et al. (1996). Intramolecular inhibition of human defensin HNP-1 by its propiece. *J Clin Invest* 97 (7): 1624–1629.

Vindrola, O., A.M. Mayer, et al. (1994). Prohormone convertases PC2 and PC3 in rat neutrophils and macrophages: parallel changes with proenkephalin-derived peptides induced by LPS *in vivo*. *Neuropeptides* 27 (4): 235–244.

Vindrola, O., M.R. Padros, et al. (1990). Proenkephalin system in human polymorphonuclear cells: production and release of a novel 1.0-kD peptide derived from synenkephalin. *J Clin Invest* 86 (2): 531–537.

Zanetti, M., R. Gennaro, et al. (1995). Cathelicidins: a novel protein family with a common proregion and a variable C-terminal antimicrobial domain. *FEBS Lett* 374 (1): 1–5.

Zhu, X., A. Zhou, et al. (2002). Disruption of PC1/3 expression in mice causes dwarfism and multiple neuroendocrine peptide processing defects. *Proc Natl Acad Sci USA* 99 (16): 10293–10298.

17 Clinical Relevance of Opioid-Induced Immunosuppression: Are All Drugs Similar?

Paola Sacerdote, Sivia Franchi, and Cataldo Martucci

CONTENTS

INTRODUCTION

In the past two decades, the interest in the immune effects of opioid drugs gained significant ground concomitantly with the spread of human immunodeficiency virus (HIV) infection.

In fact, opioids were considered to have some role in the increased incidence of infection in heroin addicts originally attributed to the use of contaminated needles, and have now been implicated as cofactors in the pathogenesis of HIV infection.[1]

Although they are common substances of abuse, opioids also represent mainstays of treatment for acute pain after surgery or injury and for many types of chronic pain including cancer and non-cancer related pain. Due to their widespread and expanding use, the immunological effects of opioids are receiving considerable attention because of concerns that opioid-induced changes of the immune system may affect the outcome of surgery or a variety of disease processes including bacterial and viral infections and cancers.

Most studies performed on the immunological effects of opioids refer to the prototype drug: morphine. While in clinical practice morphine remains the "golden standard," semisynthetic and synthetic derivatives of morphine are commonly used in the treatment of various pain conditions in humans. It is therefore necessary to present detailed analyses of the different opioid drugs in order to characterize whether they all share the same immunosuppressive properties.

MORPHINE

Well-established literature has demonstrated that the acute administration of morphine to rodents, primates, and humans leads to generalized immunosuppression.[1,2] Natural killer (NK) cells have been shown to be very sensitive to morphine modulation *in vivo*. Injections of morphine led to depressed NK activity in rats, mice, monkeys, and humans.[3-6] Considerable evidence indicates that morphine given *in vivo* modulates T cell functions. Independently of the stimulus utilized (polyclonal mitogen, CD3 activation, antigen-specific challenge), T lymphocyte proliferation is decreased by both acute and chronic morphine administration.[5,6] Morphine also decreases most cytokines such as interleukin-2 and interferon-γ.[5,6] Clear inhibitory effects of *in vivo* morphine on mono-cyte/macrophage functions have been consistently described. The impairment was evident with circulating, peritoneal, alveolar and splenic macrophages, indicating a general down-regulation of innate immunity.[3,7,8]

Although most data have been obtained from experimental animals, clear evidence points to morphine immunosuppressive effects also in humans.[1] However, it is becoming clear that not all opioid drugs share the same immunosuppressive properties. It is therefore important to check the immune properties of the different opioids used for the treatment of pain.

Obviously, in order to compare the immune properties of the different drugs, it is necessary to evaluate the effects of equianalgesic doses. Animal studies indicate, in fact, that the immune effects of opioids frequently become evident at doses higher than those necessary to produce antinociception. A second general consideration is the fact that most studies have been conducted on experimental animals, and the data obtained from healthy volunteers and patients are still scarce.

TRAMADOL

Tramadol is a centrally acting analgesic drug, used mainly for the treatment of pain of intermediate or severe intensity.[9] It binds with low affinity to opioid receptors, showing higher selectivity for the μ receptor.[9,10] It also exerts a modulatory effect on central monoaminergic pathways, inhibiting the neuronal uptake of noradrenaline and serotonin.[9,10]

The immunopharmacological profile of tramadol was explored both in experimental animals and humans. It was immediately clear that this weak opioid did not show any immunosuppressive effect. In contrast, when administered acutely to normal animals, tramadol exerted a clear immunoenhancing effect on parameters such as NK activity, lymphoproliferation, and cytokine production.[11] This peculiarity of tramadol must be ascribed to its serotoninergic component. Pretreatment with metergoline, a serotoninergic antagonist, prevented the immunostimulant effect of tramadol.[12]

It is well known that pain is a relevant stress factor leading to immunosuppression. The effects of tramadol on immune responses were therefore compared with the effects of morphine in different animal models of pain. In a rat model of neuropathic pain, the administration of tramadol preserved the NK activity, while morphine depressed it in the same model.[13]

Pain associated with surgery is clearly recognized as one factor contributing to surgical stress-induced immunosuppression. NK activity is particularly sensitive to perioperative stress, and animal studies provide convincing evidence for a causal link between low NK activity and susceptibility to metastatic outcomes.[14-16] When tramadol and morphine were compared in an experimental model of surgical-induced suppression of NK activity, tramadol was able to prevent the NK decrease as well as the tumor enhancing effect of surgery (Figure 17.1).[17] The efficacy of tramadol was clearly superior to that of morphine. While both drugs similarly relieved pain, tramadol also possessed intrinsic immunostimulating activity.

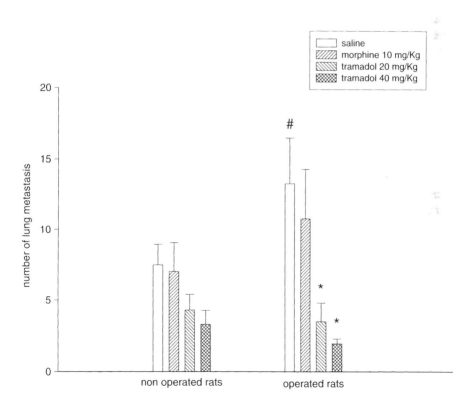

FIGURE 17.1 Effects of treatment with tramadol and morphine on the number of lung tumor metastases in rats that underwent experimental surgery. As reported by Gaspani et al.,[17] tramadol was able to prevent surgery-induced immunosuppression and related increases of metastasis numbers, while morphine, due to its intrinsic immunosuppressive properties, was not. # = p <0.05 versus saline, non-operated rats (one-way analysis of variance). * = p <0.05 versus saline-treated operated animals (one-way analysis of variance).

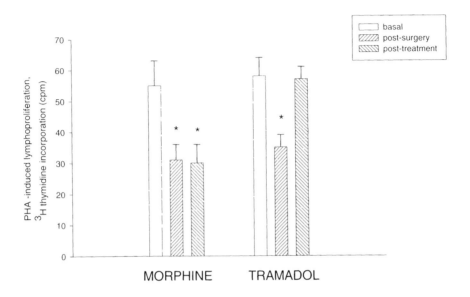

FIGURE 17.2 Phytohemoagglutinin (PHA) stimulated proliferation of lymphocytes obtained from patients before the beginning of surgery (basal), immediately after surgery (post-surgery), and 2 hours after treatment with 10 mg/Kg of morphine im or 100 mg of tramadol im (post-treatment). * = p <0.05 versus basal (one-way analysis of variance).

On the basis of these experimental results, tramadol seems to be particularly indicated for the treatment of post-operative pain. As reported in Figure 17.2, a human study confirmed the experimental observations. The comparison of morphine and tramadol in the treatment of perioperative pain in two groups of cancer patients indicated that tramadol-treated patients experienced a faster and complete recovery of immune responses depressed after surgery.[18]

In summary, as far as immunosuppression is concerned, tramadol seems to be a good alternative to morphine for the treatment of mild acute pain.

FENTANYL AND REMIFENTANIL

Fentanyl is a potent synthetic full agonist at the μ opioid receptor. Due to its short half-life, fentanyl has been for many years widely used for the management of acute pain in surgery, and only recently the development of a transdermal preparation has allowed its prescription for chronic cancer and non-cancer pain.[19]

The immunopharmacological profile of fentanyl does not seem to differ from that of morphine. When administered in experimental animals, fentanyl induced a clear dose-related immunosuppression.[20] When we analyzed the effects of continuous infusion of fentanyl on NK activity, lymphoproliferation, and cytokine production in the mouse, the suppressive effects of fentanyl appeared after 1 hour of infusion, became more evident after 24 hours, and reached a maximum after 3 days (Figure 17.3). By further increasing the duration of the infusion, however, a certain degree of tolerance started to develop to the immunosuppressive effects of fentanyl.[20] Moreover, doses of fentanyl that are clearly able to depress NK activity have also been shown to negatively impact on the development of experimental tumor metastasis.[21] However, it should be recalled that the final immune alteration emerging during an opioid treatment in the presence of pain, i.e., in a clinical situation, is due to the algebraic difference between the effects of pain and of the drug on the immune parameters. Indeed, in the presence of surgical-induced pain, low doses of fentanyl have been shown to be protective on surgery-induced immunosuppression.[22]

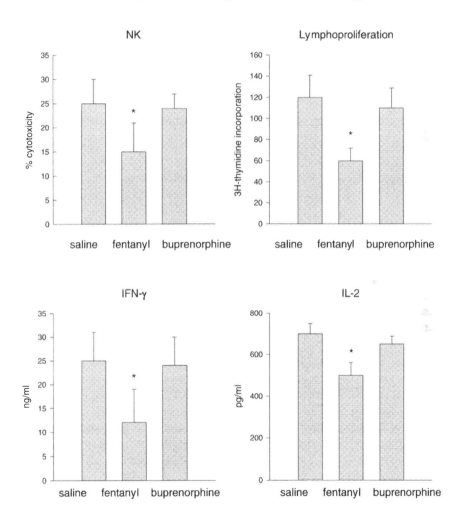

FIGURE 17.3 Immune parameters after 3 days of continuous infusion with equianalgesic doses of fentanyl or buprenorphine in mice. Spleen cells were collected and their functionality tested *in vitro* for natural killer cell activity, lymphoproliferation, and cytokine (IL-2 and IFN-γ) production. In fentanyl-treated animals, a significant decrease of all immune parameters was present, while buprenorphine did not affect immune responses. * = p <0.05 versus saline (one-way analysis of variance).

Similarly, fentanyl has been shown to affect cellular immune responses in humans, and the immune modulation seems to be dose-related.[23,24] The few studies conducted in humans, however, deal only with acute fentanyl treatment.[23,24]

In recent years, drug development has provided potent opioids possessing shorter durations of action than the classical opioids. Remifentanil is a novel μ opioid receptor agonist with an analgesic potency similar to that of fentanyl.[25] By virtue of predominant metabolism by non-specific esterases, remifentanil has a rapid systemic elimination, with a half-life of 8 to 10 minutes.[25] These pharmacokinetic characteristics make it the first choice drug for analgesia during anaesthesia.

After 1 hour continuous intravenous (iv) administration of remifentanil to rats, a significant and relevant decrease of blood as well as spleen NK activity and lymphoproliferation was observed.[26] It is important to note that, due to its metabolization by esterases, the half-life of remifentanil in rats has been estimated to be only a few minutes.[25] Immunosuppression was, however, still present 5 hours after the end of the infusion, indicating that the effects induced by opioids on immune cells are long-lasting. In contrast, a single study performed in healthy volunteers indicated that the infusion of very low doses of remifentanil did not seem to affect NK activity.[27] Again, it appears that opioid-induced immunosuppression is related to the doses utilized.

BUPRENORPHINE

Buprenorphine is a potent opioid agonist with elevated affinity for the μ opioid receptor. Although buprenorphine has always been considered a partial agonist for some opioid effects, it has been shown to possess full analgesic activity in several animal models and in humans.[28]

The analysis of the literature on the immune effects of buprenorphine points to a different profile of this molecule in comparison to morphine or fentanyl.[29-31,33] From recent work performed in experimental animals by several research groups, there emerges a comprehensive safety profile for the effect of buprenorphine on immune responses when administered both acutely and chronically.

Gomez-Flores and Weber[29] have shown in rats that following the acute injection of equianalgesic doses of buprenorphine and morphine into the mesencephalic periaqueductal gray (PAG), buprenorphine did not alter splenic NK cell activity or T cell and macrophage function, whereas morphine significantly suppressed these same parameters. Similar results were also obtained after chronic buprenorphine administration.[20,30] After 10 days of continuous infusion with buprenorphine, the immune parameters evaluated were not different from those of untreated control animals. A study performed by our group compared the effects of acute and chronic buprenorphine and fentanyl administration at equianalgesic doses on several measures of cellular immunity in mice.[20] The results are reported in Figure 17.3.

As reported above, fentanyl administration altered several immune parameters, while, in contrast, the immune responses remained consistently unaltered after continuous buprenorphine administration. After 1 week's administration of buprenorphine, the dose of infused drug was increased and the immune parameters measured. By increasing the amount of buprenorphine administered, no negative modulation of the immune responses was ever observed.

Only a single paper in the literature indicates potential immunosuppressive effects of buprenorphine.[32] This study observed decreases of two immune parameters after acute injection of buprenorphine in rats. However, the study was performed with high doses of buprenorphine and no comparison with other opioid drugs was made. Another immunotoxicological study using high repeated doses of buprenorphine in rats showed a lack of effect of the compound on leukocyte numbers and function.[33]

In conclusion, an analysis of the literature evaluating the immunomodulatory properties of buprenorphine indicates that the molecule seems devoid of the immunosuppressive effects associated with other opioids such as morphine and fentanyl. It should be emphasized that all the studies discussed were performed in experimental animals. The only study available on the effect of buprenorphine on immunity in humans involved a group of drug abusers chronically treated with buprenorphine for opioid dependence.[34] The patients had long histories of heroin intake and were switched to buprenorphine. The doses administered were obviously much higher than those used in pain treatment. However a significant amelioration of immune parameters was observed in the buprenorphine-treated subject in comparison to the measurements obtained before switching to this drug.

METHADONE

Methadone, a synthetic potent agonist, has been used for treatment of opioid addiction for many years; it is also administered for the treatment of chronic cancer pain. Surprisingly, although the first papers on the effects of methadone on the immune system date back to the 1980s,[35,36] no definitive conclusion on its immunomodulatory effects is possible. The few trials performed in drug abusers generally point to a safer immune profile in methadone patients in comparison to heroin abusers.[34] However, some studies have also evidenced an increase of HIV incidence or higher conversion rate from HIV to AIDS in methadone-treated subjects in comparison to opioid-free subjects.[37-39]

The few papers available on the effects of methadone in animals seem to indicate that at equianalgesic doses methadone and morphine exert similar immunosuppressive effects.[40]

HYPOTHESES FOR DIFFERENT IMMUNOPHARMACOLOGICAL PROFILES OF OPIOID DRUGS

The mechanisms at the basis of morphine-induced immunosuppression have been extensively studied, and it is now accepted that morphine modulates the immune response by interaction with receptors in the central nervous system and in the periphery.[1,41] It has been demonstrated that lymphocytes and mononuclear phagocytes express classical μ, κ, and δ opioid receptors functionally coupled to signal transduction mechanisms.[1] By binding to these receptors, morphine has been shown to trigger important responses in immune cells, such as the induction of apoptotic programs leading to cell death.[1] Moreover, the presence of some atypical binding sites for opioids in lymphocytes, astrocytes, microglia, and endothelial cells, referred to as μ_3 receptors, has been suggested.[1] The recognition of these non-naloxone-sensitive binding sites could be of great interest since the development of specific ligands for the μ_3 receptors may lead to a new class of immunomodulatory drugs.

The potential mechanisms by which central opioid receptors modulate peripheral immune responses may involve both the hypothalamic–pituitary–adrenal (HPA) axis and the autonomic nervous system.[42,43] Acute and chronic morphine administration can activate the HPA axis, eliciting the production of adrenocorticotropin from the pituitary that in turn stimulates the release of glucocorticoids and could eventually suppress the immune responses.

Primary (e.g., thymus and lymph nodes) and secondary (e.g., spleen) lymphoid organs are innervated by sympathetic nervous fibers that release catecholamines in the proximity of immune cells, negatively modulating their function. Direct administration of most opioids to the central nervous system produces systemic elevation of adrenaline, noradrenaline, and dopamine from the adrenal medulla as well as from the sympathetic nerve terminals in the lymphoid organs. The release of catecholamine has been demonstrated to suppress lymphoproliferation, natural killer cell activity, and macrophage functions.[42]

In conclusion, multiple mechanisms participate in the immunomodulatory properties of morphine. The reasons other opioids also binding μ opioid receptors behave differently from morphine is not clear.

For some molecules an explanation can be hypothesized. As previously reported, the immunostimulating properties of tramadol seem to depend upon its serotoninergic action. It is possible that the low μ opioid receptor binding affinity of this drug would not be sufficient to induce immunosuppression, and the serotoninergic component becomes predominant.[9,10,12]

Several hypotheses can be put forward to explain the different immune profile of buprenorphine. As already described, morphine induces immunosuppression by binding to opioid receptors in the brain, leading to HPA axis stimulation and activation of the noradrenergic fibers innervating lymphoid organs and also binding to opioid receptors expressed by leukocytes. Interestingly, buprenorphine does not seem either to activate the HPA axis or to alter the release of monoamines in the spleen.[29,30] It can therefore be hypothesized that the lack of effect of buprenorphine on immune responses derives from its lack of neuroendocrine effects. However, one must also consider the fact that buprenorphine possesses antagonistic properties at the κ opioid receptor[28] and that agonism at the κ opioid receptor has been linked to immunosuppression.[44] It is therefore possible that the agonistic activity of buprenorphine at the μ opioid receptor could be counterbalanced by an antagonistic effect at the κ opioid receptor.

CLINICAL RELEVANCE OF OPIOID-INDUCED IMMUNOSUPPRESSION

In order to assess the clinical relevance of opioid-induced immunosuppression, it is important to distinguish between transient immune alterations and actual initiation or facilitation of disease (infection, tumor metastasis, etc.). A normal healthy host can tolerate some immune perturbations and deleterious consequences are not usually dependent on disturbances in one function. However, there are clearly some times and situations when the risks derived from opioid-induced immunosuppression may become relevant. A greater vulnerability of the immune system is present in young and elderly individuals, when the immune system undergoes developmental changes: maturing in infancy and declining in old age.

Opioid-induced immunosuppression can obviously be dangerous in already immunocompromised individuals such as HIV-positive patients.[44] Another risk situation is the perioperative period, since it is well known that anesthesia and surgery affect the immune response.[14,15] It has been shown that the use of morphine in the perioperative period can slow the restoration of normal immune responses depressed by surgery.[18] In this situation, the choice of analgesics devoid of immunosuppressive activity has been shown to be especially indicated.[18]

Another clinically relevant question is whether opioid-induced immunosuppression has negative consequences in the development of cancer. Although animal studies have clearly demonstrated that the administration of morphine or fentanyl together with tumor cells seems to facilitate metastatic spread,[17,21] relevant human studies have not yet been performed.[36]

A further point that needs to be addressed is the concomitant administration of immune-modifying drugs. It is highly feasible that opioid-induced immunosuppression can be added to an immunocompromised situation due to chemotherapy or glucocorticoid treatment in cancer patients. It must also be observed that opioids, primarily the transdermal opioid preparations, are increasingly proposed for the treatment of chronic non-cancer-related pain such as arthritic pain. In rheumatoid arthritis patients, therapy with immunosuppressant drugs such as methotrexate is often used. In such cases, therefore, we do not know the potential risks of adding further immunosuppressive agents but the possibility of harm must be there.

CONCLUSION

Although many advances have been made in understanding the effects of opioid drugs on immune responses, the real clinical relevance of these effects is not completely clear. However it has definitely emerged that not all opioid drugs share the same immune profile. Indeed, it is evident that the possibility of achieving adequate and equivalent pain control by choosing either immunosuppressive drugs or drugs without effect on immune responses could represent an important point to be considered in opioid therapy.

REFERENCES

1. Vallejo R, de Leon-Casasola O, Benyamin R. Opioid therapy and immunosuppression. *Am J Therapeutics* 2004; 11: 354–365.
2. Sacerdote P, Limiroli E, Gaspani L. Experimental evidence for immunomodulatory effect of opioids. *Adv Exp Med Biol* 521: 106–112.
3. Eisenstein TK, Hillburger ME. Opioid modulation of immune responses: effects on phagocyte and lymphoid cell populations. *J Neuroimmunol* 1998; 83: 36–44.

4. Yeager MP, Colacchio TA, Yu CT, Hildebrandt L, Howell AL, Weiss J, Guyre PM. Morphine inhibits spontaneous and cytokine enhanced natural killer cell cytotoxicity in volunteers. *Anesthesiology* 1995; 83: 500–508.

5. Sacerdote P, Manfredi B, Mantegazza P, Panerai AE. Antinociceptive and immuno-suppressive effects of opiate drugs: a structure-related activity study. *Br J Pharmacol* 1997; 121: 834–840.

6. Yokota T, Urhara K, Nomoto Y. Addition of noradrenaline to intrathecal morphine augments the post-operative suppression of natural killer cell activity. *J Anaesthesth* 2004; 18: 190–195.

7. Limiroli E, Gaspani L, Panerai AE, Sacerdote P. Differential tolerance development in the modulation of macrophage cytokine production in mice. *J Leukoc Biol* 2002; 72: 43–48.

8. Risdahl JM, Khanna KV, Peterson KW, Molitor TW. Opiates and infections. *J Neuroimmunol* 1998; 83: 4–18.

9. Dayer P, Collart L, Desmeules J. Pharmacology of tramadol. *Drugs* 1994; 47: 3–7.

10. Raffa RB, Friderichs E, Reimann W, Shank RP, Codd EE, Vaught JL. Opioid and non-opioid components independently contribute to the mechanisms of action of tramadol, an atypical opioid analgesic. *J Pharmacol Exp Ther* 1992; 260: 275–285.

11. Sacerdote P, Bianchi M, Manfredi B, Panerai AE. Effects of tramadol on immune responses and nociceptive thresholds in mice. *Pain* 1997; 72: 225–230.

12. Sacerdote P, Bianchi M, Gaspani L, Panerai AE. Effects of tramadol and its enanti-omers on concanavalin-A induced proliferation and NK activity of mouse splenocytes: involvement of serotonin. *Int J Immunopharmacol* 1999; 21: 727–733.

13. Tsai YC, Wong SJ. Effects of tramadol on T lymphocyte proliferation and natural killer cell activity in rats with sciatic constriction injury. *Pain* 2001; 92: 63–69.

14. Colacchio TA, Yeager MP, Hildebrandt LW. Perioperative immunomodulation in cancer surgery. *Am J Surg* 1994; 167: 174–179.

15. Hansbrough JF, Bender EM, Zapata-Sirvent R, Anderson J. Altered helper and sup-pressor lymphocyte populations in surgical patients: a measure of postoperative immunosuppression. *Am J Surg* 1984; 148: 303–307.

16. Ben-Eliyahu S, Page GG, Yirmiya R, Shakar, G. Evidence that stress and surgical interventions promote tumor development by suppressing natural killer cell activity. *Int J Cancer* 1999; 80: 880–888.

17. Gaspani L, Bianchi M, Limiroli E, Panerai AE, Sacerdote P. The analgesic drug tramadol prevents the effect of surgery on natural killer cell activity and metastatic colonization in rats. *J Neuroimmunol* 2002; 29: 18–24.

18. Sacerdote P, Bianchi M, Gaspani L, Manfredi B, Maucione A, Terno G, Ammatuna M, Panerai AE. Effects of tramadol and morphine on immune responses and pain after surgery in cancer patients. *Anesth Analg* 2000; 90: 1411–1414.

19. Jeal W, Benfield P. Transdermal fentanyl: a review of its pharmacological properties and therapeutic efficacy in pain control. *Drugs* 1997; 53: 109–138.

20. Martucci C, Panerai AE, Sacerdote P. Chronic fentanyl or buprenorphine infusion in the mouse: similar analgesic profile but different effects on immune responses. *Pain* 2004; 110: 385–392.

21. Shavit Y, Ben-Eliyahu S, Zeidel A, Beilin B. Effects of fentanyl on natural killer cell activity and on resistance to tumor metastasis in rats. *Neuroimmunomodulation* 2004; 11: 255–260.

22. Page GG, Blakely WP, Ben-Eliyau S. Evidence that postoperative pain is a mediator of the tumor-promoting effects of surgery in rats. *Pain* 2001; 90: 191–199.

23. Karst JR, Scheinichen D, Bevilacqua C, Schneider U, Heine J, Schedlowsky M, Schmidt RE. Effects of fentanyl on cellular immune functions in man. *Int J Immunopharmacol* 1999; 21: 445–454.

24. Beilin B, Shavit Y, Hart J, Mordashov B, Cohn S, Notti I, Bessler H. Effects of anesthesia based on large versus small doses of fentanyl on natural killer cell cytotoxicity in the perioperative period. *Anesth Analg* 1996; 82: 492–497.

25. Rosow C.E. An overview of remifentanil. *Anesth Analg* 1999; 89: S1–S3.

26. Sacerdote P, Gaspani L, Rossoni G, Panerai AE, Bianchi M. Effect of remifentanil on the cellular immune responses in the rat. *Int Immunopharmacol* 2001; 1: 713–719.

27. Cronin AJ, Aucutt Walter NM, Budinetz T, Bonafide CP, DiVittore NA, Gordin V, Schuler HG, Bonneau RH. Low dose remifentanil infusion does not impair natural killer function in healthy volunteers. *Br J Anaesth* 2003; 91: 805–809.

28. Cowan A. Update of the general pharmacology of buprenorphine, in *Buprenorphine: Combating Drug Abuse with a Unique Opioid*, Cowan A, Lewis JW, Eds., Wiley-Liss, New York, 1995, pp. 31–47.

29. Gomez-Flores R, Weber R. Differential effects of buprenorphine and morphine on immune and neuroendocrine functions following acute administration in the rat mesencephalon periacqueductal gray. *Immunopharmacology* 2000; 48: 145–156.

30. D'Elia M, Patenaude J, Hamelin C, Garrel DR, Bernier J. No detrimental effect from chronic exposure to buprenorphine on corticosteroid-binding globulin and corticosensitive immune parameters. *Clin Immunol* 2003; 109: 179–187.

31. Williams W, Rice KC, Weber R. Non-peptide opioids: *in vivo* effects on the immune system. *NIDA Research Monograph* 1991; 105: 404–407.

32. Carrigan KA, Saurer TB, Ijames SG, Lysle DT. Buprenorphine produces naltrexone reversible alterations of immune status. *Int Immunopharmacol* 2004; 4: 419–428.

33. Van Loveren N, Gianotten G, Hendiksen CF, Schuurman JW, Van der Laan JW. Assessment of immunotoxicity of buprenorphine. *Lab Anim* 1994; 28: 355–363.

34. Neri S, Bruno CM, Malaguarnera M, Italiano C, Mauceri B, Abata G, Cilio D, Calvagno S, Ignaccolo S, Interlandi D, Prestianni L, Ricchena M, Noto R. Randomized clinical trial to compare the effects of methadone and buprenorphine on the immune system in drug abusers. *Psychopharmacology* 2005, 179: 700–704.

35. Lazzarin A, Mella L, Trombini M, Ubert Foppa G, Franzetti F, Mazzone G, Galli M. Immunological status in heroin addicts: effects of methadone maintenance treatment. *Drug Alcohol Depend* 1984; 13: 117–123.

36. Tubaro E, Santiangeli C, Belogi L, Boelli G, Cavallo G, Croce C, Avico U. Morphine and methadone impact on human phagocytic physiology. *Int Immunopharmacol* 1985; 7: 865–874.

37. Suzuki S, Carlos MP, Chuang LF, Torres JV, Doi RH, Chuang RY. Methadone induces CCR5 and promotes AIDS virus infection. *FEBS Lett* 2002; 519: 173–177.

38. Carballo-Dieguez AJ, Sahs J, Goetz R, el Sadr W, Sorell S, Gorman J. The effect of methadone on immunological parameters among HIV-positive and HIV-negative drug users. *Am J Drug Alcohol Abuse* 1994; 20: 317–329.

39. Quang-Cantagrel ND, Wallace MS, Ashar N, Mathews C. Long-term methadone treatment: effect on CD4 lymphocyte counts and HIV-1 plasma RNA level in patients with HIV infection. *Eur J Pain* 2001, 5: 415–417.

40. Pacifici R, Patrini G, Venier I, Parolaro D, Zuccaro P, Gori E. Effect of morphine and methadone acute treatment on immunological activity in mice, pharmacokinetics and pharmacodinamic correlates. *J Pharmacol Exp Ther* 1994; 269: 1112–1116.

41. Peterson PK, Molitor TW, Chao CC. Mechanism of morphine-induced immunomodulation. *Biochem Pharmacol* 1993; 46: 343–348.

42. Wang J, Charboneau R, Balasubramian S, Barke RA, Loh HH, Roy S. The immunosuppressive effects of chronic morphine treatment are partially dependent on corticosterone and mediated by the mu opioid receptor. *J Leukoc Biol* 2002; 71: 782–790.

43. Elenkov IJ, Wilder RL, Chrousos GP, Vizi ES. The sympathetic nerve: an integrative interface between two supersystems: the brain and the immune system. *Pharmacol Rev* 2000; 4: 595–638.

44. Alicea C, Belkowsky S, Eisenstein TK, Adler MW, Rogers TJ. Inhibition of primary murine macrophage cytokine production *in vitro* following treatment with the kappa-opioid agonist U50-488H. *J Neuroimmunol* 1996; 64: 83–90.

45. Donahoe RM, Vlahov D. Opiates as potential cofactors in progression of HIV-1 infections to AIDS. *J Neuroimmunol* 1998; 83: 77–87.

18 Human Retroviruses and the Cytokine Network

Massimo Alfano and Guido Poli

CONTENTS

ABSTRACT

Retroviruses are enveloped RNA viruses that enter host cells via binding of their surface glycoproteins to specific plasma membrane receptors. Following fusion of the viral and cellular membranes and cellular intake of the ribonucleoprotein viral complex the RNA genome is transcribed into a double-stranded DNA by the action of the viral enzyme retrotranscriptase (RT). This process initiates in the cytoplasm and is completed in the nucleus after transport of the pre-integration complex across the nuclear membrane. Then, by means of a viral integrase, the linear viral DNA is inserted stably into the host DNA as provirus whereas circular forms of viral DNA will be degraded.

All human retroviruses are characterized by common structural genes regulating the synthesis of Envelope and Gag proteins, as well as of crucial viral enzymes such as RT, integrase, and protease. On the other hand, human retroviruses, and lentiviruses in general, differ from other retroviruses for the presence of regulatory and accessory genes in their genome, which finely tune virus expression at transcriptional and post-transcriptional levels. Moreover, because of stable viral integration into the host genome, retroviral infected cells, mainly CD4+ T cells (in the case of HIV-1 and HIV-2 and, to a minimal extent, HTLV-I) or CD8+ T cells (in the case of HTLV-II), are at present impossible to eradicate, therefore representing stable viral reservoirs. Infection of T lymphocytes functionally deregulates the capacity of the immune system to respond to common pathogens ultimately resulting in increased susceptibility to otherwise benign infections (i.e., opportunistic infections) and in the emergence of B-cell lymphomas and Kaposi's sarcoma. A profound alteration in the expression of cytokines, chemokines, and their related receptors has been described even in individuals infected by HIV and HTLVs and have been implicated in different aspects of the viral-induced pathogenesis, including disorders of the central nervous system.

INTRODUCTION

Following microbial infection, the cells belonging to the innate immune system release cytokines and related factors that profoundly activate and regulate the adaptive T cell and B cell immune responses. Depending on the nature of the foreign antigen (Ag), different cells and their soluble products can orient the adaptive (clonotypic) immune response to the invading pathogen toward a Th1 (cellular, phagocyte-dependent) or Th2 (humoral, phagocyte-independent) immune response (Table 18.1). Therefore, microbial-induced disregulation of cytokine expression may bear profound effects on the quality and efficacy of the induced immune responses. As best exemplified by human immun-odeficiency virus (HIV) infection, the ultimate consequence of selective immune cell destruction and immune disregulation may lead to a profound state of immunodeficiency characterized by the emergence of deadly opportunistic infections and tumors [1,2].

In this chapter, we will analyze in particular how human retroviral infections alter the profiles of expression of host cytokines and chemokines and how these factors may in turn influence the replicative abilities of retroviruses.

HUMAN PATHOGENIC RETROVIRUSES

The human T lymphotropic viruses type I (HTLV-I) and type II (HTLV-II) and the HIV-type 1 (HIV-1) and -type 2 (HIV-2) are the currently identified exogenous human retroviruses. All of them, with the possible exception of HTLV-II, are pathogenic and cause mortal diseases in the absence of treatment. HTLV-I and HTLV-II share the same genomic organization with up to 70% of nucleotide similarity and are characterized by a high degree of genomic stability [3]. The HTLVs and the HIVs share similar features in terms of mode of transmission, genomic organization, and functions of their main proteins, particularly in the mechanism of action of key regulatory viral proteins, such as Tax and Tat and Rex and Rev, respectively, that play fundamental roles in virus expression [4].

TABLE 18.1
Innate Immune Effectors and Their Abilities to Secrete Cytokines and Chemokines

Cell Population	Secreted Factors	Regulation of Immune Response
DC	IL-2, IL-10, IL-12, IL-18, TNF-α, CCL3, CCL4, CXCL1	Triggering Th1/Th2 response
PDC	IFN-α, IL-12, IL-15	Activation of Mø, NK cells and CD8⁺ T cells, Th1/Th2 response
NK	IFN-γ, FasL, TRAIL, CCL1, CCL3, CCL4, CCL5, CCL22	Priming of CTL and Th1 response
NKT	TNF-α, IFN-γ, IL-4, IL-10, IL-13	Recruitment, activation and differentiation of DC and Mø
γδ T cells	TNF-α, IFN-γ, IL-6, CCL3, CCL4, CCL5,	Killing of infected Mø
Basophils, neutrophils	TNF-α, IL-4	Activation of NK cells

DC = dendritic cells. PDC = plasmacytoid dendritic cells. NK = natural killer cells. NKT = natural killer T cells. Mø = macrophages. For a detailed explanation of the role of cytokine-mediated regulation of immune response see references in Alfano, M. and Poli, G. *Mol Immunol* 42, 161, 2005.

HTLV-I

HTLV-I was the first recognized pathogenic exogenous retrovirus [5]. It is endemic in several countries [6] and it is the etiological agent of a severe T lymphocytic neoplastic degeneration leading to adult T cell leukemia (ATL) [5]. In addition, it causes HTLV-I-associated myelopathy/tropical spastic paraparesis (HAM/TSP) [7] as well as several chronic illnesses such as uveitis and dermatitis [8]. More than 15 million individuals are infected worldwide with asymptomatic infections and only 3 to 5% of them will develop ATL during their lifetimes although after several up to (50) years post-infection [9]. Once clinically overt, the median survival of ATL patients is <2 years [10]. HTLV-I transmission can be horizontal, via blood transfusion, and vertical (mother to child) [9].

Of note, viral transmission is mostly mediated by cell-associated virus, whereas free HTLV-I particles are characterized by very low infectivity [11]. HTLV-I preferentially infects primary CD4⁺ T cells [12], although infection of CD8⁺ T cells [13], dendritic cells (DC) [14], glial cells [15], B cells [16], monocytes/macrophages [17], natural killer (NK) cells [18], and endothelial cells [19] has also been described.

As for other retroviruses, incorporation of HTLV-I into the host genome may result in either a silent or productive infection; in this regard it has been calculated that only 1 cell out of 5000 HTLV-I infected CD4⁺ T cells productively expresses the virus [20]. HTLV-I replication alters host cell signaling pathways, particularly through the viral encoded proteins Tax and p12 (Table 18.2), thereby activating cell signaling

TABLE 18.2
Genes and Properties of Retroviral Proteins

Genes Common to All Retroviruses	Properties of Encoded Protein	Protein
Gag	p55 gag protein, precursor of structural proteins	matrix, capsid, nucleocapsid
Pro	Precursor of protease enzyme	protease
Pol	Precursor of RT and IN enzymes	RT and IN
Env	Precursor of Envelope glycoproteins	envelope surface protein, transmembrane protein

HTLV-1 Regulatory Gene	Properties of Encoded Protein	Protein
Tax	Transcriptional and post-transcriptional activator	p40 Tax
Rex	Splicing and RNA post-transcriptional regulator	pp27 Rex, pp21 Rex
ORF I	Maintenance of high viral load *in vivo*	p30, P13
ORF II	Viral replication and infectivity of primary lymphocytes *in vivo*	p12

RT = retrotranscriptase. IN = integrase [301,302].

via T cell receptor (TCR), CD28, and interleukin (IL)-2 receptor (R). In addition, HTLV-I, particularly via its Tax protein, activates transcription factors like nuclear factor-κB (NF-κB) [21], activating protein (AP-1) [22], and also the protein kinase C (PKC)-dependent pathway [23], resulting in a prolonged state of T cell activation [24].

Therefore, HTLV-I-infected cells proceed to the G_1/S transition phase [25] and are characterized by a constitutive activation of the Janus kinase (JAK) signal transducer and activator of transcription (STAT) pathway [26], leading to their survival and propagation which become progressively independent of IL-2 [27]. Of note, it has been recently described that the clonal proliferation of HTLV-I-infected cells could be mediated by the viral protein p21 that enhances STAT5 activation and decreases the IL-2 requirement for cell proliferation [28]. Moreover, HTLV-I Tax has been recently shown to bind to a mitotic checkpoint protein, suggesting that it may also regulate the G_2/M phase of the cell cycle [29].

HTLV-I infected cells proliferate spontaneously *in vitro* in the absence of exogenous growth factors [24] and are characterized by resistance to apoptosis [30], depending on expression of Tax [31] and Tax-mediated inhibition of p53 [32], contributing to the transforming capacity of the virus. Therefore, increased production of IL-2 and IL-2R expression, resulting in an autocrine IL-2-dependent T cell proliferation, is frequently detectable in T cells from HTLV-I-infected individuals [33]. Of note, even uninfected T cells of HTLV-I+ individuals express several markers of immune activation [34], a phenomenon that seems to be dependent of the interaction between the CD58 (LFA-3) [35], which is over-expressed by infected cells [36], and its R (CD2) [23]. In addition to CD58, other cell membrane molecules such as CD54 are over-expressed by infected cells [37] and have been shown to regulate the activation of uninfected cells [23].

HTLV-I-Induced Expression of Cytokines and Chemokines

A number of cytokines, chemokines, and related Rs are over-expressed in cells infected with HTLV-I both *in vivo* and *in vitro*, as well as in HTLV-I transformed cell lines and Tax-transfected cells (Table 18.3). The main determinant of HTLV-I-induced expression of cytokines, chemokines, and their Rs has always been linked to Tax-induced activation of cellular transcription factors [38]. Moreover, Tax can also *trans*-repress the gene expression of DNA polymerase α [39] and inhibitors of cyclin-dependent kinases [40], thereby disregulating the DNA repair mechanisms regulating the cell cycle.

Thus, the *in vivo* survival of infected cells and the lymphoproliferative effect associated with HTLV-I infection depend upon the up-regulation of cytokines sustaining cell proliferation, i.e., IL-2, IL-13, IL-15, and cytokines exerting anti-apoptotic effects such as IL-13 and I-309. In addition, disregulation of genes controlling cell proliferation and cell migration into different organs, including the chemokines CCL4, CCL17, and CCL22, contribute to HTLV-I induced disregulation.

Because HTLV-I free virions are poorly infective, the lymphoproliferative effect caused either by infection or by Tax is a servomechanism promoting amplification of proviral DNA via cell proliferation.

In vivo, increased levels of tumor necrosis factor (TNF)-α, granulocytes and monocytes–colony stimulating factor (GM-CSF), interferon (IFN)-γ, and IL-1 have been found in individuals with HAM/TSP in comparison to those of asymptomatic carriers [41–45]. The concentrations of sIL-2R in plasma were correlated to the HTLV-I DNA load [46], whereas either sIL-2R [47] levels or genetic polymorphisms increasing the production of TNF-α [48] are risk factors for the development of ATL among HTLV-I-infected individuals. Enhanced production of IL-5 associated with eosinophilia is frequently observed in ATL individuals [49], whereas increased expression of IFN-γ–inducible protein-10 (IP-10) has been suggested as a potential link between HTLV-I infection and the epidermal tropism of cutaneous T-cell lymphomas [50].

Cytokines produced by HTLV-I infected T cells are also responsible for intraocular inflammation in patients with HTLV-I-induced uveitis [51]. TNF-α expression from HTLV-I infected synoviocytes causes the synovial hyperplasia observed in HTLV-I-associated arthropathy [52]. Tax-induced TNF-α expression, either from infected T cells infiltrating the central nervous system (CNS) [42,53] or from infected astrocytes [54] or Tax-stimulated neurons [55], has been implicated in the development of HAM/TSP [42,48,53,55–57]. Enhanced levels of soluble TNF R (sTNFR) in the CNS have been proposed to predict HAM/TSP progression [58]. Because of the increased production of inflammatory cytokines [59], HTLV-I has been proposed as a cause of autoimmune diseases such

TABLE 18.3
**Increased Cytokines, Chemokines, and Related Receptor
Expression Following HTLV-I Infection or Tax Transfection**

Name	HTLV- Infected Cells (1) or Tax-Transfected Cells (2)	References
GM-CSF	1, 2	[303–306]
IL-1	1, 2, ATL patients	[88,307,308]
IL-2	2	[309]
IL-2R	2	[268]
IL-15	2	[310]
IL-6	1, 2, ATL patients	[311]
IL-8	1, 2	[312,313]
IL-10	1, ATL patients	[314]
IL-13	1, 2, ATL patients	[315,316]
IL-13R	1	[316]
IL-15	2, TSP patients	[317,318]
TGF-β	2, ATL patients	[319,320]
IL-17	2	[321]
TNF-α/β	1, 2	[54,92,322]
CCL3/MIP-1α	1, 2, HTLV-1 carriers	[312,313]
MIP-1αR	2	[323]
CCL1/I-309	ATL patients	[324]
CCL4/MIP-1β	2	[325]
CCR5	2	[325]
CCL20/MIP-3α	1	[326]
MIP-3αR	1	[326]
CCL5/RANTES	1, 2, HTLV-1 carriers	[312,313]
CCL2/MCP-1	1	[327]
SDF-1	1, 2	[328]
CXCR4	1, 2	[328]
IP-10	1	[327]
CCR4	1, ATL patients	[329]
G-CSFR	ATL patients	[330]
IFN-γ	1, 2	[331]
IL-3	1	[332]
IL-4	1	[332]
IL-9	1, ATL patients	[333,334]

ATL = adult T cell leukemia. TSP = tropical spastical paraparesis.

as rheumatoid arthritis (RA) although other studies have not confirmed this association [60].

In vitro, HTLV-I infection of plasmacytoid DCs (PDCs) decreased the capacity of these cells to express IFN-α, a feature resembling what is observed in peripheral blood mononuclear cells (PBMCs) of ATL patients [61]. Of interest, IFN-α producing capacity was found inversely correlated to HTLV-I DNA load in PBMCs of asymptomatic carriers [61], suggesting a functional defect of PDCs in HTLV-I-infected individuals. Depletion of PDCs and/or decreased capacity to express IFN-α may contribute to the immunodeficiency in ATL or to the development of ATL itself since IFN-α has been shown to inhibit the assembly of HTLV-I virions [62].

Therapy of HTLV-I Infection

IFN-α has been shown to decrease *in vitro* HTLV-I expression [63]. *In vivo*, IFN-α therapy caused decreased viral load and motor disability in HAM/TSP individuals [64–66], whereas it has been shown to induce cell cycle arrest and apoptosis of HTLV-I+ cells in combination with arsenite trioxide [67]. Immunosuppressive agents such as hydrocortisone, FK506, and rapamycin [68] or immunotherapy based on anti-IL-2R antibodies (Abs) [67] have also been suggested as therapeutic agents. Engineered toxins fused with IL-2 have been used to eliminate tumor cells over-expressing IL-2 R [69] and could be useful in the treatment of HTLV-I infection [70]. Of note, an "immunotoxin analogue" based on the fusion of IL-2 and human pancreatic RNase1 enzyme proved to block protein synthesis in HTLV-I-infected malignant T cells hyper-expressing high affinity IL-2R [71]. Finally, combination of Abs against IL-2 and IL-15 completely inhibited cellular proliferation of *ex-vivo* HTLV-I infected cells [72].

Of interest, molecules regulating cellular proliferation and apoptosis of HTLV-I-transformed cells have been developed. For example, the agent known as 2-benzoyl-phenyl-6,7-dichloroquinoxaline 1,4-dioxide (DCQ) has been shown to induce apoptosis and inhibit cell growth [73]. Inhibition of tumor growth was observed in mice treated with the proteasome inhibitor PS-341 [74], a combination of arsenite and IFN-α [75], capsaicin [76], or Bay 11-7082 [77], that inhibited NF-κB activation and led to apoptotic DNA fragmentation.

Finally, antiretroviral therapy with zidovudine and lamivudine, either alone or in combination, has also been tested on HTLV-I-positive individuals and proved to be effective in reducing viral load and viral transmission [78,79]. In this regard, viral resistance has been shown for the nucleoside reverse-transcriptase (RT) inhibitor lamivudine [80].

HTLV-II

HTLV-II transmission can be either vertical (mother to child) or horizontal, mainly via blood transfusion and needle sharing among intravenous drug users (IVDUs) [81], with a rate of infection in these individuals ranging from 10% to 25%, reaching 60% in IVDUs of South Vietnam [82]. The role of HTLV-II in human disease has not been defined, although there are reports that this infection may cause neurological symptoms similar to those observed in HTLV-I-infected individuals [82]. On the other hand, the relationship between HTLV-II infection and human diseases has not been definitively established either because of a state of HIV-1 co-infection or because of difficulties in differentiating distinctive features from those caused by drug abuse [82].

HTLV-II-Induced Expression of Cytokines

As demonstrated for HTLV-I and HIV infections, HTLV-II-infected PBMCs cultivated *ex-vivo* are also characterized by STAT1 activation, as a consequence of IFN-γ production [83]. Moreover, *in vitro* HTLV-II infection of CD34+ TF-1 cells has been shown to induce expression of GM-CSF and IFN-γ that, in turn, activate STAT1 and STAT5 [84]. HTLV-II-induced cell proliferation of infected TF-1 cells has been shown to depend upon autocrine release of GM-CSF [84] and increased telomerase activity [85]. Spontaneously proliferating PBMCs isolated *ex-vivo* from HTLV-II infected individuals are characterized by high levels of IFN-γ, IL-2, IL-4, IL-6, and TNF-α and decreased levels of IL-10 [86 87]. In addition, increased levels of IL-1α [88], IL-2, and IL-2R [89], IL-6 [90], leukemia inhibitory factor (LIF), GM-CSF [91], and TNF-β [92] have been reported in cell lines transformed *in vitro* with HTLV-II or transfected with its Tax protein.

As for HTLV-I infection, triple antiretroviral drug combinations such as lamivudine and protease inhibitors have been tested in HTLV-II/HIV infected individuals, resulting in undetectable plasma levels of HIV-1, but only in a slight decrease of plasma HTLV-II DNA levels [78].

HIV-1

Originally named LAV or HTLV-III [93], HIV infection currently affects >43 million individuals worldwide. Primary HIV infection is frequently associated with a clinical syndrome almost indistinguishable from acute mononucleosis that emerges approximately 2 to 6 weeks following infection [94], and determining a drop in the numbers of circulating CD4+ T cells [95] in conjunction with high levels of virus replication in peripheral blood, lymphoid organs, and the CNS [94,96]. After that, a clinically asymptomatic phase coinciding with the onset of strong adaptive cellular and humoral immune responses [97] establishes in most individuals and persists for 8 to 10 years in the absence of antiretroviral therapy [98].

A slow but progressive decline in the numbers of circulating CD4+ T lymphocytes [99] is associated with continuous viral replication [100]. The levels of viremia (HIV RNA in blood) at steady state (once the immune response has mounted) and the number of peripheral CD4+ T lymphocytes are good predictors of the rapidity of evolution of HIV disease [101]. Thus, although strong and specific anti-HIV cytotoxic T lymphocyte (CTL) and Ab responses emerge during the course of HIV infection, virus replication is only partially controlled. The progressive erosion of CD4+ T cells compromises the function of virus-specific CTLs, whereas the error-prone viral enzyme RT generates mutants that can escape their control as well as that exerted by neutralizing Abs [102].

When the number of circulating CD4+ T cells falls below to 200/μl [99], the likelihood of emergence of opportunistic infections or tumors (defining the acquired immunodeficiency syndrome [AIDS] stage of HIV disease) increases significantly [103]. It should be underscored that clearance of HIV infection has never been documented. Therefore, it is likely that manipulation of the immune system will be required to induce stronger and broader immune responses against virus-infected cells.

HIV is a 9-Kb human retrovirus belonging to the lentiviridae [104]. It infects target cells expressing the CD4 molecule [105] and a chemokine R, either CCR5 or CXCR4, on its cell surface [106–109]. Following entry into host cells, HIV-1 RNA is retrotranscribed to DNA by the RT while the so-called preintegration complex (composed of Gag-derived p17 matrix, nucleic acids, RT, and other factors) is actively imported into cell nuclei [110]. Following proviral integration, a state of microbiological latency may persist for the entire life span of the infected cell unless cellular RNA polymerase II transcription complex is assembled at the transcription start site, driving expression of viral genes.

This event can be triggered by different immunologic signals, including pro-inflammatory cytokines (such as TNF-α, and IL-1), TCR engagement and activation of co-stimulatory signaling cascades leading to nuclear factor of activated cells (NFAT), and NF-κB activation. Once triggered, HIV transcription is strongly potentiated by one of the earliest HIV gene products, the viral protein transcriptional activator (Tat) that acts as a positive servomechanism [111]. HIV transcription is also regulated by untranslated identical sequences present at both the 5′ and 3′ ends of the viral genome and named long terminal repeats (LTRs). Indeed, the LTRs contain the RNA binding sites for Tat (TAR) and the DNA recognition elements for several constitutive and inducible cellular transcription factors including Sp-1, AP-1, NF-κB, and NFAT [112]. The newly synthesized 9.2-Kb full-length mRNA undergoes a process of splicing, leading first to the synthesis of the viral proteins Tat, Rev, and Nef, and then viral structural proteins and enzymes. Through the action of Rev, partially spliced (4.5-Kb) and unspliced (9.2-Kb) mRNAs are exported from the nucleus to the cytoplasm where they can be translated into structural and accessory viral proteins.

Assembly of viral proteins and genomic RNA occurs in the inner leaflet of the plasma membrane, mostly in lipid rafts [113]. The process of new viral particle (virion) budding and release from the plasma membrane has been well characterized [114], with distinctive features of T lymphocytes and mononuclear phagocytes (MPs). In particular, infection of MPs, unlike that of lymphocytes, is characterized by virion production and accumulation in intracellular vesicles in addition to plasma membrane. The envelope composition of virions budding from macrophages has been reported to contain proteins typical of exosomes [115], subcellular organelles derived from the multivesicular endosomes [116].

Finally, Tat, and likely Tax, can be released from infected cells and affect the functions of neighboring cells after being taken up via several cell surface receptors, including chemokine receptors and particularly CXCR4 [117,118]. Tas has recently been shown to act as a facilitator of HIV infection via binding to gp120 Env [119]. In addition, VpR, a retroviral protein present in the virions, can act in the cells (including non-infected cells) as homologous of glucocorticoids via binding to their intracellular receptors [120]. Therefore, either retroviral infection or the expression and uptake of retroviral proteins can modulate the expression and secretion of several cytokines (Table 18.3 and Table 18.4).

HIV-1-Induced Expression of Cytokines and Chemokines

HIV infection *in vivo* profoundly alters cytokine and chemokine levels, therefore disregulating immune responses to viral Ags [121]. *In vivo* studies reported that the progression of HIV infection toward AIDS and the levels of plasma viremia are associated with decreased levels of IFN-α, IL-2, IL-12, and IL-13, although increased levels of IFN-γ, IL-7, and TGF-β have also been reported (Table 18.4).

TABLE 18.4
Influence of HIV-1 Infection on Cytokine Expression *in Vivo*

Cytokine	Level Modification	Cell Sources/Compartments [References]	Effect of Antiretroviral Therapy on Cytokine Levels [References]
IFN-α	Decreased	PBMC, DC, PDC, CNS [214,335,336]	Conflicting data [211–213]
IFN-γ	Increased	Peripheral blood, LN [337]	nt
IL-12	Decreased	PBMC [338–340]	nt
IL-2	Decreased	PBMC, LN [341–343]	Increased [344,345]
IL-7	Increased	Plasma and serum [346–348]	nt
IL-13	Decreased	Serum, CD4+ and CD8+ T cells [349]	Increased [350]
TGF-β	Increased	Brain, CSF, serum, PBMC, kidney [351–354]	nt

PBMC = peripheral blood mononuclear cells, DC = dendritic cells, PDC = plasmacytoid dendritic cells, CNS = central nervous system, LN = lymph nodes, CSF = cerebrospinal fluid, nt = not tested.

Effective anti-retroviral therapy decreasing plasma viremia has shown to be effective for the restoration of physiological IL-2 and IL-13 levels (Table 18.4).

HIV proteins are able to disregulate cytokine production even in uninfected cells independently of viral replication. HIV-1 gp120 envelope (Env) has been shown to induce expression of macrophage inflammatory protein-1β (CCL4/MIP-1β) and of stromal cell derived factor-1α (CXCL12/SDF-1α) in primary lymphocytes and macrophages, respectively [122]. HIV-1 Env from R5 viruses exerted chemotactic effects on DCs [123], whereas both gp120 Env and synthetic peptides encompassing the gp41 Env (the second external protein endowed with fusogenic properties) were shown to down-regulate IL-13 production from basophils [124,125] and up-regulate TGF-β expression in human PBMCs and macrophages [126,127].

HIV matrix protein Gag p17 up-regulated IL-12 and IL-15 from purified human NK cells [128], whereas the Gag precursor p55 Gag triggered expression of IL-12, CXCL8/IL-8, CCL3/MIP-1α, and CCL4/MIP-1β [129,130] in immature DCs (iDCs), therefore favoring their maturation [131]. Similar effects were seen with Nef [132]. Exogenous Tat up-regulated TGF-β secretion in different cell subsets, such as human PBMCs, macrophages, and CD8+ T cells [133–136], and induced CCL2/MCP-1 secretion in monocyte-derived macrophages (MDMs) [137], astrocytes, and endothelial cells [138,139].

HIV-1 Life Cycle Control by Cytokines, Chemokines, and Defensins

Cytokines, chemokines, and defensins can regulate the HIV life cycle by acting on distinct viral steps from viral entry to release of new progeny virions (Table 18.5).

IFN-α/β exerts potent antiviral activity *in vitro* and protect HIV-infected mice with severe combined immunodeficiency (SCID) when reconstituted with human

TABLE 18.5
Key Cytokines, Chemokines, and Defensins in HIV-1 Infection and Replication

Cytokine/Chemokine	Effect on HIV Infection/Replication
IL-2, IL-15	Up-regulation via induction of pro-inflammatory cytokines
IL-7, IL-12, CCL2, CXCL8	Enhancement of HIV transcription
CCL3, CCL4, CCL5	Inhibition of R5 HIV entry
Defensins	Inhibition of (X4) HIV entry and virion infectivity
IL-13	Post-transcriptional inhibition HIV replication in Mø
IFN-α/β	Inhibition of multiple steps of the virus life cycle
IL-4, IL-10	Bimodal: inhibition of cytokine-mediated virus replication, but enhancement of HIV expression
IFN-γ	Bimodal: enhancement of HIV transcription, but inhibition of R5 virus entry and virion release
TGF-β	Bimodal: both enhancement and suppression of HIV replication as a function of time of stimulation vs. infection (Mø)

cells or tissues from CD4$^+$ T cell depletion [140]. In this surrogate model of HIV infection, as well as in chronically infected cells, IFN-α-mediated inhibition of viral replication has been associated with trapping of new progeny virions within cells [141]. In addition, IFN-α/β can inhibit early post-entry steps in the HIV life cycle [142] or transcriptional events in infected MDMs [143].

In contrast to IFN-α/β, opposite effects have been described for IFN-γ in terms of its influence on HIV replication. Although inhibitory effects due to the activation of STAT-1 were observed in acutely infected U937 "plus" clones [144], IFN-γ induced viral expression in chronically HIV-infected promonocytic U1 cells [145]. Furthermore, IFN-γ neutralization reduced viral replication in IL-2-stimulated PBMCs infected *in vitro* [146]. In combination with TNF-α and TNF-β, IFN-γ showed potent inductive effects on both U937 and U1 cells along with a highly increased cytopathicity, resulting in an abortive HIV infection [145]. Production of IFN-γ and IL-10 increases during the interaction of infected DCs with T cells leading to HIV spread [147].

Concerning interleukins, IL-1α/β, like TNF-α, is a pro-inflammatory cytokine that has been associated with enhancement of viral replication both in U1 cells [148] and in primary PBMCs stimulated with IL-2 [146]. IL-2 strongly synergized with IL-4, causing viral production from *in vitro* infected mature thymocytes [149], an effect associated with increased expression of CCR5 and CXCR4 [150]. As mentioned, IL-2 stimulation of PBMCs led to a productive infection by both R5 and CXCR4-using viruses that was profoundly dependent upon the release of secondary cytokines including TNF-α, IL-1β, and IFN-γ [146]. However, when PBMC or lymph node-derived mononuclear cells of infected individuals were stimulated *ex vivo* with either IL-2 or IL-12, only the latter induced viral production unless CD8$^+$ T cells were removed from the culture [151]. This observation was explained by the ability of IL-2 to induce the release of "non-cytolytic antiviral factors" from CD8+ T cells. It should be underscored that IL-12 was also shown to exert suppressive effects on HIV replication linked to a down-regulation of CCR5 [152] when T lymphocytes were stimulated with this cytokine before infection.

IL-7 was quickly shown to increase HIV replication in CD8-depleted PBMCs of infected individuals stimulated with anti-CD3 Ab [153]. Furthermore, IL-7 induced HIV expression in chronically infected human cells [154] and synergized with TNF-α in sustaining HIV spreading in single CD4+ thymocytes by inducing the up-regulation of the p75 TNF R [155]. IL-7 was then reported to up-regulate CXCR4 expression in naïve T cells [156], PBMCs, and thymocytes [150,157], an effect that has been hypothesized to play a role in the emergence of CXCR4-using HIV-1 variants [158].

This hypothesis was supported by a correlation between increased plasma levels of both IL-7 and SDF-1α and up-regulated expression of CXCR4 and plasma viremia [159]. Recently, IL-7 was shown to be the strongest inducer of HIV replication in CD8+ and monocyte-depleted resting CD4+ T cells of HAART-virally suppressed individuals in comparison to phytohemagglutinin (PHA) plus IL-2. Of interest is the fact that different molecular species were induced in different patients'cells when stimulated with IL-7 versus PHA/IL-2 [163]. At the molecular level, IL-7 has been suggested to induce HIV replication via activation of STAT5 [156] although only minimal transcriptional effects were reported independently [163]. In spite of its potentiation on HIV replication, IL-7 remains a potentially important cytokine for the immunologic reconstitution of HIV-infected individuals. This is supported by its ability to contribute to CTL development [160] and the fact that in HIV+ individuals and children, highly active antiretroviral therapy (HAART) plus IL-2 treatment induced significant increases of CD4+ cells and plasma levels of IL-7 [161] and increased expression of IL-7 R (CD127) on CD8+ T cells [162].

Another common γ-chain cytokine, in addition to IL-2 and IL-7, shown to enhance HIV replication in acutely infected PBMCs or T cells with a predilection for R5 HIV strains is IL-15 [146,151,164,165]. No correlation was found between *in vitro* HIV infection of PBMCs and IL-15 production [166]. As previously shown for IL-2 [146], this effect was caused by the induction of pro-inflammatory cytokines including TNF-α, IFN-γ, and IL1-β and by the up-regulation of CCR5 [167–169]. In one study, IL-15 stimulation of PBMCs enhanced both HIV replication and secretion of CCR5-binding chemokines; however, IL-15-induced levels of CC chemokines (<10 ng/ml) were likely insufficient for causing inhibition of HIV infection and/or replication [169–171].

Less univocal information concerns the immunosuppressive cytokines, namely IL-4, IL-13, IL-10, and TGF-β. IL-4 differently regulates the expression of the main viral entry co-receptors, namely CXCR4 (up-regulation) and CCR5 (down-regulation) [172–174], thus potentially playing a role in the so-called phenotypic switch from the R5 to X4 HIV strain, an event occurring in approximately 50% of individuals infected with clade B HIV-1. Both inductive effects on freshly isolated monocytes and inhibitory effects on HIV-1 replication in MDMs, depending on the suppression of pro-inflammatory cytokines, have also been reported [175,176].

Similar in many aspects to IL-4, IL-13 inhibited HIV replication in MDMs but not in activated T cells [177,178]. This effect was consequent to IL-13-induced down-regulation of several receptors including CD4 [179], CCR5 [173,179], and CXCR4 [173].

Depending on IL-10 concentrations, either inhibitory [180,181] or inductive effects on *in vitro* HIV replication have been observed. Inhibition of viral replication in MDMs was correlated to the prevention of the synthesis and release of endogenous TNF-α and IL-6 [182], whereas lower concentrations of IL-10 resulted in the enhancement of HIV replication in MDMs. This paradox was interpreted as a consequence of the fact that IL-10 can cooperate with secreted TNF-α and IL-6 to promote viral dissemination as demonstrated in terms of induction of HIV expression in U1 cells [183]. In addition, as previously discussed for IL-4, IL-10 can up-regulate the expression of CCR5 thereby favoring R5 HIV replication in freshly isolated monocytes [184].

In vitro, TGF-β has been reported to mediate NF-κB-dependent viral transcription in cell lines [185]. Earlier studies indicated that TGF-β (like retinoic acid) could either induce or suppress HIV transcription in U1 cells and replication in MDMs as a function of whether the cells were stimulated with the cytokine before or after infection [186–190]. The observation that TGF-β can increase the expression of both CCR5 and CXCR4 [191] provides a plausible mechanism for these early discrepant findings.

Concerning chemokines, both HIV-preventive and potentiating effects have been reported. The anti-HIV activities of CCL3/MIP-1α, CCL4/MIP-1β, and CCL5/RANTES [192] shared with MCP-2 [193] were later demonstrated to reflect their binding capacities to CCR5 [192]. The CXCR4 ligand, CXCL12/SDF-1, inhibited X4 virus entry in CD4$^+$ cells [107,194]. Recently, a polymorphism of the gene coding for a minor isoform of CCL3/MIP-1α, named CCL3L1 or LD-78β, the most potent natural inhibitor of R5 HIV-1, has been shown to significantly affect susceptibility to HIV infection and its levels of viral replication *in vivo* [195]. However, CCR5-binding chemokines were also shown to up-regulate HIV expression in MDMs infected with R5 HIV-1 [196] and in DCs and PBMCs infected with X4 virus [197,198]. Up-regulation of HIV replication by CCL2/MCP-1, CXCL8/IL-8, and Gro-α/CXCL1 [199,200] has also been reported in different systems including PBMCs infected with dual-tropic HIV strains [201] and monocyte-depleted PBMCs of HIV-infected individuals [202]. A strong correlation *in vivo* between CCL2 expression and HIV replication in the CNS, leading to HIV encephalitis, has been reported by us [203] and several other groups [204,205], whereas a polymorphism of its gene is correlated to higher or lower levels of virus replication and disease progression, with special regard to the infection of the CNS [206]. Inhibitory effects on HIV replication have been also reported for CCL22/MDC [207].

In addition to cytokines and chemokines, other soluble molecules, namely defensins, participate in the innate immunity to pathogens and are involved in the control of HIV infection and replication. α-defensins have recently been shown to inhibit *in vitro* HIV infection [208]. After *in vitro* HIV stimulation of epithelial cells, the levels of expression of β-defensins 2 and 3 were found to be increased.

Moreover, β-defensins decreased CXCR4 but not CCR5 expression in PBMCs and lymphocytic cells, and therefore inhibited X4 but not R5 HIV-1 strain infections [209]. Finally, an θ-defensin known as retrocyclin has been shown to inhibit HIV entry in primary CD4+ T cells [210].

In Vivo Cytokine-Based Treatment of HIV: IFN-α and IL-2

HAART-treated HIV+ individuals exhibit decreased plasma viremia and increased numbers of IFN-α-producing PDCs, according to some authors [211,212]. However, others reported no influence of viral load and HAART on the capacity of PDCs to produce IFN-α [213]. Moreover, levels of IFN-α in the cerebrospinal fluid have been positively associated with viral load and the staging of AIDS dementia complex in humans [214].

In vivo administration of IFN-α as a therapeutic agent has been pursued since the earliest evidence of the viral nature of HIV/AIDS. Indeed, beneficial effects of IFN-α were observed in AIDS patients with Kaposi's sarcoma and high (>500 cells/μl) CD4+ T cell counts [215], as recently confirmed in an open-label randomized controlled trial [216]. In addition, IFN-α caused delayed progression, palliate symptoms, and prolonged survival in individuals with HIV-associated progressive multifocal leukoencephalopathy [217]. The polyethylene-glycol (PEG)-conjugated forms of IFN-α are characterized by prolonged half-lives and easier compliance and may lead to a re-evaluation of this classical antiviral molecule in the context of HAART regimens. In support of this hypothesis, enhanced lytic activity along with increased concentrations of perforin and granzyme A expression in NK cells was demonstrated in HIV+ individuals receiving PEG-IFN-α [218]. Finally, HIV-infected human DCs stimulated with type I IFNs induced a potent primary immune response against various HIV-1 Ags, suggesting a potential use of type I IFNs as vaccine adjuvants [219].

Co-administration of IL-2 and IFN-γ cDNA together with simian immunodeficiency virus (SIV) gag/pol or HIV env/rev enhanced Ag-specific T cell-mediated immune responses [220]. IFN-γ was shown to increase the protection of macaques previously infected with nef-deleted SIV from the challenge with wild-type SIV [221], although experimental therapy with IFN-γ reconstituted with human cells showed no inhibitory effects on viral loads in SCID mice [222].

Administration of exogenous IL-12 did not affect either the virus loads or the frequency of circulating infected lymphocytes in chronically SIV-infected rhesus monkeys [223,224], although it increased the proliferative responses to multiple HIV Ags in chimpanzees vaccinated with a DNA-based vaccine [225]. IL-12 administration to SIV-infected macaques [224] and HIV-infected individuals [225] at an early stage of infection increased the frequency and activity of circulating NK cells in contrast to an earlier report indicated a paradoxical decrease of NK cell activities in IL-12-treated HIV+ individuals [226].

Administration of exogenous IL-2 has been shown to prevent depletion of immature CD4+CD8+ and CD5+CD1+ thymocytes in the HIV-infected thymuses of SCID mice implanted with human fetal thymus and liver tissues without increasing viral load [227]. In addition, IL-2 prevented the outgrowth of human Epstein–Barr virus (EBV) lymphoproliferative disease, a typical cancer emerging in AIDS patients [228], in SCID mice engrafted with human PBMCs from EBV+

donors [229]. In this regard, IL-2 has been successfully used in humans to prevent EBV disease [230]. *In vitro,* IL-2 strongly synergized with IL-4, causing viral production from *in vitro*-infected mature thymocytes [149], an effect associated with increased expression of CCR5 and CXCR4 [150,231]. Once expressed through a vaccinia virus or following DNA vaccination IL-2 did not alter viral replication and showed adjuvant properties [220,232]. Therefore, IL-2 is currently under evaluation in phase III clinical trials (ESPRIT) for its potential therapeutic effects when administered with antiretroviral therapy to stably increase the levels of circulating CD4+ T cells up to usual [233].

IL-2 plus HAART reduced the state of immune activation and, in some studies, the HIV DNA content of PBMCs, likely as a consequence of the numerical expansion of circulating CD4+ T cells [234]. In addition, administration of IL-2 without anti-retrovirals has not resulted in the expression of a previously silent quasispecies [235].

Concerning other common-γ chain cytokines, IL-15 has been shown to exert number of immunorestoration functions including the up-regulation of Ab-dependent cellular cytotoxicity from PBMCs and several polymorphonuclear phagocyte functions in HIV+ individuals [236,237]. In addition, IL-15 induced virus-specific CTLs in primates infected with SIV and in humans [238]. IL-7, in spite of its capacity to induce and potentiate HIV replication, remains a potentially important cytokine for the immunologic reconstitution of HIV-infected individuals, given its ability to contribute to CTL development [160], and because HIV+ individuals and children, HAART plus IL-2 treatment induced significant increases of CD4+ T cells and plasma levels of IL-7 [161] and increased expression of IL-7 R (CD127) on CD8+ T cells [162]. In the future other cytokines or cytokine-like molecules are expected to enter the arena of immune-based control of HIV infection and replication.

HIV-2

Unlike HIV-1 which is widely diffused throughout the world, HIV-2 is concentrated in West African countries. HIV-2 has about 50% genetic homology to HIV-1, but in spite of structural and functional similarities and usage of CD4 and CCR5 to gain entry into host cells [239], its efficiency of transmission both horizontally and vertically, is much lower [240]. In addition, the progression of HIV-2 from the asymptomatic stage to AIDS is slower than in HIV-1-infected individuals [241]. Consistently, the rate of CD4+ T cell count erosion is less marked in HIV-2 than HIV-1 asymptomatic individuals [242]. In fact, the incubation period for immuno-logical deterioration of the infected host and development of disease is longer for HIV-2-infected individuals [243]. HIV-2 asymptomatic infection is characterized by proviral levels similar to those found in HIV-1-infected individuals [244], although viral replication is spontaneously controlled to low or undetectable levels much more frequently than observed in HIV-1-infected individuals [245].

HIV-2-Induced Expression of Cytokines

Based on the observations reported above, it has been proposed that HIV-2 infection may be controlled by stronger cellular immune responses than those observed in

HIV-1-infected individuals [246]. Indeed, HIV-2-infected individuals frequently have higher numbers of antigen-specific CD8+ T cells producing IL-2 and IFN-γ than HIV-1-infected individuals [247], although other findings did not support this observation [248].

In vitro studies have shown that HIV-2 can inhibit HIV-1 replication by interfering with viral entry (by either up-regulating expression of CCR5-binding chemokines [249,250] and consequent down-modulation of CCR5 expression [251]) or at post-entry levels [252,253]. *In vivo*, HIV-2-infected individuals experience much lower rates of HIV-1 infection [254] and it has been inferred that this would be consequent to a robust humoral and cellular cross-immunity conferred by HIV-2 infection [255].

Plasma levels of TNF-α and IL-1 are usually lower in HIV-2-infected than in HIV-1-infected individuals [256], whereas HIV-2 infection *in vitro* induces a lower percentage of apoptotic cells than HIV-1 infection [257]. These features, together with the observation that HIV-2 frequently carries mutations and deletions within the *nef* gene [258], may help explain the observation that HIV-2-infected individuals have proportionally higher CD4+ T cell counts than HIV-1-infected individuals with comparable histories of infection. *In vitro* IFN-γ inhibits HIV-2 acute and chronic infections [259] and many HIV-2 isolates can infect cells independently of CD4 [260].

Whether HAART regimens with predicted efficacy for treatment of HIV-1 infections are also efficacious for treatment of HIV-2 infections [261,262] remains a controversial issue, whereas non-nucleoside RT inhibitors (NNRTIs) are not effective against HIV-2 [263,264].

CO-INFECTIONS AND INTERACTIONS AMONG HUMAN RETROVIRUSES

HIV AND HTLV-I CO-INFECTION

This co-infection has been shown to accelerate the progression of AIDS [265,274], although other studies did not support this finding [266]. In particular, it has been suggested that the net effect of HTLV-I co-infection in HIV-infected individuals favors the transition from R5 to X4-tropic HIV phenotype, which is generally indicative of progressive HIV disease [267], although other authors proposed that HIV/HTLV-I co-infected individuals have higher prevalences of HTLV-I related outcomes [266].

In addition to its role on HTLV-I transcription, Tax has been shown to up-regulate HIV expression via activation of the cellular transcription factor NF-κB which recognizes one or two binding sites in the U3 region of the HIV-2 and HIV-1 LTRs, respectively [268]. Its mechanism mimics that operated by cytokines such as TNF-α or IL-1β (IL-1β) that converge on NF-κB-dependent triggering or potentiation of HIV transcription [269]. HIV-2 Tat can substitute HIV-1 Tat to some extent in binding to the RNA region known as TAR in close proximity of the transcription start site in the R region of the HIV-1 LTR [270]. Analogous pathways exist for the Rex/Rev axis, in which the viral proteins bind RNA regions named Rex-RRE (Rev responsive element) or RRE, thus allowing the export of partly spliced and unspliced viral transcripts in the cytoplasm to undergo translation of both structural and regulatory proteins [271]. Finally, Tat, and likely Tax, can be released from infected cells and affect the functions of neighboring cells after being taken up via several cell surface receptors [272,273]. Thus, both retroviral infection and/or the expression of retroviral proteins can modulate the expression and secretion of several cytokines (Table 18.3 and Table 18.4).

HIV AND HTLV-II CO-INFECTION

HTLV-II is present at significant rate (10% to 25%) among intravenous drug users, with 85% to 98% of these individuals co-infected by HIV-1 [275]; however, it is still unclear whether this co-infection may influence HIV disease progression [276]. *Ex vivo*, it has been shown that the replicative ability of HIV-1 was inversely correlated to the PBMC-associated HTLV-II proviral DNA load, whereas PBMCs with undetectable HTLV-II DNA efficiently propagated HIV-1 as measured by p24 Gag antigen in culture supernatant [277].

Although both HIV⁺ and HTLV-II⁺ PBMCs cultivated *ex vivo* are characterized by IFN-γ production and/or STAT1 activation [83,84] (G. Poli, unpublished observations), co-infection of PBMCs with these two retroviruses is characterized by lower levels of both IFN-γ secretion and STAT1 activation [83]. Since HTLV-II preferentially infects CD8⁺ T cells [4] that serve as major sources of HIV-inhibitory chemokines [192], it has been shown that individuals with the highest HTLV-II loads usually produced the highest levels of CC chemokines *ex vivo*, suggesting a potential linkage of HTLV-II load, chemokine secretion, and HIV replication. Indeed, PBMCs of HTLV-II/HIV co-infected individuals are characterized by increased levels of CCR5-binding chemokines, and particularly MIP-1α, and reduced/suppressed HIV replication [277,278]. Thus, it appears that HTLV-II infection may inhibit HIV infection at multiple levels via CCR5-binding chemokines and IFN expression.

CYTOKINES AND HUMAN RETROVIRUSES: CENTRAL ROLE OF IL-2

Before the discovery of the importance of certain chemokines and their receptors in HIV entry of CD4⁺ cells, HTLV-I and HTLV-II and HIV-1 and HIV-2 have shown multiple intersections with the cytokine network (Table 18.3 through Table 18.5) and/or evidence of interference with their signaling pathways. Conversely, numerous cytokines were demonstrated to either up- or down-regulate HIV expression [279].

Among other cytokines, IL-2 can be considered crucial for regulating several aspects of T cell infection by both cytopathic HIVs and transforming human retroviruses (HTLVs). IL-2 is a central regulator of T cell function and survival produced by activated T lymphocytes and, in some cases, by microbial stimulation of DCs [280]. IL-2 induces proliferation and activation of both CD4⁺ and CD8⁺

T cells [281], potentiates the cytotoxicity of CD8$^+$ T lymphocytes and NK cells, and stimulates B cell function, therefore playing a major role in the containment of viral infections and in the elimination of intracellular microorganisms [282–285].

A defect of IL-2 production from PBMCs was noted as one of the benchmarks of the immunodeficiency associated with HIV-1 infection [286]. HTLV-I infection was shown to induce the up-regulation of the IL-2R and consequent triggering of an autocrine/paracrine loop of T cell proliferation driven by the IL-2 signaling cascade [287]. It was then demonstrated that the Tax regulatory protein encoded by HTLV-I can functionally bypass the requirement for the receptor ligand, i.e., IL-2, by virtue of its capacity to directly phosphorylate the IL-2R [288].

In vitro, IL-2 leads to the propagation of HIV-1, an effect highly dependent upon the release of pro-inflammatory cytokines such as TNF-α, IL-1β, IFN-γ, and IL-6 [145,279,289,290]. However, IL-2 also strongly potentiates the ability of CD8$^+$ T cells of HIV$^+$ infected individuals to release potent soluble factors including some chemokines, thus suppressing HIV replication. This second functional component usually overcomes the previous one (in the presence of CD8$^+$ T cells, cell stimulation with IL-2 alone is frequently insufficient to induce HIV replication from *in vivo* infected cells) [146], unlike IL-7 [163]. Therefore, these findings represent a rationale for investigating the potential of IL-2 in immunological restoration of infected individuals [291]. IL-2 is currently in phase III clinical trials (ESPRIT, SIILCAT) to evaluate its potential therapeutic effects when administered with antiretroviral therapy to stably increase the levels of circulating CD4$^+$ T cells [233,292].

HUMAN RETROVIRUSES AND THE JAK/STAT PATHWAY

HTLV-I and HIV-1 infections have been correlated to the constitutive activation of the JAK/STAT pathway commonly utilized by several cytokines and interferons [293], both *in vivo* and *in vitro* [288,294,295]. Infection by HTLV-I *in vitro* of PBMCs or cord blood lymphocytes induced over time the transition from IL-2-dependent to IL-2-independent growth correlated to the constitutive activation of the JAK1 and JAK3 kinases and of the STAT3 and STAT5 transcription factors [288]. Furthermore, the study of uncultured leukemic cells of patients with adult T cell leukemia revealed that the majority of cells displayed constitutive activation of JAK3 and DNA-binding activity of STAT1, STAT3, and STAT5 [296]. On the other hand, the analysis of HTLV-II-transformed T cell lines did not demonstrate constitutive activation of either the JAK or STAT proteins in any cell line tested [294]. Not surprisingly, individuals mono-infected by HTLV-II do not show constitutive activation of their PBMC-associated STATs.

It has been observed that up to 80% of randomly selected individuals infected with HIV showed a constitutive activation of both STAT1 and STAT5 in their PBMCs [295]. In addition, the STAT5 isoform predominant in infected individuals was truncated at the C terminus, likely resulting in a transdominant negative molecule as observed in other cell systems [297]. Of interest, PBMCs freshly isolated from individuals dually infected with HIV-1 and HTLV-II did not show evidence of constitutive activation of STAT, suggesting that either HTLV-II proteins or HTLV-II-induced host factors may overcome the capacity of HIV to activate the JAK/STAT pathway (although these cells as well as cells infected with HTLV-II alone are "primed" for IFN-γ secretion and related STAT1 activation once cultivated *ex vivo*) [83].

CONCLUSIONS

Human retroviruses are potent biological weapons that induce different types and degrees of immunodeficiency, leading to either neoplastic transformation and neuro-logical disease (HTLV-I) or to CD4+ T lymphocyte depletion and immunodeficiency up to the lethal condition known as AIDS (HIV-1 and HIV-2). Of note, disregulation of the cytokine pattern of expression characterizes both HTLV and HIV infections, indicating the possibility of applying therapeutic strategies to restore the normal profile of cytokine expression. As an example, fusion proteins made in such a way to recognize and eliminate IL-2R positive cells, have been tested against different tumors as well as HIV-infected cells [298], whereas administration of IL-2 in HIV+ individuals is now showing potentially beneficial effects [299,300].

HIV-1 infection has been shown to be decreased by co-infection with HIV-2 or HTLV-II, while disease progression has been reported to be accelerated in HTLV-I co-infected individuals, at least by some studies. It is interesting to note that in all cases of co-infection by more than one retrovirus, a peculiar pattern of altered cytokine expression has been described *in vivo*, *ex-vivo*, and *in vitro*. This strongly suggests that human retroviruses are intimately related by their genetic sequences and expres-sion strategies and also in their interactions with cells of the human immune system and the cytokine network. HTLV-II and HIV-2 may actually decelerate the pace of HIV-1 disease by targeting of CD8+ T lymphocytes (at least in the case of HTLV-II), thus potentiating their capacity to synthesize a number of HIV-suppressive factors, such as CCR5-binding chemokines. These findings also suggest that HTLV-II and HIV-2 proteins may represent interesting tools for developing new strategies of intra-cellular immunization against HIV infection and spread.

In conclusion, although most of the scientific advancements have been accom-plished by studying HIV infection and its interaction with the human immune system, human retroviruses should be regarded as a family of related viruses whose genetic programs may unravel unexpected opportunities for preventing the develop-ment of AIDS and perhaps to combat neoplastic transformation.

ACKNOWLEDGMENTS

We wish to thank the many collaborators of the AIDS Pathogenesis Unit who have contributed over the years to studies of the relationships between human retroviruses and the cytokine network. In particular, we wish to acknowledge the contributions of Priscilla Biswas, Manuela Mengozzi, and Chiara Bovolenta who left our research unit to pursue their own research goals. In addition, we wish to thank Francesco Novelli (University of Turin) and Claudio Casoli (University of Parma) for their insights into IFN-γ and HTLV-II biology and co-infection, respectively. This work was supported by grants of the V° National Program of Research against AIDS of the Istituto Superiore di Sanità.

REFERENCES

1. Nunez, M. et al. Rate, causes, and clinical implications of presenting with low CD4⁺ cell counts in the era of highly active antiretroviral therapy. *AIDS Res Hum Retroviruses* 19, 363, 2003.

2. Willemot, P. and Klein, M.B. Prevention of HIV-associated opportunistic infections and diseases in the age of highly active antiretroviral therapy. *Expert Rev Anti Infect Ther* 2, 521, 2004.

3. Gessain, A. et al. Low degree of human T-cell leukemia/lymphoma virus type I genetic drift *in vivo* as a means of monitoring viral transmission and movement of ancient human populations. *J Virol* 66, 2288, 1992.

4. Franchini, G. Molecular mechanisms of human T-cell leukemia/lymphotropic virus type I infection. *Blood* 86, 3619, 1995.

5. Poiesz, B.J. et al. Detection and isolation of type C retrovirus particles from fresh and cultured lymphocytes of a patient with cutaneous T-cell lymphoma. *Proc Natl Acad Sci USA* 77, 7415, 1980.

6. Manns, A. et al. Human T-lymphotropic virus type I infection. *Lancet* 353, 1951, 1999.

7. Osame, M. et al. Blood transfusion and HTLV-I associated myelopathy. *Lancet* 2, 104, 1986.

8. Edlich, R.F. et al. Global epidemic of human T-cell lymphotrophic virus type-I (HTLV-I): an update. *J Long Term Eff Med Implants* 13, 127, 2003.

9. Mahieux, R. and Gessain, A. HTLV-1 and associated adult T-cell leukemia/lymphoma. *Rev Clin Exp Hematol* 7, 336, 2003.

10. Poiesz, B.J. et al. The human T-cell lymphoma/leukemia viruses. *Cancer Invest* 21, 253, 2003.

11. Yamamoto, N. et al. Transformation of human leukocytes by cocultivation with an adult T cell leukemia virus producer cell line. *Science* 217, 737, 1982.

12. Macchi, B. et al. Human Th1 and Th2 T-cell clones are equally susceptible to infection and immortalization by human T-lymphotropic virus type I. *J Gen Virol* 79 (Pt 10), 2469, 1998.

13. Nagai, M. et al. CD8(+) T cells are an *in vivo* reservoir for human T-cell lymphotropic virus type I. *Blood* 98, 1858, 2001.

14. Macatonia, S.E. et al. Dendritic cells from patients with tropical spastic paraparesis are infected with HTLV-1 and stimulate autologous lymphocyte proliferation. *AIDS Res Hum Retroviruses* 8, 1699, 1992.

15. Lehky, T.J. et al. Detection of human T-lymphotropic virus type I (HTLV-I) tax RNA in the central nervous system of HTLV-I-associated myelopathy/tropical spastic paraparesis patients by *in situ* hybridization. *Ann Neurol* 37, 167, 1995.

16. Dhawan, S. et al. Model for studying virus attachment. II. Binding of biotinylated human T cell leukemia virus type I to human blood mononuclear cells potential targets for human T cell leukemia virus type I infection. *J Immunol* 147, 102, 1991.

17. de Revel, T. et al. *In vitro* infection of human macrophages with human T-cell leukemia virus type I. *Blood* 81, 1598, 1993.

18. Lo, K.M. et al. Infection of human natural killer (NK) cells with replication-defective human T cell leukemia virus type I provirus. Increased proliferative capacity and prolonged survival of functionally competent NK cells. *J Immunol* 149, 4101, 1992.

19. Ho, D.D. et al. Infection of human endothelial cells by human T-lymphotropic virus type I. *Proc Natl Acad Sci USA* 81, 7588, 1984.

20. Gessain, A. et al. Human T-cell leukemia-lymphoma virus type I (HTLV-I) expression in fresh peripheral blood mononuclear cells from patients with tropical spastic paraparesis/HTLV-I-associated myelopathy. *J Virol* 65, 1628, 1991.

21. Sun, S.C. and Ballard, D.W. Persistent activation of NF-kappa-B by the Tax transforming protein of HTLV-1: hijacking cellular I-kappa-B kinases. *Oncogene* 18, 6948, 1999.

22. Mori, N. et al. Apoptosis induced by the histone deacetylase inhibitor FR901228 in human T-cell leukemia virus type 1-infected T-cell lines and primary adult T-cell leukemia cells. *J Virol* 78, 4582, 2004.

23. Hollsberg, P. Mechanisms of T-cell activation by human T-cell lymphotropic virus type I. *Microbiol Mol Biol Rev* 63, 308, 1999.

24. Hollsberg, P. et al. Characterization of HTLV-I *in vivo* infected T cell clones: IL-2-independent growth of nontransformed T cells. *J Immunol* 148, 3256, 1992.

25. Sherr, C.J. Cancer cell cycles. *Science* 274, 1672, 1996.

26. Nakamura, N. et al. Human T-cell leukemia virus type 1 Tax protein induces the expression of STAT1 and STAT5 genes in T-cells. *Oncogene*; 18, 2667, 1999.

27. Modiano, J.F. et al. Differential requirements for interleukin-2 distinguish the expression and activity of the cyclin-dependent kinases Cdk4 and Cdk2 in human T cells. *J Biol Chem* 269, 32972, 1994.

28. Nicot, C. et al. HTLV-1 p12(I) protein enhances STAT5 activation and decreases the interleukin-2 requirement for proliferation of primary human peripheral blood mononuclear cells. *Blood* 98, 823, 2001.

29. Jin, D.Y. et al. Human T cell leukemia virus type 1 oncoprotein Tax targets the human mitotic checkpoint protein MAD1. *Cell* 93, 81, 1998.

30. Copeland, K.F. et al. Inhibition of apoptosis in T cells expressing human T cell leukemia virus type I Tax. *AIDS Res Hum Retroviruses* 10, 1259, 1994.

31. Kishi, S. et al. Resistance to fas-mediated apoptosis of peripheral T cells in human T lymphocyte virus type I (HTLV-I) transgenic mice with autoimmune arthropathy. *J Exp Med* 186, 57, 1997.

32. Gatza, M.L. et al. Cellular transformation by the HTLV-I Tax protein, a jack-of-all-trades. *Oncogene* 22, 5141, 2003.

33. Kimata, J.T. et al. The mitogenic activity of human T-cell leukemia virus type I is T-cell associated and requires the CD2/LFA-3 activation pathway. *J Virol* 67, 3134, 1993.

34. Copeland, K.F. and Heeney, J.L. T helper cell activation and human retroviral pathogenesis. *Microbiol Rev* 60, 722, 1996.

35. Selvaraj, P. et al. The T lymphocyte glycoprotein CD2 binds the cell surface ligand LFA-3. *Nature* 326, 400, 1987.

36. Imai, T. et al. Enhanced expression of LFA-3 on human T-cell lines and leukemic cells carrying human T-cell-leukemia virus type 1. *Int J Cancer* 55, 811, 1993.

37. Owen, S.M. et al. Transcriptional activation of the intercellular adhesion molecule 1 (CD54) gene by human T lymphotropic virus types I and II Tax is mediated through a palindromic response element. *AIDS Res Hum Retroviruses* 13, 1429, 1997.

38. Matsuoka, M. Human T-cell leukemia virus type I and adult T-cell leukemia. *Oncogene* 22, 5131, 2003.

39. Jeang, K.T. et al. HTLV-I trans-activator protein, tax, is a trans-repressor of the human beta-polymerase gene. *Science* 247, 1082, 1990.

40. Suzuki, T. et al. Down-regulation of the INK4 family of cyclin-dependent kinase inhibitors by tax protein of HTLV-1 through two distinct mechanisms. *Virology* 259, 384, 1999.

41. Watanabe, H. et al. Exaggerated messenger RNA expression of inflammatory cytokines in human T-cell lymphotropic virus type I-associated myelopathy. *Arch Neurol* 52, 276, 1995.

42. Goon, P.K. et al. High circulating frequencies of tumor necrosis factor alpha- and interleukin-2-secreting human T-lymphotropic virus type 1 (HTLV-1)-specific CD4+ T cells in patients with HTLV-1-associated neurological disease. *J Virol* 77, 9716, 2003.

43. Kuroda, Y. and Matsui, M. Cerebrospinal fluid interferon-gamma is increased in HTLV-I-associated myelopathy. *J Neuroimmunol* 42, 223, 1993.

44. Nakamura, S. et al. Detection of tumor necrosis factor-alpha-positive cells in cerebrospinal fluid of patients with HTLV-I-associated myelopathy. *J Neuroimmunol* 42, 127, 1993.

45. Umehara, F. et al. Cytokine expression in the spinal cord lesions in HTLV-I-associated myelopathy. *J Neuropathol Exp Neurol* 53, 72, 1994.

46. Etoh, K. et al. Rapid quantification of HTLV-I provirus load: detection of monoclonal proliferation of HTLV-I-infected cells among blood donors. *Int J Cancer* 81, 859, 1999.

47. Yasuda, N. et al. Soluble interleukin 2 receptors in sera of Japanese patients with adult T cell leukemia mark activity of disease. *Blood* 71, 1021, 1988.

48. Tsukasaki, K. et al. Tumor necrosis factor alpha polymorphism associated with increased susceptibility to development of adult T-cell leukemia/lymphoma in human T-lymphotropic virus type 1 carriers. *Cancer Res* 61, 3770, 2001.

49. Yamagata, T. et al. Triple synergism of human T-lymphotropic virus type 1-encoded tax, GATA-binding protein, and AP-1 is required for constitutive expression of the interleukin-5 gene in adult T-cell leukemia cells. *Mol Cell Biol* 17, 4272, 1997.

50. Daliani, D. et al. Tumor necrosis factor-alpha and interferon-gamma, but not HTLV-I tax, are likely factors in the epidermotropism of cutaneous T-cell lymphoma via induction of interferon-inducible protein-10. *Leuk Lymphoma* 29, 315, 1998.

51. Sagawa, K. et al. Immunopathological mechanisms of human T cell lymphotropic virus type 1 (HTLV-I) uveitis: detection of HTLV-I-infected T cells in the eye and their constitutive cytokine production. *J Clin Invest* 95, 852, 1995.

52. Yin, W. et al. Synovial hyperplasia in HTLV-I associated arthropathy is induced by tumor necrosis factor-alpha produced by HTLV-I infected CD68+ cells. *J Rheumatol* 27, 874, 2000.

53. Santos, S.B. et al. Exacerbated inflammatory cellular immune response characteristics of HAM/TSP is observed in a large proportion of HTLV-I asymptomatic carriers. *BMC Infect Dis* 4, 7, 2004.

54. Mendez, E. et al. Astrocyte-specific expression of human T-cell lymphotropic virus type 1 (HTLV-1) Tax: induction of tumor necrosis factor alpha and susceptibility to lysis by CD8+ HTLV-1-specific cytotoxic T cells. *J Virol* 71, 9143, 1997.

55. Cowan, E.P. et al. Induction of tumor necrosis factor alpha in human neuronal cells by extracellular human T-cell lymphotropic virus type 1 Tax. *J Virol* 71, 6982, 1997.

56. Fox, R.J. et al. Tumor necrosis factor alpha expression in the spinal cord of human T-cell lymphotrophic virus type I associated myelopathy/tropical spastic paraparesis patients. *J Neurovirol* 2, 323, 1996.

57. Szymocha, R. et al. Human T-cell lymphotropic virus type 1-infected T lymphocytes impair catabolism and uptake of glutamate by astrocytes via Tax-1 and tumor necrosis factor alpha. *J Virol* 74, 6433, 2000.

58. Matsuda, M. et al. Increased levels of soluble tumor necrosis factor receptor in patients with multiple sclerosis and HTLV-1-associated myelopathy. *J Neuroimmunol* 52, 33, 1994.

59. Zucker-Franklin, D. et al. Prevalence of HTLV-I Tax in a subset of patients with rheumatoid arthritis. *Clin Exp Rheumatol* 20, 161, 2002.

60. Sebastian, D. et al. Lack of association of Human T-cell lymphotrophic virus type 1(HTLV-1) infection and rheumatoid arthritis in an endemic area. *Clin Rheumatol* 22, 30, 2003.

61. Hishizawa, M. et al. Depletion and impaired interferon-alpha-producing capacity of blood plasmacytoid dendritic cells in human T-cell leukaemia virus type I-infected individuals. *Br J Haematol* 125, 568, 2004.

62. Feng, X. et al. Alpha interferon inhibits human T-cell leukemia virus type 1 assembly by preventing Gag interaction with rafts. *J Virol* 77, 13389, 2003.

63. Oka, T. et al. Inhibitory effects of human interferons on the immortalization of human, but not rabbit, T lymphocytes by human T-lymphotropic virus type-I (HTLV-I). *Int J Cancer* 51, 915, 1992.

64. Nakagawa, M. et al. Therapeutic trials in 200 patients with HTLV-I-associated myelopathy/ tropical spastic paraparesis. *J Neurovirol* 2, 345, 1996.

65. Yamasaki, K. et al. Long-term, high dose interferon-alpha treatment in HTLV-I-associated myelopathy/tropical spastic paraparesis: a combined clinical, virological and immunological study. *J Neurol Sci* 147, 135, 1997.

66. Saito, M. et al. Decreased human T lymphotropic virus type I (HTLV-I) provirus load and alteration in T cell phenotype after interferon-alpha therapy for HTLV-I-associated myelopathy/tropical spastic paraparesis. *J Infect Dis* 189, 29, 2004.

67. Bazarbachi, A. and Hermine, O. Treatment of adult T-cell leukaemia/lymphoma: current strategy and future perspectives. *Virus Res* 78, 79, 2001.

68. Sagawa, K. et al. *In vitro* effects of immunosuppressive agents on cytokine production by HTLV-I-infected T cell clones derived from the ocular fluid of patients with HTLV-I uveitis. *Microbiol Immunol* 40, 373, 1996.

69. Di Venuti, G. et al. Denileukin diftitox and hyper-CVAD in the treatment of human T-cell lymphotropic virus 1-associated acute T-cell leukemia/lymphoma. *Clin Lymphoma* 4, 176, 2003.

70. Foss, F.M. and Waldmann, T.A. Interleukin-2 receptor-directed therapies for cutaneous lymphomas. *Hematol Oncol Clin North Am* 17, 1449, 2003.

71. Yamamura, T. et al. Immunosuppressive and anticancer effect of a mammalian ribonuclease that targets high-affinity interleukin-2-receptors. *Eur J Surg* 168, 49, 2002.

72. Azimi, N. et al. Involvement of IL-15 in the pathogenesis of human T lymphotropic virus type I-associated myelopathy/tropical spastic paraparesis: implications for therapy with a monoclonal antibody directed to the IL-2/15R beta receptor. *J Immunol* 163, 4064, 1999.

73. Harakeh, S. et al. Inhibition of proliferation and induction of apoptosis by 2-benzoyl-3-phenyl-6,7-dichloroquinoxaline 1,4-dioxide in adult T-cell leukemia cells. *Chem Biol Interact* 148, 101, 2004.

74. Mitra-Kaushik, S. et al. Effects of the proteasome inhibitor PS-341 on tumor growth in HTLV-1 Tax transgenic mice and Tax tumor transplants. *Blood* 104, 802, 2004.

75. Nasr, R. et al. Arsenic/interferon specifically reverses two distinct gene networks critical for the survival of HTLV-1-infected leukemic cells. *Blood* 101, 4576, 2003.

76. Zhang, J. et al. Capsaicin inhibits growth of adult T-cell leukemia cells. *Leuk Res* 27, 275, 2003.

77. Dewan, M.Z. et al. Rapid tumor formation of human T-cell leukemia virus type 1-infected cell lines in novel NOD-SCID/gammac(null) mice: suppression by an inhibitor against NF-kappa-B. *J Virol* 77, 5286, 2003.

78. Machuca, A. et al. The effect of antiretroviral therapy on HTLV infection. *Virus Res* 78, 93, 2001.

79. Zhang, J. et al. Efficacy of 3′-azido 3′deoxythymidine (AZT) in preventing HTLV-1 transmission to human cord blood mononuclear cells. *Virus Res* 78, 67, 2001.

80. Garcia-Lerma, J.G. et al. Susceptibility of human T cell leukemia virus type 1 to reverse-transcriptase inhibitors: evidence for resistance to lamivudine. *J Infect Dis* 184, 507, 2001.

81. Vandamme, A.M. et al. Evolutionary strategies of human T-cell lymphotropic virus type II. *Gene* 261, 171, 2000.

82. Araujo, A. and Hall, W.W. Human T-lymphotropic virus type II and neurological disease. *Ann Neurol* 56, 10, 2004.

83. Bovolenta, C. et al. Retroviral interference on STAT activation in individuals coinfected with human T cell leukemia virus type 2 and HIV-1. *J Immunol* 169, 4443, 2002.

84. Bovolenta, C. et al. Human T-cell leukemia virus type 2 induces survival and proliferation of CD34(+) TF-1 cells through activation of STAT1 and STAT5 by secretion of interferon-gamma and granulocyte macrophage-colony-stimulating factor. *Blood* 99, 224, 2002.

85. Re, M.C. et al. Human T cell leukemia virus type II increases telomerase activity in uninfected CD34+ hematopoietic progenitor cells. *J Hematother Stem Cell Res* 9, 481, 2000.

86. Lal, R.B. and Rudolph, D.L. Constitutive production of interleukin-6 and tumor necrosis factor-alpha from spontaneously proliferating T cells in patients with human T-cell lymphotropic virus type-I/II. *Blood* 78, 571, 1991.

87. Dezzutti, C.S. et al. Down-regulation of interleukin-10 expression and production is associated with spontaneous proliferation by lymphocytes from human T lymphotropic virus type II-infected persons. *J Infect Dis* 177, 1489, 1998.

88. Mori, N. and Prager, D. Transactivation of the interleukin-1 alpha promoter by human T-cell leukemia virus. *Leuk Lymphoma* 26, 421, 1997.

89. Greene, W.C. et al. Trans-activator gene of HTLV-II induces IL-2 receptor and IL-2 cellular gene expression. *Science* 232, 877, 1986.

90. Lal, R.B. et al. Infection with human T-lymphotropic viruses leads to constitutive expression of leukemia inhibitory factor and interleukin-6. *Blood* 81, 1827, 1993.

91. Nimer, S.D. et al. Activation of the GM-CSF promoter by HTLV-I and -II tax proteins. *Oncogene* 4, 671, 1989.

92. Nakajima, T. et al. Constitutive expression and production of tumor necrosis factor-beta in T-cell lines infected with HTLV-I and HTLV-II. *Biochem Biophys Res Commun* 191, 371, 1993.

93. Gallo, R.C. et al. Isolation of human T-cell leukemia virus in acquired immune deficiency syndrome (AIDS). *Science* 220, 865, 1983.

94. Tindall, B. and Cooper, D.A. Primary HIV infection: host responses and intervention strategies. *AIDS* 5, 1, 1991.

95. Gaines, H. et al. Immunological changes in primary HIV-1 infection. *AIDS* 4, 995, 1990.

96. Piatak, M., Jr. et al. High levels of HIV-1 in plasma during all stages of infection determined by competitive PCR. *Science* 259, 1749, 1993.

97. Phillips, A.N. Reduction of HIV concentration during acute infection: independence from a specific immune response. *Science* 271, 497, 1996.

98. Lemp, G.F. et al. Survival trends for patients with AIDS. *JAMA* 263, 402, 1990.

99. Pantaleo, G. et al. New concepts in the immunopathogenesis of human immunodeficiency virus infection. *New Engl J Med* 328, 327, 1993.

100. Simmonds, P. et al. Discontinuous sequence change of human immunodeficiency virus (HIV) type 1 env sequences in plasma viral and lymphocyte-associated proviral populations *in vivo*: implications for models of HIV pathogenesis. *J Virol* 65, 6266, 1991.

101. Vlahov, D. et al. Prognostic indicators for AIDS and infectious disease death in HIV-infected injection drug users: plasma viral load and CD4+ cell count. *JAMA* 279, 35, 1998.

102. Richman, D.D. et al. Rapid evolution of the neutralizing antibody response to HIV type 1 infection. *Proc Natl Acad Sci USA* 100, 4144, 2003.

103. Jones, J.L. et al. Surveillance for AIDS-defining opportunistic illnesses, 1992-1997. *MMWR CDC Surveill Summ* 48, 1, 1999.

104. Wain-Hobson, S. et al. Nucleotide sequence of the AIDS virus LAV. *Cell* 40, 9, 1985.

105. Klatzmann, D.R. et al. The CD4 molecule and HIV infection. *Immunodefic Rev* 2, 43, 1990.

106. Alkhatib, G. et al. CC CKR5: a RANTES, MIP-1alpha, MIP-1beta receptor as a fusion cofactor for macrophage-tropic HIV-1. *Science* 272, 1955, 1996.

107. Feng, Y. et al. HIV-1 entry cofactor: functional cDNA cloning of a seven-transmembrane, G protein-coupled receptor. *Science* 272, 872, 1996.

108. Choe, H. et al. The beta-chemokine receptors CCR3 and CCR5 facilitate infection by primary HIV-1 isolates. *Cell* 85, 1135, 1996.

109. Dragic, T. et al. HIV-1 entry into CD4+ cells is mediated by the chemokine receptor CC-CKR-5. *Nature* 381, 667, 1996.

110. Rey, M.A. et al. Characterization of the RNA dependent DNA polymerase of a new human T-lymphotropic retrovirus (lymphadenopathy associated virus). *Biochem Biophys Res Commun* 121, 126, 1984.

111. Butera, S.T. et al. Regulation of HIV-1 expression by cytokine networks in a CD4+ model of chronic infection. *J Immunol* 150, 625, 1993.

112. Pereira, L.A. et al. A compilation of cellular transcription factor interactions with the HIV-1 LTR promoter. *Nucleic Acids Res* 28, 663, 2000.

113. Ono, A. and Freed, E.O. Plasma membrane rafts play a critical role in HIV-1 assembly and release. *Proc Natl Acad Sci USA* 98, 13925, 2001.

114. von Schwedler, U.K. et al. The protein network of HIV budding. *Cell* 114, 701, 2003.

115. Gould, S.J. et al. The Trojan exosome hypothesis. *Proc Natl Acad Sci USA* 100, 10592, 2003.

116. Denzer, K. et al. Exosome: from internal vesicle of the multivesicular body to intercellular signaling device. *J Cell Sci* 113, Pt 19, 3365, 2000.

117. Xiao, H. et al. Selective CXCR4 antagonism by Tat: implications for *in vivo* expansion of coreceptor use by HIV-1. *Proc Natl Acad Sci USA* 97, 11466, 2000.

118. Ghezzi, S. et al. Inhibition of CXCR4-dependent HIV-1 infection by extracellular HIV-1 Tat. *Biochem Biophys Res Commun* 270, 992, 2000.

119. Marchio, S. et al. Cell surface-associated Tat modulates HIV-1 infection and spreading through a specific interaction with gp120 viral envelope protein. *Blood* 105, 2802, 2005.

120. Ramanathan, M.P. et al. Carboxyl terminus of hVIP/mov34 is critical for HIV-1-Vpr interaction and glucocorticoid-mediated signaling. *J Biol Chem* 277, 47854, 2002.

121. Alfano, M. and Poli, G. Role of cytokines and chemokines in the regulation of innate immunity and HIV infection. *Mol Immunol* 42, 161, 2005.

122. Liu, Q.H. et al. HIV-1 gp120 and chemokines activate ion channels in primary macrophages through CCR5 and CXCR4 stimulation. *Proc Natl Acad Sci USA* 97, 4832, 2000.

123. Lin, C.L. et al. Macrophage-tropic HIV induces and exploits dendritic cell chemotaxis. *J Exp Med* 192, 587, 2000.

124. Patella, V. et al. HIV-1 gp120 induces IL-4 and IL-13 release from human Fc epsilon RI+ cells through interaction with the VH3 region of IgE. *J Immunol* 164, 589, 2000.

125. de Paulis, A. et al. HIV-1 envelope gp41 peptides promote migration of human Fc epsilon RI+ cells and inhibit IL-13 synthesis through interaction with formyl peptide receptors. *J Immunol* 169, 4559, 2002.

126. Hu, R. et al. HIV-1 gp160 induces transforming growth factor-beta production in human PBMC. *Clin Immunol Immunopathol* 80, 283, 1996.

127. Singhal, P.C. et al. HIV-1 gp160 protein-macrophage interactions modulate mesangial cell proliferation and matrix synthesis. *Am J Pathol* 147, 1780, 1995.

128. Vitale, M. et al. HIV-1 matrix protein p17 enhances the proliferative activity of natural killer cells and increases their ability to secrete proinflammatory cytokines. *Br J Haematol* 120, 337, 2003.

129. Messmer, D. et al. Endogenously expressed nef uncouples cytokine and chemokine production from membrane phenotypic maturation in dendritic cells. *J Immunol* 169, 4172, 2002.

130. Quaranta, M.G. et al. HIV-1 Nef induces dendritic cell differentiation: a possible mechanism of uninfected CD4(+) T cell activation. *Exp Cell Res* 275, 243, 2002.

131. Quaranta, M.G. et al. HIV-1 Nef triggers Vav-mediated signaling pathway leading to functional and morphological differentiation of dendritic cells. *FASEB J* 17, 2025, 2003.

132. Maccormac, L.P. et al. The functional consequences of delivery of HIV-1 Nef to dendritic cells using an adenoviral vector. *Vaccine* 22, 528, 2004.

133. Garba, M.L. et al. HIV antigens can induce TGF-beta(1)-producing immunoregulatory CD8+ T cells. *J Immunol* 168, 2247, 2002.

134. Gibellini, D. et al. Recombinant human immunodeficiency virus type-1 (HIV-1) Tat protein sequentially up-regulates IL-6 and TGF-beta 1 mRNA expression and protein synthesis in peripheral blood monocytes. *Br J Haematol* 88, 261, 1994.

135. Lotz, M. et al. HIV-1 transactivator protein Tat induces proliferation and TGF beta expression in human articular chondrocytes. *J Cell Biol* 124, 365, 1994.

136. Sawaya, B.E. et al. Regulation of TNFalpha and TGFbeta-1 gene transcription by HIV-1 Tat in CNS cells. *J Neuroimmunol* 87, 33, 1998.

137. Mengozzi, M. et al. Human immunodeficiency virus replication induces monocyte chemotactic protein-1 in human macrophages and U937 promonocytic cells. *Blood* 93, 1851, 1999.

138. Kutsch, O. et al. Induction of the chemokines interleukin-8 and IP-10 by human immunodeficiency virus type 1 tat in astrocytes. *J Virol* 74, 9214, 2000.

139. Park, I.W. et al. HIV-1 Tat promotes monocyte chemoattractant protein-1 secretion followed by transmigration of monocytes. *Blood* 97, 352, 2001.

140. Lapenta, C. et al. Type I interferon is a powerful inhibitor of *in vivo* HIV-1 infection and preserves human CD4(+) T cells from virus-induced depletion in SCID mice transplanted with human cells. *Virology* 263, 78, 1999.

141. Sanhadji, K. et al. Experimental gene therapy: the transfer of Tat-inducible interferon genes protects human cells against HIV-1 challenge *in vitro* and *in vivo* in severe combined immunodeficient mice. *AIDS* 11, 977, 1997.

142. Pitha, P.M. Multiple effects of interferon on the replication of human immunodeficiency virus type 1. *Antiviral Res* 24, 205, 1994.

143. Gendelman, H.E. et al. Regulation of HIV1 replication by interferon alpha: from laboratory bench to bedside. *Res Immunol* 145, 679, 1994.

144. Bovolenta, C. et al. A selective defect of IFN-gamma- but not of IFN-alpha-induced JAK/STAT pathway in a subset of U937 clones prevents the antiretroviral effect of IFN-gamma against HIV-1. *J Immunol* 162, 323, 1999.

145. Biswas, P. et al. Interferon gamma induces the expression of human immunodeficiency virus in persistently infected promonocytic cells (U1) and redirects the production of virions to intracytoplasmic vacuoles in phorbol myristate acetate-differentiated U1 cells. *J Exp Med* 176, 739, 1992.

146. Kinter, A.L. et al. HIV replication in IL-2-stimulated peripheral blood mononuclear cells is driven in an autocrine/paracrine manner by endogenous cytokines. *J Immunol* 154, 2448, 1995.

147. Ludewig, B. et al. Transmission of HIV-1 from productively infected mature Langerhans cells to primary CD4+ T lymphocytes results in altered T cell responses with enhanced production of IFN-gamma and IL-10. *Virology* 215, 51, 1996.

148. Poli, G. et al. Interleukin 1 induces expression of the human immunodeficiency virus alone and in synergy with interleukin 6 in chronically infected U1 cells: inhibition of inductive effects by the interleukin 1 receptor antagonist. *Proc Natl Acad Sci USA* 91, 108, 1994.

149. Hays, E.F. et al. *In vitro* studies of HIV-1 expression in thymocytes from infants and children. *AIDS* 6, 265, 1992.

150. Pedroza-Martins, L. et al. Differential tropism and replication kinetics of human immunodeficiency virus type 1 isolates in thymocytes: co-receptor expression allows viral entry, but productive infection of distinct subsets is determined at the post-entry level. *J Virol* 72, 9441, 1998.

151. Kinter, A.L. et al. Interleukin 2 induces CD8+ T cell-mediated suppression of human immunodeficiency virus replication in CD4+ T cells and this effect overrides its ability to stimulate virus expression. *Proc Natl Acad Sci USA* 92, 10985, 1995.

152. Wang, J. et al. Inhibition of CCR5 expression by IL-12 through induction of beta-chemokines in human T lymphocytes. *J Immunol* 163, 5763, 1999.

153. Smithgall, M.D. et al. IL-7 up-regulates HIV-1 replication in naturally infected peripheral blood mononuclear cells. *J Immunol* 156, 2324, 1996.

154. Scripture-Adams, D.D. et al. Interleukin-7 induces expression of latent human immunodeficiency virus type 1 with minimal effects on T-cell phenotype. *J Virol* 76, 13077, 2002.

155. Chene, L. et al. Thymocyte-thymic epithelial cell interaction leads to high-level replication of human immunodeficiency virus exclusively in mature CD4(+) CD8(-) CD3(+) thymocytes: a critical role for tumor necrosis factor and interleukin-7. *J Virol* 73, 7533, 1999.

156. Ducrey-Rundquist, O. et al. Modalities of interleukin-7-induced human immunodeficiency virus permissiveness in quiescent T lymphocytes. *J Virol* 76, 9103, 2002.

157. Schmitt, N. et al. Positive regulation of CXCR4 expression and signaling by interleukin-7 in CD4+ mature thymocytes correlates with their capacity to favor human immunodeficiency X4 virus replication. *J Virol* 77, 5784, 2003.

158. Llano, A. et al. Interleukin-7 in plasma correlates with CD4 T-cell depletion and may be associated with emergence of syncytium-inducing variants in human immunodeficiency virus type 1-positive individuals. *J Virol* 75, 10319, 2001.

159. Shalekoff, S. and Tiemessen, C.T. Circulating levels of stromal cell-derived factor 1alpha and interleukin 7 in HIV type 1 infection and pulmonary tuberculosis are reciprocally related to CXCR4 expression on peripheral blood leukocytes. *AIDS Res Hum Retroviruses* 19, 461, 2003.

160. Kim, J.H. et al. Expansion of restricted cellular immune responses to HIV-1 envelope by vaccination: IL-7 and IL-12 differentially augment cellular proliferative responses to HIV-1. *Clin Exp Immunol* 108, 243, 1997.

161. Marchetti, G. et al. Low-dose prolonged intermittent interleukin-2 adjuvant therapy: results of a randomized trial among human immunodeficiency virus-positive patients with advanced immune impairment. *J Infect Dis* 186, 606, 2002.

162. MacPherson, P.A. et al. Interleukin-7 receptor expression on CD8(+) T cells is reduced in HIV infection and partially restored with effective antiretroviral therapy. *J Acquir Immune Defic Syndr* 28, 454, 2001.

163. Wang, F.X. et al. IL-7 is a potent and proviral strain-specific inducer of latent HIV-1 cellular reservoirs of infected individuals on virally suppressive HAART. *J Clin Invest* 115, 128, 2005.

164. Al-Harthi, L. et al. Induction of HIV-1 replication by type 1-like cytokines, interleukin (IL)-12 and IL-15: effect on viral transcriptional activation, cellular proliferation, and endogenous cytokine production. *J Clin Immunol* 18, 124, 1998.

165. Patki, A.H. et al. Activation of antigen-induced lymphocyte proliferation by interleukin-15 without the mitogenic effect of interleukin-2 that may induce human immunodeficiency virus-1 expression. *J Clin Invest* 98, 616, 1996.

166. Chehimi, J. et al. IL-15 enhances immune functions during HIV infection. *J Immunol* 158, 5978, 1997.

167. Weissman, D. et al. Interleukin-2 up-regulates expression of the human immunodeficiency virus fusion coreceptor CCR5 by CD4+ lymphocytes *in vivo*. *J Infect Dis* 181, 933, 2000.

168. Zou, W. et al. Acute upregulation of CCR-5 expression by CD4+ T lymphocytes in HIV-infected patients treated with interleukin-2. *AIDS* 13, 455, 1999.

169. Yang, Y.F. et al. IL-12 as well as IL-2 upregulates CCR5 expression on T cell receptor-triggered human CD4+ and CD8+ T cells. *J Clin Immunol* 21, 116, 2001.

170. Fehniger, T.A. et al. Natural killer cells from HIV-1+ patients produce C-C chemokines and inhibit HIV-1 infection. *J Immunol* 161, 6433, 1998.

171. Oliva, A. et al. Natural killer cells from human immunodeficiency virus (HIV)-infected individuals are an important source of CC-chemokines and suppress HIV-1 entry and replication *in vitro*. *J Clin Invest* 102, 223, 1998.

172. Valentin, A. et al. Dual effect of interleukin 4 on HIV-1 expression: implications for viral phenotypic switch and disease progression. *Proc Natl Acad Sci USA* 95, 8886, 1998.

173. Wang, J. et al. Cytokine regulation of human immunodeficiency virus type 1 entry and replication in human monocytes/macrophages through modulation of CCR5 expression. *J Virol* 72, 7642, 1998.

174. Galli, G. et al. Enhanced HIV expression during Th2-oriented responses explained by the opposite regulatory effect of IL-4 and IFN-gamma of fusin/CXCR4. *Eur J Immunol* 28, 3280, 1998.

175. Schuitemaker, H. et al. Proliferation-dependent HIV-1 infection of monocytes occurs during differentiation into macrophages. *J Clin Invest* 89, 1154, 1992.

176. Kedzierska, K. et al. The influence of cytokines, chemokines and their receptors on HIV-1 replication in monocytes and macrophages. *Rev Med Virol* 13, 39, 2003.

177. Montaner, L.J. et al. IL-13 acts on macrophages to block the completion of reverse transcription, inhibit virus production, and reduce virus infectivity. *J Leukoc Biol* 62, 126, 1997.

178. Montaner, L.J. et al. Interleukin 13 inhibits human immunodeficiency virus type 1 production in primary blood-derived human macrophages *in vitro*. *J Exp Med* 178, 743, 1993.

179. Bailer, R.T. et al. IL-13 and TNF-alpha inhibit dual-tropic HIV-1 in primary macrophages by reduction of surface expression of CD4, chemokine receptors CCR5, CXCR4 and post-entry viral gene expression. *Eur J Immunol* 30, 1340, 2000.

180. Kollmann, T.R. et al. Inhibition of acute *in vivo* human immunodeficiency virus infection by human interleukin 10 treatment of SCID mice implanted with human fetal thymus and liver. *Proc Natl Acad Sci USA* 93, 3126, 1996.

181. Schols, D. and De Clercq, E. Human immunodeficiency virus type 1 gp120 induces anergy in human peripheral blood lymphocytes by inducing interleukin-10 production. *J Virol* 70, 4953, 1996.

182. Weissman, D. et al. Interleukin 10 blocks HIV replication in macrophages by inhibiting the autocrine loop of tumor necrosis factor alpha and interleukin 6 induction of virus. *AIDS Res Hum Retroviruses* 10, 1199, 1994.

183. Rabbi, M.F. et al. Interleukin-10 enhances tumor necrosis factor-alpha activation of HIV-1 transcription in latently infected T cells. *J Acquir Immune Defic Syndr Hum Retrovirol* 19, 321, 1998.

184. Sozzani, S. et al. Interleukin 10 increases CCR5 expression and HIV infection in human monocytes. *J Exp Med* 187, 439, 1998.

185. Li, J.M. et al. Transforming growth factor beta stimulates the human immunodeficiency virus 1 enhancer and requires NF-kappa-B activity. *Mol Cell Biol* 18, 110, 1998.

186. Lazdins, J.K. et al. TGF-beta: upregulator of HIV replication in macrophages. *Res Virol* 142, 239, 1991.

187. Lazdins, J.K. et al. *In vitro* effect of transforming growth factor-beta on progression of HIV-1 infection in primary mononuclear phagocytes. *J Immunol* 147, 1201, 1991.

188. McKiel, V. et al. Inhibition of human immunodeficiency virus type 1 multiplication by transforming growth factor beta 1 and AZT in HIV-1-infected myeloid cells. *J Interferon Cytokine Res* 15, 849, 1995.

189. Poli, G. et al. Retinoic acid mimics transforming growth factor beta in the regulation of human immunodeficiency virus expression in monocytic cells. *Proc Natl Acad Sci USA* 89, 2689, 1992.

190. Poli, G. et al. Transforming growth factor beta suppresses human immunodeficiency virus expression and replication in infected cells of the monocyte/macrophage lineage. *J Exp Med* 173, 589, 1991.

191. Wang, J. et al. Synergistic induction of apoptosis in primary CD4(+) T cells by macrophage-tropic HIV-1 and TGF-beta-1. *J Immunol* 167, 3360, 2001.

192. Cocchi, F. et al. Identification of RANTES, MIP-1 alpha, and MIP-1 beta as the major HIV-suppressive factors produced by CD8+ T cells. *Science* 270, 1811, 1995.

193. Gong, W. et al. Monocyte chemotactic protein-2 activates CCR5 and blocks CD4/CCR5-mediated HIV-1 entry/replication. *J Biol Chem* 273, 4289, 1998.

194. Berger, E.A. et al. Chemokine receptors as HIV-1 coreceptors: roles in viral entry, tropism, and disease. *Annu Rev Immunol* 17, 657, 1999.

195. Gonzalez, E. et al. The influence of CCL3L1 gene-containing segmental duplications on HIV-1/AIDS susceptibility. *Science* 307, 1422, 2005.

196. Schmidtmayerova, H. et al. Chemokines and HIV replication. *Nature* 382, 767, 1996.

197. Wang, H. et al. Role of beta-chemokines in HIV-1 infection of dendritic cells maturing from CD34+ stem cells. *J Acquir Immune Defic Syndr* 21, 179, 1999.

198. Dolei, A. et al. Increased replication of T-cell-tropic HIV strains and CXC-chemokine receptor-4 induction in T cells treated with macrophage inflammatory protein (MIP)-1alpha, MIP-1beta and RANTES beta-chemokines. *AIDS* 12, 183, 1998.

199. Lane, B.R. et al. Interleukin-8 stimulates human immunodeficiency virus type 1 replication and is a potential new target for antiretroviral therapy. *J Virol* 75, 8195, 2001.

200. Lane, B.R. et al. Human immunodeficiency virus type 1 (HIV-1)-induced GRO-alpha production stimulates HIV-1 replication in macrophages and T lymphocytes. *J Virol* 75, 5812, 2001.

201. Kinter, A.L. et al. HIV replication in CD4+ T cells of HIV-infected individuals is regulated by a balance between the viral suppressive effects of endogenous beta-chemokines and the viral inductive effects of other endogenous cytokines. *Proc Natl Acad Sci USA* 93, 14076, 1996.

202. Vicenzi, E. et al. Divergent regulation of HIV-1 replication in PBMC of infected individuals by CC chemokines: suppression by RANTES, MIP-1alpha, and MCP-3, and enhancement by MCP-1. *J Leukoc Biol* 68, 405, 2000.

203. Cinque, P. et al. Elevated cerebrospinal fluid levels of monocyte chemotactic protein-1 correlate with HIV-1 encephalitis and local viral replication. *AIDS* 12, 1327, 1998.

204. Kelder, W. et al. Beta-chemokines MCP-1 and RANTES are selectively increased in cerebrospinal fluid of patients with human immunodeficiency virus-associated dementia. *Ann Neurol* 44, 831, 1998.

205. Conant, K. et al. Induction of monocyte chemoattractant protein-1 in HIV-1 Tat-stimulated astrocytes and elevation in AIDS dementia. *Proc Natl Acad Sci USA* 95, 3117, 1998.

206. Gonzalez, E. et al. HIV-1 infection and AIDS dementia are influenced by a mutant MCP-1 allele linked to increased monocyte infiltration of tissues and MCP-1 levels. *Proc Natl Acad Sci USA* 99, 13795, 2002.

207. Cota, M. et al. Selective inhibition of HIV replication in primary macrophages but not T lymphocytes by macrophage-derived chemokine. *Proc Natl Acad Sci USA* 97, 9162, 2000.

208. Mackewicz, C.E. et al. Alpha-defensins can have anti-HIV activity but are not CD8 cell anti-HIV factors. *AIDS* 17, F23, 2003.

209. Quinones-Mateu, M.E. et al. Human epithelial beta-defensins 2 and 3 inhibit HIV-1 replication. *AIDS* 17, F39, 2003.

210. Munk, C. et al. The theta-defensin, retrocyclin, inhibits HIV-1 entry. *AIDS Res Hum Retroviruses* 19, 875, 2003.

211. Siegal, F.P. et al. Interferon-alpha generation and immune reconstitution during anti-retroviral therapy for human immunodeficiency virus infection. *AIDS* 15, 1603, 2001.

212. Servet, C. et al. Dendritic cells in innate immune responses against HIV. *Curr Mol Med* 2, 739, 2002.

213. Chehimi, J. et al. Persistent decreases in blood plasmacytoid dendritic cell number and function despite effective highly active antiretroviral therapy and increased blood myeloid dendritic cells in HIV-infected individuals. *J Immunol* 168, 4796, 2002.

214. Krivine, A. et al. Measuring HIV-1 RNA and interferon-alpha in the cerebrospinal fluid of AIDS patients: insights into the pathogenesis of AIDS dementia complex. *J Neurovirol* 5, 500, 1999.

215. Lane, H.C. et al. Anti-retroviral effects of interferon-alpha in AIDS-associated Kaposi's sarcoma. *Lancet* 2, 1218, 1988.

216. Haas, D.W. et al. A randomized trial of interferon alpha therapy for HIV type 1 infection. *AIDS Res Hum Retroviruses* 16, 183, 2000.

217. Huang, S.S. et al. Survival prolongation in HIV-associated progressive multifocal leukoencephalopathy treated with alpha-interferon: an observational study. *J Neurovirol* 4, 324, 1998.

218. Portales, P. et al. Interferon-alpha restores HIV-induced alteration of natural killer cell perforin expression *in vivo*. *AIDS* 17, 495, 2003.

219. Santini, S.M. et al. Type I interferon as a powerful adjuvant for monocyte-derived dendritic cell development and activity *in vitro* and in Hu-PBL-SCID mice. *J Exp Med* 191, 1777, 2000.

220. Kim, J.J. et al. Modulation of antigen-specific cellular immune responses to DNA vaccination in rhesus macaques through the use of IL-2, IFN-gamma, or IL-4 gene adjuvants. *Vaccine* 19, 2496, 2001.

221. Giavedoni, L. et al. Expression of gamma interferon by simian immunodeficiency virus increases attenuation and reduces postchallenge virus load in vaccinated rhesus macaques. *J Virol* 71, 866, 1997.

222. Uittenbogaart, C.H. et al. Effects of cytokines on HIV-1 production by thymocytes. *Thymus* 23, 155, 1994.

223. Watanabe, N. et al. Administration of recombinant human interleukin 12 to chronically SIVmac-infected rhesus monkeys. *AIDS Res Hum Retroviruses* 14, 393, 1998.

224. Villinger, F. et al. *In vitro* and *in vivo* responses to interleukin 12 are maintained until the late SIV infection stage but lost during AIDS. *AIDS Res Hum Retroviruses* 16, 751, 2000.

225. Boyer, J.D. et al. Therapeutic immunization of HIV-infected chimpanzees using HIV-1 plasmid antigens and interleukin-12 expressing plasmids. *AIDS* 14, 1515, 2000.

226. Kohl, S. et al. Interleukin-12 administered *in vivo* decreases human NK cell cytotoxicity and antibody-dependent cellular cytotoxicity to human immunodeficiency virus-infected cells. *J Infect Dis* 174, 1105, 1996.

227. Uittenbogaart, C.H. et al. Effect of cytokines on HIV-induced depletion of thymocytes *in vivo*. *AIDS* 14, 1317, 2000.

228. Ambinder, R.F. Epstein–Barr virus associated lymphoproliferations in the AIDS setting. *Eur J Cancer* 37, 1209, 2001.

229. Khatri, V.P. et al. Immunotherapy with low-dose interleukin-2: rationale for prevention of immune-deficiency-associated cancer. *Cancer J Sci Am* 3, Suppl 1, S129, 1997.

230. Baiocchi, R.A. et al. GM-CSF and IL-2 induce specific cellular immunity and provide protection against Epstein–Barr virus lymphoproliferative disorder. *J Clin Invest* 108, 887, 2001.

231. Glushakova, S. et al. Nef enhances human immunodeficiency virus replication and responsiveness to interleukin-2 in human lymphoid tissue *ex vivo*. *J Virol* 73, 3968, 1999.

232. Ruby, J. et al. Response of monkeys to vaccination with recombinant vaccinia virus which coexpress HIV gp160 and human interleukin-2. *Immunol Cell Biol* 68 (Pt 2), 113, 1990.

233. Davey, R.T., Jr. and Capra, W.B. Viral load in treatment with antiretroviral therapy and interleukin 2. *JAMA* 284, 2055, 2000.

234. Tambussi, G. et al. Efficacy of low-dose intermittent subcutaneous interleukin (IL)-2 in antiviral drug-experienced human immunodeficiency virus-infected persons with detectable virus load: a controlled study of 3 il-2 regimens with antiviral drug therapy. *J Infect Dis* 183, 1476, 2001.

235. Kovacs, J.A. et al. Effects of intermittent interleukin-2 therapy on plasma and tissue human immunodeficiency virus levels and quasi-species expression. *J Infect Dis* 182, 1063, 2000.

236. Loubeau, M. et al. Enhancement of natural killer and antibody-dependent cytolytic activities of the peripheral blood mononuclear cells of HIV-infected patients by recombinant IL-15. *J Acquir Immune Defic Syndr Hum Retrovirol* 16, 137, 1997.

237. Mastroianni, C.M. et al. Interleukin-15 enhances neutrophil functional activity in patients with human immunodeficiency virus infection. *Blood* 96, 1979, 2000.

238. Kanai, T. et al. IL-15 stimulates the expansion of AIDS virus-specific CTL. *J Immunol* 157, 3681, 1996.

239. McKnight, A. et al. A broad range of chemokine receptors are used by primary isolates of human immunodeficiency virus type 2 as coreceptors with CD4. *J Virol* 72, 4065, 1998.

240. Adjorlolo-Johnson, G. et al. Prospective comparison of mother-to-child transmission of HIV-1 and HIV-2 in Abidjan, Ivory Coast. *JAMA* 272, 462, 1994.

241. Kanki, P.J. et al. Slower heterosexual spread of HIV-2 than HIV-1. *Lancet* 343, 943, 1994.

242. Jaffar, S. et al. Rate of decline of percentage CD4+ cells is faster in HIV-1 than in HIV-2 infection. *J Acquir Immune Defic Syndr Hum Retrovirol* 16, 327, 1997.

243. Pepin, J. et al. HIV-2-induced immunosuppression among asymptomatic West African prostitutes: evidence that HIV-2 is pathogenic, but less so than HIV-1. *AIDS* 5, 1165, 1991.

244. Alabi, A.S. et al. Plasma viral load, CD4 cell percentage, HLA and survival of HIV-1, HIV-2, and dually infected Gambian patients. *AIDS* 17, 1513, 2003.

245. Berry, N. et al. Low peripheral blood viral HIV-2 RNA in individuals with high CD4 percentage differentiates HIV-2 from HIV-1 infection. *J Hum Virol* 1, 457, 1998.

246. Whittle, H.C. et al. HIV-2 and T cell recognition. *Curr Opin Immunol* 10, 382, 1998.

247. Sousa, A.E. et al. Comparison of the frequency of interleukin (IL)-2-, interferon-gamma-, and IL-4-producing T cells in 2 diseases, human immunodeficiency virus types 1 and 2, with distinct clinical outcomes. *J Infect Dis* 184, 552, 2001.

248. Jaye, A. et al. No differences in cellular immune responses between asymptomatic HIV type 1- and type 2-infected Gambian patients. *J Infect Dis* 189, 498, 2004.

249. Akimoto, H. et al. Binding of HIV-2 envelope glycoprotein to CD8 molecules and related chemokine production. *Immunology* 95, 214, 1998.

250. Kokkotou, E.G. et al. *In vitro* correlates of HIV-2-mediated HIV-1 protection. *Proc Natl Acad Sci USA* 97, 6797, 2000.

251. Martin, R.A. and Nayak, D.P. Receptor interference mediated by the envelope glycoproteins of various HIV-1 and HIV-2 isolates. *Virus Res* 45, 135, 1996.

252. Arya, S.K. and Gallo, R.C. Human immunodeficiency virus (HIV) type 2-mediated inhibition of HIV type 1: a new approach to gene therapy of HIV-infection. *Proc Natl Acad Sci USA* 93, 4486, 1996.

253. Rappaport, J. et al. Inhibition of HIV-1 expression by HIV-2. *J Mol Med* 73, 583, 1995.

254. Sarr, A.D. et al. HIV-1 and HIV-2 dual infection: lack of HIV-2 provirus correlates with low CD4+ lymphocyte counts. *AIDS* 12, 131, 1998.

255. Bertoletti, A. et al. Cytotoxic T cells from human immunodeficiency virus type 2-infected patients frequently cross-react with different human immunodeficiency virus type 1 clades. *J Virol* 72, 2439, 1998.

256. Chollet-Martin, S. et al. Comparison of plasma cytokine levels in African patients with HIV-1 and HIV-2 infection. *AIDS* 8, 879, 1994.

257. Machuca, A. et al. HIV type 2 primary isolates induce a lower degree of apoptosis *in vitro* compared with HIV type 1 primary isolates. *AIDS Res Hum Retroviruses* 20, 507, 2004.

258. Switzer, W.M. et al. Evidence of Nef truncation in human immunodeficiency virus type 2 infection. *J Infect Dis* 177, 65, 1998.

259. Yahi, N. et al. Inhibition of human immunodeficiency virus infection in human colon epithelial cells by recombinant interferon-gamma. *Eur J Immunol* 22, 2495, 1992.

260. Lin, G. et al. CD4-independent use of Rhesus CCR5 by human immunodeficiency virus Type 2 implicates an electrostatic interaction between the CCR5 N terminus and the gp120 C4 domain. *J Virol* 75, 10766, 2001.

261. Mullins, C. et al. Highly active antiretroviral therapy and viral response in HIV type 2 infection. *Clin Infect Dis* 38, 1771, 2004.

262. Smith, N.A. et al. Antiretroviral therapy for HIV-2 infected patients. *J Infect* 42, 126, 2001.

263. Debyser, Z. et al. An antiviral target on retrotrascriptase of human immunodeficiency virus type 1 revealed by tetrahydroimidazo-[4,5,1-jk] [1,4]benzodiazepin-2 (1H)-one and -thione derivatives. *Proc Natl Acad Sci USA* 88, 1451, 1991.

264. Hightower, M. and Kallas, E.G. Diagnosis, antiretroviral therapy, and emergence of resistance to antiretroviral agents in HIV-2 infection: a review. *Braz J Infect Dis* 7, 7, 2003.

265. Bartholomew, C. et al. Progression to AIDS in homosexual men co-infected with HIV and HTLV-I in Trinidad. *Lancet* 2, 1469, 1987.

266. Harrison, L.H. and Schechter, M. Coinfection with HTLV-I and HIV: increase in HTLV-I-related outcomes but not accelerated HIV disease progression? *AIDS Patient Care STDS* 12, 619, 1998.

267. Moriuchi, H. et al. Factors secreted by human T lymphotropic virus type I (HTLV-I)-infected cells can enhance or inhibit replication of HIV-1 in HTLV-I-uninfected cells: implications for *in vivo* coinfection with HTLV-I and HIV-1. *J Exp Med* 187, 1689, 1998.

268. Leung, K. and Nabel, G.J. HTLV-1 transactivator induces interleukin-2 receptor expression through an NF-kappa B-like factor. *Nature* 333, 776, 1988.

269. Siebenlist, U. et al. Structure, regulation and function of NF-kappa B. *Annu Rev Cell Biol* 10, 405, 1994.

270. Rhim, H. and Rice, A.P. TAR RNA binding properties and relative transactivation activities of human immunodeficiency virus type 1 and 2 Tat proteins. *J Virol* 67, 1110, 1993.

271. Cullen, B.R. and Greene, W.C. Regulatory pathways governing HIV-1 replication. *Cell* 58, 423, 1989.

272. Rubartelli, A. et al. HIV-I Tat: a polypeptide for all seasons. *Immunol Today* 19, 543, 1998.

273. Jeang, K.T. et al. Multifaceted activities of the HIV-1 transactivator of transcription, Tat. *J Biol Chem* 274, 28837, 1999.

274. Lefrere, J.J. et al. Rapid progression to AIDS in dual HIV-1/HTLV-I infection. *Lancet* 336, 509, 1990.

275. Cimarelli, A. et al. Quantification of HTLV-II proviral copies by competitive polymerase chain reaction in peripheral blood mononuclear cells of Italian injecting drug users, central Africans, and Amerindians. *J Acquir Immune Defic Syndr Hum Retrovirol* 10, 198, 1995.

276. Harrison, L.H. et al. Human T cell lymphotropic virus type I does not increase human immunodeficiency virus viral load *in vivo. J Infect Dis* 175, 438, 1997.

277. Casoli, C. et al. HTLV-II down-regulates HIV-1 replication in IL-2-stimulated primary PBMC of coinfected individuals through expression of MIP-1alpha. *Blood* 95, 2760, 2000.

278. Lewis, M.J. et al. Spontaneous production of C-C chemokines by individuals infected with human T lymphotropic virus type II (HTLV-II) alone and HTLV-II/HIV-1 coinfected individuals. *J Immunol* 165, 4127, 2000.

279. Alfano, M. and Poli, G. Cytokine and chemokine based control of hiv infection and replication. *Curr Pharm Des* 7, 993, 2001.

280. Granucci, F. et al. Dendritic cell regulation of immune responses: a new role for interleukin 2 at the intersection of innate and adaptive immunity. *Embo J* 22, 2546, 2003.

281. Waldmann, T.A. T-cell receptors for cytokines: targets for immunotherapy of leukemia/lymphoma. *Ann Oncol* 11, Suppl 1, 101, 2000.

282. Brinchmann, J.E. Differential responses of T cell subsets: possible role in the immunopathogenesis of AIDS. *AIDS* 14, 1689, 2000.

283. Napolitano, L.A. Approaches to immune reconstitution in HIV infection. *Top HIV Med* 11, 160, 2003.

284. Urba, W.J. et al. Immunomodulatory properties and toxicity of interleukin 2 in patients with cancer. *Cancer Res* 50, 185, 1990.

285. Paul, W.E. and Seder, R.A. Lymphocyte responses and cytokines. *Cell* 76, 241, 1994.

286. Lane, H.C. et al. Qualitative analysis of immune function in patients with the acquired immunodeficiency syndrome: evidence for a selective defect in soluble antigen recognition. *New Engl J Med* 313, 79, 1985.

287. Waldmann, T.A. and Tagaya, Y. The multifaceted regulation of interleukin-15 expression and the role of this cytokine in NK cell differentiation and host response to intracellular pathogens. *Annu Rev Immunol* 17, 19, 1999.

288. Migone, T.S. et al. Constitutively activated Jak-STAT pathway in T cells transformed with HTLV-I. *Science* 269, 79, 1995.

289. Poli, G. et al. Interleukin 6 induces human immunodeficiency virus expression in infected monocytic cells alone and in synergy with tumor necrosis factor alpha by transcriptional and post-transcriptional mechanisms. *J Exp Med* 172, 151, 1990.

290. Poli, G. et al. Tumor necrosis factor alpha functions in an autocrine manner in the induction of human immunodeficiency virus expression. *Proc Natl Acad Sci USA* 87, 782, 1990.

291. Kovacs, J.A. et al. Increases in CD4 T lymphocytes with intermittent courses of interleukin-2 in patients with human immunodeficiency virus infection: preliminary study *New Engl J Med* 332, 567, 1995.

292. Kovacs, J.A. et al. Controlled trial of interleukin-2 infusions in patients infected with the human immunodeficiency virus. *New Engl J Med* 335, 1350, 1996.

293. Leonard, W.J. and O'Shea, J.J. Jaks and STATs: biological implications. *Annu Rev Immunol* 16, 293, 1998.

294. Mulloy, J.C. et al. Human T-cell lymphotropic/leukemia virus type 1 Tax abrogates p53-induced cell cycle arrest and apoptosis through its CREB/ATF functional domain. *J Virol* 72, 8852, 1998.

295. Bovolenta, C. et al. Constitutive activation of STATs upon *in vivo* human immunodeficiency virus infection. *Blood* 94, 4202, 1999.

296. Takemoto, S. et al. Proliferation of adult T cell leukemia/lymphoma cells is associated with the constitutive activation of JAK/STAT proteins. *Proc Natl Acad Sci USA* 94, 13897, 1997.

297. Bovolenta, C. et al. Positive selection of apoptosis-resistant cells correlates with activation of dominant-negative STAT5. *J Biol Chem* 273, 20779, 1998.

298. Zhang, L.J. et al. The interleukin-2 fusion protein, DAB389IL-2, inhibits the development of infectious virus in human immunodeficiency virus type 1-infected human peripheral blood mononuclear cells. *J Infect Dis* 175, 790, 1997.

299. Imami, N. et al. Immune responses and reconstitution in HIV-1 infected individuals: impact of anti-retroviral therapy, cytokines and therapeutic vaccination. *Immunol Lett* 79, 63, 2001.

300. Smith, K.A. Low-dose daily interleukin-2 immunotherapy: accelerating immune restoration and expanding HIV-specific T-cell immunity without toxicity. *AIDS* 15, Suppl 2, S28, 2001.

301. Johnson, J.M. et al. Molecular biology and pathogenesis of the human T-cell leukaemia/lymphotropic virus type-1 (HTLV-1). *Int J Exp Pathol* 82, 135, 2001.

302. Coffin, J.M., Hughes, S.H., and Varmus, H.E. *Retroviruses*, Cold Spring Harbor Laboratory, Cold Spring Harbor, NY, 1997.

303. Himes, S.R. et al. HTLV-1 tax activation of the GM-CSF and G-CSF promoters requires the interaction of NF-kB with other transcription factor families. *Oncogene* 8, 3189, 1993.

304. Miyatake, S. et al. Activation of T cell-derived lymphokine genes in T cells and fibroblasts: effects of human T cell leukemia virus type I p40x protein and bovine papilloma virus encoded E2 protein. *Nucleic Acids Res* 16, 6547, 1988.

305. Wano, Y. et al. Stable expression of the tax gene of type I human T-cell leukemia virus in human T cells activates specific cellular genes involved in growth. *Proc Natl Acad Sci USA* 85, 9733, 1988.

306. Sawada, M. et al. Induction of cytokines in glial cells by trans activator of human T-cell lymphotropic virus type I. *FEBS Lett* 313, 47, 1992.

307. Tsukada, J. et al. Human T-cell leukemia virus type I Tax transactivates the promoter of human prointerleukin-1beta gene through association with two transcription factors, nuclear factor-interleukin-6 and Spi-1. *Blood* 90, 3142, 1997.

308. Mori, N. and Prager, D. Transactivation of the interleukin-1alpha promoter by human T-cell leukemia virus type I and type II Tax proteins. *Blood* 87, 3410, 1996.

309. Siekevitz, M. et al. Activation of interleukin 2 and interleukin 2 receptor (Tac) promoter expression by the trans-activator (tat) gene product of human T-cell leukemia virus, type I. *Proc Natl Acad Sci USA* 84, 5389, 1987.

310. Blumenthal, S.G. et al. Regulation of the human interleukin-5 promoter by Ets transcription factors. Ets1 and Ets2, but not Elf-1, cooperate with GATA3 and HTLV-I Tax1. *J Biol Chem* 274, 12910, 1999.

311. Muraoka, O. et al. Transcriptional activation of the interleukin-6 gene by HTLV-1 p40tax through an NF-kappa B-like binding site. *Immunol Lett* 37, 159, 1993.

312. Baba, M. et al. Constitutive expression of various chemokine genes in human T-cell lines infected with human T-cell leukemia virus type 1: role of the viral transactivator Tax. *Int J Cancer* 66, 124, 1996.

313. Mori, N. et al. Human T-cell leukemia virus type I Tax transactivates human interleukin 8 gene through acting concurrently on AP-1 and nuclear factor-kappaB-like sites. *Cancer Res* 58, 3993, 1998.

314. Mori, N. and Prager, D. Interleukin-10 gene expression and adult T-cell leukemia. *Leuk Lymphoma* 29, 239, 1998.

315. Chung, H.K. et al. Activation of interleukin-13 expression in T cells from HTLV-1-infected individuals and in chronically infected cell lines. *Blood* 102, 4130, 2003.

316. Waldele, K. et al. Interleukin-13 overexpression by tax transactivation: a potential autocrine stimulus in human T-cell leukemia virus-infected lymphocytes. *J Virol* 78, 6081, 2004.

317. Azimi, N. et al. Human T cell lymphotropic virus type I Tax protein trans-activates interleukin 15 gene transcription through an NF-kappaB site. *Proc Natl Acad Sci USA* 95, 2452, 1998.

318. Azimi, N. et al. How does interleukin 15 contribute to the pathogenesis of HTLV type 1-associated myelopathy/tropical spastic paraparesis? *AIDS Res Hum Retroviruses* 16, 1717, 2000.

319. Niitsu, Y. et al. Expression of TGF-beta gene in adult T cell leukemia. *Blood* 71, 263, 1988.

320. Kim, S.J. et al. Transactivation of the transforming growth factor beta 1 (TGF-beta 1) gene by human T lymphotropic virus type 1 tax: a potential mechanism for the increased production of TGF-beta 1 in adult T cell leukemia. *J Exp Med* 172, 121, 1990.

321. Dodon, M.D. et al. Tax protein of human T-cell leukaemia virus type 1 induces interleukin 17 gene expression in T cells. *J Gen Virol* 85, 1921, 2004.

322. Twizere, J.C. et al. Interaction of retroviral Tax oncoproteins with tristetraprolin and regulation of tumor necrosis factor-alpha expression. *J Natl Cancer Inst* 95, 1846, 2003.

323. Sharma, V. and May, C.C. Human T-cell lymphotrophic virus type-I tax gene induces secretion of human macrophage inflammatory protein-1-alpha. *Biochem Biophys Res Commun* 262, 429, 1999.

324. Ruckes, T. et al. Autocrine antiapoptotic stimulation of cultured adult T-cell leukemia cells by overexpression of the chemokine I-309. *Blood* 98, 1150, 2001.

325. Sharma, V. and Lorey, S.L. Autocrine role of macrophage inflammatory protein-1 beta in human T-cell lymphotropic virus type-I tax-transfected Jurkat T-cells. *Biochem Biophys Res Commun* 287, 910, 2001.

326. Imaizumi, Y. et al. Human T cell leukemia virus type-I Tax activates human macrophage inflammatory protein-3 alpha/CCL20 gene transcription via the NF-kappa B pathway. *Int Immunol* 14, 147, 2002.

327. Yamazato, Y. et al. High expression of p40(tax) and pro-inflammatory cytokines and chemokines in the lungs of human T-lymphotropic virus type 1-related bronchopulmonary disorders. *Chest* 124, 2283, 2003.

328. Arai, M. et al. Human T-cell leukemia virus type 1 Tax protein induces the expression of lymphocyte chemoattractant SDF-1/PBSF. *Virology* 241, 298, 1998.

329. Yoshie, O. et al. Frequent expression of CCR4 in adult T-cell leukemia and human T-cell leukemia virus type 1-transformed T cells. *Blood* 99, 1505, 2002.

330. Matsushita, K. and Arima, N. Involvement of granulocyte colony-stimulating factor in proliferation of adult T-cell leukemia cells. *Leuk Lymphoma* 31, 295, 1998.

331. Brown, D.A. et al. The human interferon-gamma gene contains an inducible promoter that can be transactivated by tax I and II. *Eur J Immunol* 21, 1879, 1991.

332. Buckle, G.J. et al. HTLV-I-induced T-cell activation. *J Acquir Immune Defic Syndr Hum Retrovirol* 13, Suppl 1, S107, 1996.

333. Kubota, S. et al. Cis/trans-activation of the interleukin-9 receptor gene in an HTLV-I-transformed human lymphocytic cell. *Oncogene* 12, 1441, 1996.

334. Matsushita, K. et al. Frequent expression of interleukin-9 mRNA and infrequent involvement of interleukin-9 in proliferation of primary adult T-cell leukemia cells and HTLV-I infected T-cell lines. *Leuk Res* 21, 211, 1997.

335. Ferbas, J. et al. Selective decrease in human immunodeficiency virus type 1 (HIV-1)-induced alpha interferon production by peripheral blood mononuclear cells during HIV-1 infection. *Clin Diagn Lab Immunol* 2, 138, 1995.

336. Feldman, S. et al. Decreased interferon-alpha production in HIV-infected patients correlates with numerical and functional deficiencies in circulating type 2 dendritic cell precursors. *Clin Immunol* 101, 201, 2001.

337. Poli, G. et al. Interferons in the pathogenesis and treatment of human immunodeficiency virus infection. *Antiviral Res* 24, 221, 1994.

338. Clerici, M. et al. Restoration of HIV-specific cell-mediated immune responses by interleukin-12 *in vitro*. *Science* 262, 1721, 1993.

339. Chehimi, J. et al. Enhancing effect of natural killer cell stimulatory factor (NKSF/interleukin-12) on cell-mediated cytotoxicity against tumor-derived and virus-infected cells. *Eur J Immunol* 23, 1826, 1993.

340. Marshall, J.D. et al. The interleukin-12-mediated pathway of immune events is dysfunctional in human immunodeficiency virus-infected individuals. *Blood* 94, 1003, 1999.

341. Graziosi, C. et al. Lack of evidence for the dichotomy of TH1 and TH2 predominance in HIV-infected individuals. *Science* 265, 248, 1994.

342. Koopman, G. et al. Decreased expression of IL-2 in central and effector CD4 memory cells during progression to AIDS in rhesus macaques. *AIDS* 15, 2359, 2001.

343. Airoldi, I. et al. Cytokine gene expression and T-cell proliferative responses in lymph node mononuclear cells from children with early stage human immunodeficiency virus infection. *Haematologica* 85, 1237, 2000.

344. Andersson, J. et al. Early reduction of immune activation in lymphoid tissue following highly active HIV therapy. *AIDS* 12, F123, 1998.

345. Gray, C.M. et al. Identification of cell subsets expressing intracytoplasmic cytokines within HIV-1-infected lymph nodes. *AIDS* 10, 1467, 1996.

346. Boulassel, M.R. et al. Interleukin-7 levels may predict virological response in advanced HIV-1-infected patients receiving lopinavir/ritonavir-based therapy. *HIV Med* 4, 315, 2003.

347. Chiappini, E. et al. Interleukin-7 and immunologic failure despite treatment with highly active antiretroviral therapy in children perinatally infected with HIV-1. *J Acquir Immune Defic Syndr* 33, 601, 2003.

348. Clerici, M. et al. T-lymphocyte maturation abnormalities in uninfected newborns and children with vertical exposure to HIV. *Blood* 96, 3866, 2000.

349. Bailer, R.T. et al. IL-13 and IFN-gamma secretion by activated T cells in HIV-1 infection associated with viral suppression and a lack of disease progression. *J Immunol* 162, 7534, 1999.

350. Zanussi, S. et al. Immunological changes in peripheral blood and in lymphoid tissue after treatment of HIV-infected subjects with highly active anti-retroviral therapy (HAART) or HAART + IL-2. *Clin Exp Immunol* 116, 486, 1999.

351. Perrella, O. et al. Transforming growth factor beta-1 and interferon-alpha in the AIDS dementia complex (ADC): possible relationship with cerebral viral load? *Eur Cytokine Netw* 12, 51, 2001.

352. Alonso, K. et al. Cytokine patterns in adults with AIDS. *Immunol Invest* 26, 341, 1997.

353. Navikas, V. et al. Increased levels of interferon-gamma (IFN-gamma), IL-4 and transforming growth factor-beta (TGF-beta) mRNA expressing blood mononuclear cells in human HIV infection. *Clin Exp Immunol* 96, 59, 1994.

354. Bodi, I. et al. Renal TGF-beta in HIV-associated kidney diseases. *Kidney Int* 51, 1568, 1997.

19 Psychiatric Toxicity of Interferon-α: A Model for Understanding the Etiology of Major Depression and Chronic Fatigue Syndrome?

Gopinath Ranjith and Carmine Pariante

CONTENTS

INTRODUCTION

Interferon-α is increasingly used in therapeutics. The commonly used indications for interferon-α treatment include hepatitis C and malignant melanoma. One of the main concerns about using interferon-α in therapy is the risk of psychiatric toxicity that leads to high drop-out rates during high dose interferon therapy.[1] The psychiatric symptoms caused by interferon-α include depression, anxiety, fatigue, mania, and cognitive dysfunction. In this chapter, we review clinical studies of depression and fatigue in patients receiving interferon-α and the effects of such symptoms on response to interferon treatment. We offer a brief overview of the mechanism by which interferon-α produces psychiatric symptoms, relating this to the existing research on the neurobiology of major depression and chronic fatigue syndrome. We conclude by offering an integrative viewpoint and proposing areas for further research.

NEUROPSYCHIATRIC TOXICITY OF INTERFERON-α

The most common reason for discontinuation of interferon-α therapy is neuropsychiatric toxicity.[1] Common side effects include symptoms of depression such as low mood, insomnia, fatigue, loss of appetite, and weight loss. Cognitive side effects including memory dysfunction and executive dysfunction are also common. Rarer but reported side effects also include psychosis, mania, delirium, and suicidal behavior. Most studies reviewed in this chapter concern low dose interferon-α therapy in hepatitis C; studies of high dose therapy in melanoma where the incidence of depression is higher are also discussed where relevant.

Depression has been the most studied psychiatric side effect of interferon. Most studies show increases in the rate of depressive symptoms during interferon therapy. These studies differ in the rigor with which depressive symptoms were measured. Some studies used self-report scales such as the Beck Depression Inventory (BDI),[2] the Montgomery Asberg Depression Rating Scale (MADRS),[3] the Zung Self-Rating Depression Scale (SDS),[4] or the Inventory to Diagnose Depression (IDD),[5] while others used observer-rated scales such as the Hamilton Depression Rating Scale (HAM-D)[6] and clinical interviews. Few studies utilized a structured interview schedule, currently considered the gold standard. Most were cohort studies and a recent systematic review[7] was able to identify only one randomized study.

In a sample of 50 patients, Pariante et al.[8] found that 11 patients developed major depressive disorder, generalized anxiety disorder, or severe dysphoria as measured by the Structured Clinical Interview for DSM-IV (SCID).[9] Similar results were replicated by the same group.[10,11] Bonaccorso et al.[12] found that half the sample of 14 patients receiving interferon-α-2a scored more than 15 on the MADRS. Malaguarnera et al.[13] randomized patients into groups receiving four types of interferon-α and compared them to a control group receiving no treatment. All the active treatment groups but not the control group developed significant depressive symptoms during treatment.

An exception was the study by Mulder et al.[14] that did not find increases in depression scores in patients with hepatitis C treated with interferon-α. In terms of the course of development of depression, Maddock et al.[15] found that depression increased linearly with time and at 24 weeks, the estimated increase was 4.5 points on the BDI. Details of other studies that looked at the incidence of depression during interferon-α treatment in hepatitis C are shown in Table 19.1.[16–20]

Few studies systematically studied fatigue as a symptom during interferon therapy. Maddock et al.[15] found that fatigue and quality of life deteriorated in the first 8 weeks of treatment and remained at deteriorated levels for the duration of treatment. This was different from the course of depression and anxiety that increased steadily during the course of therapy. Capuron and colleagues[21] also noticed a differential course of symptom dimensions during interferon therapy. Neurovegetative and somatic symptoms including depression developed within 2 weeks of treatment, but mood and cognitive symptoms appeared later.

TABLE 19.1
Studies of Depression during Treatment of Hepatitis C with Interferon-α

Study	Number of Subjects	Measure	Outcome
Malaguarnera et al.[13](1998)	96	Zung SDS	Patients in interferon treatment groups but not in control group, developed statistically significant increases in SDS scores
Pariante et al.[8] (1999)	50	SCID	Eleven patients developed psychiatric adverse effects, six had major depression, and three had depressive disorders not otherwise specified
Hauser et al.[18] (2002)	39	BDI, SCID	Thirty-three percent developed interferon-induced major depressive disorder
Bonaccorso et al.[12] (2002)	18	MADRS	Significant increase in MADRS scores at week 4 and 4–6 months
Dieperink et al.[16] (2003)	55	HAM-D, BDI, Zung SDS, IDD	23% developed symptoms consistent with major depression
Horikawa et al.[19] (2003)	99	HAM-D, Zung SDS, SCID	Twenty-three percent diagnosed with major depression at least once in 24-week treatment period
Kraus et al.[20] (2003)	84	Symptom Check List 90	Significant increase in depression scores at 4 weeks, 3–4 months, and 6–8 months after treatment
Gohier et al.[17] (2003)	71	MADRS	Thirty-three percent developed psychiatric side effects of which 13% had depression
Maddock et al.[15] (2005)	29	BDI	Linear increase in depression during treatment period; significant increase in BDI scores at 24 weeks

Zung SDS = Zung Self-Rating Depression Scale. SCID = Structured Clinical Interview for DSM-IV. MADRS = Montgomery Asberg Depression Rating Scale. HAM-D = Hamilton Depression Rating Scale. BDI = Beck Depression Inventory. IDD = Inventory to Diagnose Depression.

RISK FACTORS AND CONSEQUENCES OF PSYCHIATRIC TOXICITY

Most of the studies have concentrated on demographic and clinical predictors of psychiatric symptoms in patients undergoing treatment with interferon-α. Sub-clinical depressive symptoms have been reported to predict major depression during therapy. Past history of multiple psychiatric disorders and family history of psychiatric disorder have also emerged as significant but not consistent predictors. Other risk factors studied but not found to be consistently associated with psychiatric toxicity include history of substance abuse, gender, severity of hepatitis C virus (HCV) infection, and virus genotype.

Among the studies of biological predictors, Gochee et al.[22] detected a statistically significant association between the apolipoprotein (APOE) 4 allele and neuropsychiatric symptoms. Lower activity of serum peptidases predicted symptoms of depression and anxiety during interferon therapy.[23] The peptidases are involved in the degradation of behaviorally active peptides such as arginine vasopressin (AVP), thyrotropin releasing hormone (TRH), and substance P that play roles in the regulation of emotional states.

Not all patients develop depression or other psychiatric symptoms during interferon therapy — proving that interferon is not a sufficient cause of depression. It is thus intuitively appealing to study other psychosocial factors that are implicated as risk factors for depression. Few studies specifically looked at psychological or social predictors. Capuron et al.[24] recently studied other psychosocial factors such as social support and coping. They found that a low quantity but not a poor quality of social support at baseline increased the risk of developing depressive symptoms in patients with elevated baseline depression scores.

Other variables such as coping strategies, age, and gender were not predictive of depression. We recently completed a study with similar results.[25] Number of life events in the 6 months prior to initiation of treatment, baseline social support, and perceptions regarding the time course of the illness and cure did not predict changes in scores of depression, fatigue, or quality of life during treatment with interferon-α.

Some evidence indicates that the development of psychiatric symptoms exerts effects on virologic responses during interferon-α treatment of hepatitis C. There is no consensus in the field of the nature of the effect. Loftis et al.[26] found that interferon-induced major depressive disorder was a predictor of positive response to interferon therapy. In contrast, Raison et al.[27] found that patients who developed significant increases in depressive symptoms during interferon treatment were less likely to clear the virus. Maddock et al. also found that the patients in their sample who did not respond to interferon treatment had greater deterioration in psychological variables including depression and fatigue during treatment; this reached statistical significance in the case of fatigue.[15] Maddock et al. opine that the better response in depressed patients found by Loftis et al. may be attributed to antidepressant treatment rather than depression itself.[15]

MECHANISMS OF DEPRESSION AND FATIGUE DURING INTERFERON THERAPY

Interferon-α affects multiple systems implicated in the pathophysiology of depression. Therapy with interferon-α significantly induces the cytokine network, and the therapy-related increases in some of the pro-inflammatory cytokines such as IL-6 are significantly and positively related to the increases in depression scores.[28] The mechanism of interferon-α-induced depression is uncertain, but any discussion must take into account systems involved in the pathophysiology of major depression, i.e., the hypothalamic–pituitary–adrenal (HPA) axis and the serotonergic, noradrenergic, and dopaminergic systems.

Cytokines such as IL-1, IFN-γ, and TNF-α reduce the production of serotonin (5-HT) by stimulating an enzyme called indoleamine 2, 3-dioxygenase (IDO) that converts tryptophan into kynurenine. Over-stimulation of IDO leads to depletion of plasma tryptophan and reduced synthesis of 5-HT. Kynurenine metabolites such as 3-hydroxy-kynurenine and quinolinic acid have also direct toxic effects on the brain by increasing the production of reactive oxygen species and over-stimulation of hippocampal NMDA receptors, respectively.[29] Neopterin is a pteridine derived from GTP that is released from human monocytes and macrophages on stimulation with interferons, thus acting as a marker of activated cell-mediated immunity.

Many studies in humans have investigated the serotonergic system during interferon therapy. Capuron et al. studied 26 patients with malignant melanoma who were randomly allocated to receive paroxetine or placebo beginning 2 weeks before interferon-α therapy and continuing for the first 12 weeks.[30] Among antidepressant-free patients, those who developed major depression exhibited greater increases in kynurenine and neopterin and more prolonged decreases in tryptophan concentrations than non-depressed patients. Similar changes in tryptophan concentrations were demonstrated by other groups.[31,32] Capuron et al. also found a correlation of tryptophan depletion with mood and cognitive symptoms but not with neurovegetative or somatic symptoms.

Cytokines also affect other neurotransmitter systems.[33] IL-1 has been shown to stimulate hypothalamic and preoptic noradrenergic neurotransmission in rats. IL-1 also increases the 3-methoxy-4-hydroxyphenylglycol/norepinephrine (MHPG/NE) ratio in the frontal cortex and hippocampus in mice. Dopamine has been hypothesized to play a role in depression and irritability and drugs with dopamine blocking action such as amisulpiride have been used in the treatment of interferon-induced depression.[34] Another neurotransmitter implicated in interferon-induced depression is nitric oxide.[35]

In vivo and *in vitro* administration of interferon-α activates corticotrophin releasing factor (CRF) production and/or release in animals. CRF hypersecretion is a reliable finding in patients with major depression. CRF is a key regulatory peptide of the HPA axis. Peripheral administration of interferon-α also potently induces the production of pro-inflammatory cytokines that activate the HPA axis. Cassidy et al.[36] found that following injection of interferon-α in healthy volunteers, there was an increase in IL-6 which has been shown to be a potent stimulator of the HPA axis. Capuron et al. also demonstrated a link between ACTH and cortisol responses, but not IL-6 response.[37] Pro-inflammatory cytokines may also reduce glucocorticoid receptor translocation and function,[38] which is a mechanism in the pathogenesis of depression as explained in the next section.

IMMUNE AND ENDOCRINE FINDINGS IN MAJOR DEPRESSION AND CHRONIC FATIGUE SYNDROME

It is beyond the scope of this chapter to describe the psychoneuroimmunology and psychoneuroendocrinolgy of major depression and chronic fatigue syndrome in detail. The stress–cytokine–depression model explains the relationship of stressful events, immune changes, and depression.[39] This model also takes into account the changes in the HPA axis that are the hallmarks of depression. Stress results in the release of pro-inflammatory cytokines such as IL-1, IL-6, and tumor necrosis factor (TNF) that regulate the acute phase response. These cytokines also induce a group of behavioral symptoms called sickness behavior.

Sickness behavior occurs in a variety of infections as well as during treatment with high dose cytokine therapy and includes symptoms such as fatigue, loss of appetite, sleep disturbance, social withdrawal, decreased libido, depressed mood, and general malaise. The symptoms of sickness behavior overlap with psychiatric disorders such as major depression and chronic fatigue syndrome — this has been called the malaise theory of depression.[40]

Pro-inflammatory cytokines are elevated in medically ill patients with depression and correlate with symptoms of sickness behavior. Moreover, studies have found increased levels of plasma and cerebrospinal fluid levels of pro-inflammatory cytokines such as IL-1 and IL-6 and increased *in vitro* production of cytokines from stimulated peripheral blood mononuclear cells in medically healthy depressive patients. Increased plasma concentrations of acute phase reactants such as haptoglobin, C-reactive protein, α-1-antitrypsin, and ceruloplasmin have also been reported in depression. However, the relationship between cytokines and depression has been largely correlational, without a clear indication as to the direction of causality.

Many recent reviews have examined the neuroendocrinology of depression.[41,42] Various clinical studies have demonstrated the hyperactivity of the HPA axis in patients with depression. One of the main features of this HPA axis hyperactivity is the reduced sensitivity to the inhibitory effects of dexamethasone on the production of adrenocorticotropic hormone and cortisol during the dexamethasone suppression test (DST) and its modification, the dexamethasone–corticotrophin releasing hormone (DEX-CRH) test.

The HPA axis abnormalities are thought to be a consequence of hypersecretion of CRH. The increased levels of CRH in the hypothalamus are believed to be related to altered feedback inhibition by endogenous glucocorticoids. The feedback regulation of the HPA axis by glucocorticoids is mediated through two receptor subtypes, the mineralocorticoid receptor (MR) and the glucocorticoid receptor (GR). GR is considered to be more important in the regulation of response to stress when endogenous levels of glucocorticoids are high. The involvement of GR in the pathogenesis of depression comes from a variety of studies summarized by Juruena et al.[42] that show impaired GR signaling in the absence of clear evidence for decreased GR expression. Indirect evidence also comes from studies that show direct effects of antidepressants on GR, leading to enhanced GR function.

Chronic fatigue syndrome (CFS) is a medically unexplained syndrome characterized by new onset of fatigue accompanied by multiple physical symptoms.[43] A variety of immune abnormalities have been reported in CFS but results have not been consistent. Two recent reviews have tried to critically analyze the immune findings in CFS.[44,45] The conclusion is that the available evidence does not support chronic fatigue syndrome as being due to any consistent immunological dysfunction. Among studies of interferon-α in chronic fatigue syndrome, one reported increases in interferon-α while four found no differences with regard to control groups.[44]

The role of the HPA axis in CFS developed from the finding that fatigue characterized patients with disorders with low circulating cortisol such as Addison's disease and following bilateral adrenalectomy. Studies of basal HPA axis function yielded mixed results.[46] An unpublished meta-analysis of all studies of 24-hour urinary free cortisol (UFC) and morning and afternoon plasma cortisol found a moderate overall effect size for reduced 24-hour UFC and morning cortisol but with heterogeneity between studies. Dynamic challenge tests of the HPA axis using the CRH test, the ACTH test, the insulin stress test, and the DST provide evidence for enhanced negative feedback and enhanced GR sensitivity. The finding of low circulating cortisol led to randomized controlled trials with hydrocortisone that have been successful in the short term.[47] Another development pointing to the role of the HPA axis is the description of a mutation in the cortisol-binding globulin gene in families with high prevalences of CFS-like illness.

It has been proposed that an interaction between cytokine abnormalities and neuroendocrine abnormalities may underlie symptoms seen in patients with CFS.[48] Inflammatory cytokines such as IL-6 and tumor necrosis factor-α are potent stimulants of the HPA axis. Cortisol inhibits the secretion of IL-6 and TNF-α while corticosteroid deficiency leads to elevation of plasma concentration of the above cytokines. As described earlier in the section on sickness behavior, these inflammatory cytokines give rise to symptoms common in CFS such as fatigue, somnolence, anorexia, and headache.

INTEGRATIVE VIEW

Symptoms similar to major depression and CFS occur frequently during treatment with interferon-α. The different time frames over which these symptoms develop, independently replicated by different research groups,[15,21] indicate the need to study them separately. The mechanisms involved in the development of these symptoms overlap with systems implicated in major depression and chronic fatigue syndrome such as the HPA axis, monoaminergic neurotransmitter systems, and the cytokine network.

Capuron and Miller[49] suggested a model for the differential development of mood/cognitive and neurovegetative symptoms during interferon treatment. They postulated the hyper-responsiveness of the CRF pathways as a vulnerability factor and the involvement of the serotonin pathway as a pathogenic factor in the development of interferon-induced mood/cognitive symptoms. Early life adversity and family and past histories of depression that sensitize the CRF pathways need to be studied as vulnerability factors in interferon-induced depression. These systems have been extensively investigated in major depression and further research may broaden our understanding of the pathophysiology of depression.

The dopaminergic system and the basal ganglia are implicated in the development of neurovegetative symptoms including fatigue by Capuron and Miller.[49] Preliminary findings show altered glucose metabolism in the basal ganglia of interferon-treated patients. Moreover, case reports of movement disorders during treatment with interferon treatment support the involvement of basal ganglia. Recent functional MRI findings that the motor system may be involved in the pathophysiology of chronic fatigue syndrome[50] indicate the importance of studying interferon-induced fatigue as a model for chronic fatigue syndrome.

CONCLUSION

Major depression and CFS are complex disorders with multiple risk factors.[51,52] Research into the biological underpinnings of these disorders and their interactions with psychosocial factors is essential to improve the care of patients with these disorders. Our review shows that treatment with interferon-α produces symptoms that closely resemble depression and chronic fatigue. Thus the study of psychiatric toxicity of interferon-α may give us insights into the etiology of these disorders. The HPA axis, cytokine networks, and neurotransmitter systems could be studied further. Research designs should also incorporate proximal and distal psychosocial factors to study their interactions with biological variables. Advances in pharmacogenetics and functional neuroimaging[53] may throw further light on understanding these disorders.

REFERENCES

1. Musselman, D.L. et al. Paroxetine for the prevention of depression induced by high-dose interferon alfa. *New Engl J Med*, 344, 961, 2001.
2. Beck, A.T. and Beamesderfer, A. Assessment of depression: the depression inventory. *Mod Probl Pharmacopsychiatr*, 7, 151, 1974.
3. Montgomery, S.A. and Asberg, M. A new depression scale designed to be sensitive to change. *Br J Psychiatry*, 134, 382, 1979.
4. Zung, W.W.K. et al. Self-rating depression scale in an outpatient clinic. *Arch Gen Psychiatr*, 13, 508, 1965.
5. Zimmerman, M. and Coryell, W. The Inventory to Diagnose Depression (IDD): a self report scale to diagnose major depressive disorder. *J Consult Clin Psycho.*, 55, 55, 1987.
6. Williams, J.B. A structured interview guide for the Hamilton Depression Rating Scale. *Arch Gen Psychiatr*, 45, 742, 1988.
7. Patten, S. and Barbui, C. Drug-induced depression: a systematic review to inform clinical practice. *Psychother Psychosom*, 73, 207, 2004.
8. Pariante, C.M. et al. Treatment with interferon-alpha in patients with chronic hepatitis and mood or anxiety disorders. *Lancet*, 354, 131, 1999.
9. Spitzer, R.L. et al. The Structured Clinical Interview for DSM-III-R (SCID): I. History, rationale and description. *Arch Gen Psychiatr*, 49, 624, 1992.
10. Pariante, C.M. et al. Interferon-alpha-induced psychiatric adverse effects in patients with chronic viral hepatitis and a psychiatric diagnosis: a prospective, controlled study. *New Eng J Med*, 347, 148, 2002.
11. Orru, M.G. et al. Interferon-alpha-induced psychiatric side effects in patients with chronic viral hepatitis: a prospective, observational, controlled study. *Epidemiol e Psichiatri Soc*, in press, 2005.
12. Bonaccorso, S. et al. Depression induced by treatment with interferon-alpha in patients affected by hepatitis C virus. *J Aff Disord*, 72, 237, 2002.
13. Malaguarnera, M. et al. Interferon alpha-induced depression in chronic hepatitis C patients: comparison between different types of interferon alpha. *Neuropsychobiology*, 37, 93, 1998.
14. Mulder, R.T. et al. Interferon treatment is not associated with a worsening of psychiatric symptoms in patients with hepatitis C. *J Gastroenterol Hepatol*, 15, 300, 2000.

15. Maddock, C. et al. Psychopathological symptoms during interferon-alpha treatment and ribavirin treatment: effects on virologic response. *Mol Psychiatry*, 10, 332, 2005.

16. Dieperink, E. et al. A prospective study of neuropsychiatric symptoms associated with interferon-alpha-2b and ribavirin therapy for patients with chronic hepatitis C. *Psychosomatics*, 44, 104, 2003.

17. Gohier, B. et al. Hepatitis C, alpha interferon, anxiety and depression disorders: a prospective study of 71 patients. *World J Biol Psychiatry*, 4, 115, 2003.

18. Hauser, P. et al. A prospective study of the incidence and open-label treatment of interferon-induced major depression in patients with hepatitis C. *Mol Psychiatr*, 7, 942, 2002.

19. Horikawa, N. et al. Incidence and clinical course of major depression in patients with chronic hepatitis type C undergoing interferon-alpha therapy: a prospective study. *Gen Hosp Psychiatr*, 25, 34, 2003.

20. Kraus, M.R., et al. Psychiatric symptoms in patients with chronic hepatitis C receiving interferon alfa-2b therapy. *J Clin Psychiatr*, 64, 708, 2003.

21. Capuron, L. et al. Neurobehavioral effects of interferon-alpha in cancer patients: phenomenology and paroxetine responsiveness of symptom dimensions. *Neuropsychopharmacology*, 26, 643, 2002.

22. Gochee, P.A. et al. Association between apolipoprotein E 4 and neuropsychiatric symptoms during interferon alpha treatment for chronic hepatitis C. *Psychosomatics*, 45, 49, 2004.

23. Maes, M. and Bonaccorso, S. Lower activities of serum peptidases predict higher depressive and anxiety levels following interferon-alpha-based immunotherapy in patients with hepatitis C. *Acta Psychiatr Scand*, 109, 126, 2004.

24. Capuron, L. et al. Baseline mood and psychosocial characteristics of patients developing depressive symptoms during interleukin-2 and/or inteferon-alpha cancer therapy. *Brain Behav Immun*, 18, 205, 2004.

25. Ranjith, G. et al. unpublished data, 2005.

26. Loftis, J.M. et al. Association of interferon-alpha-induced depression and improved treatment response in patients with hepatitis C. *Neurosci Lett*, 365, 87, 2004.

27. Raison, C.L. et al. Depressive symptoms and viral clearance in patients receiving interferon-alpha and ribavirin for hepatitis C. *Brain Behav Immun*, 19, 23, 2005.

28. Bonaccorso, S. et al. Immunotherapy with interferon-alpha in patients affected by chronic hepatitis C induces an intercorrelated stimulation of the cytokine network and an increase in depression and anxiety symptoms. *Psychiatr Res*, 105, 45, 2001.

29. Wichers M. and Maes M. The role of indoleamine 2,3-dioxygenase (IDO) in the pathophysiology of interferon-alpha-induced depression. *J Psychiatr Neurosci*, 29, 11, 2004.

30. Capuron, L. et al. Interferon-alpha-induced changes in tryptophan metabolism: relationship to depression and paroxetine treatment. *Biol Psychiatr*, 54, 906, 2003.

31. Van Gool, A.R. et al. Serum amino acids, biopterin and neopterin during long-term immunotherapy with interferon-alpha in high-risk melanoma patients. *Psychiatr Res*, 119, 125, 2003.

32. Bonnaccorso, S. et al. Increased depressive ratings in patients with hepatitis C receiving interferon-alpha-based immunotherapy are related to interferon alpha-induced changes in the serotonergic system. *J Clin Psychopharmacol*, 22, 86, 2002.

33. Wichers, M. and Maes, M. The psychoneuroimmunopathophysiology of cytokine-induced depression in humans. *Int J Neuropsychopharmacol*, 5, 375, 2002.

34. Maddock, C. et al. Psychopharmacological treatment of depression, anxiety, irritability and insomnia in patients receiving interferon-alpha: a prospective case series and a discussion of biological mechanisms. *J Psychopharmacol*, 18, 41, 2004.

35. Suzuki, E. et al. Nitric oxide involvement in depression during interferon-alpha therapy. *Int J Neuropharmacol*, 6, 415, 2003.
36. Cassidy, E.M. et al. Acute effects of low-dose interferon-a on serum cortisol and plasma interleukin-6. *J Psychopharmacol*, 16, 230, 2002.
37. Capuron, L. et al. Association of exaggerated HPA axis response to the initial injection of interferon-alpha with development of depression during interferon-alpha therapy. *Am J Psychiatr*, 160, 1342, 2003.
38. Pariante, C.M. et al. The proinflammatory cytokine, interleukin-1-alpha reduces glucocorticoid receptor translocation and function. *Endocrinology*, 140, 4359, 1999.
39. Maddock, C. and Pariante, C. How does stress affect you? An overview of stress, immunity, depression and disease. *Epidemiol Psichiatri Soc*, 10, 153, 2001.
40. Charlton, B.G. The malaise theory of depression: major depressive disorder is sickness behaviour and antidepressants are analgesic. *Med Hypotheses*, 54, 126, 2000.
41. Pariante, C.M., Miller, A. Glucocorticoid recertors in major depression: relevance to pathophysiology and treatment. *Biol Psychiatr*, 49, 391, 2001.
42. Juruena, M., Cleare, A.J., and Pariante, C.M. The hypothalamic pituitary adrenal axis, glucocorticoid receptor function and relevance to depression. *Rev Bras Pisquatr*, 26, 189, 2004.
43. Fukuda, K. et al. The chronic fatigue fatigue syndrome: a comprehensive approach to the study of its definition and study. *Ann Int Med*, 121, 953, 1994.
44. Natelson, B.H., Haghighi, M.H., and Ponzio, N.M. Evidence for the presence of immune dysfunction in chronic fatigue syndrome. *Clin Diagn Lab Immunol*, 9, 747, 2002.
45. Lyall, M., Peakman, M., and Wessely, S. A systematic review and critical evaluation of the immunology of chronic fatigue syndrome. *J Psychosom Res*, 55, 79, 2003.
46. Cleare, A.J. The neurobiology of chronic fatigue syndrome. *Endocrine Rev.*, 24, 236, 2003.
47. Cleare, A.J. et al. Low-dose hydrocortisone in chronic fatigue syndrome: a randomised crossover trial. *Lancet*, 353, 455, 1999.
48. Papanicolou, D.A. et al. Neuroendocrine aspects of chronic fatigue syndrome. *Neuroimmunomodulation*, 11, 65, 2003.
49. Capuron, L. and Miller, A.H. Cytokines and psychopathology: lessons from interferon-alpha. *Biol Psychiatr*, 56, 819, 2004.
50. De Lange, F.P. et al. Neural correlates of chronic fatigue syndrome: an fMRI study. *Brain*, 127, 1948, 2004.
51. Kendler, K.S., Gardner, C.O., and Prescott, C.A. Towards a comprehensive developmental model for major depression in women. *Am J Psychiatr*, 159, 1133, 2002.
52. White, P.D. What causes chronic fatigue syndrome? *Br Med J*, 329, 928, 2004.
53. Matthews, S.C., Paulus, M.P., and Dimsdale, J.E. Contribution of functional neuroimaging to understanding neuropsychiatric side effects of interferon in hepatitis C. *Psychosomatics*, 45, 28, 2004.

20 Role of Genetic Predisposition, Cytokines, and Neuroendocrine Response in Development of Thyroid Autoimmunity

Antonio Martocchia and Paolo Falaschi

CONTENTS

INTRODUCTION

Thyroid autoimmunity was described about 48 years ago with the identification of antibodies against thyroglobulin in patients with Hashimoto's thyroiditis (HT) and against the thyrotropin-stimulating hormone (TSH) receptor in patients with Graves' disease (GD).[1,2]

The clinical spectrum of the pathogenetic autoimmune mechanism may include hypofunction and hyperfunction of the gland, silent and focal thyroiditis, and cellular and humoral immune responses against the thyroid. An immune-mediated mechanism has been also demonstrated in painful subacute thyroiditis (with absence or low levels of circulating anti-thyroid autoantibodies) and in variants of autoimmune thyroid diseases (AITDs) such as postpartum thyroiditis and drug-induced thyroiditis (lithium, amiodarone, interferons).[3,4]

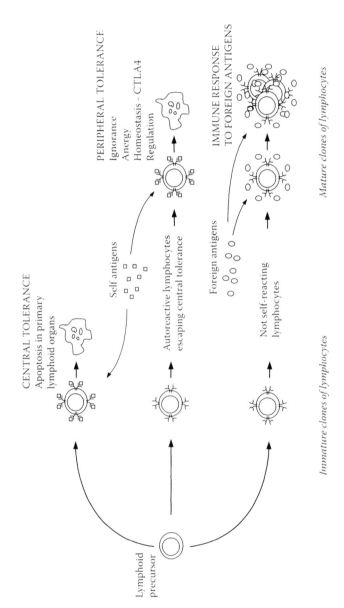

FIGURE 20.1 Normal immune response to self and foreign antigens.

The etiology of AITDs remains unknown. Increasing evidence in the literature suggests a genetic influence in the development of the autoimmune response, with the susceptibility genes, environmental triggers, and endogenous factors acting in concert in the early stages of the disease to initiate autoimmunity.[5,6]

Autoimmunity refers to the presence of autoantibodies (Abs) or T lymphocytes that react with self antigens. Autoimmunity is prevalent in healthy older subjects, in various infections, and it may usually be self-limited while the pathologic consequences resulting from self reactivity depend on the tissue damage induced by the immunologic reaction (Abs that bind and activate the TSH receptor in GD, antibody-dependent cellular cytotoxicity to thyroglobulin and thyroid peroxidase and T cell-mediated injury in HT).

Autoimmunity represents the end result of the breakdown of the basic mechanisms regulating immune tolerance in respect to self antigens. Central and peripheral processes are involved in the maintenance of the unresponsiveness to autoantigens (Figure 20.1). Autoreactive lymphocytes may undergo clonal deletion during fetal and early postnatal life. Since clones of cells responding to autoantigens are easily demonstrated in normal circulation, other peripheral mechanisms have to control the immune response to prevent autoimmunity, like the sequestration of self antigens in inaccessible sites, the specific anergy of T and B lymphocytes, regulatory mechanisms through costimulatory signals, or anti-idiotype antibodies or T cell activities.

PATHOGENETIC MECHANISMS INDUCING AUTOIMMUNITY

Derangements may derive from exogenous stimulation of the immune system as in molecular mimicry, superantigen stimulation, or microbial adjuvanticity. On the other hand, endogenous agents may predispose to the development to autoimmunity. In the central event of the immune response, the antigen-presenting cell (APC) presents the antigen bound to the human leukocyte antigen (HLA) class II to the CD4+ T cell that recognizes the antigen through the α/β T cell receptor (Figure 20.2). This interaction leads to activation of the T cell in the presence of an additional costimulation (engagement of B7 with CD28 and CD40 with CD40 ligand) and to unresponsiveness of the T cell in the presence of a negative signal (engagement of B7 with CTLA-4).

Alteration of antigen presentation may induce autoimmunity through a variety of mechanisms such as the loss of privilege, the spreading of novel or cryptic epitopes, the alteration of self antigens, the enhanced function of APCs by costimulatory molecule expression or cytokine production, the increased T cell help by costimulatory molecules or cytokine production, the increase of B cell function, the apoptosis defect, the cytokine imbalance, and the altered immunoregulation by anti-idiotype and regulatory T cells.

The evidence of a genetic susceptibility in AITD is based on the observation of thyroid Abs in siblings of probands with autoimmune thyroid disease, the association with HLA class II antigens, the concordance studies in twins, the association with CTLA-4 polymorphism, and the linkage with chromosomal locations (14q31, 18q21,

Antigen presenting cell

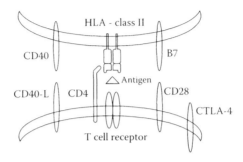

Tlymphocyte

FIGURE 20.2 Presentation of antigen by antigen-presenting cell to T lymphocyte.

20q11, Xp11, Xq21, 6p, 13q32, 12q22).[7–12] Excluding some commune genes, fluctuations between hypofunction and hyperfunction in some clinical courses, and a partially shared pathogenesis, the differences among the different models of AITDs are striking.

Environmental risk factors for AITD may include pollution (including radioactive emissions) and excess iodine intake (through jodbasedow, Wolff–Chaikoff effect, or immunological release of autoantigens). Smoking is a well-known major risk factor for thyroid-associated ophthalmopathy. Among toxins and infections, congenital rubella syndrome is frequently associated with AITD, whereas Epstein–Barr and *Yersinia enterocolitica* have been investigated as potential triggers of AITD. Allostatic load in stress response may be a condition favoring the development of AITDs. An increasing number of drugs like lithium, amiodarone, interferons (IFNs), and anti-CD52 monoclonal antibody Campath-1H may induce AITD.[13–16] In particular, preparations of leukocyte-derived IFN contaminated with γ-IFN were potent inducers *in vivo* of AITD in humans.[17]

AITD incidence clearly increases with age, resulting from extended exposure to environmental factors and possibly changes in immune regulation. Among the endogenous factors, a sexual dimorphism has been described in AITD and in other autoimmune diseases, with increased incidence in women (female:male = 4–10:1). Post-partum thyroiditis occurs in 5% of women.

Regarding the mechanisms by which sex steroids affect susceptibility to autoimmune disease, it is worth noting that the effects of sex hormones on the immune system may be directly or indirectly mediated through actions of the hypothalamic–pituitary–gonadal (HPG) or hypothalamic–pituitary–adrenal (HPA) axis. Sex hormones may directly affect immune mechanisms, including the homing of lymphocytes, the expression of adhesion molecules, the balance between Th1 and Th2 responses, the transcription and translation of cytokine genes, antigen presentation and costimulation

(B7.1, B7.2, and CD40), and T cell receptor signaling[18] To become a target of sex steroid hormones, cells of the immune system must express the cognate receptor. In fact, the presence of these receptors (respectively for androgens, estrogens, and progesterone) has been demonstrated on immune cells. A model of interactions between the initiating factors (susceptibility genes/environmental stimuli) and the modulating factors (sex hormones/neuroendocrine influences) has been proposed in the progression of the autoimmune diseases. A marked increase in hyperthyroidism was reported during the early years of World War II. More recently, the association between life events and the onset of GD was examined.[19]

At physiological concentrations, glucocorticoids inhibit Th1 (characterized by production of pro-inflammatory IL-2 and γ-IFN) and enhance Th2 cytokine production (characterized by production of IL-4 and IL-10), thus shifting immune responses from a Th1 to a Th2 pattern.[20–22] Cytokines exhibit different degrees of sensitivity to glucocorticoid suppression under physiological conditions. At lower evening cortisol levels, IL-6, tumor necrosis factor (TNF), and IL-1 are produced equally in response to a pro-inflammatory stimulus, while at higher morning levels and with stress levels produced during exercise, relative amounts of these cytokines change because IL-6 is relatively resistant to the suppression. At high stress levels of glucocorticoids, IL-6 remains elevated while IL-1 and TNF are significantly suppressed. The association between a blunted HPA axis and susceptibility to autoimmune/inflammatory disease has been clearly shown in many animal models, across species, strains, and diseases.[23]

γ-IFN is the only cytokine capable of inducing class II expression on thyroid cells *in vitro*.[24] Intrathyroidal CD4+ clones from patients with both GD and HT produce the following cytokines: γ-IFN, IL-2, IL-6 (stimulating both T and B cells), IL-8 (chemoattractant for mononuclear cell infiltration), TGF-β, TNF-α, and lymphotoxin.[25] Class II molecule expression in thyrocytes seems to be the result of the cytokine production by T cells and, in particular, of the γ-IFN release, but other factors may modify this. TNF has a synergistic effect with γ-IFN: both cytokines individually increase constitutive class I expression.[26] TSH and thyroid-stimulating antibodies can also enhance γ-IFN-induced class II molecules.[27] Transient expression of class II on thyrocytes may induce peripheral tolerance in potentially autoreactive T cells, but it induces proliferation response in previously activated T cells that do not require a costimulatory signal in the presence of thyroid autoantigens.

Autoimmunity may derive from a decrease of local production of immunosuppressive cytokines like transforming growth factor (TGF)-β and IL-10, a biased production of cytokines by Th1 phenotype cells in respect of Th2 cells or a decreased apoptosis of activated T cells (as in defects of interaction of Fas [CD95] and Fas ligand).

HCV-RELATED CHRONIC HEPATITIS, α-IFN TREATMENT, AND DEVELOPMENT OF AITD

Chronic hepatitis C virus (HCV) infection may be associated with AITD (10%) and thyroid dysfunction (3%). The hypothyroidism:hyperthyroidism ratio in HCV-related AITD approaches 2:1.[28–37] Underlying latent thyroid disorders may be exacerbated or induced by α-IFN therapy for HCV-related chronic hepatitis, increasing the incidence rates of AITD and dysfunction to 20 and 11% respectively.[28-31,33-35,37,38] The α-IFN therapy is associated with the *de novo* appearance of thyroid Abs and overt dysfunctions in pre-existing euthyroid subjects. This suggest that α-IFN is a direct inducer of AITD.[28,29,33-35,37,38]

Age, female gender, and pre-existing positive Abs are well known risk factors for the development of AITD in IFN-treated HCV patients.[28,29,31,33,39] The human leukocyte antigen (HLA) may be an independent risk factor for liver and thyroid diseases, suggesting a genetic predisposition to immune-mediated organ damage.[40,41]

In the next section, we describe our experience with AITD during α-IFN treatment for viral chronic hepatitis. This appears to be an interesting clinical model for autoimmunity, since it includes interactions of both environmental and endogenous factors.

The aim of our first observation was to investigate the effect of recombinant human α-IFN (rhα-IFN) on hypothalamic–pituitary–thyroid (HPT) axis secretion.[42] It is noteworthy that α-IFN administration in humans may induce increases of endogenous γ-IFN and IL-6, thus supporting a well-defined sequence in the cascade of cytokines able to modulate neuroendocrine axis secretion.[43] At thyroid level, IFNs (α, β, and γ) inhibit TSH-induced thyroid functions (iodide uptake and hormone release) on human thyrocyte cultures.[44] At pituitary level, γ-IFN and IL-6 do not induce any change in TSH release.[45] At hypothalamic level, γ-IFN stimulates soma-tostatin release[46] that causes TSH suppression.

The effect of rhα-IFN (3 million international units [IU] intramuscularly [im] 3 times weekly) on the HPT axis was studied in 12 patients with viral chronic hepatitis, selected on the basis of negative anti-thyroid Abs. A slight and not statis-tically relevant decrease of thyroid hormones and TSH blood levels was observed after rhα-IFN administration. TSH response to TRH was in the normal range either before or after the therapy. At the end of the treatment, the absence of anti-thyroid Abs was confirmed in all the patients, and none developed thyroid disorders after the therapy. It was therefore assumed that rhα-IFN does not induce development of autoimmunity, but it enhances the levels of pre-existing thyroid Abs and exacerbates subclinical autoimmunity.

We described an interesting case of subacute thyroiditis during α-IFN therapy for HCV-related chronic hepatitis, confirmed by laboratory, ultrasonography, radio-iodine scanning, and fine needle aspiration findings.[47] The interesting feature of the case was the persisting negative results of anti-thyroid Abs after α-IFN therapy. A possible viral infection (Coxsackie virus, mumps, Epstein–Barr virus, adenovirus, cytomegalovirus) is commonly suggested in De Quervain thyroiditis[48] and an asso-ciation with HLA-Bw35 has been described.[49] Our patient had no viral disease other than chronic hepatitis C; the HLAB-35 was positive.

α-IFN has a regulatory role in the differentiation of human CD4+ T cells by favoring their development on Th1 cells.[50] During viral infection, macrophages may process and present antigens to Th cells in the presence of cytokines (i.e., α-IFN, IL-12) that induce them to differentiate toward the Th1 phenotype. The Th1-type-specific immune response may cause cellular damage along with a direct action of viruses on cells. In a subject with an unusual susceptibility to viral infections (such as our patient with HLAB-35 antigen), the process that led to thyroiditis and thyroid damage may be facilitated by α-IFN therapy.

It has been recently hypothesized that HCV may exert direct extrahepatic effects, both on the immune system and thyroid cells, interfering with their functions and with the fundamental mechanisms of self recognition.[33,51] Therefore, HCV may start autoimmune thyroid disease by directly destroying thyroid tissue or mimicking the structure of some component of the thyroid gland. In a second case report from this group, a euthyroid patient with HCV infection and negative anti-thyroid Abs before α-IFN treatment developed Hashimoto's disease during treatment.[52] The study of HLA antigen showed the typical association for Hashimoto's disease (HLA-DR5) in Caucasians.[53] This second case suggested that the study of HLA antigens may be a useful tool for detecting patients with predispositions to developing AITDs.

Therefore, we decided to start a preliminary longitudinal study in 15 patients (10 females and 5 males, 38 to 74 years of age) with chronic hepatitis C. All patients were negative for thyroid disorders at the baseline. The genotype of the virus was determined according to Simmonds' classification.[54] Eleven patients were treated with rhα-IFN 2a (3 to 6×10^6 IU im 3 times weekly). No treatments were given to the other four patients.

Every patient's HLA system was examined to evaluate the antigens (n = 40) of the loci A, B, and Cw (by the complement-dependent lymphocyte cytotoxicity test) and the alleles (n = 19) of the loci DRB1* and DQB1* (by the polymerase chain reaction [PCR] method with sequence-specific primers [SSPs]). The HLA-DR3 and HLA-DR5 antigens correspond to the HLA-DRB1.03 and to the HLA-DRB1.11/HLA-DRB1.12 alleles, respectively.

The relationship between the HLA and thyroid disorders during the α-IFN treatment was evaluated, with particular attention to the well-known association between the HLA system and thyroid disorders. HLA-A2 has been demonstrated in thyroid disorders (with clinical features of either thyrotoxicosis/hyperthyroidism or hypothyroidism) presented during α-IFN therapy in patients with chronic hepatitis C.[41] The immune-mediated subacute thyroiditis has been associated with HLA-B35.[49,55] HLA-DR3 (HLA-DRB1.03) has been found in autoimmune thyrotoxicosis/hyperthyroidism,[56-60] while HLA-B35 and HLA-DR5 (HLA-DRB1.11/HLA-DRB1.12) have been found in autoimmune hypothyroidism.[61-63] The antigen/allele HLA frequency was also evaluated in healthy subjects (n = 107) as a control group. The HCV genotypes in the whole group of patients were 1b (20%), 2a (60%), and 3a (20%). The genotype distribution (1b:2a:3a) was 1:3:1; no patient presented a mixed HCV genotype.

Eleven of fifteen patients received the rhα-IFN 2a treatment (duration of treatment: 3 to 12 months; duration of follow-up after α-IFN therapy: 18 to 42 months). Four patients entered the follow-up protocol without receiving the α-IFN treatment (duration of follow-up: 12 to 38 months). Six of fifteen patients (40%) presented double positive HLA results (HLA-A2/B-35, HLA-A2/DRB1.03, HLA-A2/DRB1.11, or HLA-B35/DRB1.11). Five of six patients with double-positive HLA received α-IFN treatment. Four double-positive HLA patients treated with α-IFN developed clinical thyroid disorders, including two cases of autoimmune hypothyroidism, one case of transient thyrotoxicosis in autoimmune hypothyroidism before treatment, and one case of subacute thyroiditis.

The mean ages of patients with thyroid disorders were lower but not significantly different with respect to patients who had no thyroid diseases. All the patients presenting thyroid disorders were females. These patients had the HLA system susceptibility to the development of thyroid diseases and the HLA system was specifically associated with the particular kind of the thyroid disorder the patient had. The patient with subacute thyroiditis was HLA-B35-positive; the patient with thyrotoxicosis was HLA-DRB1.03-positive. The two patients with autoimmune hypothyroidism were HLA-DRB1.11-positive. In addition, these patients presented double-positive HLA susceptibilities (HLA-A2/DRB1.11, HLA-A2/DRB1.03, HLA-A2/B35, and HLA-B35/DRB1.11). The HLA-A2 was not specific for the kind of thyroid disorder; it was present in hypothyroidism, in thyrotoxicosis, and in thyroiditis.

The development of thyroid disorders in the α-IFN-treated patients with HCV chronic hepatitis was significantly associated with presence of the double-positive HLA (p <0.05; see Table 20.1). The analysis of the relationship between the development of thyroid disorders and the HCV genotype did not reveal significant association.

This preliminary study showed that α-IFN treatment induced the development of thyroid disorders in 36% (4 of 11) of patients with HCV-related chronic hepatitis and in 30% (3 of 10) of patients with pre-treatment negative anti-thyroid Abs.

Previous studies showed that female gender, older age, pre-existing positive anti-thyroid Abs, and mixed genotype infections were associated with the higher frequencies of AITDs in α-IFN-treated patients with HCV-related chronic hepatitis.[28,40,32,33,36,37] Our results suggest that the HLA system is an additional and very strong susceptibility factor to the development of AITD. In particular, in the patients who presented two antigens together, the double association seemed to increase the risk of AITD.

TABLE 20.1

Association of Double-Positive HLA System and Development of AITD during α-IFN Treatment for HCV-Related Chronic Hepatitis

	Patients who developed AITD		Patients who did not develop AITD		Total patients		
	HLA pos.	HLA neg.	HLA pos.	HLA neg.	HLA pos.	HLA neg.	
Treated patients	4	0	1	6	5	6	p<0.05
Untreated patients	0	0	1	3	1	3	

Double positive HLA system: HLA-A2/B35
HLA-A2/DRB1.03
HLA-A2/DRB1.11
HLA-B35/DRB1.11

AITD = autoimmune thyroid disease. IFN = interferon. HCV = hepatitis C virus.

The HLA-A2 antigen is involved in the I class molecule-restricted presentation of viral peptides by APCs to cytotoxic T lymphocytes (CTLs) during HCV chronic infection.[64] APCs may induce an HLA-A2-restricted CTL immune response against viral peptides in order to cleave the infected cells, and the response is strongly increased by α-IFN treatment.[65] The CTL-mediated mechanism may be involved in the recognition and in response against I class HLA-restricted viral and cross-reacting self peptides, the final outcome of the response being the disruption of the target cells (both at the liver and thyroid gland levels).[66,67] The HLA-A2 antigen was not specific for this kind of thyroid disorder and, in fact, was associated with cases of hypothyroidism, thyrotoxicosis, and thyroiditis [41].

The HLA-B35, HLA-DR3 and HLA-DR5 antigens may play a different and more relevant role in α-IFN induced AITDs, being specifically associated with these kinds of thyroid disorders.[41,49,55–63] In our study, the HLA system was associated with thyroid disease and, in particular, when two (I and/or II class) HLA antigens were associated in a single patient, their potential role in the susceptibility to the development of thyroid disorders became significant.

In conclusion, our preliminary results on the occurrence of AITD during α-IFN treatment for HCV-related chronic hepatitis suggest that the HLA system may be an important risk factor for the appearance of AITD, particularly in patients with double-positive HLA genetic backgrounds. Further studies are necessary to confirm the useful predictive value of HLA system typing as part of basal assessments in a larger group of patients.

REFERENCES

1. Adams, D.D. and Purves H.D., Abnormal responses in the assay of thyrotrophin, *Proc. Univ. Otago Med. School*, 34, 11, 1956.
2. Roitt, I.M. et al., Autoantibodies in Hashimoto's disease (lymphoadenoid goitre), *Lancet* II, 820, 1956.
3. Martino, A. et al., The effects of amiodarone on the thyroid, *Endocr. Rev.*, 22, 240, 2001.
4. Stagnaro-Green, A., Postpartum thyroiditis, *J. Clin. Endocrinol. Metab.*, 87, 4042, 2002.
5. Tomer, Y. and Davies, T.F., Searching for the autoimmune thyroid disease susceptibility genes: from gene mapping to gene function, *Endocr. Rev.*, 24, 694, 2003.
6. Weetman, A.P., Autoimmune thyroid disease: propagation and progression, *Eur. J. Endocrinol.*, 148, 1, 2003.
7. Bech, K. et al., HLA antigens in Graves' disease, *Acta Endrocrinol.* 86, 510, 1977.
8. Brix, T.H., Kyvik, K.O., and Hegedus, L., What is evidence of genetic factor in the aetiology of Graves' disease? A brief review, *Thyroid*, 8, 727, 1998.
9. Hall, R., Owen, S.G., and Smart, G.S., Evidence for genetic predisposition to formation of thyroid autoantibodies, *Lancet*, II, 187, 1964.
10. Hunt, P.J. et al., Histocompatibility leukocyte antigens and closely linked immunomodulatory genes in autoimmune thyroid disease, *Clin. Endocrinol.* 55, 491, 2001.
11. Tomer, Y. et al., A new Graves' disease susceptibility locus maps to chromosome 20q11.2, *Am. J. Hum. Gen.*, 63, 1749, 1998.

12. Yanagawa, T. et al., CTLA-4 gene polymorphism associated with Graves' disease in Caucasian population, *J. Clin. Endocrinol. Metab.*, 80, 41, 1995.

13. Chiovato, L. and Pinchera, A., Stressful life events and Graves' disease, *Eur. J. Endocrinol.*, 134, 680, 1996.

14. Coles, A. et al., Pulsed monoclonal antibody treatment and autoimmune thyroid disease in multiple sclerosis, *Lancet*, 354, 183, 1999.

15. Ruwhof, C. and Drexhage, H.A., Iodine and thyroid autoimmune disease in animal models, *Thyroid*, 11, 427, 2001.

16. Weetman, A.P. and McGregor, A.M., Autoimmune thyroid disease: further developments in our understanding, *Endocrinol. Rev.*, 15, 788, 1994.

17. Burman, P. et al., Thyroid autoimmunity in patients on long-term therapy with leukocyte-derived interferon, *J. Clin. Endocrinol. Metab.*, 63, 1086, 1986.

18. Whitacre, C.C., Sex differences in autoimmune disease, *Nature Immunol.*, 2, 777, 2001.

19. Lidman, K. et al., Stressful life events and Graves' disease, *Lancet*, 338, 1475, 1991.

20. Elenkov, I.J. and Chrousos G.P., Stress hormones, TH1/TH2 patterns, pro/anti-inflammatory cytokines and susceptibility to disease, *Trends Endocrinol. Metab.*, 10, 359, 1999.

21. Franchimont, D. et al. Inhibition of TH1 immune response by glucocorticoids: dexamethasone selectively inhibits IL-12-induced Stat4 phosphorylation in T lymphocytes, *J. Immunol.*, 164, 1768, 2000.

22. McGregor, A.M., Immunoendocrine interactions and autoimmunity, *New Engl. J. Med.*, 322, 1739, 1990.

23. Sternberg, E.M., Neuroendocrine regulation of autoimmune/inflammatory disease, *J. Endocrinol.*, 169, 429, 2001.

24. Iwatani, Y. et al., Thyrocyte HLA-DR expression and interferon-γ production in autoimmune thyroid disease, *J. Clin. Endocrinol. Metab.*, 63, 695, 1986.

25. Grubeck-Loebenstein, B. et al., CD4+ T-cell clones from autoimmune thyroid tissue cannot be classified according to their lymphokine production, *Scand. J. Immunol.*, 32, 433, 1990.

26. Bucsema, M. et al., Influence of tumour necrosis factor-α on the modulation by interferon-γ of HLA class II molecules in human thyroid cells and its effect on interferon-γ binding, *J. Clin. Endocrinol. Metab.*, 69, 433, 1990.

27. Todd, I. et al., Enhancement of thyrocyte HLA Class II expression by thyroid stimulating hormone, *Clin. Exp. Immunol.*, 69, 524, 1987.

28. Broussolle, C. et al., Hepatitis C virus infection and thyroid diseases, *Rev. Med. Int.*, 20, 766, 1999.

29. Carella, C. et al. Long-term outcome of interferon-alpha-induced thyroid autoimmunity and prognostic influence of thyroid autoantibody pattern at the end of treatment, *J. Clin. Endocrinol. Metab.*, 86, 1925, 2001.

30. Deutsch, M. et al., Thyroid abnormalities in chronic viral hepatitis and their relationship to interferon alpha therapy, *Hepatology*, 26, 206, 1997.

31. Fernandez-Soto, L. et al., Increased risk of autoimmune thyroid disease in hepatitis C vs hepatitis B before, during, and after discontinuing interferon therapy, *Arch. Int. Med.*, 158, 1445, 1998.

32. Ganne-Carrie, N. et al., Latent autoimmune thyroiditis in untreated patients with HCV chronic hepatitis. Case-control study, *J. Autoimmun.*, 14, 189, 2000.

33. Hsieh, M.C. et al., Virologic factors related to interferon-alpha-induced thyroid dysfunction in patients with chronic hepatitis C, *Eur. J. Endocrinol.*, 142, 431, 2000.

34. Marazuela, M. et al., Thyroid autoimmune disorders in patients with chronic hepatitis C before and during interferon-alpha therapy, *Clin. Endocrinol.*, 44, 635, 1996.

35. Marcellin, P., Pouteau, M., and Benahamou, J.P., Hepatitis C virus infection, alpha interferon therapy and thyroid dysfunction, *J. Hepatol.*, 22, 364, 1995.

36. Oppenheim, Y., Ban, Y., and Tomer, Y. Interferon induced autoimmune thyroid disease (AITD): a model of human autoimmunity, *Autoimmun. Rev.*, 3, 388, 2004.

37. Prummel, M.F. and Laurberg, P., Interferon-alpha and autoimmune thyroid disease, *Thyroid*, 13, 547, 2003.

38. Rocco, A. et al., Incidence of autoimmune thyroiditis in interferon-alpha treated and untreated patients with chronic hepatitis C virus infection, *Neuroendocrinol Lett.*, 22, 39, 2001.

39. Huang, M.J. et al., Prevalence and significance of thyroid autoantibodies in patients with chronic hepatitis C virus infection: a prospective controlled study, *Clin. Endocrinol.*, 50, 503, 1999.

40. Czaja, A. et al., Immunologic features and HLA associations in chronic viral hepatitis, *Gastroenterology*, 108, 157, 1995.

41. Kakizaki, S. et al., HLA antigens in patients with interferon-α-induced autoimmune thyroid disorders in chronic hepatitis C, *J. Hepatol.*, 30, 794, 1999.

42. Falaschi, P. et al., Effect of r-interferon alpha administration on hypothalamus–pituitary–thyroid axis in chronic hepatitis, *Life Sci.*, 60, 43, 1997.

43. Gisslinger, H. et al., Thyroid autoimmunity and hypothyroidism during long-term treatment with recombinant interferon-alpha, *Clin. Exp. Immunol.*, 90, 363, 1992.

44. Yamazaki, K. et al., Reversible inhibition by interferons alpha and beta of 125I incorporation and thyroid hormone release by human thyroid follicles in vitro, *J. Clin. Endocrinol. Metab.*, 77, 1439, 1993.

45. McCann, S.M. et al., Mechanism of action of cytokines to induce the pattern of pituitary hormone secretion in infection, *Ann. NY Acad. Sci.*, 29, 386, 1995.

46. Ryu, S.Y. et al., Somatostatin and substance P induced *in vivo* by lipopolysaccharide and in peritoneal macrophages stimulated with lipopolysaccharide or interferon-gamma have differential effects on murine cytokine production, *Neuroimmunomodulation*, 8, 25, 2000.

47. Falaschi, P. et al., Subacute thyroiditis during interferon-alpha therapy for chronic hepatitis C, *J. Endocrinol. Invest.*, 20, 24, 1997.

48. Hall, R., Subacute (De Quervain's) thyroiditis, in *Fundamentals of Clinical Endocrinology*, Hall, R. and Besser, G.M., Eds., Churchill Livingstone, Edinburgh, 1989, p. 101.

49. Nyulassy, S. et al., Subacute (De Quervain's) thyroiditis: association with HLA-Bw35 antigen and abnormalities of the complement system, immunoglobulins and other serum proteins, *J. Clin. Endocrinol. Metab.*, 45, 270, 1977.

50. Romagnani, S., Induction of Th1 and Th2 response: a key role for the "natural" immune response? *Immunol. Today*, 13, 379, 1992.

51. Lunel, F., Hepatitis C virus and autoimmunity: fortuitous association or reality? *Gastroenterology*, 107, 1550, 1994.

52. Martocchia, A. et al., Hashimoto's disease during interferon-alpha therapy in a patient with pre-treatment negative anti-thyroid autoantibodies and with the specific genetic susceptibility to the thyroid disease, *Neuroendocrinol Lett.*, 22, 49, 2001.

53. Defots, L.J. and Catherwood, B.D., Genetic aspects of autoimmune disorders, in *Basic and Clinical Endocrinology*, 2nd ed., Greenspan, F.S. and Forsham, P.H., Eds., Lange Medical Publications, Los Altos, CA, 1990, p. 655.

54. Simmonds, P., Variability of hepatitis C virus, *Hepatology*, 21, 570, 1995.

55. Ohsako, N. et al., Clinical characteristics of subacute thyroiditis classified according to human leukocyte antigen typing, *J. Clin. Endocrinol. Metab.*, 80, 3653, 1995.

56. Chen, Q.Y. et al., HLA-DRB1*08, DRB1*03/DRB3*0101, and DRB3*0202 are susceptibility genes for Graves' disease in North American Caucasians, whereas DRB1*07 is protective, *J. Clin. Endocrinol. Metab.*, 84, 3182, 1999.

57. Dalton, T.A. and Bennett, J.C., Autoimmune disease and the major histocompatibility complex: therapeutic implications, *Am. J. Med.*, 92, 183, 1992.

58. Heward, J.M. et al., Linkage disequilibrium between the human leukocyte antigen class II region of the major histocompatibility complex and Graves' disease: replication using a population case control and family-based study, *J. Clin. Endocrinol. Metab.*, 83, 3394, 1998.

59. Kinney, J.S. et al., Community outbreak of thyrotoxicosis: epidemiology, immunogenetic characteristics, and long term outcome, *Am. J. Med.*, 84, 10, 1988.

60. Zamani, M. et al., Primary role of the HLA class II DRB1*00301 allele in Graves' disease, *Am. J. Hum. Genet.*,18, 432, 2000.

61. Bogner, U. et al., HLA-DR/DQ gene variation in non-goitrous autoimmune thyroiditis at the serological and molecular level, *Autoimmunity*,14, 155, 1992.

62. Farid, N.R. et al., The association of goitrous autoimmune thyroiditis with HLA-DR5, *Tissue Antig.*, 17, 265, 1981.

63. Pocecco, M., Barbi, E., and De Campo, C., Autoimmune thyroid pathology: study and follow-up of pediatric case reports, *Pediat. Med. Chir.*, 6, 691, 1986.

64. Sarobe, P. et al., Characterization of an immunologically conserved epitope from the hepatitis C virus E2 glycoprotein recognized by HLA-A2 restricted cytotoxic T lymphocytes, *J. Hepatol.*, 34, 321, 2001.

65. Vertuani, S. et al., Effect of interferon-alpha therapy on epitope-specific cytotoxic T lymphocyte responses in hepatitis C virus-infected individuals, *Eur. J. Immunol.*, 32, 144, 2002.

66. Brazillet, M.P. et al., Induction of experimental autoimmune thyroiditis by heat-denatured porcine thyroglobulin: a CTL-mediated disease, *Eur. J. Immunol.*, 29, 1342, 1999.

67. Iwatani, Y. et al., Decrease in alpha beta T cell receptor negative T cells and CD8 cells, and an increase in CD4+CD8+ cells in active Hashimoto's disease and subacute thyroiditis, *Clin. Exp. Immunol.*, 87, 444, 1992.

21 Gender Differences, Stress, and Immunity*

Nicholas P. Plotnikoff and Robert E. Faith

CONTENTS

INTRODUCTION

It has long been known that there is a sexual dichotomy in immune function. Males produce less antibody and are more susceptible to infectious disease than are females (Batchelor & Chapman, 1965; Goble & Konopka, 1973; Michaels & Rogers, 1971; Stein & Davidsohn, 1955; Terres et.al. 1968; Washburn et al., 1965; Wheaton & Hurst, 1961; Willoughby & Watson, 1964). This dichotomy is apparently exhibited in all aspects of the immune system. Females have higher plasma concentrations of immunoglobulin (Eidinger & Garret, 1972; McCruden & Stimson, 1991; Rawley & McKay, 1969, Tartokovsky et al., 1981) and greater primary and secondary antibody responses to a number of antigens (Batchelor & Chapman, 1965; Kalland, 1980; London & Drew, 1977; Spencer et al., 1977; Terres et al., 1968). Some aspects of cell-mediated immunity are weaker in females than in males (Inman, 1978; Kalland, 1980; Santoli et al., 1976; Trinchieri & Zinijewski, 1976).

The difference in immune responses of men and women extends to autoimmunity. There is a greater prevalence of autoimmune diseases in women. These include rheumatoid arthritis, systemic lupus erythematosus (SLE), autoallergic thyroiditis, and multiple sclerosis (Chiovato et. al., 1993; Duquette et al., 1992; Grossman et. al., 1991;

---

* This chapter represents the views solely of the authors and no government agency. No official endorsement by the National Cancer Institute is intended or should be inferred.

Hockberg, 1981; Masi, 1984; McCruden & Stimson, 1981). Large amounts of information support the view that hormones of the endocrine system are involved in the sexual dichotomy of immune function. They include the gonadal steroids, the adrenal glucocorticoids, growth hormone, prolactin, and thymic hormones (Grossman, 1989). Both *in vivo* and *in vitro* evidence supports the role of these hormones in the sexual dichotomy of immunity.

Mathur et al. (1979) reported cyclic variations in circulating white blood cell subpopulations in the human menstrual cycle. These changes were correlated with levels of progesterone and estradiol. A negative correlation between estradiol levels and lymphocytes was reported, with minimum lymphocyte counts coinciding with peak estradiol levels. It was also observed that these cyclic changes do not occur in males or in females in non-ovulatory cycles (Mathur et al., 1979). The authors speculate that the drop in lymphocyte counts, especially T cells, around midcycle, i.e., at the time of ovulation, may play a role suppressing immunoreactivity at the time of possible impregnation, thus enhancing the survival of a fertilized egg. Similarly, Krzych et al. (1978) reported that the immune responsiveness of female BALB/c mice was cyclic in harmony with estrus cyclic variations in the responses of isolated splenic lymphocytes from female BALB/c mice to mitogen stimulation depending upon when in the estrus cycle the cells were harvested.

Leslie & Dubey (1994) studied the production of prostaglandins by human monocytes. They found that when stimulated *in vitro* by bacterial lipopolysaccharide (LPS), monocytes isolated from females produced on average significantly more prostaglandin than did monocytes isolated from males. When changes coincident with the female menstrual cycle were studied, it was found that significantly more prostaglandin was produced by LPS-stimulated monocytes isolated during the luteal phase of the cycle than during the early follicular phase (Leslie & Dubey, 1994). The authors suggested that *in vivo* hormonal changes associated with the menstrual cycle modulated monocyte synthesis of prostaglandins and other immune modulators such as interleukin-1. They further suggest that this could be a key to understanding differences in vulnerability between males and females, as well as changes in females in different phases of the menstrual cycle, to immune and inflammatory insult.

The above studies indicate that the sex hormones, especially estrogens, are involved in the regulation of immune functions. For the sex hormones to function as immune modulators, one would expect the receptors for these hormones to exist within the immune system. Indeed, a number of studies have demonstrated the presence of such receptors. Estrogen binding sites have been demonstrated in four human thymomas (Ranelletti et al, 1980). Estrogen binding sites have been shown to exist and have been characterized in normal human mononuclear, spleen, and thymus cells (Cohen et al., 1983; Daniel et al., 1982; Kawashima et al., 1990). Receptors for estrogen have also been identified in mouse thymus (Detlefson et al., 1978) and in rat thymus (Barr et al., 1979; Imanishi et al., 1980; Malacarne et al., 1980). The bursa of Fabricius of the chicken has been shown to contain estrogen receptors (Sullivan & Wira, 1979). Finally, estrogen receptors have been shown to occur on the suppressor/cytotoxic subsets of human T cells, but not on the helper subsets (Cohen et al., 1983; Stimson, 1988).

Receptors for androgens and progestagens have also been demonstrated to exist within the immune system. While no androgen receptors have been demonstrated in any class of lymphocyte, androgen receptors have been shown to occur in the epithelial portion of the thymus (Grossman et al., 1979; McCruden & Stimson, 1980; Raveche et al., 1980; Sasson & Mayer, 1981). Androgen receptors have also been demonstrated to occur in the bursa of Fabricius of chickens (Sullivan & Wica, 1979). The epithelial position of the thymus has been shown to possess a specific high-affinity receptor for progesterone (Pearce et al., 1983; Sakabe et al., 1986).

Androgens have been shown to have the ability to modify immune function. Testosterone was observed to suppress the reactivity of passively transferred lymphocytes (Rifkind et al., 1973) and increase susceptibility to infection (Levine & Madin, 1961). It has been indicated that the testes exert a regulatory effect upon the growth of the thymus, particularly at the time of puberty (Goldstein et al., 1974) when the growth of the testes is correlated with thymic involution. It has been shown that testosterone can inhibit the *in vitro* immune response against sheep red blood cells (SRBCs), with a complete inhibition of the response obtained with a testosterone concentration of 100Fg/ml (Deschaux et al., 1980). This study also showed that testosterone inhibits the stimulatory effects of thymosin. The authors speculate that testosterone may suppress immune function by interfering with the mode of action of thymosin; thus thymosin-induced amplification of immune response may be less efficient when androgen levels are increased.

Testosterone appears able to directly affect lymphocyte population interactions with other compounds. It significantly inhibits the plaque forming cell responses of human peripheral blood mononuclear cells (PBMCs) stimulated by pokeweed mitogen (Sthoeger et al., 1988). This response was observed in cells obtained from normal men and women and appears to be an early event because testosterone had to be added to the cultures in the first 12 hours for the effect to be observed. Athreya et al. (1993) showed testosterone to significantly increase the percentage of CD4+ cells following *in vitro* interleukin-2 (IL-2) stimulation of human PBMCs. Finally, there is some indication that androgens may inhibit development of autoimmune disease in males (Kappas et al., 1963). Androgens have been used to treat human systemic lupus erythematosus patients with some success, whereas estrogen has been shown to exacerbate the condition (Amor et al., 1983; Horowitz et al., 1977; Morimoto, 1978).

Progesterone has been shown to influence various aspects of immune function. It appears to function as an agonist for the rat thymocyte glucocorticoid receptor (Kaiser et al., 1979) and progesterone metabolizing enzymes occur in the thymus (Weinstein et al., 1977). *In vitro* studies have shown that progesterone has the ability to inhibit blast transformation by lymphocytes stimulated with purified protein derivative (PPD) (Wyle & Kent, 1977) or phytohemagglutinin (PHA) (Tomada et al., 1976). The suppression of the PHA responsiveness of lymphocytes by progesterone has been reversed by the addition of IL-2 (Scambia et al., 1988). Chao et al. (1995) have shown progesterone to significantly stimulate a maximal release of tumor necrosis factor (TNF) from male rat peritoneal macrophages in a dose-dependent manner. *In vivo* progesterone has been shown to prolong the survival of skin grafts in animals (Kind & Ciacio, 1980; Sekiya et al., 1975) and to promote the generation of suppressor cell activity (Holdstock et al., 1982).

The most important of the sex hormone interactions leading to immunological dimorphism are the effects elicited by estrogens elaborated at elevated levels from the ovary after puberty (Grossman, 1989). The elevated levels of estrogens that follow puberty lead to increased prolactin levels, increased thymosin release, and basal growth hormone secretion (Grossman, 1989). All these hormones are hypothesized to effect lymphocyte development and stimulate adult T and B cell functions in females. It is also thought that interactions of hormonal regulatory axes involving the hypothalamus, pituitary, gonads, adrenals, and thymus are involved in these processes.

Estrogens have mixed effects on immune function. They have been shown to generally depress cell-mediated immunity (Ablin et al., 1988; Ablin et al., 1979; Comsa et al., 1982; Kuhl et al., 1983) while they have the ability to elevate antibody responses to T-dependent antigens (Brick et al., 1985; Stern & Davidson, 1955; Stimson & Hunter, 1980). Diethylstilbestrol (a synthetic estrogen) has been shown to cause depressed mitogen responsiveness and peripheral lymphopenia in female mice following neonatal treatment (Kalland et al., 1979). Estrogens have also been shown to reduce natural killer (NK) cell activity (Seaman & Ginhart, 1979). Kenny et al. (1976) studied the effects of estradiol on *in vivo* and *in vitro* antibody responses to Swiss Webster mice to heat-killed *Escherichia coli*. They found that a single dose of estradiol given from 1 day through 3.5 days after the administration of antigen significantly increased numbers of splenic antibody-producing cells in male mice sacrificed 4 days after receiving antigen. Administration of estradiol early in the proliferative phase of antibody production, i.e., 1 day before or 1 day after antigen administration, appeared to increase numbers of antibody-producing cells more than when estradiol was administered at a later time. Estradiol had a biphasic effect on *in vitro* antibody responses, with high concentrations enhancing responses while low concentrations were inhibiting (Kenny et al., 1976).

Estrogen at physiologic concentrations is able to elicit the production of immunoregulatory factors from thymic epithelial cultures, and these factors are different in character from those elicited by androgens (Stimson & Crilly, 1981). Supernatants from estrogen-treated thymic epithelial cell cultures inhibited the mitogen responsiveness of bone marrow cells, while supernatants from androgen-treated thymic epithelial cell cultures enhanced the mitogen responsiveness of bone marrow cells (Stimson & Crilly, 1981). The proliferation of thymocytes was similarly affected. These studies showed that physiologic concentrations of sex steroids may modify the production of thymic epithelial immunoregulatory factors (Stimson & Crilly, 1981). Sthoeger et al. studied the *in vitro* effects of physiologic concentrations of estradiol on the antigen non-specific differentiation of human peripheral blood mononuclear cells (PBMCs). Cells from normal male and female volunteers were cultured in the presence of pokeweed mitogen. When estradiol was added to the cultures, the mitogen responsiveness of cells from both sexes was enhanced. These types of processes must play a role in the *in vivo* response to sex steroids.

As mentioned above, the CD8+ set of lymphocytes has receptors for estrogen. There is evidence that estrogens can directly affect this subpopulation of lymphocytes both *in vivo* and *in vitro*. Estrogen inhibition of T cell-mediated suppression has been shown to enhance the pokeweed mitogen-stimulated immunoglobulin synthesis of B cells (Paavonen et al., 1981). Athreya et al. (1983) studied the proliferative responses of PBMCs from normal adult males to various stimuli in the presence or absence of estradiol. They showed estradiol to significantly enhance the percentage of CD8+ cells following stimulation with phytohemagglutinin (PHA).

Not only do estrogens affect lymphocytes, but they have also been shown to have effects on macrophages. Phagocytosis of IgG-coated erythrocytes by guinea pig macrophages was shown to be reduced by estradiol administered in levels similar to those found in pregnancy (Friedman et al., 1985). The clearance of circulating colloidal carbon in mice has been shown to be enhanced by estrogen (Nicol et al., 1964). Macrophages treated *in vitro* with physiological concentrations of estrogens increased lysosomal enzyme activity and phagocytosis (Stimson, 1983). The effects of estrogens on macrophages are most likely direct as macrophages have been shown to possess estrogen receptors. (Gulshan et al., 1990).

In addition to gender differences in immune function, there are also gender differences in response to stressors. The mechanisms involved in these gender differences may be similar or related. The following discussion focuses on depression as a stressor that exhibits gender differences in responses. Other gender differences are also explored.

Clinical depression occurs more frequently in females than in males. Is this tendency toward depression related to neuroendocrine influences? Review of other chapters in this book lends insight to the answer. Since depression is more common in females, it can be assumed that estrogen and progesterone influence mood states. (Perkins et al., 1991; Andrianopoulos & Flaherty, 1991).

Of specific interest is the finding that clinical depression may be accompanied by reduced immunocompetence (Stein et al., 1991). Thus, clinical depression accompanying loss of spouse (bereavement) or divorce may be correlated with reduced immunocompetence in clinical depression (Schleifer et al., 1983). Are there gender differences in reduced immunocompetence present in clinical depression? The available clinical data have not been compared in this manner. Most of the clinical studies cited were carefully matched as to age, sex, and clinical diagnosis but did not analyze the data in terms of possible gender differences. One such study was reported with multiple analysis of variance but no differences were apparent (Schleifer et al., 1989). However, since clinical depression is one of the more common symptoms in many disease states, it can be considered as an important variable for study.

Because clinical depression is more prevalent in women than in men, it may be clinically relevant to consider immunological differences between genders. Decreases in cytotoxic cell activity and reductions in NK cell activity were reported in women, particularly with advancing age (Pung et al., 1986). Since estrogen receptors are found on CD8+ suppressor/cytotoxic cells, down-regulation of function would be expected (Cohen et al., 1983; Stimson, 1988). Reduced CD8+ cell activity (particularly cytotoxic activity) could make a major impact on tumor surveillance and viral infections.

It is possible that breast cancer development is related to breast estrogen receptors and also to estrogen down-regulation of CD8+ cell activity. In addition, we are faced with a growing array of estrogenic environmental toxins (DDT, PCB, dioxins, and others) that may also depress the immune system. Strangely, there are no androgen or progesterone receptors on CD8+ cells. Many believe that possibly, binding that takes place on the glucocorticoid receptors that also have down-regulatory functions. The most important area of research today is probably the effect of sex steroids on cytokine production. Reports indicate that estrogens may depress IL-2 production, leading to autoimmunity disorders (McCruden & Stimson, 1991).

The complexity of the problem can be further illustrated by the fact that clinical depression is accompanied by hypercorticism in many patients (Kronfol et al., 1986). Thus, gonadotropin secretion from the pituitary can be reduced by cortisol (stress) (Berczi, 1986). Clinical depression has been considered to be an expression of "accumulative stress," resulting in reduced immunocompetence. Exaggerated cortisol elevation has been observed in many depressive patients by the use of the dexamethasone suppression test. Since cortisol depresses both IL-1 and IL-2, cellular immunity is reduced (DeSouza, 1993), gender dimorphism on the basis of estrogen binding to CD8+ cells in women (plus hypercortisol levels in clinical depression) would suggest additive immunosuppression (Irwin & Jones, 1991). Direct comparative studies are lacking in terms of estrogen levels, elevated cortisol (dexamethasone non-suppression), and diagnosis of clinical depression (Schleifer & Keller, 1991).

Several reports indicate that postmenopausal women have increased incidence of depression, elevated cortisol levels, and lowered estrogen levels. This apparent dichotomy between increased cortisol and reduced estrogen may not be contradictory in terms of suppression of cell-mediated immunity via CD8+ cells and cytokines. Thus, low postmenopausal levels of estrogens may reduce CD8 activity by virtue of high specific activity on CD8+ receptors (Perkins et al., 1991; McCruden & Stimson, 1991; Pung et al., 1986).

Of great interest are the reports that clinical depression may be related to serotonin dysfunction. Estrogens have been shown to increase binding and uptake of serotonin in the brain and periphery (platelets). Clinically, estrogen replacement therapy reduces clinical depression. What does such therapy do to immunocompetence? Is there an increase in autoimmune disorders? Reductions in rheumatoid arthritis have been reported with the use of oral contraceptives (OCs) ascribed to the progesterone content that enhances T suppressor CD8+ activity. Rheumatoid arthritis responds favorably to pregnancy. In contrast OCs (estrogens) exacerbate patients with SLE (McCruden & Stimson, 1991; McCann et al., 1994; Scarborough, 1990).

Future research will show greater definition of mechanisms involved in clinical depression and "depressed immunity," particularly in females. More exciting comparative studies of gender in clinical depression appear appropriate. Such studies may reveal the importance of cytokines as they relate to immune functions and endocrine and central nervous system effects. Are there gender differences in cytokine production? Are cell-mediated immune responses reduced in females because of estrogen effects on CD8+ cells (IL-2 and other cytokines)? Is recurrence of genital herpes and progression of HIV infection related to reduced cell mediated immunity? Yes! (Kemeny, 1991; McCann et al., 1994; Rivest & Rivier, 1993; DeSouza, 1993).

One might ask why there is such selectivity of estrogen on CD8+ cells. Perhaps it is an evolutionary development of reproduction (pregnancy). Progesterone generates CD8+ suppressor cell activity, perhaps through binding on the glucocorticoid receptor.

Humoral immunity (antibodies) increases during pregnancy while cell-mediated immunity is reduced; thus graft rejection is reduced (Hillhouse et al., 1991; Schleifer & Keller, 1991).

All of the above immunological events are interrelated with pituitary and adrenal hormones and represent modulatory activity to maintain homeostatic balance. It is not all together clear why certain individuals succumb to clinical depression and various autoimmune disorders. Perhaps genetic differences in light of environmental insult (estrogenic toxins) contribute to selectivity of response. Certainly it would be informative to review the incidence of cell-mediated immune disorders in terms of gender (Levy et al., 1987; Irwin et al., 1987; Kiecolt-Glaser et al., 1987).

AUTOIMMUNE DISEASES

The tendency for gender differences becomes more apparent in relation to autoimmune diseases, e.g., frequencies of rheumatoid arthritis, SLE, and thyroiditis are much higher in females. What common denominator can explain these differences? We can speculate that estrogens diminish CD8+ suppressor/cytotoxic activities (progesterone enhances T suppressor activity). What are the consequences of depressing or enhancing suppressor/cytotoxic activities? Significant increases in antibody production have been observed. The consequences of such increases in antibody production against nuclear components and native double-stranded DNA forming soluble complexes, are filtered out in kidneys and become trapped in glomeruli (lupus erythematosus) (Grossman et al., 1991; Horowitz et al., 1977).

In the case of rheumatoid arthritis, inflammatory processes result from immune complexes (rheumatoid factor and IgG). Pregnancy and oral contraceptives reduce the symptomatology of rheumatoid arthritis. Since progesterone has been reported to increase T suppressor activity (luteal phase of the menstrual cycle), it is probable that cell-mediated immunity is more relevant to rheumatoid arthritis. Although the incidence of arthritis is more frequent in women than men (7:1 in the 15- to 35-year age range), it is possible that other hormonal factors are involved (Nelson & Steinberg, 1987).

ENDOMETRIOSIS

This disease is characterized by ectopic growth of endometrium and is accompanied by depressed immunity. Endometriosis patients have impaired NK cytotoxicity. Women in advanced stages of the disease have elevated serum levels of estrogen and decreased NK cytotoxicity. Although estrogen has been shown to impair IL-2 and interferon-enhancing effects on NK cells, such is not the case in this disease state, suggesting other factors may be involved (Stefano et al., 1994).

INFECTIONS

Infections, like other stress factors, cause increases in adrenocorticotropic hormone (ACTH), prolactin (PRL), and growth hormone (GH). Infection suppresses the release of thyrotropin, follicle stimulating hormone (FSH), and luteinizing hormone (LH).

The interleukins (IL-1, IL-2, IL-6, IFN) stimulate ACTH, PRL, and GH release and inhibit TSH and LH (but not FSH). It is possible that the reduction of LH from the pituitary may lower the levels of estrogens, thus reducing the effects on CD8+ cells (Berczi, 1986; McCann et al., 1994).

During pregnancy, various parasitic diseases such as malaria, babesiosis, trypa-nosomiasis, and toxoplasmosis flare up. These are all examples of diseases in which cell-mediated immunity instead of humoral immunity is the important host defense mechanism. Women who take oral contraceptives have increased frequency of gen-itourinary infections caused by *Candida albicans* and trichomonads. Men are much more prone to liver diseases, active hepatitis, post-necrotic sclerosis, and hepatocel-lular carcinoma and are carriers of the hepatitis B virus. Men have much higher incidences of hepatitis b virus and cancer of the liver. Pregnant women have decreased resistance to viral and fungal infections (Bray & Anderson, 1979).

CHRONIC FATIGUE SYNDROME

Women are more frequently affected by chronic fatigue syndrome than men (3:1). The syndrome is characterized by lethargy, painful lymph nodes, sore throat, and depression. Alterations in IgG subclasses, abnormal NK cells, and depressed IL-2 and interferon production have been reported. Allergies to common molds and pollens are common. Patients show depressed responses to mitogenic stimulation. The above pattern of immune responses may be related to estrogen hyperactivity in concert with elevated cortisol due to the stress reactions seen in these patients (Gratzner et al., 1991).

HERPES INFECTIONS AND HIV

Studies of the recurrence rates of genital herpes lesions predominantly among women (30 females, 6 males) indicated that depressed mood was highly correlated to recurrence rate. Depressed mood was also correlated to lower levels of CD8+ cells. In a second study of 58 women, increased anxiety was associated with herpes simplex virus recurrence (Kemeny, 1991). In three separate studies of HIV-infected homo-sexual individuals, Kemeny (1991) found a correlation between depressed mood and lower percentages of CD4 helper cells. Thus, individuals with high levels of depres-sion are subject to a cofactor for progression of disease.

CANCER

The fact that the immune system plays an important role in controlling tumor growth and metastasis is well known. Behavioral and hormonal factors can modulate the immune response and tumor growth (Plotnikoff et al., 1991). Gender differences in the immune response may play a role in the development of a variety of neoplastic disorders.

Carcinoma of the breast occurs in men with an incidence about 1% of that in women. Although hyperestrogenism appears to be involved in the development of breast cancer in men, it is not clear why men with lymph node-positive breast cancers have poorer prognoses than similarly staged women (Heller et al., 1978). Kaposi's sarcoma, including the Mediterranean, African, AIDS-related, and iatrogenic varieties, occurs more frequently in men than in women (Groopman & Broder, 1989). Acute myelogenous and lymphoblastic leukemia are slightly more common in men than in women (Linet & Devesa, 1990). The incidence of B cell chronic lymphocytic leukemia in men is about twice that in women (Linet & Devesa, 1990). Some studies have shown that survival in female patients with acute (Henderson et al., 1990) or chronic (Han & Rai, 1990) lymphocytic leukemia is longer than in male patients. Numerous studies have shown that women with malignant melanoma have better survival rates than men (Balch et al., 1985). Further study is needed to determine whether gender dichotomy in the immune response plays a role in the development and progression of these and other malignancies.

SUMMARY

Gender dichotomy in immune function may be explained, at least in part, by the differential effects of sex hormones on the immune response. Sex hormones can influence both the development and function of cells of the immune system. Binding sites for estrogens have been found on cells of the thymus, spleen, and bursa of Fabricius. Estrogen-binding sites are also found on macrophages and suppressor/cytotoxic T cells, but not on helper T cells. Binding sites for androgens and progestagens are found in the bursa of Fabricius and epithelial cells of the thymus but not on mature lymphocytes including CD8+ T cells.

Testosterone inhibits the stimulatory effects of thymosin and suppresses antibody formation. Estrogens mostly inhibit cell-mediated responses and enhance antibody formation. These differential effects may account for the higher incidence of autoimmune disorders in women compared to men. Additional studies are needed to better explain the gender dichotomy present in autoimmunity, behavior disorders, and cancer. Further elucidation of these gender differences is required for developing pharmacological, immunological, and behavioral interventions to treat and prevent these disorders.

REFERENCES

Ablin, R.J., Barthus, J.M., and Gonder, M.J. (1988). *In vitro* effects of diethylstilbestrol and the LHRH analogue leuprolide on natural killer cell activity. *Immunopharmacology*, 15, 95–101.

Ablin, R.J., Bhalti, R.A., Guinan, P.D., and Khin, W. (1979). Modulatory effects of estrogen on immunological responsiveness. II. Suppression of tumor-associated immunity in patients with prostate cancer. *Clin Exp Immunol*, 38, 83–91.

Amor, B., Bougados, M., Benhamou, L., Kuhn, J.M., and Laudat, M.H. (1983). Achec de l'anrogesotherspic an course l'une poussu e lupus erythemateux. *Presse Med*, 12, 1726–1734.

Andrianopoulos, G.D., and Flaherty, J.A. (1991). Bereavement: effects on immunity and risk of disease, in *Stress and Immunity*, Plotnikoff, N., Murgo, A., Faith, R., and Wybran, J., Eds., CRC Press, Boca Raton, FL, pp. 129–156.

Athreya, B.H., Pletcher, J., Zulian, F., Weiner, D.B., and Williams, W.V. (1993). Subset-specific effects of sex hormones and pituitary gonadotropins on human lymphocyte proliferation *in vitro*. *Clin Immunol Immunopathol*, 66, 201–211.

Balch, C.M., Soong, S.J., and Shaw, H.M. (1985). A comparison of worldwide melanoma data, in *Cutaneous Melanoma: Clinical Management and Treatment Results World-wide*, Balch, C.M., and Milton, G.W., Eds., Lippincott, Philadelphia, p. 507.

Barr, I.G., Pyke, K.W., Peace, P., Toh, P.H., and Funder, J.W. (1984). Thymic sensitivity to sex hormones develops post-naturally: an *in vivo* and *in vitro* study. *J Immunol*, 132, 1095–1099.

Batchelor, J.R. and Chapman, B.A. (1965). The influence of sex upon the anitbody response to an incompatible tumor. *Immunology*, 9, 553–564.

Berczi, I. (1986). Gonadotropins and sex hormones, in *Pituitary Function and Immunity*, Berczi, I., Ed., CRC Press, Boca Raton, FL, pp. 185–212.

Berczi, I. (1986). The influence of hormones on infectious and parasitic disease. In I. Berczi (Ed.), *Pituitary Function and Immunity* (pp. 273-282), Boca Raton, FL.: CRC Press.

Bray, R.S. and Anderson, M.J. (1979). Falciparum malaria and pregnancy. *Trans Roy Soc Trop Med Hyg*, 73, 427–431.

Brent, L. and Medawar, P.B. (1966). Quantitative studies on tissue transplantation immunity. *Proc Roy Soc Ser B*, 165, 413–423.

Brick, J.E., Wilson, D.A., and Walker, S.E. (1985). Hormonal modulation of responses to T-dependent and T-independent antigens in autoimmune NZB/NZW mice. *J Immunol*, 134, 3693–3698.

Brodie, I.Y., Hunter, I.C., Stimson, W.H., and Green, B. (1980): Specific oestradiol binding in cytosols from the thymus glands from normal and homone-treated male rats. *Thymus*, 1, 337–345.

Chao,T.C., Van Alten, P.J., Greager, A., and Walter, R.J. (1995). Steroid sex hormones regulate the release of tumor necrosis factor by macrophages. *Cell Immunol*, 160, 43–49.

Chiovato, L., Lapi, P., Fiore, E., Tonacchera, M., and Pinchera, A. (1993). Thyroid autoimmunity and female gender. *J Endocrinol Invest*, 16, 384–391.

Cohen J.H.M., Danel, L., Cordier, G., Saez, S., and Revillar, J.P. (1983). Sex steroid receptors in peripheral T-cells: absence of androgen receptors and restriction of estrogen receptors to OKT8-positive cells. *J Immunol*, 131, 2767–2771.

Comsa, J., Leonhardt, H., and Wekerle, H. (1982). Hormonal coordination of the immune response. *Physiol Biochem Pharmacol*, 92, 115–191.

Daniel, L. Souweine, G., Manier, J.C., and Saez, S. (1993). Specific estrogen binding sites in human lympoid cells and thymic cells. *J Steroid Biochem*, 18, 559–563.

De Souza, E. (1993). Corticotropin-releasing factor and interleukin-1 receptors in the brain–endocrine–immune axis. *Ann NY Acad Sci*, 679, 9–27.

Deschaux, P., Ulrich, T., and Goldstein, A.L. (1980). *In vitro* effects of thymosin, testosterone and growth hormone on antibody formation in murine spleen cells. *Thymus*, 1, 287–291.

Desquetti, P., Pleines, J., Girarad, M., Charest, L., Senecal-Quevillan, M., and Masse, C. (1992). The increased susceptibility of women to multiple scleroisis. *Can J Neurol Sci*, 19, 466–471.

Detlefson, M.A., Smith, B.C., and Dickerman, H.W. (1978). A high affinity and low capacity receptor for estradiol in normal and anaemic mouse spleen cytosols. *Biochem Biophys Res Commun*, 76, 1151–1158.

Eidinger D. and Garret, T.J. (1972). Studies of the regulatory effects of sex hormones on antibody formation and stem cell differentiation. *J Exp Med*, 136, 1098–1116.

Ferin, M. (1993). Neuropeptides, the stress response, and the hypothalamo–pituitary–gonadal axis in the female rhesus monkey. *Ann NY Acad Sci*, 697, 106–116.

Freidman, D., Netti, F., and Schreiber, A. (1985). Effect of estradiol and steroid analogs on the clearance of immunoglobulin-G coated erythrocytes. *J Clin Invest*, 75, 162–167.

Goble, F.C. and Konopka, E.A. (1973). Sex as a factor in infectious diseases. *Trans NY Acad Sci*, 35, 325–346.

Goldstein, A.L., Hooper, J.A., Schulof, R.S., Cohen, G.H., Thurman, G.H., McDaniel, M.C. White, A., and Dardenne, M. (1974). Thymosin and the immunology of aging. *Fed Proc*, 33, 2053.

Graff, R.J., Hildemann, W.H., and Snell, G.D. (1966). Histocompatibility genes of mice. *Transplantation*, 4, 425–437.

Graff, R.J., Lappe, M.A., and Snell, G.D. (1969). The influence of gonads and adrenal glands on the immune response to skin grafts. *Transplantation*, 7, 105–111.

Gratzner, H.G., Johnson, T.S., Hermann, W.J., Steinbach, T.L., and De Herrera, R. (1991). Assessment of stress-induced immune function in chronic fatigue syndrome patients, in *Stress and Immunity*, Plotnikoff, N., Murgo, A., Faith, R., and Wybran, J., Eds., CRC Press, Boca Raton, FL, pp. 247–257.

Groopman, J.E. and Broder, S. (1989). Cancer in AIDS and other immunodefiency states, in *Cancer: Principles and Practice of Oncology*, 3rd ed., De Vita, E. et al., Eds., Lippincott, Philadelphia, 1953–1970.

Grossman, C. (1989). Possible underlying mechanisms of sexual dimorphism in the immune response, fact and hypothesis. *J Steroid Biochem*, 34, 241–251.

Grossman, C.J. Nathan, P., Taylor, B.B., and Sholiton, L.J. (1979). Rat thymic dihydrotestosterone receptor: preparation; location and physicochemistry properties. *Steroids*, 34, 539–553.

Grossman, C.J., Roselle, G.A., and Mendenhall, C.L. (1091). Sex steroid regulation of autoimmunity. *J Steroid Biochem Mol Biol*, 40, 649–659.

Grossman, C.J., Sholiton, L.J., and Nathan, P. (1979). Rat thymic estorgen receptor. I. Preparation, location and physicochemical properties. *J Steroid Biochem*, 11, 1233–1240.

Gulshan, S., McCruden, A.B., and Stimson, W.H. (1990). Estrogen receptors in macrophages. *Scand J Immunol*, 31, 691–697.

Han, T. and Rai, K.R. (1990). Chronic lymphocytic leukemia, in *Leukemia*, 5th ed., Henderson and Lister, Eds., W.B. Saunders, Philadelphia, p. 574.

Heller, K.S., Rosen, P.P., and Schottenfeld, D. (1978). Male breast cancer: a clinicopathologic study of 97 cases. *Ann Surg*, 188, 60–65.

Henderson, E.S., Hoelzer, D., and Freeman, A.L. (1990). The treatment of acute lymphoblastic leukemia, in *Leukemia*, 5th ed., Henderson and Lister, Eds., W.B. Saunders, Philadelphia, p. 468.

Hillhouse, J.E., Kiecolt-Glaser, J.K., and Glaser, R. (1991). Stress-associated modulation of the immune response in humans, in *Stress and Immunity*, Plotnikoff, N., Murgo, A., Faith, R., and Wybran, J., Eds., CRC Press, Boca Raton, FL, pp. 3–27.

Hockberg, M.C. (1981). Adult and juvenile rheumatoid arthritis: current epidemiological concepts. *Epidemiol Rev*, 3, 27–44.

Holdstock, G., Chastenay, B.J., and Krawitt, E.L. (1982). Effects of testosterone, estradiol and progesterone on immune reaction. *Clin Exp Immunol*, 47, 449–456.

Horowitz, S., Brocherding, W., Vishnu Moorthy, A., Chesney, R., Schulti-Wisserman, H., and Hong, L. (1977). Induction of suppressor T-cells in systemic lupus erythematosus by thymosin and cultured thymic epithelium. *Science*, 197, 999–1001.

Imanishi, Y., Seiki, K., and Haruki, Y. (1980). Cytoplasmic estrogen receptor in castrated rat thymus. *Endocrinol Jpna*, 27, 395–399.

Inman, R.D. (1978). Immunologic sex differences and the female predominance in systemic lupus erythematosus. *Arthr Rheumat*, 21, 849–852.

Irwin, M. Daniels and Jones, L. (1991). Life stress, depression, and reduced natural cytotoxicity: clinical findings and putative mechanisms, in *Stress and Immunity*, Plotnikoff, N., Murgo, A., Faith, R., and Wybran, J., Eds., CRC Press, Boca Raton, FL, pp. 109–128.

Irwin, M., Daniels, M., Smith, T.L., Bloom, El, and Weiner, H. (1987). Imparted natural killer cell activity during bereavement. *Brain Behav Immun*, 1, 98–104.

Kaiser, N., Mayer, M., Milholland, R.J., and Rosen, F. (1979). Studies of the antiglucocorticoid action of progesterone in rat thymocytes: early *in vitro* effects, *J Steroid Biochem*, 10, 379–386.

Kalland, T. (1980). Decreased and disproportionate T-cell population in adult mice after maternal exposure to diethylstilbestrol. *Cell Immunol*, 51, 55–63.

Kalland, T., Strand, O., and Forsberg, J.G. (1979). Long term effects of neonatal estrogen treatment on mitogen responsiveness of mouse spleen lymphocytes. *J Clin Invest*, 63, 413–421.

Kawashima, I., Sakabe, K., Seiki, K., and Fujii-Hanamoto, H. (1990). Hormone and immune response, with special reference to steroid hormone. 3. Sex steroid effect on T-cell differentiation. *Takai J Exp Clin Med*, 15, 213–218.

Kemeny, M.E. (1991). Psychological factors, immune processes, and the course of herpes simplex and human immunodeficiency virus infection, in *Stress and Immunity*, Plotnikoff, N., Murgo, A., Faith, R., and Wybran, J., Eds., CRC Press, Boca Raton, FL, pp. 199–211.

Kenny, J.F., Pangburn, P.C., and Trail, G. (1976). Effect of estradiol on immune competence: *in vivo* and *in vitro* studies. *Infect Immun*, 13, 448–456.

Kiecolt-Glaser, J.K., Fisher, L., Ogrocki, P., Stout, J.C., Speicher, C.E., and Glaser, R. (1987). Marital quality, marital disruption, and immune function. *Psychosom Med*, 49, 13–34.

Kiecolt-Glaser, J.K., Kennedy, S., Malkoff, S., Fisher, L., Speicher, C.E., and Glaser, R. (1988). Marital discord and immunity in males. *Psychosom Med*, 50, 213–229.

Kincl, F.H. and Ciaccio, L.A. (1980). Suppression of the immune response by progesterone. *Endrocrinol Exp*, 14, 27–33.

Koppas, A., Jones, H.E.S., and Roitt, J.M. (1963). Effects of steroid sex hormones on immunological phenomenon. *Nature*, 198, 902–904.

Kronfol, A. and Schlechte, J. (1986). Depression, hormones and immunity, in *Enkephalins and Endorphins: Stress and the Immune System*, Plotnikoff, N.P., Faith, R.E., Murgo, A.J., and Good, R.A., Eds., Plenum Press, New York, pp. 69–80.

Kryzch, U., Stausser, H.R., Breasler, J.P., and Goldstein, A.R. (1978). Quantitative differences in immune responses during the various stages of the estrous cycle in female BALB/c mice. *J Immunol*, 121, 1603–1605.

Kuhl, H., Gross, M., Schneider, M., Veber, W, Mehlis, W., Stegmuller, M., and Taubert, M. (1983). The effect of sex steroids and hormonal contraceptives upon thymus and spleen in intact female rats. *Contraception*, 28, 587–601.

Leslie, C.A. and Dubey, D.P. (1994). Increased PGE2 from human monocytes isolated in the luteal phase of the menstrual cycle: implications for immunity? *Prostaglandins*, 47, 41–54.

Levine, H.B. and Madin, S.H. (1962). Enhancement of experimental coccidioidomycosis in mice with testosterone and estradiol, *Sabouraudia*, 2, 47–52.

Levy, S., Herberman, R., Lippman, M., and d'Angelo, T. (1987). Correlation of stress factors with sustained depression of natural killer cell activity and predicted prognosis in patients with breast cancer. *J Clin Oncol*, 5, 348–353.

Linet, M.S. and Devesa, S.S. (1990). Descriptive epidemiology of the leukemias, in *Leukemia*, 5th ed., Henderson and Lister, Eds., W.B. Saunders, Philadelphia, pp. 209–212.

London, W.I. and Drew, J.R. (1977). Sex differences in the response to hepatitis B infections among patients receiving chronic dialysis treatment. *Proc Natl Acad Sci USA*, 74, 2561–2563.

Malacarine, P., Piffanelli, A., Indelli, M., Fumero, S., Mondino, A., Gionchiglia, E., and Silvestri, S. (1980). Estradiol binding in rat thymus cells. *Hormone Res*, 12, 224–232.

Masi, A.T. (1984). Clinical epidemiologic perspective of systemic lupus erythematosus, in *Epidemiology of the Rheumatic Diseases*, Lawrence, R.C. and Shulman, L.E., Eds., Gower Medical, New York, pp. 145–163.

Mathur, S., Mathur, R.S., Goust, J.M., Williamson, H.O., and Fudenberg, H.H. (1979). Cyclic variations in white cell subpopulations in the human menstrual cycle: correlations with progesterone and estradiol. *Clin Immunol Immunopathol*, 13, 246–253.

McCruden, A.B. and Stimson, W.H. (1991). Sex hormones and immune function, in *Psychoneuroimmunology*, Adler, R., Felten, D.L., and Cohen, N., Eds., Academic Press, San Diego, pp. 475–493.

McCann, S.M., Lyson, K., Karanth, S., Gimeno, M., Belova, N., Kamat, A., and Rettori, V. (1994). Role of cytokines in the endocrine system. *Ann NY Acad Sci*, 741, 50–63.

Morimoto, C. (1978). Loss of suppressor T-lymphocyte function in patients with systemic lupus erythematosus. *Clin Exp Immunol*, 32, 125–133.

Michaels, R.H. and Rogers, K.D. (1971). A sex difference in immunologic responsiveness. *Pediatrics*, 47, 120–122.

Nelson, J.L. and Steinberg, A.D. (1987). Sex steroids, autoimmunity, and autoimmune diseases, in *Hormones and Immunity*, Berczi, I. and Kalman, K., Eds., MPT Press, Norwell, MA, pp. 93–119.

Nicol, T.D., Bilbey, D.L.J, Charles, L.M., Cordingley, J.L., and Vernon-Roberts, B. (1964). Oestrogen: the natural stimulant of body defense. *J Endocrinol*, 30, 277–291.

Paavonen, T., Andersson, L.C., and Adlercreutz, H. (1981). Sex hormone regulation of *in vitro* immune responses: estradiol enhances human B-cell maturation via inhibition of suppressor T-cells in pokeweed mitogen-stimulated cultures. *J Exp Med*, 154, 1935–1945.

Pearce, P.T., Khalid, P.A.K., and Funder, J.W. (1983). Progesterone receptors in rat thymus. *Endocrinology*, 13, 1287–1291.

Perkins, D.O., Leserman, J., Gilmore, J.H., Petitto, J.M., and Evans, D.L. (1991). Stress, depression and immunity: research findings and clinical implications, in *Stress and Immunity*, Plotnikoff, N., Murgo, A., Faith, R., and Wybran, J., Eds., CRC Press, Boca Raton, FL, pp. 167–188.

Pung, O.J., Tucker, A.N., and Luster, M.I. (1986). Estrogen-mediated immunomodulation, in *Enkephalins and Endorphins: Stress and the Immune System*, Plotnikoff, N.P., Faith, R.E., Murgo, A.J., and Good, R.A., Eds., Plenum Press, New York, pp. 173–188.

Ranelletti, F.O., Carmignai, M., Marchetti, P., Natoli, C., and Iacobelli, S. (1980). Estrogen binding by neoplastic human thymus cytosol. *Eur J Cancer*, 16, 951–955.

Raveche, E.S. Vigersky, R.A., Rice, M.K., and Steinberg, A.D. (1980). Murine thymic androgen receptors. *J Immunopathol*, 2, 425–434.

Rawley, M.J. and MacKay, I.R. (1969). Measurement of antibody producing capacity in man. *Clin Exp Immunol*, 5, 407–418.

Rifkind, D., Frey, J.A., and Davis, J.R. (1973). Influence of gonadal factors on skin test reactivity of CFW mice to *Candida albicans*. *Infect Immun*, 7, 322–328.

Rivest, S. and Rivier, C. (1993). Central mechanisms and sites of action involved in the inhibitory effects of CRF and cytokines on LHRH neuronal activity. *Ann NY Acad Sci*. 697, 117–141.

Sakabe, K., Kawashina, I., Seiki, K., and Fujii-Hanamoto, H. (1990). Hormone and immune response, with special reference to steroid hormone. 2. Sex steroid receptors in rat thymus. *Tokai J Exp Clin Med*, 15, 201–211.

Sakabe, K., Seiki, K., and Fujii, H. (1986). Histochemical localization of progestin receptor in the rat thymus. *Thymus*, 8, 97–107.

Santoli, D., Trinchieri, G. and Zinijewski, C.M. (1976). HLA-related control of spontaneous and antibody-mediated cell mediated cytotoxic activity in humans. *J Immunol*, 117, 765–770.

Sasson, S. and Mayer, M. (1981). Effect of androgenic steroids on rat thymus and thymocytes in suspension. *J Steroid Biochem*, 14, 509–517.

Scambia, G., Panici, P.B., Maccio, A., Castilli, P., Serri, F., Mantovani, G., Massida, B., Jacobelli, S., Del Giacco, S., and Mancuso, P. (1988). Effects of antiestrogen and progestin on immune function in breast cancer. *Cancer*, 61, 2214–2218.

Scarborough, D.E. (1990). Cytokine modulation of pituitary hormone secretion. *Ann NY Acad Sci*, 594, 169–187.

Schleifer, S.J., Keller, S.E., Camerino, M., Thornton, J.C., and Stein, M. (1983). Supression of lymphocyte stimulation following bereavement. *JAMA*, 250, 374–377.

Schleifer, S.J., Keller, S.E., Bond, R.N., Cohen, J., and Stein, M. (1989). Depression and immunity: role of age, sex and severity, *Arch Gen Psych* 46, 81–87.

Schleifer, S.J. and Keller, S.E. (1991). Depressive disorders and immunity, in *Stress and Immunity*, Plotnikoff, N., Murgo, A., Faith, R., and Wybran, J., Eds., CRC Press, Boca Raton, FL, pp. 157–165.

Seaman, W.E. and Gindhart, T.D. (1979). Effect of estrogen on natural killer cells. *Arth Rheum*, 22, 1234–1240.

Sekiya, S., Kamiyama, M., and Takomizawa, H. (1975). *In vivo* and *in vitro* tests of inhibitory effect of progesterone on cell-mediated immunity in rats bearing a syngeneic uterine adenocarcinoma. *J Natl Cancer Inst*, 54, 769–771.

Spencer, M.J., Cherry, J.D., Powell, K.R., Mickey, M.R., Teraski, P., Marey, S.M., and Sumaya, C.V. (1977). Antibody responses following Rubella immunization analyzed by HLA and ABO types. *Immunogenetics*, 4, 365–372.

Stefano, G.D., Provinciali, M., Muzzioli, M., Garzetti, G.G., Ciavattini, A., and Fabris, N. (1994). Correlation between estradiol serum levels and NK cell activity in endometriosis. *Ann NY Acad Sci*, 741, 197–203.

Stein, M., Miller, A.H., and Trestman, R.L. (1991). Depression and the immune system, in *Psychoneuroimmunology*, Adler, R., Felten, D.L., and Cohen, N., Eds., Academic Press, San Diego, pp. 897–930.

Stern, K. and Davidsohn, I. (1955). Effects of estrogen and cortisone or immune hemoantibodies in mice of inbred strains. *J Immunol*, 74, 479–484.

Sthoeger, Z.M., Chiorazzi, N. and Lohita, L.G. (1988). Regulation of the immune response by sex hormones. I. *In vitro* effects of estradiol and testosterone on pokeweed mitogen-induced human B-cell differentiation. *J Immunol*, 141, 91–98.

Stimson, W.H. (1983). Serum proteins, steroids and the maternal immune response, in *Immunology of Reproduction*, Wagman, T.G. and Gill, T.J., Eds., Oxford University Press, Oxford, U.K., pp. 281–301.

Stimson, W.H. (1988). Oestrogen and human T-lymphocytes: presence of specific receptors in the T-suppressor/cytotoxic subset. *Scand J Immunol*, 28, 345–350.

Stimson, W.H. and Crilly, P.J. (1981). Effects of steroids on the secretion of immunoregulatory factors by thymic epithelial cell cultures. *Immunology*, 44, 401–407.

Stimson, W.H. and Hunter, J.C. (1980). Oestrogen-induced immunoregulation mediated through the thymus. *J Clin Lab Immunol*, 4, 27–33.

Sullivan, D.A. and Wica, C.R. (1979). Sex hormone and glucocorticoid receptors in the bursa of Fabricius of immature chicks. *J Immunol*, 122, 2617–2623.

Tartakovsky, B., DeBaetselies, P., Feldman, M., and Segal, S. (1981). Sex associated differences in the immune response against fetal major histocompatibility antigens. *Transplantation*, 32, 395–397.

Terres G., Morrison, S.L. and Halicht, G.S. (1968). A quantitative difference in the immune response between male and female mice. *Proc Soc Exp Biol Med*, 127, 664–667.

Tomada, Y., Fuma, J., Mina, T., Saiki, N., and Ishraka, N. (1976). Cell mediated immunity in pregnancy. *Gynecol Invest*, 7, 280–292.

Washburn, T.C., Madearis, D.N., and Childs, B. (1965). Sex differences in susceptibility to infections. *Pediatrics*, 35, 57–64.

Weinstein, Y., Lindner, H.R., and Eckstein, B. (1977). Thymus metabolizes progesterone: possible enzymic marker for T-lymphocytes. *Nature*, 266, 632–633.

Wheaton, D.W. and Hurst, E.W. (1961). The effect of sex on bacterial infections in mice and the chemotherapy of one of them. *J Pathol Bacteriol*, 82, 117–139.

Willoughby, D.S. and Watson, D.W. (1964). Host-parasite relationships among group A streptococci. II. Influence of sex on the susceptibility of inbred mice toward streptococcal infection. *J Bacteriol*, 87, 1457–1461.

Wyle, F.A. and Kent, J.R. (1977). Immunosuppression by sex hormones: the effect upon PHA and PPD stimulated lymphocytes. *Clin Exp Immunol*, 27, 407–415.

Index